WP 870 JAC £99

This book is due for return on or before the last date shown below.

Early Diagnosis and
Treatment of Cancer:
Breast Cancer

EARLY DIAGNOSIS AND TREATMENT OF CANCER

Series Editor: Stephen C. Yang, MD

Breast Cancer

Edited by

Lisa Jacobs, MD

Associate Professor
Department of Surgery
Johns Hopkins University School of Medicine
Baltimore, Maryland

Christina A. Finlayson, MD

Professor
Department of Surgery
University of Colorado School of Medicine
Aurora, Colorado

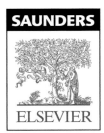

SAUNDERS

ELSEVIER

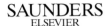

SAUNDERS
ELSEVIER

1600 John F. Kennedy Blvd.
Ste 1800
Philadelphia, PA 19103-2899

Notices

Knowledge and best practice in this field are constantly changing. As new research and experience broaden our understanding, changes in research methods, professional practices, or medical treatment may become necessary.

Practitioners and researchers must always rely on their own experience and knowledge in evaluating and using any information, methods, compounds, or experiments described herein. In using such information or methods they should be mindful of their own safety and the safety of others, including parties for whom they have a professional responsibility.

With respect to any drug or pharmaceutical products identified, readers are advised to check the most current information provided (i) on procedures featured or (ii) by the manufacturer of each product to be administered, to verify the recommended dose or formula, the method and duration of administration, and contraindications. It is the responsibility of practitioners, relying on their own experience and knowledge of their patients, to make diagnoses, to determine dosages and the best treatment for each individual patient, and to take all appropriate safety precautions.

To the fullest extent of the law, neither the Publisher nor the authors, contributors, or editors, assume any liability for any injury and/or damage to persons or property as a matter of products liability, negligence or otherwise, or from any use or operation of any methods, products, instructions, or ideas contained in the material herein.

Library of Congress Cataloging-in-Publication Data

Early diagnosis and treatment of cancer : breast cancer / edited by Lisa Jacobs and Christina A. Finlayson
    p. ; cm.—(Early diagnosis and treatment of cancer series)
  Includes bibliographical references.
  ISBN 978-1-4160-4932-6
  1. Breast—Cancer. I. Jacobs, Lisa. II. Finlayson, Christina A. III. Series: Early diagnosis and treatment of cancer series.
  [DNLM: 1. Breast Neoplasms—diagnosis. 2. Breast Neoplasms—therapy. 3. Early Diagnosis. WP 870 B6205 2010]
    RC280.B8B6655626   2011
    616.99′449—dc22

                                                                                    2010012922

Acquisitions Editor: Dolores Meloni
Design Direction: Steven Stave

Printed in the United States of America

Last digit is the print number: 9 8 7 6 5 4 3 2 1

Series Preface

Seen on a graph, the survival rate for many cancers resembles a precipice. Discovered at an early stage, most cancers are quickly treatable, and the prognosis is excellent. In late stages, however, the typical treatment protocol becomes longer, more intense, and more harrowing for the patient, and the survival rate declines steeply. No wonder, then, that one of the most important means in fighting cancer is to prevent or screen for earlier stage tumors.

Within each oncologic specialty, there is a strong push to identify new, more useful tools for early diagnosis and treatment, with an emphasis on methods amenable to an office-based or clinical setting. These efforts have brought impressive results. Advances in imaging technology, as well as the development of sophisticated molecular and biochemical tools, have led to effective, minimally invasive approaches to cancer in its early stages.

This series, *Early Diagnosis and Treatment of Cancer*, gathers state-of-the-art research and recommendations into compact, easy-to-use volumes. For each particular type of cancer, the books cover the full range of diagnostic and treatment procedures, including pathologic, radiologic, chemotherapeutic, and surgical methods, focusing on questions like these:

■ What do practitioners need to know about the epidemiology of the disease and its risk factors?
■ How do patients and their families wade through and interpret the myriad of testing?
■ What is the safest, quickest, least invasive way to reach an accurate diagnosis?
■ How can the stage of the disease be determined?
■ What are the best initial treatments for early-stage disease, and how should the practitioner and the patient choose among them?

■ What lifestyle factors might affect the outcome of treatment?

Each volume in the series is edited by an authority within the subfield, and the contributors have been chosen for their practical skills as well as their research credentials. Key Points at the beginning of each chapter help the reader grasp the main ideas at once. Frequent illustrations make the techniques vivid and easy to visualize. Boxes and tables summarize recommended strategies, protocols, indications and contraindications, important statistics, and other essential information. Overall, the attempt is to make expert advice as accessible as possible to a wide variety of health care professionals.

For the first time since the inception of the National Cancer Institute's annual status reports, the 2008 "Annual Report to the Nation on the Status of Cancer," published in the December 3 issue of the *Journal of the National Cancer Institute*, noted a statistically significant decline in "both incidence and death rates from all cancers combined." This mark of progress encourages all of us to press forward with our efforts. I hope that the volumes in *Early Diagnosis and Treatment of Cancer* will make health care professionals and patients more familiar with the latest developments in the field, as well as more confident in applying them, so that early detection and swift, effective treatment become a reality for all of our patients.

Stephen C. Yang, MD
The Arthur B. and Patricia B. Modell
Professor of Thoracic Surgery
Chief of Thoracic Surgery
The Johns Hopkins Medical Institutions
Baltimore, Maryland

Preface

Breast cancer is the most common malignancy to occur in women. It is estimated that in 2009 approximately 192,500 women were diagnosed with invasive breast cancer and 62,300 were diagnosed with in situ disease. Breast cancer is the second most common cause of cancer death in women, with an estimated 40,000 women dying of the disease in 2009. The combination of the high incidence of the disease, strong grass-roots advocacy, and consistent, focused research has resulted in numerous advances in the treatment of breast cancer over the past several decades. In this book we provide a comprehensive review of current recommendations for the clinical management of early breast cancer, including prevention, diagnosis, and treatment. We also include some of the new and innovative interventions on the horizon that have not yet become standard.

The battle against breast cancer mortality begins with prevention. The decision to pursue breast cancer prevention must be based on an accurate assessment of risk, and this risk assessment is aided by risk assessment models. For patients at very high risk, genetic assessment with germ-line gene mutation testing such as BRCA becomes important. Even for those patients without a genetic mutation or at low risk for a mutation, interventions for breast cancer prevention may still be desirable. Previously, surgery was the only option for risk reduction, but now hormonal therapies are available. In addition, evidence is building for lifestyle changes that each individual woman can adopt to reduce her personal risk of developing breast cancer. These options provide the patient and the physician with a range of effective risk reduction strategies that can then be selected to meet the patient's desired level of risk reduction while taking into consideration the risks and process involved in the strategy. It is possible that new biomarkers will be developed that will further improve risk assessment for individual patients and further allow us to tailor our recommendations for prevention based on the degree of risk

and potentially to select the mechanism of prevention most effective for a given patient.

Diagnostic evaluations of patients at risk for breast cancer are also evolving, and controversial changes in screening recommendations have recently been published. The goal of screening is to diagnose and treat patients with breast cancer before there has been systemic spread. The biggest challenge with our current screening techniques is the high rates of false positives. These result in a large number of women undergoing biopsies for benign disease. Another challenge in our screening process is the diagnosis and management of ductal carcinoma in situ (DCIS). Although we are able to identify DCIS as a very early breast cancer, the natural history of this disease process is not well understood, and the need to pursue aggressive treatment is being questioned. This has prompted some groups to recommend changes in the screening recommendations to reduce the number of patients with DCIS who are diagnosed and treated. Methods of screening and diagnostic imaging are included in this text to further define the current standard of care.

Pathologic assessment of diagnostic tissue and surgical specimens is critical to understanding the prognosis for the patient and for making treatment recommendations to the patient. Stage of diagnosis based on the Tumor, Node, Metastasis (TNM) staging system provides basic prognostic information on which many treatment recommendations are made. We fortunately now have other prognostic markers such as grade and Ki-67 and genetic markers such as oncotype DX that provide further prognostic accuracy and allow more informed treatment recommendations. The importance of pathologic assessment in the treatment recommendations for patients supports the extensive review of pathologic assessment included in this text.

The treatment of breast cancer continues to be based on surgery, chemotherapy, hormonal therapy, and radiation therapy: each approach remains a mainstay in the overall treatment plan. Modifications in the recommendation for each of these components are based on estimates of local, regional, or systemic recurrence. Each of these therapies has become more targeted. Surgical management now involves improved selection for breast preservation by using improved diagnostic tests and neoadjuvant therapy to encourage patients to seek breast preservation. The broad improvements in screening, diagnosis, and systemic therapies have allowed surgeons to decrease the extent of surgical therapies both in the regional nodal basin and in the breast. The same concepts apply to the use of radiation therapy. The selection of patients for elimination of radiation therapy or reduction in the extent of radiation therapy has become possible through research in patient selection and improvements in radiation therapy techniques that reduce complications, field of exposure, and time commitment required for treatment. Systemic adjuvant therapies have also become more targeted, with far more patients avoiding chemotherapy with the use of hormonal therapy. In addition, newer systemic agents that provide improved systemic control with reduced risk are being utilized. The selection of patients for systemic hormonal

therapy now has many additional possibilities, and patients and their physicians are able to select their treatment choices based on therapeutic benefit and side effect profile in a much more informed manner.

Prevention, diagnosis, and management of breast cancer are all continually evolving, and we include each of these subjects in this book. One of the most satisfying aspects of caring for patients with breast disease is that in each step of the process we are able to offer a variety of options with differing levels of risk and benefit. Patients and their health care providers are able to weigh the risks and benefits of their options and then make well-informed decisions. This is the result of an extensive research effort into all aspects of breast cancer prevention, diagnosis, and treatment. Fortunately, even with the array of options currently available, even more are on the horizon that promise further reductions in risk by more targeted therapies, better predictors of risk of disease development or progression through biomarkers, and improved diagnostic accuracy.

Lisa Jacobs, MD
Christina A. Finlayson, MD

Contents

Contributors

Benjamin O. Anderson, MD
Professor of Surgery and Global Health-Medicine, University of Washington; Joint Member, Division of Public Health Sciences, Fred Hutchinson Cancer Research Center; Director, Breast Health Clinic, Seattle Cancer Care Alliance, Seattle, Washington

Erica D. Anderson, BS, MD
Assistant Professor, Emory University School of Medicine, Atlanta, Georgia

Jennifer E. Axilbund, MS
Research Associate in Oncology, Johns Hopkins University; Senior Genetic Counselor, Johns Hopkins Hospital, Baltimore, Maryland

Brian Bagrosky, MD
Department of Diagnostic Radiology, University of Colorado School of Medicine, Aurora, Colorado

Virginia F. Borges, MD
Associate Professor, Department of Medicine, University of Colorado School of Medicine; Director, Young Women's Breast Cancer Translational Program, University of Colorado Cancer Center, Aurora, Colorado

James P. Borgstede, MD
Professor and Vice Chairman, Department of Radiology, University of Colorado School of Medicine, Aurora, Colorado

Daniel Bowles, MD
Fellow in Hematology and Medical Oncology, University of Colorado School of Medicine, Aurora, Colorado

Susanne Briest, MD
Director, Breast Cancer Program, University of Leipzig, Leipzig, Germany

Kristine E. Calhoun, MD
Assistant Professor, Department of Surgery, Division of General Surgery, Section of Surgical Oncology, University of Washington School of Medicine, Seattle, Washington

Judy L. Chavez, RT(R)(M)(BS), RDMS
Supervisor, Breast Procedure Suite, Centrum Surgical Center, In affiliation with Invision/Sally Jobe Breast Care Network and Radiology Imaging Associates, Greenwood Village, Colorado

Chin-Yau Chen, MD
Department of Surgery, Taipei City Hospital Zhong Xing Branch, Taipei, Taiwan

Alex Colque, MD
Plastic Surgery Fellow, The Methodist Hospital, Houston, Texas

Lisa Ware Corbin, MD
Associate Professor, Department of Medicine, University of Colorado School of Medicine, Aurora; Medical Director, The Center for Integrative Medicine, University of Colorado School of Medicine, Aurora, Colorado

Donald C. Doll, MD
Staff Physician, Division of Hematology, Oncology Section, James A. Haley Veterans Hospital, Tampa, Florida

Anthony D. Elias, MD
Martha Cannon Dear Professor, Department of Medicine, University of Colorado School of Medicine, University of Colorado Cancer Center, Aurora, Colorado

Christina A. Finlayson, MD
Professor, Department of Surgery, University of Colorado School of Medicine, Aurora, Colorado

Michael Ford, MD
Department of Surgery, University of Colorado School of Medicine, Aurora, Colorado

Timothy George, MD
Fellow, Johns Hopkins University School of Medicine; Department of Surgery, Johns Hopkins Hospital, Baltimore, Maryland

Nancy S. Goldstein, DNP, CRNP, RNC
The Johns Hopkins University School of Nursing, Baltimore, Maryland

Amy L. Gross, MHS
Johns Hopkins School of Public Health, Baltimore, Maryland

Lara Hardesty, MD
Associate Professor, Department of Radiology, University of Colorado School of Medicine; Director, Breast Imaging, University of Colorado Hospital, Aurora, Colorado

Lisa Jacobs, MD
Associate Professor, Department of Surgery, Johns Hopkins University School of Medicine, Baltimore, Maryland

Peter Kabos, MD
Assistant Professor, Department of Medicine, University of Colorado School of Medicine, Aurora, Colorado

Terese I. Kaske, MD
Radiologist, Breast Imaging Specialist, RIA/Invision Sally Jobe, Englewood, Colorado

M. Catherine Lee, MD
Assistant Professor of Surgery, Division of Oncologic Sciences, University of South Florida School of Medicine, Tampa; Assistant Member, Comprehensive Breast Program, Moffit Cancer Center and Research Institute, Tampa, Florida

John M. Lewin, MD
Section Chief, Breast Imaging, Diversified Radiology of Colorado, PC; Medical Director, Rose Breast Center, Denver, Colorado

Scott W. McGee, MD
Assistant Clinical Professor, Northeastern Ohio Universities, College of Medicine; Akron General Partners Physician Group, Oncology, Akron General Medical Center, Akron, Ohio

Lee Myers, PhD
Senior Clinical Physicist, Johns Hopkins University, Baltimore, Maryland

Samia Nawaz, MD
Associate Professor, Department of Pathology, University of Colorado School of Medicine, Aurora; Staff Pathologist, VA Medical Center, Denver, Colorado

Steve H. Parker, MD
Staff Pathologist, Sally Jobe Breast Center, Greenwood Village, Colorado

Elizabeth Prier, MD
General Surgeon, Private Practice, Boise Surgical Group, Boise, Idaho

Rachel Rabinovitch, MD
Professor, Department of Radiation Oncology, University of Colorado School of Medicine, University of Colorado Cancer Center, Aurora, Colorado

Jon V. Rittenbach, MD
Clinical Laboratory Director and Pathologist (AP/CP), Providence Saint Mary Medical Center; Pathologist, Walla Walla General Hospital; Pathologist, Walla Walla VA Medical Center; Davis-Sameh-Meeker Laboratories, Walla Walla, Washington

Michael S. Sabel, MD
Associate Professor of Surgery, University of Michigan, Ann Arbor, Michigan

Edward R. Sauter, MD, PhD, MHA
Professor of Surgery and Associate Dean for Research, University of North Dakota School of Medicine and Health Sciences, Grand Forks; Surgical Oncologist and General Surgeon, Meritcare Health System, Fargo, North Dakota, and Thief River Falls, Minnesota

Meenakshi Singh, MD
Professor and Vice Chair for Anatomic Pathology, Department of Pathology, Stonybrook University Medical Center, State University of New York at Stonybrook, Stonybrook, New York

Hanjoon Song, MD
Associate, Prima Center for Plastic Surgery, Duluth, Georgia

Michael D. Stamatakos, MD
Assistant Professor, Anatomic Pathology, George Washington University Hospital, Washington, DC

Vered Stearns, MD
Associate Professor of Oncology, Medical Oncology, Johns Hopkins School of Medicine, Johns Hopkins Hospital, Baltimore, Maryland

Kala Visvanathan, MD
Associate Professor of Epidemiology and Oncology, Johns Hopkins Medical Institutions, Baltimore, Maryland

Anna Voltura, MD
Medical Director, Christus St. Vincent Breast Institute; Breast Oncology Surgeon, Christus St. Vincent Hospital, Santa Fe, New Mexico

Richard Zellars, MD
Associate Professor, Department of Radiation Oncology, Sidney Kimmel Comprehensive Cancer Center at Johns Hopkins, Baltimore, Maryland

Constance R. Ziegfeld, RN
Clinical Nurse Specialist, Johns Hopkins University, Baltimore, Maryland

1

The Normal Breast and Benign Diseases of the Breast

Samia Nawaz

KEY POINTS

- The functional unit of the female breast is the terminal duct lobular unit (TDLU).
- The entire ductal system is lined by two cell layers: inner epithelial cells and outer myoepithelial cells.
- Ectopic breast tissue in the axilla may raise clinical concern for metastasis.
- Inverted nipples may be congenital or may be associated with breast carcinoma.
- Acute mastitis and inflammatory carcinoma may look alike clinically.
- Chronic mastitis and fat necrosis can result in a hard irregular mass and mimic malignancy.
- Fibroadenoma is the most common benign neoplasm of the female breast, composed of benign proliferation of stroma and epithelium.
- Sclerosing adenosis is a proliferation of the stroma and the smallest tubules within the TDLU. It may mimic carcinoma clinically, radiologically, and histologically. The presence of myoepithelial cells confirms the benign nature of the lesion.
- Ductal hyperplasia (proliferation of the ductal epithelial lining cells) may be of the usual type (mild, moderate, or florid) or atypical and may have varying degrees of risk for future cancer.
- Atypical lobular hyperplasia (proliferation of the epithelium lining the lobules) is associated with an increased risk of future carcinoma. There is no such entity as lobular hyperplasia of the usual type.

The Normal Breast

The breast is a modified, specialized apocrine gland located in the superficial fascia of the anterior chest wall (Fig. 1-1). The nipple projects from the anterior surface and is hyperpigmented. It is composed of dense fibrous tissue covered by skin and contains bundles of smooth muscle fibers, which assist with milk expression. The skin adjacent to the nipple is also hyperpigmented and is called the areola.

The breast parenchyma consists of 15 to 20 lobules, which drain secretions into a ductal system that converges and opens into the nipple.[1] The functional unit of the breast is the terminal duct lobular unit (TDLU) (Fig. 1-2), which is composed of the terminal (intralobular) duct, and its ductules/acini (also referred to as lobules). The terminal ducts join together to form the larger ducts, which have a dilatation (lactiferous sinus) just before they open into the nipple. The TDLUs are embedded in loose specialized, hormonally responsive connective tissue stroma, the intralobular stroma. The dense fibrous tissue between the breast lobules is called interlobular stroma, which is not responsive to hormones (Fig. 1-3).

Lymphatic drainage of the breast is to the *axillary*, *supraclavicular*, and *mediastinal* lymph nodes.

Histology

The entire ductal system, extralobular large and intermediate ducts, as well as the intralobular (terminal ducts and ductules/lobules), is lined by two cell layers: inner epithelial cells and an outer interrupted layer of myoepithelial cells.[1] The latter cells have contractile properties and assist in expelling milk. Special techniques can be used to highlight the myoepithelial cells. Immunohistochemical stains for muscle-specific actin (MSA), S100, p63, and calponin can be used to detect the myoepithelial cell layer (Fig. 1-4).

The largest ducts change from a columnar epithelial lining to a squamous epithelial lining just distal to the lactiferous sinus, beyond which it becomes stratified squamous epithelium and merges with the surface skin.

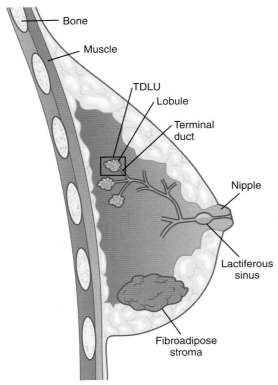

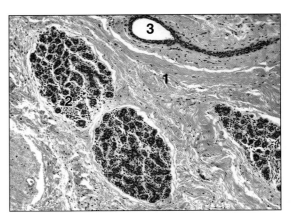

Figure 1-3. Normal female breast.   Lobules (2) scattered within interlobular stroma (1). A larger duct is also seen (3) (H&E, ×100).

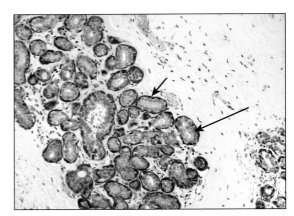

Figure 1-4. Two-cell lining of the ductal system.   The inner layer consists of epithelial cells (*long arrow*), and the calponin stain highlights the outer myoepithelial cells (*short arrow*) (Calponin stain, ×200).

Figure 1-1. Normal breast.   Diagram of breast composition and location. TDLU, terminal ductal lobular unit.

Labels on Figure 1-1: Bone, Muscle, TDLU, Lobule, Terminal duct, Nipple, Lactiferous sinus, Fibroadipose stroma

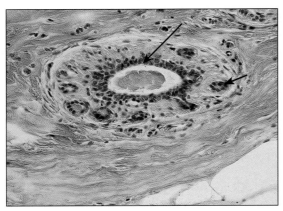

Figure 1-2. The terminal ductal lobular unit (TDLU) is the functional unit of the breast. The large arrow indicates the terminal (intralobular) duct. The short arrow identifies the ductules (lobules) (H&E, ×200).

Physiologic Changes in Female Breast Histology

During childhood and before puberty, the female breast is composed of a branching ductal system that lacks lobular units. At puberty, female glan-dular tissue proliferates under stimulation of estrogen and progesterone. Once formed, the lactiferous ducts and interlobular duct system are stable and unaffected by fluctuating hormone levels during the menstrual cycle, pregnancy, and lactation. The TDLUs, however, are dynamic and undergo changes with alterations in hormone levels. These changes involve both the epithelium and the intralobular stroma.

Menstrual Cycle

The following are pre- and postmenstrual phases of the menstrual cycle:

Follicular phase: During the follicular phase of the menstrual cycle, the TDLUs are at rest and do not show any growth. The intralobular stroma is dense and indistinct from the dense interlobular stroma.

Luteal phase: After ovulation, the terminal duct epithelium proliferates, and the number of terminal ducts within a lobule increases and the basal epithelial cells become vacuolated. The intralobular stroma is edematous and loose and becomes distinct from the interlobular stroma. These changes manifest as progressive fullness, heaviness, and tenderness of the breast.

Menses: As the levels of estrogen and progesterone fall with the onset of menstruation, there is an increase in apoptosis in the TDLU. Lymphocytes infiltrate the intralobular stroma, which becomes dense. The TDLU finally regresses to its resting appearance.

Pregnancy: During pregnancy, there is a striking increase in the number of terminal ducts, and the TDLUs are enlarged in response to the rising sex hormone levels.

Lactation: In the lactating breast, the individual terminal ducts form acini, which show epithelial vacuolization as a result of the presence of secretions that also fill their lumina (Fig. 1-5). After lactation, the units involute and return to their old structure.

Postmenopause: After menopause, the TDLUs atrophy owing to the low hormone levels so that only small residual foci remain. The lactiferous ducts and interlobular duct system remain, but the interlobular stroma is reduced in amount accompanied by a relative increase in fatty tissue.

The normal male breast differs in structure from the female breast in that there are no

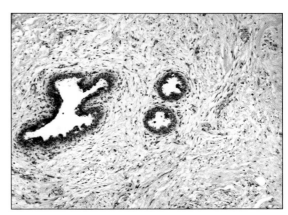

Figure 1-6. Normal male breast consists of a few ductal structures and stroma. There are no lobules (H&E, ×100).

lobules. The male breast consists of ductal structures surrounded by fibroadipose tissue (Fig. 1-6).

Abnormalities of Breast Development

The following are abnormalities that can occur in breast development:

Mammary heterotopia (accessory breasts or nipples) may occur anywhere along embryonic mammary ridges, the most common sites being the chest wall, axilla, and vulva. It may manifest as polythelia (supernumerary nipples) or polymastia (aberrant breast tissue).[2] The accessory breast tissue responds to hormonal changes and, if located in the axilla, it may enlarge and raise concern for metastases.

Congenital inverted nipples are clinically significant, since a similar change may be produced by underlying cancer.

Juvenile hypertrophy (virginal hypertrophy) is a rare condition in adolescent girls in which the breasts (usually both; rarely only one) markedly enlarge owing to hormonal stimulation. No endocrine abnormality is detected. Patients present with embarrassment, pain, and discomfort. Reduction mammoplasty improves the quality of life.

Hamartoma is a well–circumscribed, often encapsulated mass composed of varying combinations of benign epithelial and stromal elements including fat.[3] Hamartoma is usually asymptomatic. It may manifest as a palpable mass, or it may be detected by mammography. Hamartoma may cause breast deformity if it is very large.

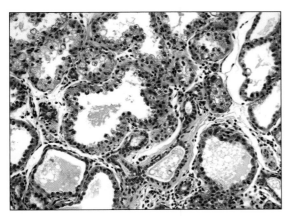

Figure 1-5. Lactating breast. Increased number of lobules with cytoplasmic vacuoles and intraluminal secretion (H&E, ×200).

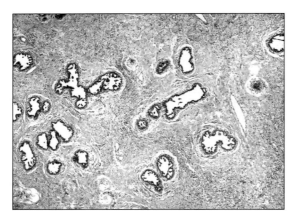

Figure 1-7. Gynecomastia. Stromal and ductal proliferation in the male breast (H&E, ×100).

Gynecomastia

Gynecomastia is defined as enlargement of one or both breasts in a male.[4] Many cases are idiopathic. In some cases, gynecomastia may be caused by excessive estrogen stimulation. Predisposing factors include the following:

- Hormonal imbalance, as may occur in puberty or old age
- Exogenous hormones
- Drugs, including dilantin, digitalis, and marijuana
- Klinefelter syndrome (testicular feminization)
- Testicular tumors
- Liver disease

On palpation, a firm disc-shaped subareolar mass is noted. Microscopic features of gynecomastia include ductal epithelial hyperplasia, stromal edema, and fibrosis around ducts (Fig. 1-7).

Inflammatory and Reactive Breast Lesions

The following are inflammatory and reactive breast conditions of various causes:

Acute inflammation of the breast (acute mastitis) is associated with redness, swelling, pain, and tenderness and may occur during the early postpartum months as a result of lactation (puerperal mastitis).[5] *Staphylococcus aureus* is the most common infecting agent. There are two general categories of predisposing factors:

- Cracks in the nipple and stasis of milk due to improper nursing technique
- Stress and sleep deprivation, which may lower the immune status and cause engorgement by inhibiting milk flow

At the microscopic level, cellulitis of the interlobular connective tissue is seen. Diagnosis is made on clinical grounds, and antibiotics lead to complete resolution. Delay in treatment may lead to abscess formation and requires drainage of pus.

Inflammatory breast carcinoma should be ruled out when there is no response to antibiotic therapy.

Chronic mastitis may be idiopathic[6–8] or in response to infection (tuberculosis), foreign material (silicone), or systemic disease (sarcoidosis). Diagnosis requires microbiologic, immunologic, and histologic evaluation. Idiopathic granulomatous mastitis[7] is diagnosed after exclusion of specific etiologic agents. Microscopically, chronic mastitis shows granulomas with or without caseation. Surgical excision may be followed by recurrence, abscess formation, or fistula formation.

Mammary duct ectasia is a distinct entity that usually occurs in perimenopausal women as a result of obstruction of the lactiferous ducts by inspissated luminal secretions. Obstruction leads to dilatation of the ducts and periductal chronic inflammation (Fig. 1-8). Grossly, chronic mastitis may produce irregular masses with induration that closely mimic breast carcinoma, and biopsy may be required to exclude carcinoma.

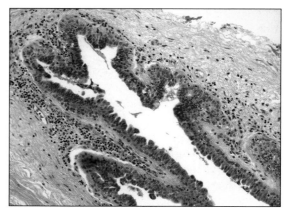

Figure 1-8. Mammary duct ectasia. A dilated duct and periductal chronic inflammation (H&E, ×200).

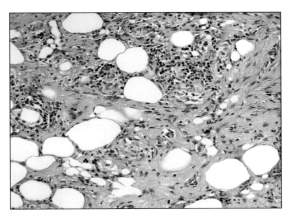

Figure 1-9. Fat necrosis. Necrotic fat cells with inflammatory cells (H&E, ×200).

Fat necrosis is a benign disease involving adipose tissue in the supporting stroma of the breast.[9] The cause may be related to ischemia and trauma (accidental or surgical). In the early phase, it is characterized by collection of neutrophils and histiocytes around the necrotic fat cells (Fig. 1-9). Later, histiocytes join to form giant cells, and fibrosis and calcification occur. The clinical importance of fat necrosis is that this may present as a hard mass that can be suggestive of carcinoma on physical examination as well as radiologic studies. Microscopic examination confirms the benign nature of the lesion.

Silicone granuloma is formed as a result of leakage of silicone gel from breast augmentation prosthesis.[10] The lesion is composed of numerous microcysts, some of which coalesce to form larger spaces that may be empty or contain refractile material. Foamy histiocytes and foreign body giant cells are also present (Fig. 1-10A and B).

Diabetic mastopathy is an uncommon condition seen in patients with type 1 diabetes.[11] Patients present with solitary or multiple ill-defined, painless nodules. Diabetic mastopathy mimics carcinoma on clinical examination and radiologic studies. Histologic examination shows dense fibrosis and lymphocytic mastitis. The latter includes B-lymphocyte infiltration surrounding the ducts, lobules, and blood vessels (Fig. 1-11). This is considered an immune response to the abnormal deposits of extracellular matrix due to hyperglycemia.

Pseudoangiomatous stromal hyperplasia (PASH) is a benign condition characterized by proliferation of interlobular stroma, which may

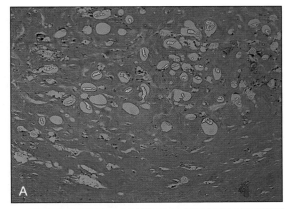

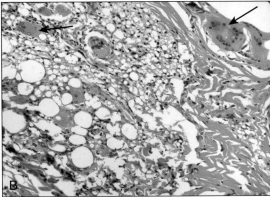

Figure 1-10. Silicone granuloma. **A,** Microcysts, some of which have coalesced around refractile foreign material. **B,** Foamy histiocytes and foreign body giant cells (*arrows*). (H&E, ×200.)

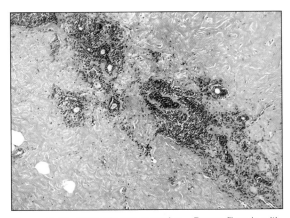

Figure 1-11. Diabetic mastopathy. Dense fibrosis with lobulitis (lobules surrounded by chronic inflammatory cells) (H&E, ×100).

manifest as a discrete palpable mass (nodular PASH) or by multifocal PASH, which may be found incidentally in benign or malignant breast biopsies.[12] Histologically, the lesion consists of complex slitlike pseudovascular spaces within a dense collagenous stroma. These spaces do not have an endothelial lining compared with true endothelial spaces. Thus, immunohistochemical stains for endothelial markers are negative, which is helpful in differentiating PASH from angiosarcoma.

Radial scar or complex sclerosing lesion is a localized nonencapsulated stellate lesion, which can mimic a carcinoma in a mammogram and a tubular carcinoma in histologic sections. Microscopic sections show a core of fibroelastic tissue with radiating bands of collagen, and within this connective tissue are foci of sclerosing adenosis, ductal hyperplasia, cysts, and apocrine metaplasia[13] (Fig. 1-12A and B).

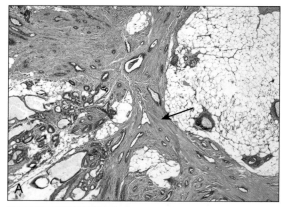

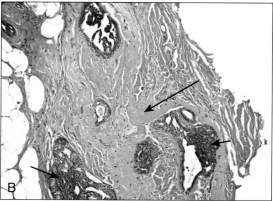

Figure 1-12. Radial scar. A, Core of fibroelastic tissue (*arrow*) and ducts with varying degrees of usual hyperplasia. **B,** Radiating bands of dense fibroelastic tissue (*long arrow*) and ductal hyperplasia (*medium and short arrows*). (H&E, ×100.)

Fibroepithelial Lesions

A **fibroadenoma** is a benign neoplasm often found in young women between the ages of 15 and 35, but it may occur at any age.[14] Clinically, it is seen as a single, discrete, mobile nontender mass composed of proliferating ducts (*adenoma*) and proliferating specialized intralobular fibroblastic stroma (*fibro*) (Fig. 1-13). Fibroadenoma is not associated with an increased risk of the development of breast cancer. It is cured by excision.

A **lactating adenoma** is a benign lesion in which lactational changes have supervened.[15] It may be associated with rapid increase in size during pregnancy, raising a suspicion of carcinoma.

Phyllodes tumors are rare tumors composed of intralobular stroma and ductal epithelium.[16] There is a spectrum of aggressiveness from benign to malignant (low grade and high grade). Most are benign, remain localized, and are cured by excision. Low-grade malignant phyllodes tumors may recur after excision. High-grade malignant phyllodes tumors can metastasize to distant sites (e.g., lungs).

Most phyllodes tumors grow to a massive size of up to 16 cm. A cut section shows leaflike architecture and clefts (*phyllodes* comes from the Greek word for leaves). Microscopically, the leaflike structures are lined by benign epithelium overlying a stromal overgrowth (Fig. 1-14). Many criteria are used to differentiate benign from malignant phyllodes tumors. Benign phyllodes tumors have no cytologic atypia and less than 5 mitoses/10 HPF. Low-grade malignant

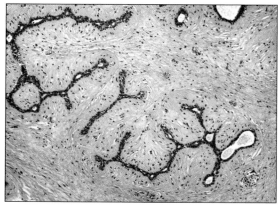

Figure 1-13. Fibroadenoma composed of benign proliferation of ducts and fibroblastic stroma (H&E, ×100).

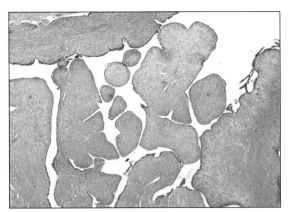

Figure 1-14. Phyllodes tumor. Leaflike structures of stromal overgrowth, lined by benign epithelium (H&E, ×100).

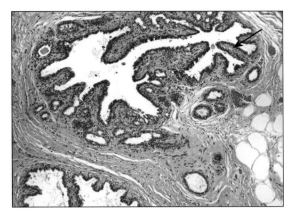

Figure 1-15. Papilloma. Intraductal epithelial proliferation composed of fibrovascular cores (*arrow* denotes the fibrovascular core) (H&E, ×100).

phyllodes tumors have 5 to 10 mitoses/10 HPF. High-grade malignant phyllodes tumors are hypercellular, with nuclear atypia and a higher number of mitoses—more than 10 mitoses/10 HPF.

Papillary Lesions

Intraductal papillomas are of two types: central papillomas, commonly originating in a major duct near the nipple, and peripheral papillomas, which arise from the TDLU.[17]

Central papillomas commonly are associated with a bloody nipple discharge. Most ductal papillomas are small—about 1 cm in diameter. Large tumors are palpable as a subareolar mass. Grossly, the tumor appears as a papillary mass projecting into the lumen of a large duct. Histologically, there are numerous delicate papillae composed of a fibrovascular core, covered by a layer of epithelial and myoepithelial cells (Fig. 1-15). Based on the cytologic and architectural features, a papilloma may be benign, atypical, or malignant (intraductal carcinoma).

Peripheral papillomas (papillomatosis) are often multiple, arise in the TDLU, and may extend into adjacent ducts. They are clinically and mammographically occult. Their histologic appearance is the same as that of central papillomas, but peripheral papillomas are more likely to be associated with various types of ductal proliferations, such as sclerosing adenosis, radial scar, usual ductal hyperplasia, atypical ductal hyperplasia, ductal carcinoma in situ, and invasive ductal carcinoma.

Fibrocystic Change

Fibrocystic change (FCC) encompasses a group of morphologic changes that often produce palpable lumps and are characterized by various combinations of cysts, fibrous overgrowth, and epithelial proliferation.[18-20] FCC has been found at autopsy in up to 50% of women who had no symptoms of breast disease during life, suggesting that these changes may be physiologic variations rather than disease. Thus, the term "fibrocystic change" rather than "fibrocystic disease" is preferred.[19] Some of these changes are entirely innocuous, whereas others are associated with increased risk of subsequent carcinoma. A diagnosis of FCC should therefore specify the components of the morphologic changes present.

The cause of FCC is not known. It is the single most common disorder of the breast. The condition is diagnosed frequently between the ages of 20 and 55 and decreases progressively after menopause. FCC consists of asymptomatic masses in the breast, which are discovered by palpation. The masses vary from diffuse small irregularities (lumpy, bumpy breast) to a discrete mass or masses. These changes may also be associated with pain, which may be cyclical with midcycle or premenstrual discomfort. Pain may be focal or diffuse and may or may not be associated with the lumps.

Cysts in the breast, which arise in the TDLU, are usually unilocular. Smaller cysts are not discernible on gross examination, but clusters of small cysts may be palpable. Large cysts often contain turbid or semitranslucent fluid, which

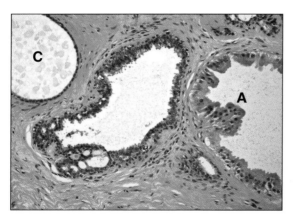

Figure 1-16. Fibrocystic change. Apocrine metaplasia (A), cysts (C), and a duct in the center with mild hyperplasia of the usual type (H&E, ×100).

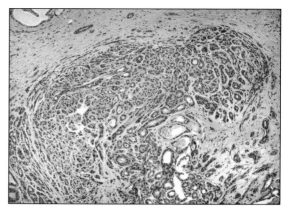

Figure 1-17. Columnar cell change without atypia (H&E, ×100).

gives a blue color to the intact cyst, the *blue-domed cyst*. Histologically, cysts may be lined by flattened epithelium or by columnar epithelium with features of apocrine cells, or they may completely lack an epithelial lining (Fig. 1-16).

Apocrine metaplasia refers to a histologic alteration of the epithelium of TDLUs in which the cells resemble apocrine sweat gland epithelium.[21] Embryologically, the breast arises from the same anlage that produces apocrine glands. However, apocrine glands are not part of the normal histologic components of the breast. Nevertheless, any benign proliferative lesion may contain cells with the cytologic features of apocrine cells.

No specific gross features are associated with apocrine metaplasia. The condition is seen most frequently in the epithelial lining of cysts. It consists of cuboidal to tall columnar cells with fine granular, eosinophilic cytoplasm, and round, uniform, basally placed nuclei with single central, small nucleoli. "Snouts" or blebs protrude from the apical surface into the glandular lumen (Fig. 1-16).

Columnar cell change (CCC) and **columnar cell hyperplasia (CCH)** involve dilated terminal duct-lobular units, which are lined by uniform, ovoid-to-elongate, nontypical columnar cells, and these frequently exhibit prominent apical snouts.[22] CCC is one or two cell layers thick, and CCH shows a lining more than two cells thick. These cells differ from apocrine metaplasia as the cytoplasm is not abundant and not pink and granular, while the nuclei are bland and oval and lack prominent nucleoli (Fig. 1-17).

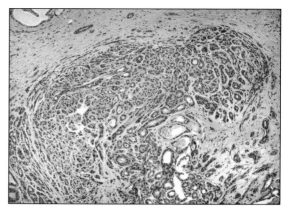

Figure 1-18. Sclerosing adenosis. Proliferation of acinar structures and stroma with distortion of the terminal duct lobular unit (H&E, ×100).

If CCC is associated with atypia (enlarged ovoid nuclei, marginated chromatin, prominent nucleoli, lack of basal polarization of nuclei), then the term **CCC with atypia** or **flat epithelial atypia** is used. This lesion is more often associated with atypical ductal proliferations and in situ carcinomas.

Sclerosing adenosis most often occurs as an incidental microscopic finding but may manifest as a palpable mass that may be mistaken clinically for cancer. It is almost always associated with other forms of fibrocystic change. Diffuse microcalcifications are commonly seen in the lesion, which may mimic carcinoma on mammography. Microscopically,[23] sclerosing adenosis consists of proliferation of acinar structures and stroma with distortion of the TDLU (Fig. 1-18). Multiple altered lobules may be seen. The pro-

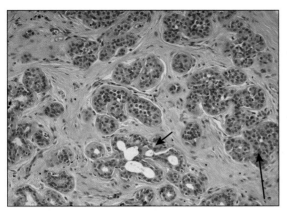

Figure 1-19. Atypical lobular hyperplasia. Less than 50% of lobules show epithelial proliferation (*long arrow*) compared with normal lobules (*short arrow*) (H&E, ×100).

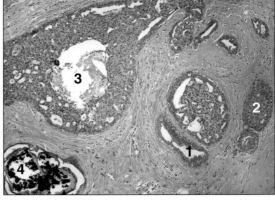

Figure 1-20. Ductal hyperplasia of the usual type: mild (1), moderate (2), and florid (3) hyperplasia of the usual type. Microcalcifications are also present (4) (H&E, ×100).

liferated acini may be compressed and deformed, producing whorls and cords that may mimic infiltrating carcinoma, particularly in the center of the lesion.

Epithelial or **ductal hyperplasia** describes a proliferative condition that is manifested histologically as an increase in the cellularity of the epithelium of the TDLU.[24–26] It is a microscopic finding that cannot be predicted clinically or by mammographic examination. The lesion may coexist with other features of fibrocystic change, but in some cases it may form the predominant pattern. Epithelial hyperplasia may involve the terminal duct epithelium (ductal hyperplasia) or the acinar epithelium (lobular hyperplasia).

Lobular hyperplasia is an increased number of cells within the lobules. The two types are:

- Atypical lobular hyperplasia (ALH), in which less than 50% of the lobules are filled with epithelial cell proliferation (Fig. 1-19)
- Lobular carcinoma in situ (LCIS), in which more than 50% of the lobules are filled and distended by epithelial proliferation

Ductal hyperplasia represents a spectrum of changes that extends from hyperplasia of the usual type to atypical hyperplasia to carcinoma in situ.

- **Ductal hyperplasia of the usual type** consists of an increase in the epithelial layer lining with more than two cell layers, which distend the terminal ducts. Either the epithelial proliferation may form papillary tufts projecting into the lumen (mild hyperplasia), or epithelial cells may proliferate to bridge and create arcades (moderate hyperplasia) or form solid masses that fill and distend the lumen and may have irregular fenestrations (florid hyperplasia) (Fig. 1-20). Individual cell borders are inconspicuous so that the cell mass has a syncytial appearance. Nuclear spacing is uneven, leading to overcrowding and nuclear overlap in areas, and nucleoli are inconspicuous or absent. Often two distinct cell populations—epithelial and myoepithelial cells—may be discerned.[24,25]
- **Atypical ductal hyperplasia** has some of the architectural and cytologic features of carcinoma in situ but lacks the complete criteria for that diagnosis.[26]
- **Ductal carcinoma in situ** consists of malignant cells confined within the basement membranes of ducts without invasion of the surrounding stroma.

The risk of breast cancer in benign and premalignant epithelial proliferation is summarized in Box 1-1.

Conclusion

The breast is a complex organ that contains hormonally responsive and hormonally unresponsive tissue elements. Normal maturational changes occur over the lifetime of the individual. Some of these changes result in clinical findings that lead to a tissue biopsy. Discriminating between benign, atypical, and malignant changes

---

Box 1-1. Risk of Breast Cancer in Benign and Premalignant Epithelial Proliferation

Studies have shown that there is a relationship between fibrocystic change and the relative risk of developing subsequent invasive carcinoma.[27] This risk is variable, depending on the type of histologic change, and is summarized below.

No increased risk

Cyst, apocrine metaplasia, sclerosing adenosis, fibrosis, and mild hyperplasia (>2 but <4 cells thick)

Slightly increased risk (1.5 to 2×)

Hyperplasia—moderate or florid (refers to extensive degrees of epithelial proliferation)
Papilloma

Moderately increased risk (4×)

Atypical ductal hyperplasia (ADH)
Atypical lobular hyperplasia (ALH)

Markedly increased risk (10×)

Ductal carcinoma in situ (DCIS)
Lobular carcinoma in situ (LCIS) is a *marker* for increased risk of developing invasive carcinoma. Risk is equal for both breasts, and subsequent carcinoma may be either ductal or lobular (see Chapter 2).

---

is important to appropriately direct therapy. Most of these benign changes do not indicate a significant increased risk for the future development of breast cancer. Some of these changes, however, do serve as a warning of a significant increased risk for the future development of breast cancer. Accurate identification of these patients can lead to appropriate interventions in screening and therapy, which will be discussed in Chapters 6 and 9.

References

1. Tucker JA, McCarty KS: Breast. In Sternberg SS (ed): Histology for Pathologists. New York, Raven Press, 1992, p 893–896.
2. Rosen PP: Abnormalities of mammary growth and development. In Rosen PP (ed): Rosen's Breast Pathology, 2nd ed. Philadelphia: Lippincott Williams & Wilkins, 2001, pp 23–27.
3. Tse GMK, Law BKB, Ma TKF, et al: Hamartoma of the breast: a clinicopathological review. J Clin Pathol 55:951–954, 2002.
4. Devilee P, Prechtel K, Levi F, et al: Tumors of the male breast. In World Health Organization Classification of Tumors: Tumors of the Breast and Female Genital Organs. Washington, DC: IARC Press, 2003, pp 110–111.
5. Barbosa-Cesnik C, Schwartz K, Foxman B: Lactation mastitis. JAMA 289:1609–1612, 2003.
6. Diesing D, Axt-Fliedner R, Hornung D, et al: Granulomatous mastitis. Arch Gynecol Obstet 269:233–236, 2004.
7. Erhan Y, Veral A, Kara E, et al: A clinicopathologic study of a rare clinical entity mimicking breast carcinoma: idiopathic granulomatous mastitis. Breast 9:52–56, 2000.
8. Azlina AF, Ariza Z, Arni T, et al: Chronic granulomatous mastitis: diagnostic and therapeutic considerations. World J Surg 27:515–518, 2003.
9. Pullyblank AM, Davies JD, Basten J, et al: Fat necrosis of the female breast: Hadfield re-visited. Breast 10:388–391, 2001.
10. Van Diest PJ, Beekman WH, Hage JJ: Pathology of silicone leakage from breast implants. J Clin Pathol 51:493–497, 1998.
11. Haj M, Weiss M, Herskovits T: Diabetic sclerosing lymphocytic lobulitis of the breast. J Diabetes Complications 18:187–191, 2004.
12. Castro CY, Whitman GJ, Sahin AA: Pseudoangiomatous stromal hyperplasia of the breast. Am J Clin Oncol 25:213–216, 2002.
13. Kennedy M, Masterson AV, Kerin M, et al: Pathology and clinical relevance of radial scars: a review. J Clin Pathol 56:721–724, 2003.
14. Bellocq JP, Magro G: Fibroepithelial tumors. In World Health Organization Classification of Tumors: Tumors of the Breast and Female Genital Organs. Washington, DC: IARC Press, 2003, pp 99–100.
15. Bellocq JP, Magro G: Fibroepithelial tumors. In World Health Organization Classification of Tumors: Tumors of the Breast and Female Genital Organs. Washington, DC: IARC Press, 2003, p 84.
16. Bellocq JP, Magro G: Fibroepithelial tumors. In World Health Organization Classification of Tumors: Tumors of the Breast and Female Genital Organs. Washington, DC: IARC Press, 2003, pp 100–101.
17. Oyama T, Koerner FC: Noninvasive papillary proliferations. Semin Diagn Pathol 21:32–41, 2004.
18. Rosai J: Breast. In Rosai and Ackerman's Surgical Pathology, 9th ed. Philadelphia: Mosby, 2004, pp 1763–1876.
19. Love SM, Gelman RS, Silen W: Fibrocystic "disease" of the breast—a non-disease? N Engl J Med 307:1010–1014, 1982.
20. Guray M, Sahin AA: Benign breast diseases: classification, diagnosis, and management. The Oncologist 11(5):435–449, May 2006; doi:10.1634/theoncologist.11-5-435.
21. O'Malley FP, Bane AL: The spectrum of apocrine lesions of the breast. Adv Anat Pathol 11:1–9, 2004.
22. Schnitt SJ, Vincent-Salomon A: Columnar cell lesions of the breast. Adv Anat Pathol 10:113–124, 2003.
23. Rosen PP: Adenosis and microglandular adenosis. In Rosen PP (ed): Rosen's Breast Pathology, 2nd ed. Philadelphia: Lippincott Williams & Wilkins, 2001, pp 139–151.
24. Dupont WD, Parl FF, Hartmann WH, et al: Breast cancer risk associated with proliferative breast disease and atypical hyperplasia. Cancer 71:1258–1265, 1993.
25. Koerner FC: Epithelial proliferations of ductal type. Semin Diagn Pathol 21:10–17, 2004.
26. Tavassoli FA: Ductal intraepithelial neoplasia. In Tavassoli FA (ed): Pathology of the Breast, 2nd ed. Norwalk, CT: Appleton & Lange, 1999, pp 205–323.
27. Fitzgibbons PL, Henson DE, Hutter RVP: Benign breast changes and the risk for subsequent breast cancer: an update of the 1985 consensus statement. Arch Pathol Lab Med 122:1053–1055, 1998.

2 Ductal and Lobular Proliferations: Preinvasive Breast Disease

Meenakshi Singh and Jon V. Rittenbach

KEY POINTS

- Epithelial proliferative diseases of the breast most commonly arise adjacent to or from the terminal duct lobular units (TDLU) of the breast and are generally classified as ductal or lobular, based on the histologic appearance.
- The current view is that breast epithelial proliferations are best viewed as a histologic and possible biologic continuum, with diagnostic criteria separating the proliferative processes into risk/prognostic groups.
- Ductal lesions include ductal hyperplasia of the usual type (DHUT), atypical ductal hyperplasia (ADH), and ductal carcinoma in situ (DCIS).
- Based on studies by the Vanderbilt group, the relative risk (RR) of invasive carcinoma increases from 2 times normal for well-established ductal hyperplasia of the usual type, to 4 times for ADH, and increases to 10 times for DCIS.
- The spectrum of proliferative lobular disease is classified as atypical lobular hyperplasia (ALH) and lobular carcinoma in situ (LCIS); both are also referred to as lobular neoplasia (LN). They have been shown to have a relative risk of 5 to 12 times the general population and an almost equal risk of ductal or lobular carcinoma in both breasts.
- Estrogen receptors are nearly uniformly present in ductal hyperplasia of the usual type and ADH and are less expressed through progressive grades of DCIS.
- Even among experienced pathologists, the interobserver diagnostic variability for intraductal and lobular proliferative processes is high, especially between ADH and low-grade DCIS.
- Correct categorization of epithelial proliferations of the breast is important for accurate risk assessment for individual patients and for therapy decisions regarding the use of chemoprevention.

Introduction

The environmental and biologic factors involved in the development of epithelial proliferations of the breast and invasive breast carcinoma have been studied extensively. Despite this effort, a unified explanation of the relationship between preinvasive breast disease and invasive carcinoma remains, at best, partially answered. One hypothesis of breast cancer development holds that a sequential progression of proliferative changes places the breast at progressively increased risk for invasive carcinoma. Application of specific diagnostic criteria ensures correct categorization of these proliferative changes. Interaction between pathologists and clinicians in breast multidisciplinary conferences results in clinical-radiographic-pathologic correlation, and this should be a gold standard for the care of patients with breast disease. Although the concept of a linear model of progression is an attractive one, it is not true for all cases. In some patients, proliferative lesions appear to stabilize or even regress, and in other patients invasive carcinoma is the first indication of disease. Fortunately, however, the latter scenario is less common, and in general the progression through the preinvasive stages of breast disease is linear and continues slowly over many years, providing ample time to make a diagnosis and treat the patient.[1]

Epithelial proliferative diseases such as atypical ductal hyperplasia (ADH) and low-grade ductal carcinoma in situ (DCIS) are lesions of interest to pathologists, since they need to be differentiated from each other and diagnosed accurately. Clinicians have an interest because they have to manage and follow up lesions that are benign but that increase the risk for breast cancer. Although patients may not have a sophisticated understanding of all the clinical implications, they have to make decisions about therapy and rely on advice from their physicians. Finally, these preinvasive diseases are of great interest to researchers as targets for reducing the incidence of breast cancer. All concerned parties can agree that the classification of breast disease should correlate with clinical outcome and their treatment tailored accordingly. Risk is categorized as relative risk and absolute risk. Relative risk is used when comparisons are made between two groups. Thus, when it is stated that DCIS has a relative risk of 10, the comparison is assumed to be the general population (women), which has its own risk of disease. This point can by illustrated by a woman with a baseline risk of 5 in 100. The addition of DCIS would give her an added relative risk of 10. Thus, her risk of invasive carcinoma increases to 50 in 100 and does not refer in any way to risk of death from this disease.[2]

Absolute risk, on the other hand, identifies the risk of an individual or group of individuals to develop cancer over a unit of time (expressed as percent), independent of risks associated with other populations.[3] In discussions of proliferative breast disease, it is customary to refer to the relative risk.[2]

The two patterns of advanced in situ proliferative lesions in the human female breast are ductal and lobular patterns. DCIS and lobular carcinoma in situ (LCIS) were recognized as being associated with invasive carcinoma 50 years ago. Although the histologic patterns of proliferative diseases are amazingly diverse, their clinical presentation is often the same (i.e., mammographically detected calcifications).[4]

Ductal proliferations have been divided into three groups based on histologic criteria, and these have been associated with differences in prognosis. These are ductal carcinoma in situ, ductal hyperplasia of the usual type, and atypical ductal hyperplasia (Fig. 2-1).

Ductal Carcinoma in Situ

DCIS is a cytologically malignant epithelial cell proliferation that is confined within the breast epithelial structures and does not cross the basement membrane, as does invasive carcinoma.[5] The distinction between DCIS and invasive carcinoma is made through histologic examination of standard hematoxylin and eosin (H&E)–stained sections and in some cases with the adjunctive use of immunohistochemical stains for delineating the myoepithelial layer that invests all the breast epithelial structures (but is

absent or breached in invasive carcinoma). The ideal marker for myoepithelial cells is p63 because it stains the nuclei. Cytoplasmic immunostains include smooth muscle myosin heavy chain, calponin, and muscle-specific actin (MSA), which is less specific since myofibroblasts can also be stained.

DCIS is common and has been reported in 25% of screen-detected breast carcinoma. It may arise in any location throughout either breast.[6] DCIS does not always progress to invasive carcinoma.

Many classification schemes have been proposed for DCIS. The commonly used ones are three-tiered, based on architectural features, the presence or absence of central necrosis, and nuclear characteristics.[5] In current practice, the nuclear grade is emphasized because it is a more consistent finding compared with architectural features, which can be multiple within one patient. The nuclear grade is reported as high, intermediate, or low. Additional features that correlate with outcome include size, margin status, and the presence or absence of necrosis.[5,7,8] The nuclear grade has been associated with significant prognostic differences, and in the event that more than one grade is present, the disease is classified based on the highest grade seen (Fig. 2-2). The surgical report therefore should include the nuclear grade, the presence of any necrosis, the architectural type, the size of the DCIS, the status of the margin, and the presence and location of calcifications.[7]

The histologic patterns of DCIS are varied, and most cases include a combination of several of the patterns. These include cribriform, solid, papillary, micropapillary, apocrine, and comedo types (see Fig. 2-3). Although additional patterns have been described, they are not common and do not convey prognostic significance. Because of the variable nature of the architectural pattern expression within the breast and the frequent overlap within these patterns, they are no longer used as the primary means of classification.[5,7,8] It is important to note that central necrosis can be present in intermediate- and high-grade lesions. The term "comedo necrosis" is applied only to high-grade disease.[9]

High-Grade DCIS

High-grade DCIS contains large neoplastic cells with markedly pleomorphic, poorly polarized

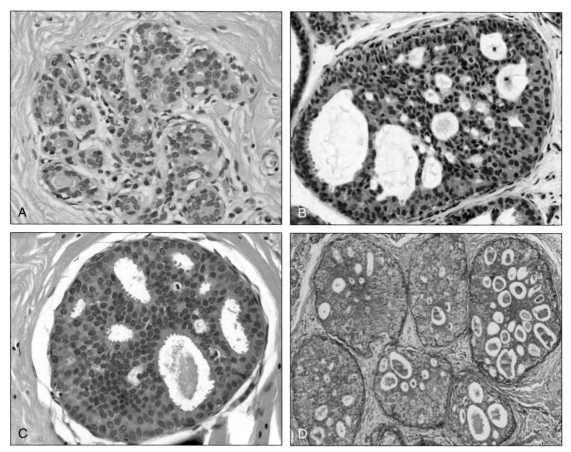

Figure 2-1. The spectrum from normal breast to ductal hyperplasia of the usual type (DHUT) to atypical ductal hyperplasia (ADH) to ductal carcinoma in situ (DCIS). **A,** The normal breast tissue illustrates a terminal duct lobular unit (×100). **B,** In this case of florid DHUT, variable-sized epithelial cells show overlap and streaming of the cells in an expanded duct. The lumina are irregular and haphazardly distributed (×400). **C,** ADH with a more monotonous cell population, occasional punched-out lumina, and part of the duct is lined by normal epithelial cells (×400). **D,** In this case of DCIS, multiple duct cross-sections are expanded by neoplastic cells, which fully replace the normal ductal epithelium, and the secondary lumina have a punched-out appearance (×100).

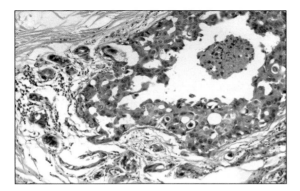

Figure 2-2. High-grade ductal carcinoma in situ (DCIS) with central necrosis. The cells in this duct display marked nuclear and cytologic pleomorphism (×100).

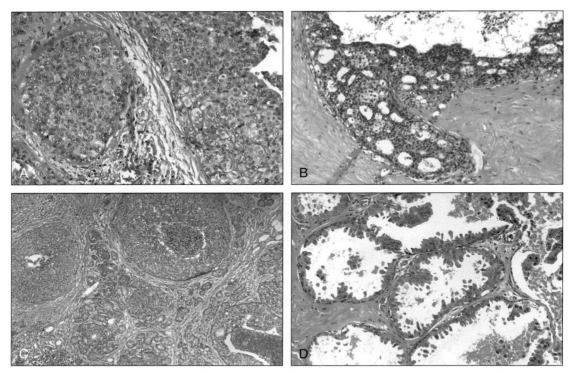

Figure 2-3. Architectural patterns of DCIS.   Solid (**A**), cribriform (**B**), central necrosis (**C**), and micropapillary (**D**) patterns (×100).

nuclei with irregular contours and a coarse, clumped chromatin with prominent nucleoli (see Fig. 2-2). Mitotic figures and central necrosis are frequently present, but are not necessary for the diagnosis. Severe anaplasia of even a single layer of duct lining cells can be sufficient for a diagnosis of high-grade DCIS. High-grade DCIS is often associated with extension into the lobules, periductal desmoplasia and an inflammatory response. Although these lesions are typically larger than 5 mm, with the appropriate histologic features, the diagnosis can be rendered on lesions of any size, even less than 1 mm, particularly in needle core biopsies[8] (Table 2-1).

Low-Grade DCIS

Low-grade DCIS is composed of uniform small cells that can grow in solid/cribriform, micropapillary, or arcade patterns. The cells are characterized by nuclear uniformity, rounded nuclear contours, finely granular chromatin, and inconspicuous nucleoli (Fig. 2-4). There is frequent nuclear polarity of the cells around the secondary lumina and the basement membrane of the

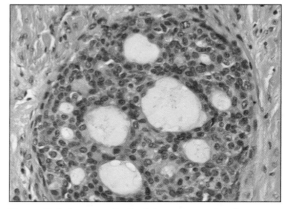

Figure 2-4. Low-grade ductal carcinoma in situ (DCIS).   This illustrates round, or ovoid, monotonous cells with hyperchromatic nuclei characteristic of this lesion. The cells are evenly spaced with well-defined borders without swirls or streaming. The extracellular lumina are smooth, round, and punched-out extracellular lumina (×400).

duct. In contrast to high-grade DCIS, mitotic activity is low. By definition, necrosis is absent. The presence of necrosis indicates a more aggressive behavior than lesions with similar cytomorphologic features, but lacking necrosis.[5–8]

Table 2-1. Comparative Features of Ductal Carcinoma in Situ of Different Grades

	Ductal Carcinoma in Situ		
	Low Grade	**Intermediate Grade**	**High Grade**
Clinical identification	Generally radiographic	Generally radiographic	Generally radiographic
Gross findings	May have pinpoint speckles	Pinpoint speckles or none	Often pinpoint speckles
Size	>2 mm	>2 mm	Usually >5 mm but can be any size
Cell distribution	Evenly spaced	With some polarization	Lacking polarization
Nucleus:cytoplasm ratio	Subtle increase	Mild increase	Marked increase
Nuclear pleomorphism and outlines	Monomorphic, round	Mild to moderate	Marked with irregular border
Nucleoli	Inconspicuous	1–2 small	Prominent
Mitotic activity	Minimal	Focal mild	High
Architectural pattern	Cribriform, micropapillary, rarely solid	Cribriform, micropapillary, solid	Solid, cribriform, micropapillary
Extracellular lumina	Usual lining cell polarization	Some polarization of lining cells	Lining cells lack polarization
Central necrosis	Not present	Can be present	Frequent
Calcifications	Generally psammomatous	Psammomatous, occasionally amorphous	Amorphous
Relative risk of carcinoma	————————————————	Generally increases with grade	————————————————

Intermediate-Grade DCIS

Intermediate-grade DCIS can have essentially the same cytology as low-grade disease with the addition of necrosis, or the nuclear and cytologic pleomorphism can be intermediate between high-grade and low-grade DCIS with or without necrosis. Finally, intermediate-grade DCIS generally has some areas of retained nuclear polarity, around either lumina or the basement membrane.[6]

Radiology

Calcifications within DCIS and in the surrounding benign breast tissue are common (see Fig. 2-3B) and can be radiographically detected in up to 70% of DCIS cases.[7] The radiographic size and characteristics of the calcifications may not accurately predict the size or histologic type. Nevertheless, coarsely granular and linear calcifications are generally associated with high-grade DCIS, whereas laminated and finely granular calcifications are more likely in low-grade lesions. Either type of calcification can be present in intermediate-grade DCIS.[5,8]

Differential Diagnosis

The differentiation of low-grade DCIS and ADH is based primarily on the extent of the disease because the lesions have similar histologic and cytologic characteristics. The two criteria for differentiating low-grade DCIS from ADH that have been proposed in the past are size greater than 2 mm and complete involvement of more than two duct cross-sections by the uniform cellular proliferation[5,10] (Table 2-2).

Receptors

Hormone receptors play a key role in regulating the growth and differentiation of breast epithelium and hormone receptor status is a prognostic indicator in invasive carcinoma. The expression of hormone receptors as determined by immunohistochemical stains indicates that the cells retain the ability to be manipulated by exogenous hormone therapy.

Estrogen receptors (ER) and progesterone receptors (PR) are uniformly expressed in normal breast tissue, ductal hyperplasia of the usual type, and ADH. In DCIS, there is less

Table 2-2. Comparative Features of Proliferative Ductal Lesions

	DHUT	ADH	Low-Grade DCIS
Clinical identification	Incidental	Incidental, mammographic	Mammographic calcifications, occasionally incidental
Gross findings	Not specific	Not specific	Not specific
Size	Generally small, <1–2 mm	<2 mm	>2 mm
Cell type	At least two types	At least focally uniform	Uniform, single cell type
Nuclear pleomorphism	Moderate	Mild to moderate with uniform areas	Minimal
Extracellular lumina	Irregular, slitlike with cells parallel to lumina	Irregular, slitlike, focally rigid	Uniformly rigid, punched out with cells perpendicular to lumina
Extracellular lumina location in duct	Primarily peripheral	Peripheral with a few central rigid spaces	Uniform distribution
Calcifications	Present or absent	Usually present	Frequent, psammomatous type
Relative risk of carcinoma	2× normal at 14–20 years	5× normal at 8–10 years, bilateral	8–11× normal, generally near lesion

ADH, atypical ductal hyperplasia; DCIS, ductal carcinoma in situ; DHUT, ductal hyperplasia of unusual type.

uniform expression, particularly in the higher-grade lesions. The overall expression of estrogen receptors in DCIS is about 75%.[8] In current practice in the United States, estrogen receptor is reported for cases of DCIS. Although HER2/neu is not assessed currently in cases of DCIS, it is known to be overexpressed in high-grade DCIS.

Patients with DCIS have a relative risk of 8 to 11 for developing invasive breast carcinoma—more so in the ipsilateral breast.[8]

Atypical Ductal Hyperplasia

ADH was first described by Dr. David Page in 1985 as having some, but not all, of the characteristics of low-grade DCIS (Fig. 2-5). One should not entertain the diagnosis of ADH unless DCIS is being considered in the differential diagnosis. ADH can have all of the cytologic features seen in low-grade DCIS. Architecturally, too, the lesions are similar, with ADH occasionally showing a few less rigid and less punched-out extracellular lumina than low-grade DCIS. The differentiating feature, however, is the extent of the process.[4] Essentially, the larger the lesion, the greater the likelihood that it is DCIS. ADH is favored when only part of a duct is involved or less than two contiguous complete ducts are involved or when the lesion is less than 2 mm in greatest dimension.[8] Even among

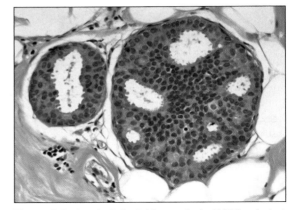

Figure 2-5. Atypical ductal hyperplasia (ADH). A duct space nearly but not completely replaced by a uniform population of cells. The secondary lumina have irregular outlines (×400).

experts, consensus for these criteria is still lacking.

ADH is considered an intermediate form of epithelial proliferation between low-grade DCIS and ductal hyperplasia of the usual type. The two primary features that separate ADH from ductal hyperplasia of the usual type are at least focal uniform cell population, and the architectural patterns (cribriform, micropapillary, solid), which ADH has and shares with low-grade DCIS and not with ductal hyperplasia of the usual type.[4]

ADH can be seen in varied locations including within fibroadenomas, papillomas, and radial scars. The clinical importance of ADH at these locations is unclear. It is appropriate to be conservative in making the diagnosis at these locations, but if the criteria of ADH are present, the diagnosis should be made. When evaluating the extent and size of the lesion, it is important to keep in mind that larger lesions are more likely to represent DCIS and that subsequent lumpectomy specimens following a diagnosis of ADH on a needle biopsy yield DCIS about 15% of the time.[5,7,8,11] In a recent large prospective study, patients with ADH had a relative risk of 4.2 for invasive carcinoma with an excess occurring in the same breast as the ADH.[12]

Ductal Hyperplasia of the Usual Type

Ductal hyperplasia of the usual type is the most common form of hyperplasia in the breast and is described in nearly 25% of benign breast biopsies (Fig. 2-6).[1] This lesion occurs primarily in the same location as other preinvasive lesions—the terminal duct lobular unit.[4]

This intraductal cellular proliferation is characterized by increased numbers of cell layers (more than two) above the basement membrane. The degree to which this occurs has been categorized as mild (three to four cells above the basement membrane), moderate, and florid hyperplasia (more than four cells above the basement membrane).[4] It may not be important to subclassify ductal hyperplasia of the usual type because there is a relatively small difference in prognosis among these categories and because even the most florid forms of ductal hyperplasia of the usual type hold very little increased risk. It is, however, significant to diagnose florid ductal hyperplasia of the usual type correctly and not to misclassify it as ADH or DCIS. The architectural features of ductal hyperplasia of the usual type include irregular extracellular/secondary lumina located at the duct periphery. The cells appear stretched and twisted with uneven nuclear distribution and some nuclear overlap. The key architectural feature is this streaming nature of the cells, especially where they form lumina and bridges, with the cells oriented parallel with the spaces.[4,8] This last feature differentiates ductal hyperplasia of the usual type from ADH and DCIS in which the cells do not show streaming, respect

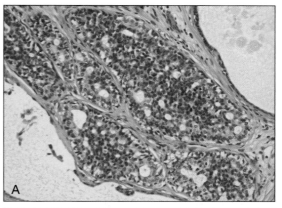

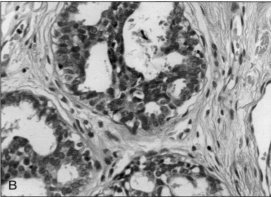

Figure 2-6. Florid ductal hyperplasia of the usual type (DHUT). Several ducts adjacent to fibrocystic changes contain proliferative epithelium (**A**) with variable cell appearance, nuclear overlap, stretched cells, streaming/swirling, and irregular secondary lumina (**B**) (×100).

each other's borders, and may be perpendicular to the luminal bridges imparting a comparison to Roman arches. One more feature helpful in differentiating ductal hyperplasia of the usual type from ADH is the presence of two or more cell types. Other features include variable-shaped nuclei and cell contours and indistinct cell margins.[8]

Ductal hyperplasia of the usual type does not have a classic clinical presentation, and the relative risk of invasive carcinoma is low at less than 2 for moderate and florid hyperplasia, whereas in mild hyperplasia it is essentially not increased. The average progression interval is 14 years with a greater occurrence in the ipsilateral breast, compared with 8.3 years for ADH in which the risk is considered to extend to both breasts.[8,10,12] It is also interesting to note that clinical risk factors such as family history, parity, menstrual history, and contralateral carcinoma all have significantly higher relative risks than ductal hyperplasia of the usual type.[9] For this reason, clinical follow-up is the preferred management strategy for these patients.

Lobular Neoplasia

In much the same way in which preinvasive ductal lesions are thought to progress from hyperplasia of the usual type to atypical ductal hyperplasia to ductal carcinoma in situ, lobular proliferations appear to follow a histologic progression from atypical lobular hyperplasia (ALH) (Fig. 2-7) to lobular carcinoma in situ (LCIS) (Fig. 2-8). Lobular hyperplasia without atypia generally is not considered a significant risk for subsequent disease and is not a well-defined entity.[1]

The term "lobular neoplasia" encompasses atypical lobular hyperplasia (ALH) and lobular carcinoma in situ (LCIS). The cell type is the same in both lesions. Lobular neoplasia, like most proliferative breast diseases, primarily involves the terminal duct lobular unit.[9] It is an important diagnostic entity found in 2% of all breast biopsies, particularly in perimenopausal women. Appropriate classification of lobular neoplasia requires application of strict diagnostic criteria.[3,7]

The cells of classic lobular neoplasia are dyscohesive, monotonous, round, cuboidal, or polygonal with clear/pale cytoplasm and round, bland nuclei. Intracytoplasmic vacuoles, when present, are a helpful feature.[13]

Architectural features are the key to differentiating ALH from LCIS (Table 2-3). LCIS is characterized by complete filling, distortion, and distention of at least one half of the terminal ducts and acini in one or more lobular units by the characteristic cells (see Fig. 2-8). ALH fails to meet at least one of the criteria for LCIS. In ALH, less than 50% of the acini are distended and distorted by the typical neoplastic cells. Neoplastic cell filling is incomplete with some central spaces remaining within acini. Other cell types may be intermixed in ALH.[3,9,14]

Morphologic clues of ADH include a compact arrangement of cells, cell borders, and a cohesive arrangement. This contrasts with LCIS, which can show intracytoplasmic vacuoles, generally

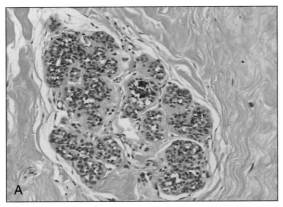

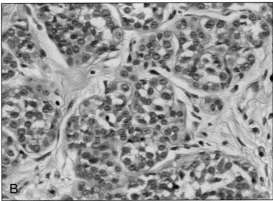

Figure 2-7. Atypical lobular hyperplasia (ALH).
Classic cells are present within the lobule, but do not significantly distend the lobule. **A,** Occasional lumina are still evident (×200). **B,** Intracytoplasmic vacuoles are present and help differentiate ALH from a ductal proliferation (×400).

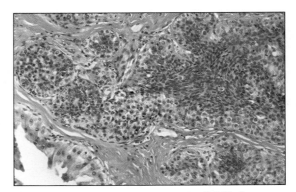

Figure 2-8. Lobular carcinoma in situ (LCIS) that resembles solid ductal carcinoma in situ (DCIS).
Neoplastic cells distend and distort a majority of the acini in a terminal duct lobular unit. Note: To differentiate this from DCIS an E-cadherin immunohistochemical stain was performed and revealed no expression, thereby confirming the diagnosis (×200).

Table 2-3. Comparative Features of Classic ALH and LCIS

	Lobular Neoplasia	
	ALH	**LCIS**
Clinical identification	Incidental, multifocal, bilateral, premenopause	Incidental, multifocal, bilateral, premenopause
Gross findings	None	None
Size	Generally <1 mm	Generally >1 mm
Cell type	Generally single-cell population, uniform size, clear cytoplasm, occasional additional cell types	Single-cell population, uniform size, clear cytoplasm
Nucleus:cytoplasm ratio	Low to moderate	Low to moderate
Nuclear pleomorphism	Minimal	Minimal
Nucleoli	Occasional, small	Occasional, small
Mitotic activity	Rare	Rare
Architectural pattern	<1/2 acini of a lobular unit filled and distended by the classic cells, intercellular spaces remain, or other cell types present	>1/2 acini of a lobular unit filled and distended by cells
Extracellular lumina	Irregular spaces can be present	Not present
Immunohistochemistry	E-cadherin-negative	E-cadherin-negative
Calcifications	May be present	May be present
Relative risk of carcinoma	5×, bilateral, any histologic type	10×, bilateral, any histologic type

ALH, atypical lobular hyperplasia; LCIS, lobular carcinoma in situ.

low-grade nuclei, dyscohesive cells, and a lack of discernible cell borders.[3]

Occasionally, morphologic overlap is seen between small cell solid ADH, in which duct spaces are filled with a uniform population of small cells, and lobular neoplasia. Therefore, if ADH extends to involve terminal duct lobules, it may be indistinguishable from LCIS on hematoxylin and eosin–stained sections. Some report such lesions as combined ADH and LCIS. This is a rare event when strict cytologic, architectural, and immunohistochemical criteria are used.[7]

Adhesion protein molecules are expressed in cells of epithelial lineage. These are calcium-dependent cell–cell adhesion proteins. One of these adhesion molecules that is important in breast cancer is E-cadherin. Loss of E-cadherin is considered to be a fundamental defect in invasive lobular carcinoma of the breast, and it is not surprising that its protein is not fully expressed in preinvasive as well as invasive lobular disease. This adhesion molecule can be useful in differentiating preinvasive ductal lesions such as solid-type DCIS in which E-cadherin is strongly expressed, from LCIS in which E-cadherin is not expressed.[7,14]

LCIS has been thought to be a marker for increased cancer risk in both breasts and not an obligate precursor. This belief underlies the clinical practice of not necessarily re-excising more tissue when LCIS is at the margin of an excision specimen (unlike with DCIS in which a negative margin is a surgical goal). However, the frequent association of LCIS with invasive lobular carcinoma and the genetic similarities suggest a possible precursor–product relationship between LCIS and invasive lobular carcinoma, and this highlights the importance of ensuring by radiologic, clinical, and pathologic correlation that the presence of LCIS at margins does not indicate additional invasive disease in the breast.[8]

LCIS and invasive lobular carcinomas often do not express E-cadherin protein. These cases often show mutations and loss of heterozygosity of wild-type CDH1 allele of the E-cadherin gene (located on Ch16q22.1).[13] This reiterates that lobular neoplasia is both a precursor lesion for invasive carcinoma and a risk factor.

Recently, a pleomorphic form of lobular carcinoma in situ (PLCIS) has been described and is often associated with a pleomorphic variant of invasive lobular carcinoma. This lesion is considered histologically similar to DCIS. In contrast to classic LCIS, pleomorphic LCIS has dyscohesive cells with larger nuclei (three to four times the size of a lymphocyte), marked nuclear pleomorphism, frequent prominent nucleoli, increased nucleus:cytoplasm ratio, and increased mitoses. Additional findings can include central necrosis and calcifications, which are generally not a feature of classic LCIS.[9,14] The primary clinical implication of this diagnosis is its common association with invasive carcinoma. Thus, it may require excision/re-excision of local tissue at margins to mitigate the risk of associated invasive carcinoma and would therefore be treated in much the same manner as DCIS.

The risk of invasive carcinoma associated with ALH and LCIS has been shown to range from 7 to 12 times that of the general population.[8] This risk doubles with a family history of breast cancer in a patient with ALH and approaches that of LCIS. The greatest risk for developing malignancy is in the first 10 to 15 years after the diagnosis. The invasive cancers associated with lobular neoplasia can be of any histologic type and may occur in either breast.[7,8,10,14]

Note that the characterization of hyperplastic lesions of the human female breast by modern molecular markers and indicators of specific biologic activity is still in its infancy. More studies are needed for the full picture to unfold; however, some of the data generated thus far raise questions about current dogmas in clinical practice, particularly those related to lobular neoplasia.

Acknowledgment: Some of these and many additional pictures of breast pathology are available online in the "Digital Atlas of Breast Pathology," by Meenakshi Singh© at www.hsc.stonybrook.edu/breast-atlas.

References

1. Arpino G, Laucirica R, Elledge RM: Premalignant and in situ breast disease: biology and clinical implications. Ann Intern Med 143(6):446–457, 2005.
2. Elmore JG, Gigerenzer G: Benign breast disease: the risks of communicating risk. N Engl J Med 353(3):297–299, 2005.
3. Simpson JF, Page DL: Lobular neoplasia. In Elston CW, Ellis IO (eds): The Breast. Bath, UK: The Bath Press, 1998, pp 91–106.
4. Jensen R, Page DL: Epithelial hyperplasia. In Elston CW, Ellis IO (eds): The Breast. Bath, UK: The Bath Press, 1998, pp 65–90.
5. Ellis IO, Elston CW, Poller DN: Ductal carcinoma in situ. In Elston CW, Ellis IO (eds): The Breast. Bath, UK: The Bath Press, 1998, pp 249–282.
6. Pinder SE, O'Malley FP: Morphology of ductal carcinoma in situ. In O'Malley FP, Pinder SE (eds): Foundations in Diagnostic Pathology: Breast Pathology. Philadelphia: Churchill Livingstone/Elsevier, 2006, pp 191–200.
7. Rosen PP, Hoda SA: Breast Pathology: Diagnosis by Needle Core Biopsy. Philadelphia: Lippincott Williams & Wilkins, 2006, pp 85–123; pp 209–223.
8. Tavassoli FA, Schnitt SJ, Hoefler H, et al: Intraductal proliferative lesions. In Tavassoli FA, Devilee P (eds): WHO Classification: Tumors of the Breast and Female Genital Organs. Lyon: IARC Press, 2003, pp 63–73.
9. Carter D: Interpretation of Breast Biopsies, 4th ed. Philadelphia: Lippincott Williams & Wilkins, 2003, pp 96–197.
10. Carter BA, Page DL, O'Malley FP: Usual epithelial hyperplasia and atypical ductal hyperplasia. In O'Malley FP, Pinder SE (eds): Foundations in Diagnostic Pathology: Breast Pathology. Philadelphia: Churchill Livingstone/Elsevier, 2006, pp 159–168.
11. Tayal S, Singh M, Lewin J: A comparative analysis of atypical hyperplasia diagnosed with core needle biopsy with corresponding surgical specimen. Breast J 9(6):511–512, 2003.
12. Hartmann LC, Sellers TA, Frost MH, et al: Benign breast disease and the risk of breast cancer. N Engl J Med 353(3):229–237, 2005.
13. Tavassoli FA, Millis RR, Boeker W, Lakhani SR: Lobular neoplasia. In Tavassoli FA, Devilee P (eds): WHO Classification: Tumors of the Breast and Female Genital Organs. Lyon: IARC Press, 2003, pp 60–62.
14. Jacobs TW: Atypical lobular hyperplasia (ALH) and lobular carcinoma in situ (LCIS) including "pleomorphic variant." In O'Malley FP, Pinder SE (eds): Foundations in Diagnostic Pathology: Breast Pathology. Philadelphia: Churchill Livingstone/Elsevier, 2006, pp 169–184.

3

Invasive Breast Cancer

Michael D. Stamatakos

KEY POINTS

- Diagnosis of invasive breast cancer requires a complex assessment of the gross features, histologic features, and occasionally special stains.
- A number of benign lesions can mimic invasive breast cancer.
- Specific features of the tumor and nodes must be included in the pathology report of an invasive breast cancer.
- Special stains can be used to distinguish the various types of breast cancer and to distinguish breast cancer from other malignancies.

Introduction

This chapter discusses the pathology of invasive breast carcinoma. It is divided into four parts. Part 1 is a discussion of the criteria necessary to make the diagnosis of invasive breast carcinoma. This includes a discussion of the histologic criteria of invasive carcinoma, the mimics of invasive carcinoma, and the various methods used to distinguish invasive carcinoma from its mimics. Part 2 is a description of the items that need to be included in a pathology report of invasive breast carcinoma. Part 3 covers the various histologic types of invasive breast carcinoma and their significance. Part 4 includes a discussion of testing for adjuvant hormone therapy.

PART 1. MAKING THE DIAGNOSIS OF INVASIVE BREAST CARCINOMA

Biopsy Procedures

A variety of methods are available for the evaluation of breast lesions. Fine-needle aspirations (FNA) can be performed in the office by either the surgeon or the pathologist, and the only equipment required includes disposable needles, disposable plastic syringes, glass slides, and proper fixative. Proper and rapid fixation is imperative on an FNA specimen, and if the surgeon is to perform the procedure in the office, coordination with and assistance from the laboratory are important. The results can generally be interpreted in a matter of hours. Although FNA cytology has many advantages (it is inexpensive and noninvasive and can be interpreted within a matter of hours), the procedure has several drawbacks. First, the architecture of the lesion is not preserved, and the pathologist cannot make a definitive assessment of the presence or absence of invasion. The assessment of the various types of proliferative lesions such as typical ductal hyperplasia and atypical ductal hyperplasia is also limited in aspirates. In addition, tumors with significant amounts of fibrous tissue frequently provide low cellularity on needle aspirations. The amount of tissue sampled and the pathologist's experience with aspiration biopsies are also factors to consider. In fact, misinterpretations of breast FNAs have been a leading cause of malpractice lawsuits for pathologists. A National Cancer Institute–sponsored consensus conference on FNA of the breast recommended a so-called triple test approach in which the needle aspiration diagnosis is correlated with the clinical and radiologic findings.[1]

Needle core biopsy offers greater sampling accuracy than FNA because the architecture of the areas of concern is preserved, and this allows the pathologist to assess invasion. In addition, ancillary studies such as hormone receptor and human epidermal growth hormone receptors (HER2/neu) studies can be performed on material from needle core biopsies, although these studies are probably best performed on larger specimens such as excisional biopsies as the amount of invasive carcinoma may be limited in a core biopsy. While more accurate than FNA, core biopsy also has several limitations:

1. The diagnosis is dependent upon sampling, and all core biopsies must be correlated with the clinical and radiographic studies to ensure that the lesion in question has been adequately sampled.
2. The procedure may be traumatic for fragile tumor cells, resulting in "crush artifact," and may limit the pathologist's ability to render a diagnosis.

Although the National Comprehensive Cancer Network (NCCN) guidelines now recommend core biopsy before surgery, in cases with discordant results the definitive method for obtaining tissue is excisional biopsy. Good cooperation between the operating room staff and the histopathology laboratory is required to optimize handling of the surgical specimen. The specimen should be provided to pathology oriented and in the fresh state (Fig. 3-1). On receipt of the specimen, the pathology staff inks the margins for orientation.

Breast is one of the most difficult specimens to process in the histopathology laboratory because of its high adipose tissue content. Proper fixation is crucial to optimize the quality of the slides. Ideally, the specimen should be serially sectioned at 2- to 3-mm intervals within several hours of receipt and placed in an adequate amount of fixative. Leaving an unsliced specimen in fixative can lead to poor tissue preservation and ultimately suboptimal histologic sections. It has also been shown that a delay in fixation of as little as 6 hours can result in a decline in the number of mitotic figures and thus lead to inaccuracy in grading.[2] Recently, the American Society of Clinical Oncology/College of American Pathologists recommended that for optimal results for HER2/neu testing in breast cancer tissue from excisional biopsies, the specimen should be fixed in neutral buffered formalin for no less than 6 hours and more than 48 hours.[3] Needle core biopsies should be fixed for at least one hour.

Histopathologic Appearance of Invasive Breast Cancer

Microscopic Appearance

There is considerable variation in the macroscopic appearance of invasive breast carcinoma, based on the histologic type. In the most common type of invasive breast carcinoma—

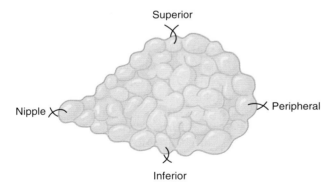

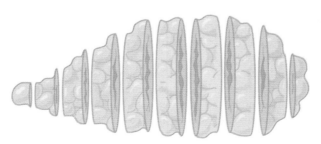

Figure 3-1. Optimal orientation and sectioning of an excisional breast biopsy. (From Tavassoli FA: Pathology of the Breast, 2nd ed. New York: McGraw-Hill, 1999, Fig. 4–5.)

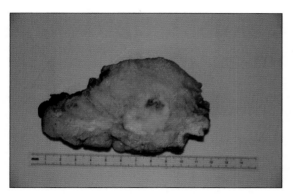

Figure 3-2. Gross photo of invasive carcinoma showing a firm, spiculated, tan-colored mass with slightly irregular borders. (Photograph courtesy of Dr. Nikki Moutsinos.)

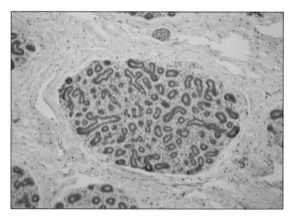

Figure 3-3. Hematoxylin and eosin stain of benign breast terminal duct lobular unit showing a prominent layer of myoepithelial cells between the epithelial cells and the stroma. The myoepithelial cells appear in this photograph as cells with clear cytoplasm owing to the presence of intracytoplasmic glycogen.

invasive ductal carcinoma not otherwise specified (NOS)—the macroscopic appearance is a firm, white mass that is denser than the surrounding fibroadipose breast tissue. The mass typically has a stellate appearance, and the borders of the nodule are generally somewhat irregular. Frequently, small white-colored spicules and occasionally foci of calcification are identified. Carcinomas frequently have a coarsely granular texture when cut or scraped with the edge of a blade (Fig. 3-2).

Histologic Appearance

The diagnosis of invasive breast carcinoma is one of the most challenging and clinically important diagnoses for the pathologist. This is explained by the numerous histologic variants of breast carcinoma as well as the numerous benign mimickers of invasive carcinoma, such as sclerosing adenosis, papillomas, sclerosing papillomas, and radial scars. Establishing the diagnosis of invasive breast carcinoma requires the demonstration of individual neoplastic cells or groups of neoplastic cells extending beyond the borders of the ducts and lobules and invading the surrounding stroma or adipose tissue. A haphazard arrangement of the groups of cells is generally the first clue at low power. The stroma frequently shows a fibrotic or desmoplastic response.

In the normal breast, myoepithelial cells can be easily identified as a flattened layer of cells or as clear cells between the epithelial cells and the stroma (Figs. 3-3 and 3-4A and B). Demonstration of the myoepithelial layer is very helpful for a differentiation of invasive breast cancer

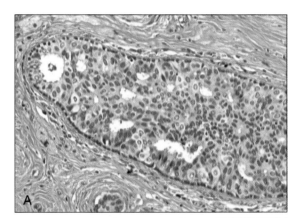

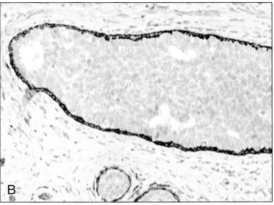

Figure 3-4. Breast duct with hyperplasia. A, The myoepithelial cell layer consists of flattened to cuboidal cells between the epithelial cells and the stroma (H&E stain). **B,** Immunoperoxidase stain for smooth muscle myosin heavy chain highlights the myoepithelial cell layer in brown.

from in situ carcinoma. With the exception of the rare entity, microglandular adenosis, the mimickers of invasive carcinoma can usually be separated from invasive breast carcinoma by the presence or absence of the myoepithelial cell layer. Invasive carcinoma also shows breaks in the basement membrane. The presence or absence of the myoepithelial cell layer can usually be determined on hematoxylin and eosin (H&E)–stained sections. However, the myoepithelial cell layer may become obscured as the ductules and acini become distorted by ductal hyperplasia and carcinoma in situ or compressed by stromal sclerosis, thus making identification of the myoepithelial cell layer difficult on H&E stain.

A variety of immunoperoxidase stains, including high-molecular-weight cytokeratin (34βE12), cytokeratin 5/6, CD10, S-100, smooth muscle actin, calponin, smooth muscle myosin heavy chain (SMMHC), and p63, can be used to highlight myoepithelial cells. Although the use of these antibodies can be of tremendous assistance, a word of caution is prudent in the interpretation of these stains. The pathologist must always correlate the immunohistochemical findings with the H&E findings, because there are several pitfalls that can lead to an erroneous diagnosis. High-molecular-weight cytokeratins such as cytokeratin 34βE12, cytokeratin 5/6, S-100, and CD10 are not very specific stains for myoepithelial cells because they frequently react with epithelial cells as well. Smooth muscle actin had been regarded as the preferred stain for myoepithelial cells for many years, but the antibody does react with desmoplastic myofibroblasts immediately surrounding the invasive ducts, and this can lead to a false interpretation of myoepithelial cells, resulting in failure to identify an invasive carcinoma.

Newer stains such as calponin and smooth muscle myosin heavy chain are more specific for myoepithelial cells than smooth muscle actin and do not demonstrate as much staining of the background myofibroblasts. Stains for basement membrane material (laminin and type IV collagen) can also be used but in practice are difficult to use and the results are difficult to interpret.

Recently, p63, a homologue of the tumor suppressor protein p53, has gained widespread popularity as a marker for myoepithelial cells. The advantage of using p63 is that it is present only in the nuclei and thus does not show cross-reactivity with myofibroblasts. Two limitations of using p63 have been described in the literature: (1) it occasionally demonstrates an apparently discontinuous myoepithelial layer, particularly around ductal carcinoma in situ (DCIS), and (2) it reacts with a small subset of breast carcinoma tumor cells that show basaloid and squamoid differentiation.[4] Figure 3-5A to E illustrates a focus of invasive carcinoma adjacent to noninvasive breast cancer and the use of various immunoperoxidase stains.

The author's preference is to use a panel of stains that includes p63 and either smooth muscle myosin heavy chain or calponin. Some laboratories use cocktails with dual-staining for smooth muscle myosin heavy chain and p63. Even with most optimal immunoperoxidase stains, there will still be a very small number of cases (around 5%) of DCIS that completely lack myoepithelial cells.[5] This underscores the importance of correlating immunohistochemical results with the H&E-stained sections.

Mimickers of Invasive Carcinoma

The most common problem for the pathologist in the differential diagnosis of invasive carcinoma is distinguishing invasive carcinoma from the various forms of adenosis and sclerosing lesions such as sclerosing adenosis, tubular adenosis, microglandular adenosis, radial scars, and sclerosing papillomas. Adenosis by definition consists of a proliferative lesion composed of small tubules lined by epithelial and myoepithelial cells arising from the terminal duct-lobular unit. The various forms of adenosis are generally observed along with fibrocystic changes. In all forms of adenosis, the proliferation lacks the haphazard appearance of invasive carcinoma. With the exception of the rare microglandular adenosis, a layer of myoepithelial cells is present between the epithelial cells and the stroma.

Sclerosing adenosis is the most common form of adenosis and consists of a proliferation of tightly packed ductules. On occasion, sclerosing adenosis may form a mass—a lesion referred to as nodular adenosis. The ductules are closely packed owing to compression of the background collagenous stroma. The compressed and elongated shape of the ductules closely resembles invasive carcinoma. In contrast to the appearance of invasive carcinoma, the ductules maintain a lobulocentric rather than the haphazard

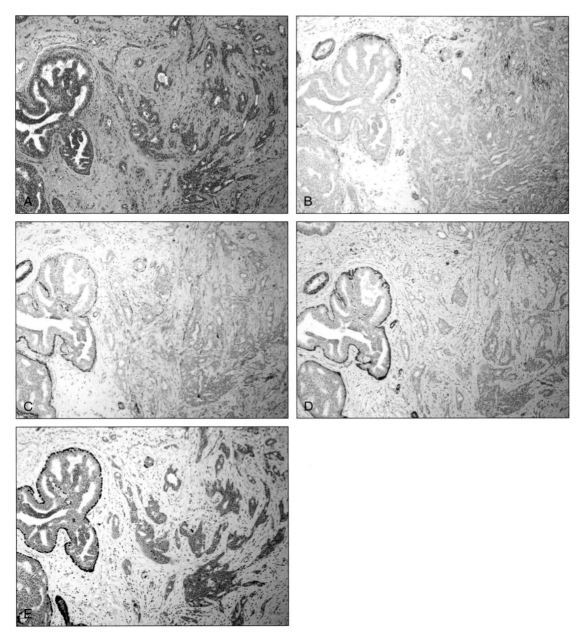

Figure 3-5. The use of several different immunoperoxidase stains demonstrating the absence of myoepithelial cells in invasive carcinoma. A, H&E stain of ductal carcinoma in situ is shown on the left and invasive carcinoma is shown on the right. The more rounded contours of the noninvasive ducts contrast with the haphazard, more angulated pattern of invasive carcinoma. In addition, a layer of cuboidal to flattened myoepithelial cells, some with clear cytoplasm, are present in the noninvasive areas, but are not present in the invasive areas. **B,** The smooth muscle actin stain highlights the layer of myoepithelial cells in the noninvasive foci and shows an absence of myoepithelial cells in the noninvasive foci. However, the background stromal cells show some staining with actin, which may lead to misinterpretation. **C,** A stain for calponin shows a bit less background staining than does smooth muscle actin, but a bit more than the smooth muscle myosin heavy chain stain seen in **D**. **E,** p63 stain with strong nuclear staining of the myoepithelial cells. p63 does stain a few of the epithelial cells.

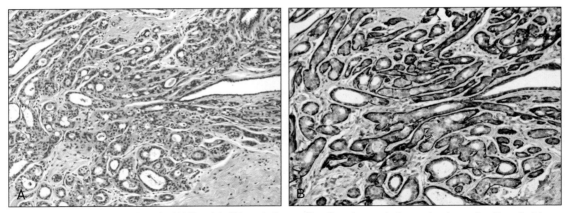

Figure 3-6. A, Sclerosing adenosis (H&E stain). Although the proliferation does not show a haphazard pattern that is suggestive of invasive carcinoma, the myoepithelial cell layer is obscured owing to compression of the small ductules. **B,** An immunoperoxidase stain for smooth muscle myosin heavy chain highlighting a layer of myoepithelial cells between the epithelial cells and the stroma.

distribution that characterizes invasive carcinoma. These features are usually appreciated at low-power microscopic magnification. In addition, a layer of myoepithelial cells and a prominent basement membrane are present between the epithelial cells and the stroma in sclerosing adenosis. The diagnosis can usually be made without the assistance of immunoperoxidase stains, but stains for myoepithelial cells are helpful in difficult cases (Fig. 3-6A and B).

Radial scars (larger forms are sometimes referred to as a complex sclerosing lesion) are closely related to sclerosing adenosis and are composed of entrapped tubules arranged around a central scar (Fig. 3-7). As with sclerosing adenosis, the absence of an invasive pattern and the presence of a layer of myoepithelial cells facilitate the distinction between radial scar and invasive carcinoma.

Microglandular adenosis is a rare condition that consists of very compact rounded tubules that are lined by a single layer of cuboidal epithelial cells (Fig. 3-8). The tubules have open lumens and are filled with a colloid-like secretory material. A layer of myoepithelial cells is not present, and the distinction between invasive carcinoma and microglandular adenosis is usually very difficult. The pathologist is able to distinguish microglandular adenosis from invasive tubular carcinoma by the recognition of the characteristic pattern of microglandular adenosis and the absence of a desmoplastic stroma. Fortunately for the pathologist, microglandular adenosis is a rare lesion.

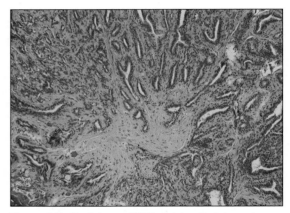

Figure 3-7. Radial scar (H&E stain).   Radial scar is characterized by a proliferation of compressed tubules arranged in a radial configuration around a central scar. On close inspection, a myoepithelial cell layer can be identified between the epithelial cells and the stroma.

Another benign lesion that can be misinterpreted as invasive carcinoma is pseudoangiomatous stromal hyperplasia (PASH), which consists of interanastomosing, angulated, and slit-like spaces lined by slender spindle cells in a dense collagenous stroma. PASH typically has a distinct H&E morphology; difficult cases may require the use of immunoperoxidase stains (Fig. 3-9A to C). PASH shows immunoreactivity for CD34 but not for cytokeratins. This is illustrated in Figure 3-9B and C.

Occasionally, groups of epithelial cells are mechanically displaced into the surrounding adipose tissue or stroma during a previous biopsy.

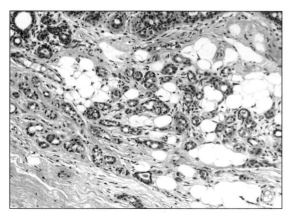

Figure 3-8. Microglandular adenosis (H&E stain).
This is characterized by a proliferation of round tubules with open lumens lined by one cell layer. Colloid-like secretory material is generally present in the center of the tubules. This is the one form of adenosis that lacks a myoepithelial cell layer. The stromal layer lacks the desmoplastic response that is commonly seen in invasive carcinoma.

This is commonly seen after needle core biopsies of papillary lesions[6] and can cause difficulty in the assessment of invasion on subsequent excisional biopsy. The absence of a desmoplastic stroma, the absence of adjacent breast structures, the similarity of the cells to a main lesion elsewhere in the excision, and the history are all helpful in distinguishing displaced epithelial cells from invasive carcinoma. Evidence of trauma in the form of blood or hemosiderin immediately adjacent to the suspicious focus is also helpful.

An additional problem has recently been described in large intracystic (in situ) papillary carcinomas. Intracystic papillary carcinomas have traditionally been considered a variant of DCIS. As illustrated in Figure 3-10A and B, the lesions typically have smooth and well-rounded borders and lack the haphazard pattern of invasive carcinoma. However, despite the use of multiple antibodies, a layer of myoepithelial cells between the epithelial cells and the stroma cannot be demonstrated in many instances. Whether or not these lesions are in situ lesions in which the myoepithelial cell layer has become markedly attenuated or represent circumscribed, encapsulated nodules of invasive papillary carcinoma has been the subject of some discussion in the literature.[7,8] Currently available outcome data indicate that these lesions have a good prognosis with adequate local therapy alone. One

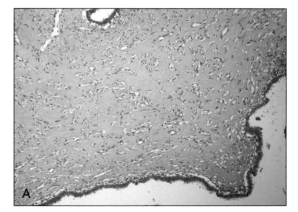

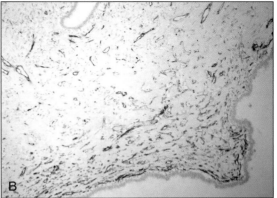

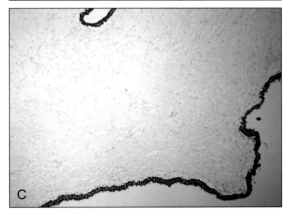

Figure 3-9. A, Pseudoangiomatous stromal hyperplasia (PASH) (H&E, ×100). The lesion consists of interanastomosing, angulated, and slit-like spaces lined by slender spindle cells in a dense collagenous stroma. **B,** CD34 stain, ×100, highlighting the slit-like spaces. **C,** Pancytokeratin stain showing staining of the overlying epithelium but an absence of staining by the slit-like spaces.

reference recommended that these lesions be referred to as "encapsulated papillary carcinoma" and that they continue to be managed as DCIS until further evidence indicates otherwise.[8]

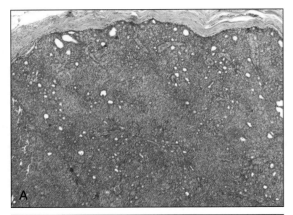

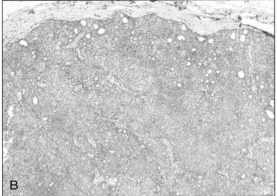

Figure 3-10. A, Large intracystic (in situ) papillary lesion (H&E stain). The absence of an invasive pattern and the well-defined, rounded contours of the lesion favor an in situ lesion. However, myoepithelial cells are not highlighted by an immunoperoxidase stain for smooth muscle myosin heavy chain as illustrated in **B**.

PART 2. THE SURGICAL PATHOLOGY REPORT

To standardize reporting of breast carcinoma and ensure that all relevant information for the clinician is included in the pathology report, the College of American Pathologists (CAP) provides a series of surgical pathology cancer protocols and checklists on all organ sites. These are based on the *AJCC Cancer Staging Manual*, 7th edition.[9] CAP protocols are periodically updated and can be accessed via the internet at www.cap.org. An additional article that addresses many of the problematic areas in staging was recently written by Connolly.[10]

Information that must be in the surgical pathology report includes the specimen type (e.g., excision, mastectomy), the specific site

of the tumor, laterality, specimen size, size of the invasive component (may be in one, two, or three dimensions), histologic type, histologic grade, margin status, presence or absence of venous and lymphatic space invasion, presence and localization of microcalcifications (involving invasive carcinoma, in situ carcinoma, or in non-neoplastic tissue), and lymph node staging.

The type of specimen, the location, and the laterality are generally provided by the submitting physician. While these factors may seem trivial, it is important that they be verified before the report is finalized.

The single most important parameter in the staging of an invasive carcinoma is the T stage, which is based on the size of the tumor. Pathologic tumor size is a measurement of the invasive component only. In most cases of invasive breast carcinoma, establishing the size of the tumor is a rather simple measurement performed at the grossing table while the specimen is being sectioned. The tumor should be measured in at least two dimensions, and the single greatest dimension of the invasive component is used for determining tumor stage. The gross measurement of the tumor must be verified by microscopic examination. When there is a discrepancy between gross and microscopic tumor measurement, the microscopic tumor measurement of the invasive component takes precedence and should be used for tumor staging. This discrepancy may be a factor in instances in which foci of invasive carcinoma extend beyond the grossly visible lesion, as in many invasive lobular carcinomas or adenoid cystic carcinoma. It is also a factor when a significant portion of the gross tumor is in situ. In other instances, an invasive tumor may be apparent only on microscopic examination.

When two or more distinct invasive tumors are present, each is separately measured and reported; they are not combined into a single larger size. For cases of multiple simultaneous ipsilateral primary carcinomas, the largest primary carcinoma is used to designate the T classification. It is not appropriate to assign a separate T classification for the smaller tumor(s); however, the pathologist should record that this is a case of multiple simultaneous ipsilateral primary carcinomas.

In patients who have undergone multiple core biopsies, the original tumor size should be reconstructed on the basis of a combination of imaging and all histologic findings. Measuring only the residual lesion or the largest size on the core biopsy may result in significant under-classification of the T component.

If a tumor is grossly cut across during surgery and there is significant tumor in a subsequent excision, an accurate pT classification cannot be assigned. Since the relationship between the two masses is unknown, summing up the two specimens may overestimate the size of the lesion. Correlation with imaging studies may be helpful in such cases.

Grading

An association between tumor grade and sur-vival has been noted since the 1920s and 1930s.[11,12] The current system of grading is the modification of the early works of Patey and Scarff[13] and Bloom and Richardson[14] and most recently the modification by Elston and Ellis.[15] In this system, also known as the Nottingham system, the following three parameters are assessed: (1) the degree of tubule formation, (2) the degree of nuclear pleomorphism, and (3) the total number of mitoses per 10 high-power fields (hpf). A score between 1 and 3 is assigned to each of the parameters. The three scores are added together, and a grade is assigned on the basis of the total number. Tumors that show greater than 75% tubule formation are assigned a score of 1; tumors that show between 10% and 75% tubule formation are assigned a score of 2;

and tumors that show less than 10% tubule for-mation are assigned a score of 3.

The nuclear grade is probably the most sub-jective aspect of the scoring. Nuclei that are of uniform size and shape are scored as 1. Bizarre nuclei showing marked variation are scored as 3, and a score of 2 is given when there are inter-mediate variations in nuclear characteristics. Mitotic counts are evaluated as the number of mitotic figures found in 10 consecutive hpf in the most mitotically active part of the tumor. Field selection for mitotic counting should be from the peripheral leading edge of the tumor. Only clearly identifiable mitotic figures should be counted; hyperchromatic, karyorrhectic, or apoptotic nuclei are excluded. Since the area of the microscopic field may vary according to the microscope used, mitotic counts require stan-dardization by converting the number of mitoses per 10 hpf into the number of mitoses per set area (such as a square millimeter), as described by Kuopio and Collan[16] or by using a grid system (Fig. 3-11). Examples of the various grades of invasive carcinoma are illustrated in Figure 3-12A to C.

It is generally recommended that final grading be performed on excisional biopsies rather than core biopsies because the core biopsy may not be representative of the entire tumor. Clinicians treating the patient should be aware that the grade of the tumor on core biopsy may differ from the final grade of the tumor assigned on the excisional biopsy as a result of sampling issues.

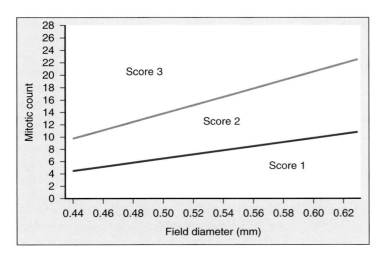

Figure 3-11. Graph of number of mitotic figures per 10 hpf by field diameter. (Reproduced with permission of authors and publisher from NHSBSP Publication, NHS Breast Screening Programme, 1997.)

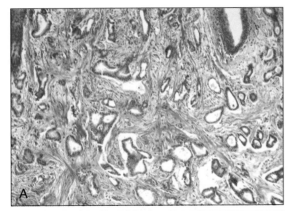

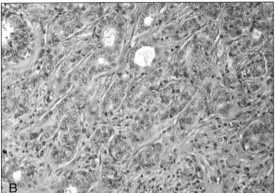

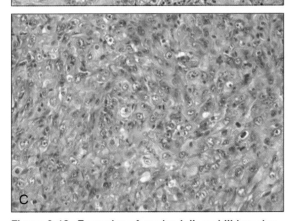

Figure 3-12. Examples of grades I, II, and III invasive ductal carcinoma. See the discussion on Nottingham grade in the text. **A,** Grade I invasive ductal carcinoma (H&E). The tumor shows abundant tubule formation, minimal nuclear atypia, and minimal mitotic activity. **B,** Grade II invasive ductal carcinoma, NOS (H&E). The tumor shows a moderate amount of tubule formation, moderate nuclear atypia, and moderate mitotic activity. **C,** Grade III invasive ductal carcinoma. The tumor shows minimal tubule formation, high-grade nuclear atypia, and abundant mitotic activity.

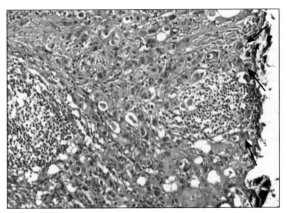

Figure 3-13. Tumor at inked margin (H&E stain). The tumor cells (*arrows*) are present at the red-inked margin on the left side.

Margin Status

Pathologic evaluation of the margin status is accomplished by the use of inked margins. In most instances, particularly with the advent of breast-conserving surgery, the surgeon identifies the various margins through the use of sutures or clips. This should be documented in the surgical report. The pathologist then uses different colors of ink to label the six margins and section the specimen along the longest axis of the specimen. In some instances, the surgeon does not provide any sutures or clips to orient the specimen. The pathologist then inks the entire outer surface of the specimen in one color. A positive margin can be identified when there is tumor against the ink (Fig. 3-13). It is also recommended that the pathologist provide the closest distance of the tumor to the inked margins on each of the six sides of the specimen.

The use of ink to identify margins presents several technical challenges. First, the surface of a breast surgical specimen is generally not flat and smooth but frequently irregular with numerous small crevices that ink may run into. In addition, ink frequently runs and can mark tissue edges for which it was not intended. The use of various mordants such as Bouin's solution helps to bind the inks to the tissue surfaces. Ink seeping into crevices or running off the surface can result in a falsely reported positive margin. The recommended distance between the tumor and the inked surface to classify it as a negative margin varies from no tumor at the inked surface up to 1 cm. There is no national consensus on the acceptable distance for classification of a negative margin. However, all groups agree that margins should be assessed and that there should be no tumor at the inked surface as a minimum standard.

Invasive Carcinoma with an Extensive in Situ Component

CAP recommends that for breast carcinomas that have both an invasive and an in situ component, the pathology report should specify whether an extensive in situ (intraductal) component (EIC) is present. EIC is present when DCIS comprises more than 25% of the main tumor and extends beyond the boundaries of the invasive tumor and into the surrounding breast parenchyma. This finding is associated with an increased risk of local recurrence when the surgical margins are positive.[17] EIC appears to have less significance when DCIS does not extend close to any of the margins after careful histologic evaluation.[18] The significance of this finding relates to the fact that in situ lesions, unlike most invasive lesions, frequently do not form a grossly apparent fibrous mass. Thus, the notation "EIC" serves to inform the treating physician that in situ carcinoma may extend beyond the boundaries of the grossly apparent tumor mass and may require more extensive excision. Correlating mammograms with the pathologic findings and assessing surgical margins are particularly important steps when treating patients with EIC.

Lymphovascular Space Invasion

Peritumoral vascular invasion should be noted because this condition has been associated with local failure and reduced overall survival (Fig. 3-14). Distinguishing between lymphatic channels and blood vessels is not necessary. However, it is important for lymphovascular space invasion to be distinguished from tissue retraction, as is commonly seen in invasive micropapillary carcinoma. The use of various stains for endothelial cells such as CD31 can be of assistance.

Lymph Nodes

Lymph node metastases consist of collections of tumor cells in either solid or tubular arrangement within the lymph node tissue (Fig. 3-15).

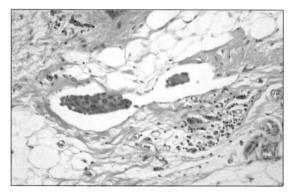

Figure 3-14. Lymphovascular space invasion (H&E stain). Tumor is present within a lymphovascular space.

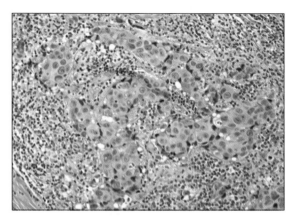

Figure 3-15. Metastatic carcinoma to a lymph node (H&E stain). The large, pleomorphic tumor cells surrounded by lymphocytes are easy to identify in this example.

These are mostly identified just beneath the lymph node capsule and are generally easily identified on H&E sections. The pathology report should clearly state the total number of lymph nodes examined, the total number of nodes involved, and the greatest dimension of the largest metastatic focus. Grossly uninvolved nodes should be submitted in their entirety for histologic evaluation. Representative sections of grossly positive nodes may be submitted, with a single microscopic section from each lymph node considered sufficient. Extranodal tumor extension, if present, should be included in the pathology report.

Recently, there has been considerable discussion on the significance of very minute metastatic foci and the use of immunohistochemistry to identify metastatic foci. As illustrated in Figure 3-16A and B, cytokeratin stains can greatly assist in the identification of lymph node metastasis. This is particularly true for invasive

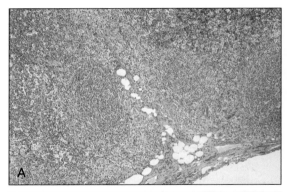

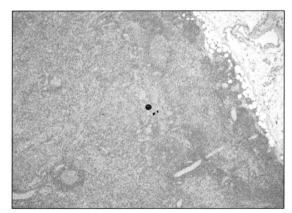

Figure 3-17. Isolated tumor cells in a lymph node identified by cytokeratin staining (brown color) pN0(i+).

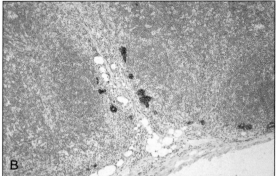

Figure 3-16. The use of immunoperoxidase stains in identifying metastatic carcinoma in lymph nodes. A, The metastatic carcinoma is subtle and has the appearance of histiocytes. **B,** Immunoperoxidase stain for pancytokeratin highlights the metastatic carcinoma cells in the lymph node.

lobular carcinoma, in which the metastatic foci can be very subtle. However, the significance of these microscopic foci, particularly those identified only with the assistance of immunohistochemical stains, has been the subject of considerable debate.

The current AJCC staging manual defines isolated tumor cells (ITCs) as single cells or small clusters of cells not larger than 0.2 mm, usually with no histologic evidence of malignant activity such as a stromal reaction[9] (Fig. 3-17). Because isolated tumor cells are sometimes dispersed throughout the entire node rather than in a single focus, making a measurement virtually impossible, the recent AJCC manual has expanded the definition of ITCs to also include cases in which there are fewer than 200 individual tumor cells in a single histologic section of a lymph node.[9] If morphologic techniques (including immunohistochemistry) are used to detect isolated tumor cells, the regional lymph nodes should be designated as pN0(i+) or pN0(i-), depending on whether the immuno-

histochemical stains are positive. If nonmorphologic (molecular) methods are used, the nodes are designated as pN0(mol-) or pN0(mol+) as appropriate.

Micrometastases are defined as tumor deposits larger than 0.2 mm but not larger than 2.0 mm. When only micrometastases are detected, tumors are classified as pN1mi. The prognosis for patients with a solitary micrometastasis has been reported to be better than for those with larger metastatic deposits; however, the significance of multiple micrometastases in one or more lymph nodes is unknown and they are still classified as pN1mi. The number of nodes that contain micrometastases should be specified in the surgical pathology report.

PART 3. HISTOLOGIC TYPES OF INVASIVE BREAST CARCINOMA

Invasive carcinomas are divided into two large categories based on the histology: *invasive ductal* and *invasive lobular*. Many of the histologic subtypes, such as tubular carcinoma, mucinous (colloid) carcinoma, medullary carcinoma, invasive papillary carcinoma, invasive micropapillary carcinoma, and invasive apocrine carcinoma, are considered special variants of invasive ductal carcinoma. As with in situ lesions, the designations invasive ductal and invasive lobular refer to a growth pattern and do not necessarily imply a site of origin. A morphologic study by Wellings and colleagues[19] demonstrated that most breast carcinomas—both ductal and lobular—originate in the terminal duct lobular unit.

Invasive Ductal Carcinoma

By far the largest group of invasive carcinomas is ductal carcinoma not otherwise specified (NOS). A synonym for this group is invasive ductal carcinoma, no special type. This heterologous group of tumors cannot be classified into any particular subtype of invasive carcinoma. Estimates are that from 50% to 75% of invasive breast carcinomas fall into this category. These tumors vary in size from a few millimeters to more than 10 cm. The tumor cells may be arranged in cords, clusters, or tubules. A solid pattern may also predominate. The tumors may show pushing or infiltrative margins or a combination of these. Nuclei vary according to the grade of the lesion. Invasive ductal carcinomas are frequently associated with DCIS.

The current World Health Organization (WHO) classification requires that for a tumor to be typed as invasive ductal carcinoma, NOS, it must have a nonspecialized pattern in over 50% of its mass. If the ductal NOS component makes up between 10% and 49% of the tumor, with the rest of the tumor composed of one recognized histologic variant, then the tumor is to be classified as mixed ductal carcinoma and special type.[20]

Invasive Lobular Carcinoma

WHO defines invasive lobular carcinoma as an invasive carcinoma usually associated with lobular carcinoma in situ and composed of non-cohesive cells individually dispersed or arranged in single-file linear pattern in a fibrous stroma. Pure invasive lobular carcinomas represent about 4% to 5% of all invasive breast carcinomas.[20] There has been an increase in the incidence of invasive lobular carcinoma in women over 50,[21] and a causal relationship with hormone replacement therapy has been suggested.[22-24]

The macroscopic appearance of invasive lobular carcinoma varies. It typically presents as a firm mass. However, in contrast to infiltrating ductal carcinoma that tends to be well circumscribed, most invasive lobular carcinomas have a diffuse, irregular, and sometimes discontinuous growth pattern that may extend into normal-appearing adipose tissue. In some instances, a grossly visible tumor may not be present. Invasive lobular carcinoma may present as multiple small masses.

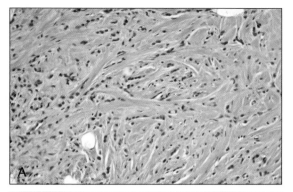

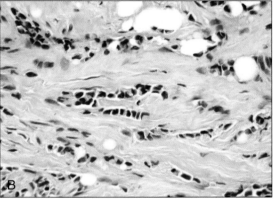

Figure 3-18. Invasive lobular carcinoma (H&E stain). This carcinoma is composed of small cells with a single cell pattern of invasion and an absence of tubule formation. **A,** ×100; **B,** ×400.

The classic pattern of invasive lobular carcinoma is illustrated in Figure 3-18A and B. The most recognizable feature is the single-file pattern of invasion. The cells are generally small, with a mild to moderate degree of nuclear pleomorphism (grade 1 or 2). The nucleus is round and regular with small to inconspicuous nucleoli. Intracytoplasmic lumens are present in some of the cells with intracytoplasmic mucin, which is highlighted by special stains (Fig. 3-19). Invasive lobular carcinoma is frequently encountered in biopsies with lobular intraepithelial neoplasia (LIN), particularly the higher-grade LIN lesions.[25]

The pathologist must be very careful not to overlook small foci of invasive lobular carcinoma, because the desmoplastic stromal response and lymphocytic response that frequently accompany other forms of invasive carcinoma are often not present. In about 25% of all cases of invasive lobular carcinoma, a palpable mass or mammographic abnormality may not be detected. In

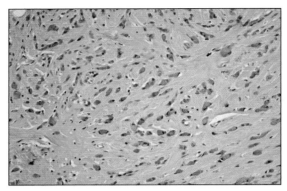

Figure 3-19. Invasive lobular carcinoma, mucicarmine stain. Mucicarmine stain stains the intracytoplasmic mucin of some invasive lobular carcinomas red.

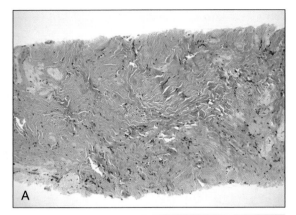

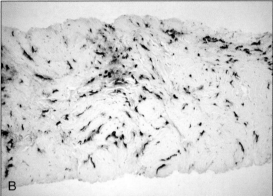

Figure 3-20. Subtle case of invasive lobular carcinoma in which the diagnosis is facilitated by the use of immunoperoxidase stains for cytokeratin. **A,** The H&E stain, the small size of the cells, the presence of crush artifact, and the absence of a desmoplastic stroma make the diagnosis of invasive carcinoma difficult. **B,** An immunoperoxidase stain for cytokeratin highlights the malignant cells.

addition, the small size and shape of the cells in many cases of invasive lobular carcinoma may resemble lymphocytes. Immunoperoxidase stains for cytokeratins may be helpful in selected cases. Figure 3-20A and B illustrates a very difficult and subtle case of invasive lobular carcinoma in which immunoperoxidase staining for cytokeratin facilitates the diagnosis.

Unlike invasive ductal carcinomas, the cells of classic invasive lobular carcinomas lack cell-to-cell cohesion and are described as having a discohesive or loosely cohesive pattern of growth. This is related to the lack of expression of the transmembrane adhesion molecule E-cadherin. Recent genetic data have noted deletions at chromosomal region 16q22 in a high percentage of invasive lobular carcinoma. This genetic locus harbors the E-cadherin molecule.[26] Whether E-cadherin staining should be used in distinguishing invasive lobular from invasive ductal carcinomas is the subject of considerable debate, particularly in cases that show the classic pattern of invasive lobular carcinoma. In a small percentage of tumors, it will be impossible to make a definitive distinction between invasive ductal or invasive lobular carcinoma.

In addition to the classic pattern, a few variant patterns of invasive lobular carcinoma have been described. In the trabecular variant, the cells grow in broader bands of cells rather than the single-file pattern of invasion. In the alveolar form, discrete alveolar groups of carcinoma cells are separated by thin bands of fibrous stroma. The solid pattern consists of solid sheets of cells. CAP currently recommends that the classic pattern of invasive lobular carcinoma be diag-

nosed only when the tumor exhibits a single-file growth pattern, a monotonous population of small cells with very low-grade nuclei, and low cell density. Tumors with a diffuse infiltrative growth pattern that do not fulfill these criteria should be reported by histologic grade with the suffix "with lobular features" (or lobular variant).

In the pleomorphic pattern of invasive lobular carcinoma, the cells maintain their single-file pattern of invasion and lack of cohesion, but show significantly more pleomorphism than in the classic variant (Fig. 3-21). Pleomorphic invasive lobular carcinoma tends to occur in older women and is generally associated with a more aggressive clinical course than the classic pattern of invasive lobular carcinoma.[27–29] One study

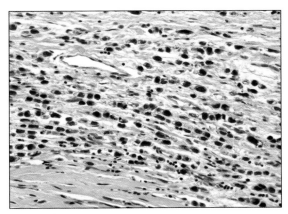

Figure 3-21. Pleomorphic pattern of invasive lobular carcinoma (H&E stain). The single-file growth pattern of pleomorphic lobular carcinoma is maintained, but the cells show considerably more nuclear pleomorphism.

noted a greater incidence of expression with markers for aggressive behavior such as p53 and HER2 in the pleomorphic pattern of invasive lobular carcinoma than in the classic variant.[30]

Invasive lobular carcinoma has traditionally been regarded as having a higher rate of multicentricity than invasive ductal carcinoma,[31,32] and a higher rate of bilaterality,[31,33–35] although not all studies support these findings.[36–39] Studies note a lower rate of lymph node metastasis for invasive lobular carcinoma than for invasive ductal carcinoma.[35,37] Lymph node involvement by invasive lobular carcinoma may be subtle and difficult to detect, because often the tumor foci in the nodes are small and resemble histiocytes. Immunoperoxidase stains for epithelial cells such as cytokeratins are often very useful in detecting minute foci of metastatic invasive lobular carcinoma.

It is difficult to state with certainty whether the prognosis of invasive lobular carcinoma differs from that of invasive ductal carcinoma, NOS, independent of stage. Some studies note a more favorable outcome for the classic and solid patterns of invasive lobular carcinoma than for invasive ductal carcinoma, NOS.[40–43] Other studies found no significant difference in survival for those with invasive lobular carcinoma compared with those with invasive ductal carcinoma.[35,44,45]

There is agreement that the metastatic pattern of invasive lobular carcinoma differs from that of invasive ductal carcinoma, with invasive lobular carcinoma showing a higher incidence of metastasis to the bone, peritoneal surface, gastrointestinal tract, and gynecologic tract. This is an important reason for distinguishing invasive lobular carcinoma from other histologic variants of invasive carcinoma.

There is some debate as to whether invasive lobular carcinomas should be graded in a manner similar to that of invasive ductal carcinoma. Studies indicate that the histologic grade of invasive lobular carcinoma correlates with prognosis.[46,47] Since invasive lobular carcinomas by definition lack tubule formation, the tubule score is 3. Thus, the grade of invasive lobular carcinoma depends on the degree of nuclear pleomorphism and mitotic activity. A study by Toikkanen and colleagues of 217 invasive lobular carcinomas noted that 34% were grade I, 54% grade II, and 12% grade III.[43] It has been pointed out by the Nottingham group that the classic pattern of invasive lobular carcinomas is usually designated grade II and the overall survival curve of invasive lobular carcinomas overlaps that of grade II tumors.[44,47] It is logical that the pleomorphic variant of invasive lobular carcinoma would be assigned a higher grade, which correlates well with their more aggressive clinical behavior. In a recent study by Bane and colleagues[46] of 50 cases of invasive lobular carcinoma using the Nottingham combined histologic grading system, grade correlated with overall tumor size and the American Joint Committee on Cancer (AJCC) nodal status.

One final and important point in the staging of invasive lobular carcinoma is the measurement of the tumor. As previously stated, unlike invasive ductal carcinomas, which typically form a well-circumscribed mass, most invasive lobular carcinomas have a diffuse, irregular, and not infrequently discontinuous growth pattern. In a substantial amount of invasive lobular carcinomas, the tumor may not be identified on gross examination. Since a desmoplastic stroma is sometimes lacking, there may be a substantial difference between the gross and microscopic measurement of the tumor. CAP favors a microscopic measurement.[47] A recent study of 74 cases noted that gross measurements alone may underestimate the T stage in 40% to 50% of cases.[48]

Invasive Tubular Carcinoma

Invasive tubular carcinoma is a very well-differentiated type of invasive ductal carcinoma. The current WHO classification defines tubular

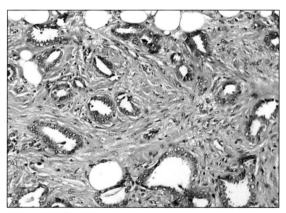

Figure 3-22. Invasive tubular carcinoma (H&E stain).
This carcinoma is characterized by a haphazard
proliferation of round to angulated open tubules in a
desmoplastic stroma. The cells often show apical snouts.

carcinoma as a special type of breast carcinoma
composed of distinct well-differentiated tubular
structures with open lumens lined by a single
layer of epithelial cells.[20] Tubular carcinoma has
a particularly favorable prognosis. This type of
breast cancer accounts for about 2% of all invasive ductal carcinomas and occurs more commonly in older patients. There are no distinctive
macroscopic features of infiltrating tubular
carcinoma, although the tumors are generally
smaller than other forms of invasive carcinoma,
with the majority being less than 1 cm.

Microscopically, invasive tubular carcinomas
consist of open, angulated tubules lined by one
layer of cells with clear lumen in a desmoplastic
stroma (Fig. 3-22). A layer of myoepithelial cells
is not identified between the tubules and the
sclerotic stroma. The cells often show apical
snouts. Because invasive tubular carcinomas are
often small and have minimal cytologic atypia,
they can be easily overlooked on a biopsy specimen. In addition, lesions such as sclerosing adenosis, radial scar, and microglandular adenosis
frequently mimic invasive tubular carcinoma.
The presence of an invasive pattern and a desmoplastic stroma is helpful in distinguishing
invasive tubular carcinoma from these lesions.
As described earlier, immunoperoxidase stains
for myoepithelial cells are often useful in difficult cases to confirm the presence of myoepithelial cells in sclerosing adenosis and radial
scars.

Although all forms of adenosis can mimic
invasive tubular carcinoma on H&E sections, the
distinction between invasive tubular carcinoma

and microglandular adenosis can be particularly
difficult. Since microglandular adenosis also
lacks a myoepithelial cell layer, immunoperoxidase stains are not helpful in distinguishing
microglandular adenosis from tubular carcinoma.
There are a few histologic differences that facilitate the distinction, however. In tubular carcinoma, the ducts are haphazard and angulated in
contrast to the rounded and more regular contours of microglandular adenosis. The tubules in
microglandular adenosis are surrounded by a
thick basement membrane, which is lacking in
invasive tubular carcinoma. In microglandular
adenosis, the surrounding stroma is collagenous
and hypocellular rather than the desmoplastic
and cellular stroma of invasive tubular carcinoma. In addition, the cells of invasive tubular
carcinoma frequently show apical snouts rather
than the colloid-like secretion noted in the
lumens of microglandular adenosis.

DCIS or atypical ductal hyperplasia is noted
in the adjacent ducts in most cases of tubular
carcinoma. Low-grade DCIS showing cribriform
or micropapillary pattern is noted in the adjacent duct in most cases of tubular carcinoma.
Lobular intraepithelial neoplasia (atypical
lobular hyperplasia or lobular carcinoma in situ)
is identified in a small minority of cases.
Recently, an association between flat epithelial
atypia and invasive tubular carcinoma has been
described.[49,50]

There is some lack of standardization with
regard to how much of the tumor should be
composed of a tubular pattern before a diagnosis
of invasive tubular carcinoma is made. WHO
recommends that at least 90% of the tumor
must show tubular features and that tumors
exhibiting between 50% and 90% be regarded as
mixed types of carcinoma.[20]

Pure tubular carcinoma is associated with an
excellent prognosis. One large study noted 5-
year disease-free survival and overall survival
rates of 94% and 88%, respectively, which
were similar to those of the age-matched
controls.[51] In a study of 50 patients with pure
invasive tubular carcinoma, Winchester and colleagues[52] noted a 5-year disease-free survival
rate of 88%. A large review of 20 studies (680
patients) noted an overall frequency of nodal
metastasis of 6.6% for pure tubular carcinoma
and 25% for mixed tubular carcinoma.[53] The
rate of nodal metastasis is considerably less for
tumors smaller than 1 cm.[53,54]

Due to the good prognosis of pure invasive tubular carcinoma, affected patients may be successfully treated with more conservative therapy. Patients with mixed tubular carcinoma should receive treatment appropriate for the grade of the carcinoma. Pure invasive tubular carcinoma and the mixed types are invariably grade 1. Tubular carcinomas tend to be estrogen and progesterone receptor–positive and generally do not show overexpression of HER2/*neu*. Given its good prognosis, it is important for pathologists to adhere to strict criteria in making the diagnosis of invasive tubular carcinoma.

Tubulolobular Carcinoma

Tubulolobular carcinoma is a recognized histologic type of invasive carcinoma that consists of an admixture of tubular structures and cords of small cells arranged in a linear pattern (Fig. 3-23A and B). One study noted staining with both E-cadherin in 100% of cases and with cytokeratin 34βE12 in 93% of cases.[55] This pattern of immunoperoxidases staining indicates that most tubulolobular carcinomas maintain immunoperoxidase features of both invasive ductal and invasive lobular carcinoma. Studies show that these tumors have a favorable prognosis, especially when they are unilateral and less than 2 cm. The tumors seem to have a rate of lymph node metastasis and recurrence that is between these rates for invasive tubular carcinoma and invasive lobular carcinoma.[55–57]

Mucinous (Colloid) Carcinoma

Mucinous (colloid) carcinoma accounts for approximately 2% of all invasive breast carcinomas. Mucinous carcinomas generally occur in older patients with mean age over 60 years. Rosen and colleagues[58] noted that mucinous carcinoma accounts for 7% of breast carcinomas in women older than 75 years of age, but for only 1% of carcinomas in women under 35 years of age. Mucinous carcinomas tend to be large tumors owing to the amount of mucin within the tumors, with a mean size about 2 cm. They typically show a gelatinous gross appearance.

Microscopically, mucinous carcinoma is characterized by islands and nests of tumor cells floating in pools of mucin (Fig. 3-24). The pools of mucin dissect through fibrous septa of the

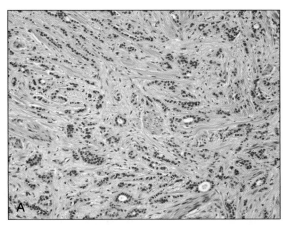

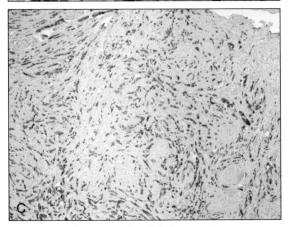

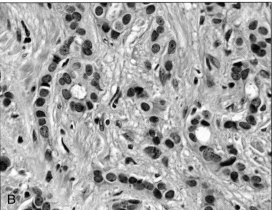

Figure 3-23. Invasive tubulolobular carcinoma.
A and **B,** Low- and high-power views of invasive tubulolobular carcinoma that consists of an admixture of tubular structures and cords of small cells arranged in a linear pattern. **C,** E-cadherin staining showing red, brown cytoplasmic staining by the tumor cells. (Photographs courtesy of Dr. Darren Wheeler.)

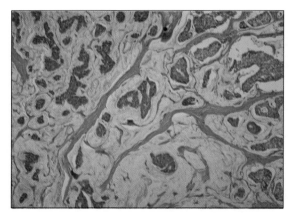

Figure 3-24. Invasive mucinous carcinoma (H&E stain). The tumor consists of islands of cells floating in a pool of mucin dissecting through fibrous septa.

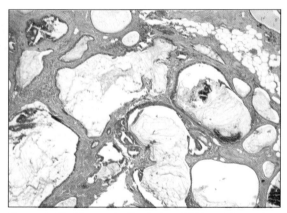

Figure 3-25. Mucocele-like lesion (H&E stain). Lesion consists of large, dilated cysts filled with mucin extruding from the ducts. The presence of detached strips of epithelial cells as opposed to islands of cells helps distinguish a mucocele-like lesion from invasive mucinous carcinoma.

mammary stroma. It is generally recommended that a tumor be regarded as invasive mucinous carcinoma only when at least 50% of the tumor is composed of extracellular mucin.[59] Tumors that show this pattern throughout 90% or more of the tumor are typically regarded as "pure" mucinous carcinoma. Tumors with less extensive mucin production should be classified as invasive ductal carcinoma with the suffix "with mucinous features" and graded in a manner similar to invasive ductal carcinoma. The amount of cellularity may vary from tumor to tumor and within the same tumor.

Pure mucinous carcinomas are associated with a good prognosis. A recent report noted an axillary lymph node metastasis rate of only 4% for pure mucinous carcinoma and 33% for mixed type.[60] Another study noted a 5-year disease-free survival rate of 90% for mucinous carcinoma compared with 80% for invasive carcinoma, NOS.[51] The study also noted that node positivity for mucinous carcinomas confers a substantially worse prognosis with a 5-year survival rate of 76%, similar to the prognosis of node-positive infiltrating ductal carcinoma.[51] Another study noted a 10-year survival rate of 90.4% for pure mucinous carcinoma and 66.0% for mixed type.[61] Mucinous carcinomas are generally estrogen receptor (ER)–positive and show less degree of progesterone receptor (PR) positivity.

The differential diagnosis of invasive mucinous carcinoma includes a mucocele-like lesion and the myxoid stroma of a fibroadenoma. A mucocele-like lesion is analogous to a mucocele of a salivary gland and consists of large, dilated cysts containing mucin with mucin extruding

outside the ducts and into the surrounding stroma[62] (Fig. 3-25). The presence of myoepithelial cells adhering to the strips of cells floating in the mucin as opposed to the islands of pure epithelial cells in a mucinous carcinoma is an important clue in differentiating a mucocele from a mucinous carcinoma. DCIS in the surrounding breast tissue is another feature that would favor the diagnosis of mucinous carcinoma over a mucocele-like lesion. Myxoid fibroadenoma can be separated from mucinous carcinoma by the presence of both epithelial and myoepithelial cells in compressed ductal spaces.

Invasive Cribriform Carcinoma

Invasive cribriform carcinoma accounts for 0.8% to 3.5% of breast carcinomas. The mean age of patients with this type of carcinoma is 53 to 58 years. The tumor typically presents as a mass but may be occult. On microscopic examination, invasive cribriform carcinoma consists of angulated nests of invasive tumor showing a prominent cribriform morphology (Fig. 3-26). The surrounding stroma typically shows a desmoplastic response. The tumor cells are small and typically show only mild to moderate nuclear pleomorphism with rare mitoses. Apical snouts are frequently seen in the epithelial cells. For a tumor to be classified as a pure cribriform carcinoma, the cribriform pattern must make up at least 90% of the lesion. Invasive cribriform car-

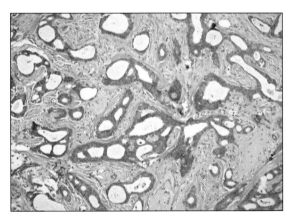

Figure 3-26. Invasive cribriform carcinoma (H&E stain).   A haphazard proliferation of tubules is seen with many of the tubules showing a cribriform architectural pattern. The tumor may blend with areas of invasive tubular carcinoma.

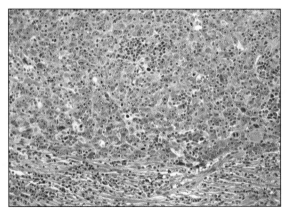

Figure 3-27. Medullary carcinoma (H&E stain).   The carcinoma (upper portion of picture) is composed of high-grade nuclei with prominent nucleoli in a syncytial growth pattern with pushing margins. The characteristic lymphocytic response is noted in the surrounding stroma (lower portion).

cinoma is also frequently seen in association with invasive tubular carcinoma. Carcinomas with more than 50% of the tumor composed of invasive cribriform carcinoma may be classified as invasive cribriform carcinoma if the remainder of the tumor is composed of a tubular carcinoma. Carcinomas that show between 50% and 90% cribriform pattern with a second component composed of another type of invasive carcinoma consisting of between 10% and 40% of the tumor should be classified as mixed-type carcinoma and graded appropriately.

Pure invasive cribriform carcinoma has a favorable prognosis, with studies showing survival rates of 100%.[63,64] The reported survival is not as good for patients who show a mixed pattern composed of invasive cribriform carcinoma and a less well-differentiated invasive carcinoma. However, the adjusted 10-year survival rate for patients with mixed carcinoma was significantly better than that for patients with invasive ductal carcinoma, NOS. Venable and colleagues[64] reported a 5-year survival rate of 100% for pure invasive cribriform carcinoma and tumors showing more than 50% invasive cribriform carcinoma. The 5-year survival rate for cases showing less than 50% cribriform was 88% in this study compared with a 5-year survival rate of 78.3% for patients with invasive ductal carcinoma, NOS.

The differential diagnosis of cribriform carcinoma includes DCIS showing a cribriform pattern and adenoid cystic carcinoma. Invasive cribriform carcinoma can be distinguished from

ductal carcinoma by the absence of a myoepithelial cell layer between the epithelial cells and the stroma.

Medullary Carcinoma

The most recent WHO classification lists five morphologic traits that characterize medullary carcinoma: (1) a syncytial architecture in over 75% of the tumor; (2) absence of glandular or tubular structures, even as a minor component; (3) a diffuse and conspicuous lymphoplasmatic stromal infiltrate; (4) carcinoma cells that are usually round with abundant cytoplasm and vesicular nuclei containing one to several nucleoli with grade 2 to 3 nuclear pleomorphism and abundant mitotic figures (atypical giant cells may be observed); and (5) complete histologic circumscription of the tumor (Fig. 3-27).[10]

The WHO reports that medullary carcinoma is reported to account for 1% to 7% of all invasive breast carcinomas. However, using the current WHO criteria as outlined above, the frequency of medullary carcinoma is very low, with medullary carcinoma comprising less than 1% of all invasive breast carcinomas as many previously published reports in the literature did not adhere to stringent criteria. The mean age is between 45 and 52 years. Clinically, the tumor is well circumscribed on mammography, palpation, and gross examination. The median diameter varies from 2.0 to 2.9 cm.

The presence of an intraductal component (DCIS) is considered a criterion for exclusion by some authors but acceptable by others. Some have recommended classifying tumors showing a predominantly syncytial architecture with only two or three of the other criteria as "atypical medullary carcinoma." Subsequent series, however, note no significant survival difference between patients with atypical medullary carcinoma and invasive ductal carcinoma, NOS, and recommend abolishing the category of atypical medullary carcinoma. Currently, the WHO recommends maintaining the category of medullary carcinomas but emphasizes the importance of adhering to strict diagnostic criteria.

The overall 10-year survival rate of medullary carcinoma is reported to be between 50% and 90%. Some studies indicate that patients with medullary carcinoma have a better prognosis than those with invasive ductal carcinoma, NOS,[65–70] but this has been questioned by others who report no significant increase in survival for patients with medullary carcinoma compared with ductal carcinoma.[42,71,72] Other studies note an improved survival but also note the importance of adhering to strict diagnostic criteria.[73,74] Currently, both WHO and CAP recommend maintaining the category of medullary carcinoma but emphasize the importance of adhering to strict diagnostic criteria.

Much of the controversy and difficulty in making the diagnosis of medullary carcinoma is related to grading the tumor. As a rule, medullary carcinoma should not be graded in the same manner as other types of invasive carcinoma. Typical medullary carcinoma is regarded as being associated with a better survival rate than invasive carcinoma. However, if one were to grade medullary carcinoma, the tumor would invariably be a high-grade tumor because the tumor lacks tubules, has significant nuclear pleomorphism, and has abundant mitotic figures. This is a unique problem for patients with medullary carcinoma, and it has potential implications for treatment. In virtually all other histologic variants of invasive carcinoma—even if one did not subclassify the carcinoma based on histologic type and merely designated the case as invasive carcinoma, NOS, and accurately graded the tumor—there would probably be little difference in treatment. For example, calling an invasive tubular carcinoma or an invasive cribriform carcinoma a well-differentiated invasive ductal carcinoma, NOS, would probably result in minimal difference in treatment. This principle does not apply to invasive medullary carcinoma.

Invasive Papillary Carcinoma

Invasive papillary carcinoma is a very rare histologic type of invasive carcinoma that accounts for less than 1% of all invasive breast carcinomas. In fact, the term *invasive papillary carcinoma* is somewhat confusing because most carcinomas showing a papillary pattern are in situ lesions. Generally, when an in situ papillary carcinoma (intraductal papillary carcinoma) demonstrates areas of invasion, the invasive component shows a pattern of invasive carcinoma, NOS. The current CAP guidelines recommend that the diagnosis of papillary carcinoma always be qualified as invasive or noninvasive. On very rare occasions, the invasive component may consist of malignant cells surrounding a fibrovascular core. Of 1603 breast cancers reviewed in the National Surgical Adjuvant Breast Project (NSABP) Protocol No. 4, only 35 examples of invasive papillary carcinoma were identified and in only 3 were the invasive papillary carcinomas pure and not admixed with other histologic types of invasive carcinoma.[75]

Invasive Micropapillary Carcinoma

Invasive micropapillary carcinoma was first described by Siriaunkgul and Tavassoli[76] in 1993 and is defined by WHO as a carcinoma composed of small clusters of tumor cells lying within clear stromal spaces resembling dilated vascular channels. Pure invasive micropapillary carcinomas are rare and make up less than 2% of all invasive breast carcinomas. However, a focus showing an invasive micropapillary pattern is identified in 3% to 7% of invasive breast carcinomas. Invasive micropapillary carcinoma typically presents as a palpable mass, and the reported age of presentation is from 25 to 92 years, with an average age of presentation basically the same as for invasive ductal carcinoma, NOS.

Microscopically, the tumor consists of small nests of about 10 to 20 malignant cells within well-defined clear spaces (Fig. 3-28). The nests of cells have either a tubular or a solid configuration. True papillary structures are rare and often are not identified. The cells typically have eosin-

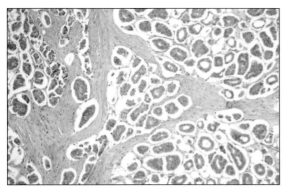

Figure 3-28. Invasive micropapillary carcinoma (H&E stain). This carcinoma is characterized by small groups of cells lying within clear spaces dissecting through the stroma.

ophilic and somewhat granular cytoplasm, and the nuclei are grade 2 to grade 3 (moderate to poorly differentiated). DCIS showing micropapillary, solid, or cribriform patterns is identified in over 50% of cases. The clear spaces are due to artifactual stromal retraction, which can be easily confused with lymphovascular space invasion. However, foci of true lymphovascular space invasion are seen in about 60% of cases. Immunoperoxidase stains for endothelial markers such as CD31 can be helpful in this distinction.

Invasive micropapillary carcinomas are considered to be high-grade tumors, with studies showing that between 37% and 59% of patients are dead of disease within the follow-up periods ranging from 1 to 12 years.[76–82] Sixty to seventy percent of patients present with lymph node metastasis. It is interesting that the micropapillary pattern is maintained in the lymph node metastasis. Studies are conflicting regarding the percentage of ER- and PR-positive cases, with some studies noting an increased percentage of ER and PR staining,[78,82] some noting no significant difference[81] and others noting a decreased percentage of cases showing ER and PR staining.[77,80] Multiple studies indicate an increased number of cases showing immunoreactivity for HER2 and an increased staining of the tumor suppressor gene product p53 compared with other forms of invasive breast carcinoma. One study noted that although the invasive micropapillary pattern is a more aggressive histologic type of invasive breast carcinoma, breast cancer patients with pure invasive micropapillary carcinoma histology show survival rates similar to those of other patients with equivalent numbers of lymph node metastases.[79] A study by Thor and colleagues[83] noted that 16 of 16 cases of invasive micropapillary carcinoma demonstrated loss of the short arm of chromosome 8 and speculated that this may explain the lymphotrophic phenotype associated with this histologic pattern.

Invasive Apocrine Carcinoma

By definition, invasive apocrine carcinomas show cytologic and immunohistochemical features of apocrine cells as characterized by an abundant, granular eosinophilic cytoplasm in more than 90% of the tumor cells (Fig. 3-29). The cytoplasmic granules stain with periodic acid-Schiff and maintain positive staining after diastase digestion. Apocrine cells typically stain with gross cystic disease fluid protein-15 (GCDFP15). They also express androgen receptor and typically do not express estrogen or progesterone receptors. Adherence to a strict definition is necessary, since apocrine differentiation can be identified in up to one third of all invasive carcinomas. WHO estimates that between 0.3% and 4.0% of invasive carcinomas would be classified as invasive apocrine carcinoma using the latter definition.[20] There is no statistically significant survival difference between invasive apocrine carcinoma and invasive ductal carcinoma, NOS, after accounting for tumor grade and stage.[84,85]

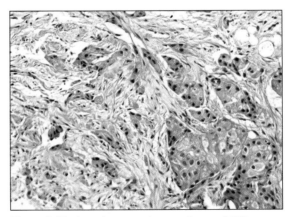

Figure 3-29. Invasive apocrine carcinoma (H&E stain). The tumor consists of sheets of apocrine cells with abundant, eosinophilic, and granular cytoplasm invading through the stroma.

Adenoid Cystic Carcinoma

Adenoid cystic carcinoma represents about 0.1% of all breast carcinomas. Adenoid cystic carcinoma has similar clinical characteristics to other histologic types of breast carcinoma because the tumors typically present as a mass with a similar age distribution to other forms of invasive breast carcinoma. The reported size varies from 0.7 to 12 cm, with an average size of 1.9 to 2.5 cm.

Adenoid cystic carcinomas are morphologically identical to adenoid cystic carcinomas in the salivary gland, lung, and skin. The tumor is composed of proliferating glands and stroma with basement membrane elements (Fig. 3-30A and B). Adenoid cystic carcinomas are composed of two basic cell populations: a basaloid population, which is usually the predominant population, and a population of smaller cells with bright eosinophilic cytoplasm. A third pop-

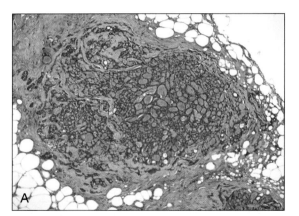
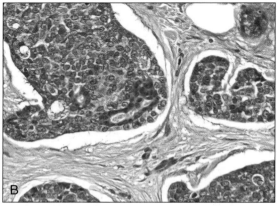

Figure 3-30. Adenoid cystic carcinoma (H&E stain). The carcinoma is composed of basaloid cells invading the stroma, which is appreciated at low power (**A**). A basaloid population, which is usually the predominant population, and a population of smaller cells with bright eosinophilic cytoplasm are identified on the higher magnification (**B**).

ulation of sebaceous cells with characteristic vacuoled cytoplasm has also been reported by Tavassoli and Norris.[86] Two or more morphologic patterns frequently exist within the same tumor. Quite often, eosinophilic basement membrane–like material, mucoid secretory material, or a bright thick eosinophilic band is deposited on the lining of the cells. Despite the well-circumscribed gross appearance, adenoid cystic carcinomas generally show an irregular, infiltrating growth pattern; a nest of cells or a cord-like arrangement is frequently present at the periphery. Unlike adenoid cystic carcinomas in the salivary gland, perineural invasion is found in only a minority of cases. Adenoid cystic carcinomas typically stain with cytokeratin 5/6, cytokeratin 34βE12 (keratin 903) and p63, and do not stain for ERs, PRs, and HER2/neu.

Patients with adenoid cystic carcinoma of the breast have a very favorable prognosis. Two studies noted 100% survival of patients, with follow-up ranging from 1 month to 15 years.[87,88] A recent study of 28 patients with adenoid cystic carcinoma of the breast in which 22 were treated with simple or modified radical mastectomy and 6 were treated with lumpectomy noted 100% 5-year disease-free survival and an overall survival rate of 85%.[89] A rare case of axillary lymph node metastasis has been reported.[90] Treatment of adenoid cystic carcinoma should include attention to complete excision because the tumor can be more infiltrative than the well-circumscribed gross appearance of the tumor.

The differential diagnosis of adenoid cystic carcinoma includes invasive cribriform carcinoma and collagenous spherulosis. Invasive cribriform carcinoma does not show the two-cell population that characterizes adenoid cystic carcinoma and does not stain with p63. Collagenous spherulosis lacks the two-cell population and generally shows a well-formed layer of myoepithelial cells between the epithelial cells and the stroma. Immunoperoxidase stains for calponin and smooth muscle myosin heavy chain can assist in highlighting the myoepithelial cells. In general, p63 is not useful in this differential diagnosis, since the tumor cells of adenoid cystic carcinoma typically stain with p63.

Metaplastic Carcinoma

Metaplastic carcinomas are a heterogeneous group of neoplasms generally characterized by an intimate admixture of adenocarcinoma, with dominant areas of spindle cell, squamous, and/or mesenchymal differentiation; the metaplastic spindle cell and squamous cell carcinomas may present in a pure form.[20] Metaplastic carcinomas of the breast comprise about 1% of all invasive breast carcinomas, with an average age at presentation of 55 years. The typical clinical presentation is a palpable mass, and on mammography these carcinomas are usually well-delineated densities.

The term metaplastic carcinoma describes a variety of lesions. WHO divides metaplastic carcinoma into two large categories, purely epithelial and mixed epithelial and mesenchymal. The purely epithelial tumors are divided into squamous, adenocarcinoma with spindle cell differentiation, and adenosquamous, including mucoepidermoid. The mixed epithelial and mesenchymal category is subdivided into carcinoma with chondroid metaplasia, carcinoma with osseous metaplasia, and carcinosarcoma.

Squamous cell carcinoma of the breast is by definition composed of metaplastic squamous cells that may be keratinizing, nonkeratinizing, spindle cell, and acantholytic histologic types. To qualify as a primary squamous cell carcinoma of the breast, the tumor must be arising in the breast parenchyma and must not be from the overlying skin or a metastasis from another site. The tumors are composed of squamous cells and have a morphology virtually identical to that of squamous cells of other organ sites such as the skin and lung (Fig. 3-31). The tumor cells are positive with cytokeratin 5/6 and cytokeratin 34βE12 (keratin 903) and are negative for ER, PR, and HER2. Reports differ somewhat on prognosis, but the tumors probably have a clinical behavior similar to that of adenocarcinomas of the breast of similar stage. The acantholytic variant is regarded as being more aggressive.[91] The origin of the squamous cells has not been established, since they may arise from epithelial cells, myoepithelial cells, or undifferentiated stem cells.

Adenocarcinoma with spindle cell metaplasia is defined as an invasive carcinoma with abundant spindle cell transformation. The spindle cells are believed to be glandular and neither squamous nor mesenchymal in origin. These tumors typically show immunoreactivity with epithelial markers such as cytokeratin 7 but do not show immunoreactivity to cytokeratin 5/6 or other markers of squamous or mesenchymal differentiation. Given the rarity of this category, it is difficult to make a statement on prognosis.

Adenosquamous carcinomas consist of invasive carcinomas (generally invasive ductal carcinomas), with areas of well-developed tubule/gland formation intimately admixed with often widely dispersed solid nests of squamous differentiation. The squamous component of adenosquamous carcinoma ranges from well-differentiated keratinizing to poorly differentiated nonkeratinizing areas. A small number of these tumors show histologic features that are virtually identical to low-grade mucoepidermoid carcinoma of the salivary gland. There are few reports of these tumors in the literature, but the prognosis seems to depend on the grade of the tumor.

The category of mixed epithelial/mesenchymal metaplastic carcinomas encompasses a wide variety of metaplastic tumors and includes tumors that show chondroid metaplasia (Fig. 3-32A), osseous metaplasia (Fig. 3-32B), spindle cell metaplasia, and carcinosarcoma.[92] Tumors that show both a malignant epithelial and mesenchymal component are designated carcinosarcoma. Tumors that show chondroid metaplasia and osseous metaplasia are frequently grouped into the category of "matrix producing" carcinomas. About 0.2% of all breast carcinomas have a focus of chondroid or osseous differentiation. They are generally well-circumscribed masses that are several centimeters in diameter.

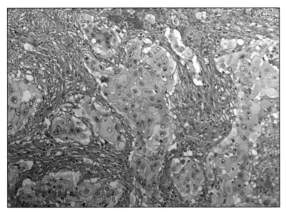

Figure 3-31. Invasive squamous cell carcinoma (H&E stain). The tumor consists of sheets of squamous cells.

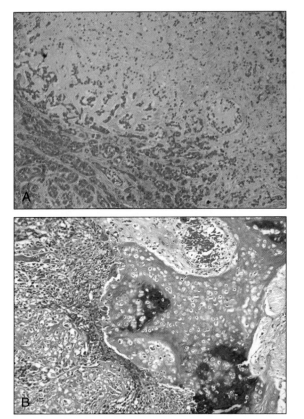

Figure 3-32. **A,** Invasive carcinoma with chondroid metaplasia. The tumor consists of an invasive carcinoima (lower right) with a chondromyxoid area in the upper right. (Photograph courtesy of Dr. Claudine Morcos.) **B,** Invasive carcinoma with osseous metaplasia showing carcinoma adjacent to an area of bone formation.

Occasionally, a breast carcinoma consists of spindle cells but without an easily recognizable invasive carcinoma seen on H&E stain. These tumors can be difficult to recognize and can be confused with a benign mesenchymal process such as stromal fibrosis, fibromatosis, or nodular fasciitis (Fig. 3-33A). In fact, spindle cell carcinoma (sarcomatoid carcinoma) is a major pitfall in breast pathology, and the pathologist must consider a spindle cell carcinoma when examining a spindle cell lesion of the breast. Immunoperoxidase stains for a panel of cytokeratins that includes both high- and low-molecular-weight cytokeratins and p63 are essential in establishing the diagnosis (Fig. 3-33B and C).

Most of the metaplastic carcinomas, particularly the spindle cell and sarcomatoid carcinomas, show a similar pattern of staining to

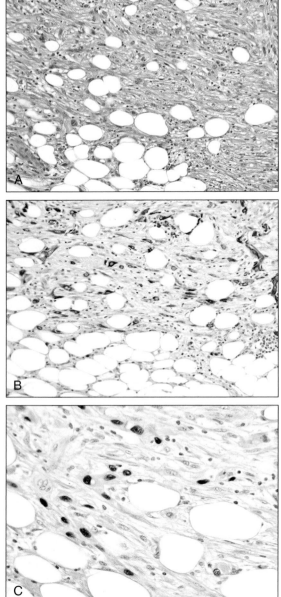

Figure 3-33. **Spindle cell (metaplastic) carcinoma. A,** H&E stain shows a population of spindle cells infiltrating through the stroma and into the adipose tissue. These tumors can be difficult to recognize as a carcinoma. **B,** A high-molecular-weight cytokeratin stain (34βE12) showing cytoplasmic staining by the tumor cells. **C,** A p63 stain demonstrating nuclear staining by the tumor cells. (Photographs courtesy of Dr. Ross Barner.)

myoepithelial cells with staining for cytokeratin 34βE12, CK5/6, CD10, smooth muscle actin, S-100, and p63,[93,94] and some researchers have proposed that these tumors are myoepithelial in origin.[93] Studies indicate that metaplastic carcinomas are generally negative for ER, PR, and HER2/neu.[95,96]

The prognosis of patients with metaplastic carcinomas has not been firmly established as these are rare tumors and there are not many large series on them. Recent studies indicate that metaplastic carcinomas, particularly the spindle cell/sarcomatoid carcinomas, are aggressive.[94,95] Other studies indicate that there is no significant difference in recurrence or survival rates compared with matched typical breast cancer cases.[96,97] One recent study suggests that metaplastic sarcomatoid carcinomas that lack or have only a minimal overt invasive carcinomatous component have a biologic behavior similar to that of sarcomas.[98]

Neuroendocrine Tumors

Focal neuroendocrine differentiation is not uncommon in both in situ and invasive breast carcinomas, with about 10% to 18% of primary breast carcinomas demonstrating some neuroendocrine differentiation.[99] Primary neuroendocrine tumors of the breast show similar morphologic features to neuroendocrine tumors in the lung or gastrointestinal tract.[20] For a primary breast carcinoma to be classified as a neuroendocrine carcinoma, it must show histologic and immunohistochemical evidence of neuroendocrine differentiation in at least 50% of the cells. Immunohistochemical stains for neuroendocrine differentiation include neuron-specific enolase, chromogranin, synaptophysin, and CD56. Although the presence of neuroendocrine changes in breast carcinomas has not been exhaustively studied, reports indicate that neuroendocrine differentiation does not have a significant impact on established prognostic factors or patient outcome.[99]

A few cases have been reported of primary small cell carcinoma of the breast showing a morphology identical to that of small cell carcinoma of the lung (Fig. 3-34). One must be careful to exclude the possibility of a metastatic lesion, and clinical correlation is extremely important in this instance. Immunoperoxidase stains are of limited value in distinguishing a primary small cell of the breast from a metastatic lesion from the lung because thyroid transcription factor-1 (TTF-1) may be positive in both a primary lung and primary breast small cell carcinoma. Although early reports noted

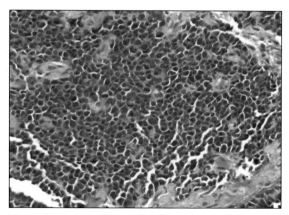

Figure 3-34. Invasive small cell carcinoma (H&E stain). This carcinoma of the breast consists of sheets of cells with small, round nuclei with neuroendocrine features and minimal cytoplasm. The morphology is identical to small cell carcinoma of the lung.

poor survival for patients with primary small cell carcinoma of the breast, a recent report indicated that the prognosis in these patients may not be as poor as previously suggested.[100]

Primary Malignant Lymphoma

Involvement of the breast by lymphoma, either primary or secondary, is rather uncommon. The reader is directed to more detailed texts on the diagnosis and treatment of hematopoietic disease. The purpose of briefly mentioning lymphomas in this chapter is to make the clinician and pathologist aware that, while rare, this may occur in the breast. In addition, the clinical presentation as well as the H&E morphology may resemble a carcinoma. WHO criteria for primary breast lymphoma are (1) availability of adequate histologic material, (2) presence of breast tissue in or adjacent to the lymphoma infiltrate, (3) no concurrent nodal disease except for the involvement of ipsilateral axillary lymph nodes, and (4) no previous history of lymphoma involvement of other organs or tissue.[101]

The lesion typically presents as a mass either on clinical examination or mammography. On macroscopic examination, the lesions tend to have a gray-white nodular appearance. The H&E microscopic morphology depends on the type of lymphoma. Diffuse large B-cell lymphoma, which is the most common type of lymphoma in the breast, consists of sheets of large cells with oval, indented, or lobulated nuclei without significant cell-to-cell cohesion (Fig. 3-35A and

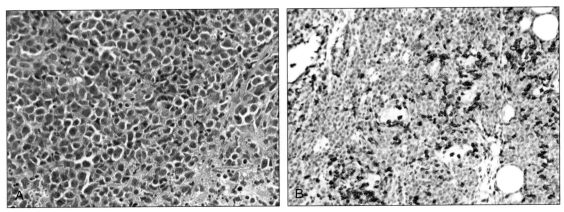

Figure 3-35. A, Diffuse large B-cell lymphoma (H&E stain). Shown are sheets of large cells with oval to indented nuclei without significant cell-to-cell cohesion. Prominent nucleoli are seen. **B,** An immunoperoxidase stain for the B-cell marker CD20.

B). Immunoperoxidase stains are essential in confirming the diagnosis of lymphoma and correctly classifying the lesion.

Inflammatory Carcinoma

Inflammatory carcinoma is a clinicopathologic entity characterized by diffuse erythema and edema involving most of the skin of the breast, often without an underlying palpable mass. The clinical presentation results from tumor emboli in dermal lymphatics, although these may not be seen on skin biopsy. The diagnosis is established by the combination of clinical findings and a biopsy showing carcinoma, either within dermal lymphatics or in the breast parenchyma (Fig. 3-36A and B). Involvement of dermal lymphatics alone does not indicate inflammatory carcinoma. For the purposes of staging, CAP and AJCC recommend the following: If the skin biopsy is negative and there is not localized measurable primary cancer, the T category is pTX; when pathologically staging a clinical inflammatory carcinoma the T category is T4d. Dimpling of the skin, nipple retraction, or other skin changes, except those in T4b and T4d, may occur in T1, T2, or T3 tumors without affecting the classification.

Paget Disease

When an invasive carcinoma is accompanied by Paget disease, the pathologist should include this in the report. (A more detailed discussion of Paget disease can be found in Chapter 11.)

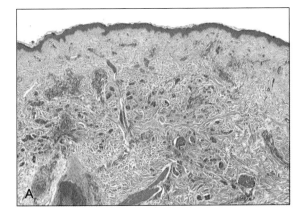

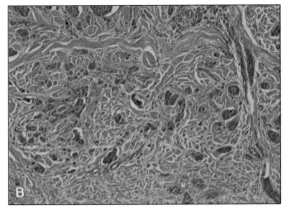

Figure 3-36. Invasive carcinoma involving dermal lymphatics (H&E stain). These photographs are low-power (**A**) and high-power (**B**) views of small groups of invasive carcinoma involving dermal lymphatics. In the appropriate clinical setting, this would be consistent with inflammatory carcinoma.

Microinvasive Carcinoma

Both CAP and AJCC define microinvasion as the extension of cancer cells beyond the basement membrane into the adjacent tissue, with no focus more than 0.1 cm in greatest dimension.[9] When there are multiple foci of microinvasion, the size of *only* the largest focus is used to classify the microinvasion. The sum of all the individual foci is not to be used. The presence of multiple foci of microinvasion should be noted and/or qualified, as it is with multiple larger invasive carcinomas. WHO defines microinvasive carcinoma as a tumor in which the dominant lesion is noninvasive but in which there are one or more clearly separate small, microscopic foci of infiltration into nonspecialized interlobular stroma.[102] WHO recommends a size limited to 1 mm, but note that the size limit does vary somewhat in the published literature.

In actual practice, making a definitive diagnosis of microinvasion can at times be very difficult, if not impossible. This is especially true for large, multifocal DCIS, particularly when the tumor is high grade. On histologic examination, microinvasion consists of small groups of cells or individual cells budding off the involved focus of DCIS and invading into the stroma (Fig. 3-37). The cells designated as microinvasive must be distributed in a haphazard pattern that does not represent tangential sectioning of a duct or lobular unit. Additional sections are often helpful in making this determination. Immunoperoxidase stains may be helpful in demonstrating a break in the myoepithelial cell layer. Nevertheless, there will be a subset of tumors in which the determination of microinvasion cannot be accurately made. In addition, small foci of invasive carcinoma can be missed in routine sampling, either as tissue that is not submitted for histologic examination or microscopic foci in tissue blocks in which the plane of tissue is not sectioned for histologic examination. As a result, some limited sampling of axillary nodes may be necessary in cases of DCIS. The use of a sentinel node biopsy may prove to be of some benefit in these cases.

Studies on microinvasion indicate that the incidence of metastatic disease is low. However, given the absence of a standard definition in the past, it is difficult to make definitive conclusions based on previous studies. Using a definition of a single focus of less than 2 mm or up to 3 invasive foci, none exceeding 1 mm, none of 38

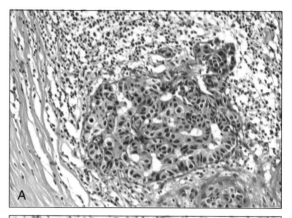

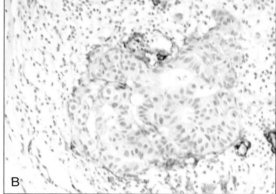

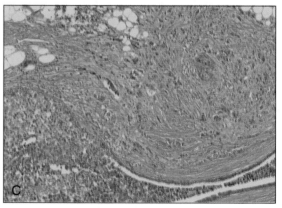

Figure 3-37. Ductal carcinoma in situ with microinvasion (H&E stain).   A, The photomicrograph shows small groups and individual epithelial cells breaking off from the duct and into the surrounding stroma. **B,** An immunoperoxidase stain for calponin highlights breast in the myoepithelial layer. **C,** Focus of more definitive microinvasion in the central portion adjacent to ductal carcinoma in situ in the lower left portion of the screen. The invasive component consists of nests and cords of cells in a fibrous, desmoplastic stroma.

women who had undergone mastectomy and axillary node dissection were noted to have lymph node metastasis.[103] Other studies have shown that a small percentage of cases (5% to 20%) will show axillary node metastasis.[104,105]

Presentation as an Axillary Lymph Node Metastasis

Though rare, with estimates of less than 1% of all invasive breast carcinoma, the initial presentation of invasive breast carcinoma may be an axillary lymph node metastasis without an identifiable breast mass by clinical examination or radiographic imaging. Even after mastectomy, there may still be a small but significant number of patients in which a primary breast tumor is not identified.[106–108] Rosen and Kimmel[106] note that the tumors follow one of three patterns. In the first pattern, which accounts for about two thirds of cases, the tumor cells show a pattern of large cells with abundant eosinophilic cytoplasm (apocrine-like features) diffusely distributed throughout the lymph node (see Fig. 3-36). Minimal gland formation is identified. In the second pattern, the tumor cells are spread individually or in small groups throughout the lymph node and can be easily confused with a diffuse lymphoma. In the third pattern, which accounts for about 20% of cases, the metastasis shows a growth pattern similar to those commonly encountered in primary breast carcinomas.

Immunoperoxidase stains provide helpful information in the differential diagnosis of a metastatic tumor from an unknown primary site. Immunoperoxidase stains should be interpreted carefully and with close attention to the clinical information. Primary breast carcinomas typically stain with cytokeratin 7 and show less diffuse and less intense staining with cytokeratin 20. Breast carcinomas do not stain for TTF-1 or melanocytic stains such as HMB45, melanin A, tyrosinase, or microophthalmic transcription factor-1. A limited amount of S-100 staining may be noted in breast carcinoma. Gross cystic fluid disease protein-15 (GCDFP-15) stains breast as well as tumors of skin adnexal origin. The specificity of the antibody is quite high (around 99%); however, the sensitivity is significantly lower (around 60% to 70%). The sensitivity is even lower in the less well-differentiated tumors, which make up many of the occult primary tumors. A newer antibody, mammoglobin, shows a similar specificity to GCDFP-15

but also shows a similar problem with a lack of sensitivity. Immunoperoxidase stains for ER and PR can be helpful, but problems with sensitivity arise because the primary breast tumor may not express ER or PR. In addition, a limited amount of staining for ER and PR can be seen in tissue that is not of breast or gynecologic tract origin.

Tumors of the colon and rectum typically stain with cytokeratin 20 and do not stain with cytokeratin 7. Thus, immunoperoxidase stains are quite helpful in excluding a metastatic tumor from the colon or rectum. However, cytokeratin 7 and cytokeratin 20 staining not so consistent in other parts of the gastrointestinal tract, particularly the stomach, and the use of immunoperoxidase stains to exclude a metastatic carcinoma from a gastrointestinal primary tumor besides the colon and rectum is limited. Similar problems are encountered with tumors of pancreatic origin. Melanomas typically do not stain with cytokeratins but stain with S-100 protein, HMB45, melanin A, and tyrosinase. Metastatic breast carcinomas typically stain for cytokeratins but do not stain for HMB45, melanin A, or tyrosinase. As previously stated, S-100 may stain epithelial cells and is of less use in distinguishing between metastatic carcinoma and melanoma.

Primary lung carcinomas show a pattern identical to cytokeratin 7 and cytokeratin 20 staining to primary breast carcinomas. TTF-1 is generally very useful in distinguishing between a metastatic breast carcinoma and metastatic lung carcinoma. Carcinomas of lung origin typically stain with TTF-1, whereas carcinomas of breast origin do not. Thus, although a panel of immunoperoxidase stains provides helpful information in the differential diagnosis in excluding melanocytic tumors, primary tumors of the colon and rectum, and adenocarcinoma of the lung, they may not provide conclusive evidence for a breast primary tumor owing to the lack of sensitivity of GCDFP-15 and mammoglobin and the lack of ER and PR.

In addition to the immunoperoxidase staining pattern, correlation with clinical and radiographic findings is crucial. Knowledge of the metastatic patterns of various primary malignancies provides significant information in determining a primary site. A large study on metastatic patterns of adenocarcinoma noted that metastatic breast carcinoma accounted for 97% of all metastatic carcinomas to axillary lymph nodes.[109] Thus, the presence of metastatic carcinoma to an axillary lymph node, particularly when the tumor shows one of the three patterns described by Rosen and

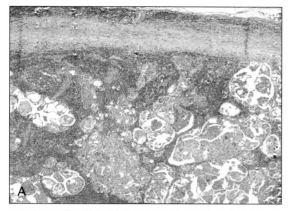

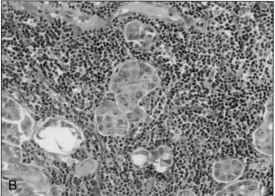

Figure 3-38. Breast carcinoma presenting as an axillary lymph node metastasis (H&E stain). The tumor consists of groups of large cells with abundant eosinophilic cytoplasm throughout the lymph node. This morphology is common for invasive breast carcinoma that presents as an axillary lymph node metastasis without a breast mass noted on clinical examination or radiographic imaging studies.

Kimmel,[106] should be considered a metastasis from the breast until proven otherwise.

The literature is not definitive on the optimal treatment for these patients. One study noted no differences in survival between patients treated with immediate surgery and radiation therapy and patients who were followed up without treatment to the breast.[107] A recent study noted improved survival for patients who received a modified radical mastectomy over those patients who did not undergo mastectomy.[108]

PART 4. REPORTING OF ESTROGEN AND PROGESTERONE STATUS

It has been known for many years that hormones, particularly estrogen, play a major role in breast cancer tumorigenesis. Increased sur-

vival for premenopausal patients after oophorectomy was reported over 100 years ago.[110] Subsequent reports of adrenalectomy and hypophysectomy were found to be effective for some postmenopausal patients.[111] In addition, many factors that contribute to the development of breast cancer, such as early menarche, late menopause, null parity, and increased body fat content, suggest that prolonged exposure to estrogen contributes to the development of breast cancer.

Estrogen receptor is a regulatory steroid protein that is located in the cell nucleus and functions as a transcription regulator of breast epithelial growth and proliferation. It is necessary for proper breast development and function. The function is mediated by complex cellular interactions of ligands, cofactors, and protein kinases. The presence of ER is not unique to the breast since it has been detected in the endometrium, myometrium, ovary, prostate, testis, pituitary, kidney, thymus, bone, and central nervous system.

Two ERs have been identified: ERα and ERβ. The two proteins are structurally similar and show high homology within the DNA and hormone-binding domains, respectively. However, the overall sequence homology is only approximately 30% and seems to indicate that their effects may be different.[112] The existence of the ERβ was noted only in 1996, and its role in breast carcinoma is still being investigated and debated.[113] There are no well-established data on whether the ERβ status provides clinical useful information. As a result, current testing is performed on the ERα receptor only. As more data are collected and analyzed, testing for ERβ may in the future become an integral part of hormone receptor analysis.[114,115]

A percentage of normal (non-neoplastic) breast epithelial cells express ER. The expression is dependent on the phase of the menstrual cycle. The expression of ERα seems to be higher during the luteal phase than during the follicular phase of the menstrual cycle. During pregnancy, expression of ERα appears to be low, but expression of ERα and ERβ appears to return during lactation. In the proliferating breast, approximately 60% to 70% of cells express neither ERα receptor nor ERβ receptor. Apocrine metaplastic cells typically do not express ER but do express androgen receptor.

The method for detection of ER has changed over the last 10 to 15 years. Initially, testing was

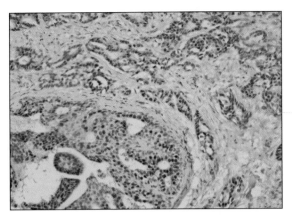

Figure 3-39. Invasive carcinoma, estrogen receptor stain. The nuclei of the invasive carcinoma cells show strong staining with estrogen receptor.

performed using a biochemical assay–based uptake binding of radioactive ligand to the receptor and quantitation of the amount of radioactivity that is bound. Even though the method is accurate and provides a rather precise quantitative number of the hormone receptor status, it has several drawbacks. First, fresh tissue or snap-frozen tissue is required for the assay. Thus, there is no confirmation that the tissue being tested is indeed carcinoma or necrotic tumor cells, scar tissue, or normal breast tissue. Second, a significant portion of the tumor is required. This markedly consists of diagnosis, staging, and grading of the tumor, particularly of tumors less than 2 cm.

Over the last 10 to 15 years, the ligand-binding assay method has been replaced by immunoperoxidase staining. Since the hormone receptor is located on the cell nucleus, only nuclear staining is regarded as positive; cytoplasmic staining is generally regarded as background and is disregarded (Fig. 3-39). Staining of surrounding "normal" breast tissue serves as an adequate internal control. The testing can be done on formalin-fixed paraffin-embedded tissue. Thus, there is visual confirmation that the cells being tested are indeed invasive carcinoma.

While there are clear advantages with immunohistochemical methods, a few drawbacks exist. First, obtaining standardization among laboratories is difficult. As with any immunohistochemical test, the type of fixative, the duration of fixation, the method of antigen retrieval, and the staining method all have an effect on the outcome. Neutral buffered formalin is used almost universally given the current American Society of Clinical Oncology (ASCO) guidelines for HER2/neu testing. Alcohol fixative may also be used. However, acidic fixative such as Bouin's and B-5 and decalcifying solutions destroy estrogen receptors. Because estrogen degrades in unfixed tissue, it is important that the tissue be adequately fixed within several hours of removal. Fixation times between 6 and 18 hours generally provide optimal results. Significantly shorter or longer fixation times may provide false negative results. Daily use of positive and negative control slides is essential in maintaining laboratory quality.

Additional problems with the use of immunohistochemical stains include the method of scoring and quantifying the amount of ER present in the carcinoma. The commonly performed method is to regard a test as positive when more than 10% of the tumor cells stain, as low positive when 1% to 10% of tumor cells stain, and as negative when 0% of tumor cells stain. This approach, which is probably used by most laboratories, does not take into account the intensity of the staining. An alternative is to use a semiquantitive approach combining both staining intensity and the number of cells staining. The best-known example of this is the Allred score, which is based on the number of cells staining and the staining intensity. Other laboratories use computed image analysis to quantify the results.

There is some debate as to the clinical value of quantitative immunohistochemistry. Harvey and colleagues[115] demonstrated a linear relationship between hormone receptor levels and ER levels using ligand binding and a difference in disease-free outcome. Other studies suggest a bimodal distribution (strongly and diffusely positive or negative) in the vast majority of cases and conclude that quantitative reporting is unimportant. Currently, NIH consensus guidelines are to treat women with any degree of hormone receptor staining with tamoxifen or aromatase inhibitors.[116]

In addition to response to ER, progesterone status is a good indicator of response to therapy. The PR gene is also a member of the nuclei receptor family. Two isoforms of PR, PRA, and PRB, are known. They are encoded by the same gene. Both PRA and PRB are expressed in normal breast tissue. However, PRB protein concentration is elevated in breast carcinoma. It is believed that the decrease in the PRA:PRB ratio is an important parameter for progesterone-mediated functions. ER is a key transcription factor for the activation of PR. Thus, positive PR staining, at least in theory, is a test for an intact estrogen response pathway. ER-positive/PR-negative tumors are less responsive to therapy. More than 50% of all ER-positive tumors are positive for PR. This suggests that PR may be necessary for positive therapeutic outcomes with hormone therapy. An alternative explanation is that because ER is a key transcription factor in the activation of PR, lack of PR expression in the ER-positive/PR-negative cells also could suggest that estrogen response pathway may not be functional in these tumors.[114]

As with ER, testing for PR is routinely performed on invasive tumors. As expected, tumors that are ER-positive and PR-positive have a better response to endocrine therapy and are less aggressive tumors than ER-negative/PR-negative and ER-positive/PR-negative tumors. ER-positive/PR-positive tumors represent a small fraction (about 1% to 2%) of invasive carcinomas and demonstrate a variable response to hormone therapy. There is some debate as to whether ER-negative/PR-positive tumors exist. It has been proposed that with the use of more sensitive estrogen antibodies, the presence of ER-negative/PR-positive breast carcinomas is virtually nonexistent.

Conclusion

Surgical pathology specimens for breast carcinoma are among the most challenging specimens for the laboratory and for pathologists in cancer treatment. Breast specimens are more difficult to process than most other surgical pathology laboratory specimens because of the high content of adipose tissue in the breast. Thus, the importance of adequate fixation cannot be overemphasized. In addition, multiple lesions such as sclerosing adenosis and radial scars clinically, radiographically, and pathologically closely resemble invasive breast carcinoma. The great variety of histologic types of invasive breast carcinomas supports the fact that breast carcinomas are indeed a biologically diverse group of diseases. The pathology report for invasive carcinoma continues to become more complicated in order to include factors that influence clinician decisions such as size, type, grade, margin status, lymph node status, and hormone receptor status.

The diagnosis of invasive breast carcinoma is based on the demonstration of malignant cells beyond the confines of the duct and terminal lobular units and into the surrounding stroma. Additional studies such as immunoperoxidase stains can be helpful; however, the diagnosis remains dependent on H&E morphology. Although the knowledge of microscopic anatomy has significantly increased over the last 50 years, the diagnostic techniques have changed remarkably little. We are at a time when we are reaching the limits of microscopic anatomy, and future advances will be in the fields of molecular biology, biochemistry, and immunology. Further advances in these newer fields will probably not replace microscopic anatomy for quite a while, but they will inevitably increase our knowledge and understanding of the disease and ultimately improve patient care. Most important, cooperation and teamwork among the involved medical disciplines are essential today and will be even more important as future advances are made.

References

1. Tabbara SO, Frost AR, Stoler MH, et al: Changing trends in breast fine-needle aspiration: results of the Papanicolaou Society of cytopathology survey. Diagn Cytopathol 22(2): 126–130, 2000.
2. Start RD, Flynn MS, Cross SS, et al: Is the grading of breast carcinomas affected by a delay in fixation? Virchows Arch 419:475–477, 1991.
3. Wolff AC, Hammond EH, Schwartz JN, et al: American Society of Clinical Oncology/College of American Pathologists Guideline Recommendations for Human Epidermal Growth Factor Receptor 2 Testing in Breast Cancer. Arch Pathol Lab Med 131:18–43, 2007.
4. Werling RW, Wang H, Yaziji H, et al: Immunohistochemical distinction of invasive from noninvasive breast lesions: a comparison study of p63 versus calponin and smooth muscle myosin heavy chain. Am J Surg Pathol 27(1):82–90, 2003.
5. Bhargava R, Esposito NN, Dabbs DJ: Immunohistology of the breast. In Dabbs DJ (ed): Diagnostic Immunohistochemistry: Theranostic and Genomic Applications, 3rd ed. Philadelphia: Saunders, 2009, p 766.
6. Nagi C, Bleiweiss I, Jaffer S: Epithelial displacement in breast lesions. Arch Pathol Lab Med 129:1465–1469, 2005.
7. Hill CB, Yeh IT: Myoepithelial cell staining patterns of papillary breast lesions: from intraductal papillomas to invasive papillary carcinoma. Am J Clin Pathol 123(1):36–44, 2005.
8. Collins LC, Carlo VP, Hwang H, et al: Intracystic papillary carcinomas of the breast: a reevaluation using a panel of myoepithelial cell markers. Am J Surg Pathol 30:1002–1007, 2006.
9. American Joint Committee on Cancer: AJCC Cancer Staging Manual, 7th ed. New York: Springer, 2010, pp 347–376.
10. Connolly JL: Changes and problematic areas in interpretation of the AJCC Cancer staging manual, 6th edition for breast cancer. Arch Pathol Lab Med 130:287–291, 2006.
11. Greenough RB: Varying degrees of malignancy in cancer of the breast. Cancer Res 9:452–463, 1925.
12. Haagensen CD: The basis for histologic grading of carcinoma of the breast. Am J Cancer 19:285–327, 1933.
13. Patey DH, Scarff RW: The position of histology in the prognosis of carcinoma of the breast. Lancet 211:801–804, 1928.
14. Bloom HJG, Richardson WW: Histological grading and prognosis in breast cancer: a study of 1409 cases of which 359

have been followed for 15 years. Br J Cancer 11:359–377, 1957.

15. Elston CW, Ellis IO: Pathological prognostic factors in breast cancer I. The value of histological grade in breast cancer: experience from a large study with long-term follow-up. Histopathology 19:403–410, 1991.

16. Kuopio T, Collan Y: Still more about counting mitoses. Hum Pathol 27:1110–1111, 1996.

17. Hurd TC, Sneige N, Allen PK, et al: Impact of extensive intraductal component on recurrence and survival in patients with stage I or II breast cancer treated with breast conservation therapy. Ann Surg Oncol 4(2):119–124, 1997.

18. Connolly JL, Boyages J, Nixon AJ, et al: Predictors of breast recurrence after conservative surgery and radiation therapy for invasive breast cancer. Mod Pathol 11:134–139, 1998.

19. Wellings SR, Jensen HM, Marcum RG: An atlas of subgross pathology of the human breast with special reference to possible precancerous lesions. J Natl Cancer Inst 55:231–273, 1975.

20. Ellis IO, Schnitt SJ, Sastre-Garau X, et al: Invasive breast carcinoma. In Tavassoli FA, Devilee P (eds): Tumours of the Breast and Female Genital Organs. Lyon: IARC Press, 2003, pp 13–59.

21. Li CI, Anderson BO, Porter P, et al: 2000 Changing incidence rate of invasive lobular breast carcinoma among older women. Cancer 88:2561–2569, 2000.

22. Bonnier P, Romain, S, Giacalone PL, et al: Clinical and biological prognostic factors in breast cancer diagnosed during postmenopausal hormone replacement therapy. Obstet Gynecol 85:11–17, 1995.

23. Li CI, Weiss NS, Stanford JL, et al: Hormone replacement therapy in relation to risk of lobular and ductal breast carcinoma in middle-aged women. Cancer 88:2570–2577, 2000.

24. O'Connor IF, Shembekar MV, Shousha S: Breast carcinoma developing in patients on hormone replacement therapy: a histological and immunohistological study. J Clin Pathol 51:935–938, 1998.

25. Bratthauer GL, Tavassoli FA: Lobular intraepithelial neoplasia: previously unexplored aspects assessed in 775 cases and their clinical implications. Virchows Arch 440(2):134–138, 2002.

26. Cleton-Jansen A-M: E-cadherin and loss of heterozygosity at chromosome 16 in breast carcinogenesis: different genetic pathways in ductal and lobular breast cancer? Breast Cancer Res 4:5–8, 2002.

27. Eusebi V, Magalhaes F, Azzopardi JB: Pleomorphic lobular carcinoma of the breast: an aggressive tumor showing apocrine differentiation. Hum Pathol 23:655–662, 1992.

28. Weidner N, Semple JP: Pleomorphic variant of invasive lobular carcinoma of the breast. Hum Pathol 23:1167–1171, 1992.

29. Bentz JS, Yassa N, Clayton F: Pleomorphic lobular carcinoma of the breast: clinicopathologic features of 12 cases. Mod Pathol 11(9):814–822, 1998.

30. Middleton LP, Palacios DM, Bryant BR, et al: Pleomorphic lobular carcinoma: morphology, immunohistochemistry, and molecular analysis. Am J Surg Pathol 24(12):1650–1656, 2000.

31. DiCostanzo D, Rosen PP, Gareen I, et al: Prognosis in infiltrating lobular carcinoma: an analysis of "classical" and variant tumors Am J Surg Pathol 14(1):12–23, 1990.

32. Lesser ML, Rosen PP, Kinne DW: Multicentricity and bilaterality in invasive breast carcinoma. Surgery 91:234–240, 1982.

33. du Toit RS, Locker AP, Ellis IO, et al: Invasive lobular carcinomas of the breast—the prognosis of histopathological subtypes. Br J Cancer 60(4):605–609, 1989.

34. Horn PL, Thompson WD: Risk of contralaeral breast cancer: associations with histologic, clinical, and therapeutic factors. Cancer 62:412–424, 1988.

35. Silverstein MJ, Lewinsky BS, Waisman JR, et al: Infiltrating lobular carcinoma: is it different from infiltrating duct carcinoma? Cancer 73:1673–1677, 1994.

36. De la Rochefordiere A, Asselain B, Scholl S, et al: Simultaneous bilateral breast carcinoma: a retrospective review of 149 cases. Int J Radiat Oncol Biol Phys 30:35–41, 1994.

37. Sastre-Garau X, Jouve M, Asselain B, et al: Infiltrating lobular carcinoma of the breast: clinicopathologic analysis of 975 cases with reference to data on conservative therapy and metastatic patterns. Cancer 77:113–120, 1996.

38. Healey EA, Cook EF, Orav EJ, et al: Contralateral breast cancer: clinical characteristics and impact on prognosis. J Clin Oncol 11:1545–1552, 1993.

39. Parker RG, Grimm P, Enstrom JE: Contralateral breast cancers following treatment for initial breast cancers in women. Am J Clin Oncol 12:213–216, 1989.

40. Dixon JM, Anderson TJ, Page DL, et al: Infiltrating lobular carcinoma of the breast. Histopathology 6:149–161, 1982.

41. du Toit RS, Locker AP, Ellis IO, et al: An evaluation of differences in prognosis, recurrence patterns and receptor status between invasive lobular and other invasive carcinomas of the breast. Eur J Surg Oncol 17(3):251–257, 1991.

42. Ellis IO, Galea M, Broughton N, et al: Pathological prognostic factors in breast cancer. II. Histologic type. Relationship with survival in a large study with long-term follow-up. Histopathology 20:479–489, 1992.

43. Toikkanen S, Pylkkanen L, Joensuu H: Invasive lobular carcinoma of the breast has better short-and long-term survival than invasive ductal carcinoma. Br J Cancer 76(9):1234–1240, 1997.

44. Pereira H, Pinder SE, Sibbering DM, et al. Pathological prognostic factors in breast cancer. IV. Should you be a typer or a grader? A comparative study of two histological prognostic features in operable breast carcinoma. Histopathology 27:219–226, 1995.

45. DiConstanzo D, Rosen PP, Garreen I, et al: Prognosis of infiltrating lobular carcinoma: an analysis of "classical" and variant tumors. Am J Surg Pathol 14:12–23, 1990.

46. Bane AL, Tujan S, Parkes RK, et al: Invasive lobular carcinoma: to grade or not to grade. Mod Pathol 18:621–628, 2005.

47. Fitzgibbons PL, Page DL, Weaver D, et al: Prognostic factors in breast cancer. College of American Pathologists Consensus Statement 1999. Arch Pathol Lab Med 124:966–978, 2000.

48. Moatamed NA, Apple SK: Extensive sampling changes T-staging of infiltrating lobular carcinoma of breast: a comparative study of gross versus microscopic tumor sizes. Breast J 12(6):511–517, 2006.

49. Goldstein NS, O'Malley BA: Cancerization of small ectatic ducts of the breast by ductal carcinoma in situ cells with apocrine snouts: a lesion associated with tubular carcinoma. Am J Clin Pathol 107:561–566, 1997.

50. Moinfar F, Man YG, Bratthauer GL, et al: Genetic abnormalities in mammary ductal intraepithelial neoplasia-flat type ("clinging ductal carcinoma in situ"): a simulator of normal mammary epithelium. Cancer 88(9):2072–2081, 2000.

51. Diab SG, Clark GM, Osborne CK, et al: Tumor characteristics and clinical outcome of tubular and mucinous breast carcinomas. J Clin Oncol 17:1442–1448, 1999.

52. Winchester DJ, Sahin AA, Tucker SL, et al: Tubular carcinoma of the breast: predicting axillary nodal metastases and recurrence Ann Surg 223(3):342–347, 1996.

53. Papadatos G, Rangan AM, Psorianos R, et al: Probability of axillary node involvement in patients with tubular carcinoma of the breast. Br J Surg 88:860–864, 2001.

54. Bradford WZ, Christensen WN, Fraser H, et al: Treatment of pure tubular carcinoma of the breast. Breast J 4(6):437–440, 1998.

55. Wheeler DT, Tai LH, Bratthauer GL, et al: Tubulolobular carcinoma of the breast: analysis of 27 cases of a tumor with a hybrid morphology and immunoprofile. Am J Surg Pathol 28:1587–1593, 2004.

56. Green I, McCormick B, Cranor M, et al: A comparative study of pure tubular and tubulolobular carcinoma of the breast. Am J Surg Pathol 21(6):653–657, 1977.

57. Fisher ER, Gregorio RNM, Redmond C, Fisher B: Tubulolobular invasive breast cancer: a variant of lobular invasive cancer. Hum Pathol 8(6):679–683, 1977.

58. Rosen PP, Lesser ML, Kinne DW: Breast carcinoma at the extremes of age: a comparison of patients younger than 35 years and older than 75 years. J Surg Oncol 28(2):90–96, 1985.

59. Silverberg SG, Kay S, Chiatale AR, et al: Colloid carcinoma of the breast. Am J Clin Pathol 55:355–363, 1971.

60. Anan K, Mitsuyama K, Tamea K, et al: Pathological features of mucinous carcinoma of the breast are favourable for breast-conserving therapy. Eur J Surg Oncol 27:459–463, 2001.

61. Komaki K, Sakamoto G, Sugano H, et al: Mucinous carcinoma of the breast in Japan: a prognostic analysis based on morphologic features. Cancer 61:989–996, 1988.

62. Rosen PP: Mucocele-like tumors of the breast. Am J Surg Pathol 10(7):464–469, 1986.

63. Page Dl, Dixon JM, Anderson TJ, et al: Invasive cribriform carcinoma of the breast. Histopathology 7:525–536, 1983.

64. Venable JG, Schwartz AM, Silverberg SG: Infiltrating cribriform carcinoma of the breast: a distinctive clinicopathologic entity. Hum Pathol 21:333–338, 1990.

65. Jensen ML, Kiaer H, Andersen J, et al: Prognostic comparison of three classifications for medullary carcinoma of the breast. Histopathology 30:523–532, 1997.

66. Maier WP, Rosemond GP, Goldman LI, et al: A ten year study of medullary carcinoma of the breast. Surg Gynecol Obstet 144:695–698, 1977.

67. Pedersen L, Zedeler K, Holck S, et al: Medullary carcinoma of the breast. Prevalence and prognostic importance of classical risk factors in breast cancer. Eur J Cancer 31A:2289–2295, 1995.

68. Reinfuss M, Stelmach A, Mitus J, et al: Typical medullary carcinoma of the breast: a clinical and pathologic analysis of 52 cases. J Surg Oncol 60:89–94, 1995.

69. Rapin V, Contesso G, Mouriesse H, et al: Medullary breast carcinoma. A reevaluation of 95 cases of breast cancer with inflammatory stroma. Cancer 61:2503–2510, 1988.

70. Ridolfi RL, Rosen PP, Port A, et al: Medullary carcinoma of the breast: a clinicopathologic study with 10 year follow-up. Cancer 40:1365–1385, 1977.

71. Black CL, Morris DM, Goldman LL, McDonald JC: The significance of lymph node involvement in patients with medullary carcinoma of the breast. Surg Gynecol Obstet 157:497–499, 1983.

72. Fisher ER, Kenny JP, Sass R, et al: Medullary cancer of the breast revisited. Breast Cancer Res Treat 16:215–229, 1990.

73. Wargotz ES, Silverberg SG: Medullary carcinoma of the breast: a clinicopathologic study with appraisal of current diagnostic criteria. Hum Pathol 19:1340–1346, 1988.

74. Rubens JR, Lewandrowski KR, Kopans DB, et al: Medullary carcinoma of the breast. Overdiagnosis of a prognostically favorable neoplasm. Arch Surg 125(5):601–604, 1990.

75. Fisher ER, Palekar AS, Redmond C, et al: Pathologic findings from the National Surgical Adjuvant Breast Project (protocol No. 4). VI. Invasive papillary cancer. Am J Clin Pathol 73:313–322, 1980.

76. Siriaunkgul S, Tavassoli FA: Invasive micropapillary carcinoma of the breast. Mod Pathol 6(6):660–662, 1993.

77. Middleton LP, Tressera F, Sobel ME, et al: Infiltrating micropapillary carcinoma of the breast. Mod Pathol 12(5):499–504, 1999.

78. Walsh MM, Bleiweiss IJ: Invasive micropapillary carcinoma of the breast: eighty cases of an underrecognized entity. Hum Pathol 32:583–589, 2001.

79. Paterakos M, Watkin WG, Edgerton SM, et al: Invasive micropapillary carcinoma of the breast: a prognostic study. Hum Pathol 30:1459–1463, 1999.

80. De la Cruz C, Moriya T, Endoh M, et al: Invasive micropapillary carcinoma of the breast: clinicopathological and immunohistochemical study. Pathol Int 54:90–96, 2004.

81. Nassar H, Wallis T, Andrea A, et al: Clinicopathologic analysis of invasive micropapillary differentiation in breast carcinoma. Mod Pathol 14(9):836–841, 2001.

82. Zekioglu O, Erhan Y, Ciris M, et al: Invasive micropapillary of the breast: high incidence of lymph node metastasis with extranodal extension and its immunohistochemical profile compared with invasive ductal carcinoma. Histopathology 44:18–23, 2004.

83. Thor AD, Eng C, Devries S, et al: Invasive micropapillary carcinoma of the breast is associated with chromosome 8 abnormalities detected by comparative genomic hybridization. Hum Pathol 33:628–631, 2002.

84. Abati AD, Kimmel M, Rosen PP: Apocrine mammary carcinoma. A clinico-pathologic study of 72 cases. Am J Clin Pathol 94:371–377, 1990.

85. d'Amore ES, Terrier-Lacombe MJ, Travagli JP, et al: Invasive apocrine carcinoma of the breast: a long-term follow-up study of 34 cases. Breast Cancer Res Treat 12:37–44, 1988.

86. Tavassoli FA, Norris HJ: Mammary adenoid cystic carcinoma with sebaceous differentiation. A morphologic study of the cell types. Arch Pathol Lab Med 110:1045–1053, 1986.

87. Rosen PP: Adenoid cystic carcinoma of the breast. A morphologically heterogeneous neoplasm. Pathol Annu 24(2):237–254, 1989.

88. Kleer CG, Oberman HA: Adenoid cystic carcinoma of the breast. Value of histologic grading and proliferative activity. Am J Surg Pathol 22(5):569–575, 1998.

89. Arpino G, Clark GM, Mohin S, et al: Adenoid cystic carcinoma of the breast. Molecular markers, treatment, and clinical outcome. Cancer 94:2119–2127, 2002.

90. Wells CA, Nicoll S, Ferguson DJ: Adenoid cystic carcinoma of the breast: a case with axillary lymph node metastasis. Histopathology 10:415–424, 1986.

91. Eusebi V, Lamovec J, Cattani MG, et al: Acantholytic variant of squamous-cell carcinoma of the breast. Am J Surg Pathol 10(12):855–861, 1986.

92. Wargotz ES, Norris HJ: Metaplastic carcinomas of the breast. I. Matrix-producing carcinoma. Hum Pathol 20:628–635, 1989.

93. Leibl S, Gogg-Kammerer M, Sommersacher A, et al: Metaplastic breast carcinomas: are they of myoepithelial differentiation? Immunohistochemical profile of the sarcomatoid subtype using novel myoepithelial markers. Am J Surg Pathol 29:347–353, 2005.

94. Carter MR, Hornick JL, Lester S, et al: Spindle cell (sarcomatoid) carcinoma of the breast. A clinicopathologic and immunohistochemical analysis of 29 cases. Am J Surg Pathol 30:300–309, 2006.

95. Barnes JD, Boutilier R, Chiasson D, et al: Metaplastic breast carcinoma: clinical-pathologic characteristics and HER2/neu expression. Breast Cancer Res Treat 91:173–178, 2005.

96. Beatty JD, Atwood CTR, Tickman R, et al: Metaplastic breast cancer: clinical significance. Am J Surg 191:657–664, 2006.

97. Dave G, Cosmatos H, Do T, et al: Metaplastic carcinoma of the breast: a retrospective review. Int J Radiat Oncol Biol Phys 64:771–775, 2006.

98. Davis WG, Hennessy B, Babiera G, et al: Metaplastic sarcomatoid carcinoma of the breast with absent or minimal overt invasive carcinomatous component: a misnomer. Am J Surg Pathol 29:1456–1463, 2005.

99. Miremadi A, Pinder SE, Lee AHS, et al: Neuroendocrine differentiation and prognosis in breast adenocarcinoma. Histopathology 40:215–222, 2002.

100. Shin SJ, DeLellis RA, Ying L, Rosen PP: Small cell carcinoma of the breast: a clinicopathologic and immunohistochemical study of nine patients. Am J Surg Pathol 24(9):1231–1238, 2000.

101. Lamovec J, Wotherspoon A, Janquermier J: Malignant lymphoma and metastatic tumours. In Tavassoli FA, Devilee P (eds): Tumours of the Breast and Female Genital Organs. Lyon: IARC Press, 2003, pp 107–109.

102. Ellis IO, Tavassoli FA: Microinvasive carcinoma. In Tavassoli FA, Devilee P (eds): Tumours of the Breast and Female Genital Organs. Lyon: IARC Press, 2003, pp 74–75.

103. Silver SA, Tavassoli FA: Mammary ductal carcinoma in situ with microinvasion. Cancer 82:2382–2390, 1998.

104. Prasad ML, Osborne MP, Giri DD, et al: Microinvasive carcinoma (T1mic) of the breast: clinicopathologic profile of 221 cases. Am J Surg Pathol 24(3):422–428, 2000.

105. De Mascarel I, MacGrogan G, Mathoulin-Pelissier S, et al: Breast ductal carcinoma in situ with microinvasion: a definition supported by long-term study of 1248 serially sectioned ductal carcinoma. Cancer 94:2134–2142, 2002.

106. Rosen PP, Kimmel M: Occult breast carcinoma presenting with axillary lymph node metastases: a follow-up study of 48 patients. Hum Pathol 21:518–523, 1990.

107. Merson M, Andreola S, Galimberti V, et al: Breast carcinoma presenting as axillary metastases without evidence of a primary tumor. Cancer 70:504–508, 1992.

108. Blanchard DK, Farley DR: Retrospective study of women presenting with axillary metastases from occult breast carcinoma. World J Surg 28:535–539, 2004.

109. Hess RK, Varadhachary GR, Taylor SH, et al: Metastatic patterns in adenocarcinoma. Cancer 106:1624–1633, 2006.

110. Beatson GT: On the treatment of inoperable cases of carcinoma of the mamma: suggestions for a new method of treatment, with illustrative cases. The Lancet 2:104–107, 1896.

111. Keen JC, Davidson NE: The biology of breast carcinoma. Cancer 97(3Suppl):825–833, 2003.

112. Kuiper GG, Enmark E, Pelto-Huikko M, et al: Cloning a novel estrogen receptor expressed in rat prostate and ovary. Proc Natl Acad Sci USA 93:5925–5930, 1996.

113. Honma N, Horii R, Iwase T, et al: Clinical importance of estrogen receptor-b evaluation in breast cancer patients treated with adjuvant tamoxifen therapy. J Clin Oncol 26:3727–3734, 2008.

114. Speirs V, Carder PJ, Lane S, et al: Oestrogen receptor? What it means for patients with breast cancer. Lancet Oncol 5: 174–181, 2004.

115. Harvey JM, Clark GM, Osborne K, Allred DC: Estrogen receptor status by immunohistochemistry is superior to the ligand-binding assay for predicting response to adjuvant endocrine therapy in breast cancer. J Clin Oncol 17:1474–1481, 1999.

116. Eifel P, Axelson JA, Costa J, et al: National Institutes of Health Consensus Development Conference Statement: Adjuvant Therapy for Breast Cancer, November 1–3, 2000. J Natl Cancer Inst 93:979–989, 2001.

4

Risk Factors and Risk Assessment

Nancy S. Goldstein and Constance R. Ziegfeld

KEY POINTS

- Lifetime risk of breast cancer in the United States is 12.5% (1 woman in 8), but individual differences in age, family history, reproductive history, and other factors dramatically reduce or increase a woman's risk.
- Age is by far the most common risk factor for breast cancer; half of a woman's lifetime risk is incurred after the age of 60.
- Only 5% to 10% of breast cancers are thought to be due to a genetic predisposition.
- Long-term exposure to estrogen increases risk. Early menarche, late menopause, hormone replacement therapy, and bone density stand as markers for exposure. Obesity, alcohol consumption, and lack of exercise all increase risk, possibly because they affect the metabolism of estrogen.
- Proliferative breast disease increases risk, and women with atypical hyperplasia require vigilant follow-up.
- The Gail model is the most validated and widely used tool for assessing risk, although the use of several models together provides a more complete perspective on risk.
- A person with a Gail model score of 1.67% or greater for 5 years is considered high risk.

Breast Cancer and Risk

Breast cancer is the most common non–skin cancer and is second only to lung cancer as a leading cause of cancer death in women. An estimated 192,370 women were diagnosed with invasive breast cancer, and an estimated 41,170 women died of this disease in 2009.[1]

As a result of increased longevity, the incidence of breast cancer has been growing since the 1980s.[2] In the 1970s, a woman's lifetime risk of being diagnosed with breast cancer in the United States was just under 10% (1 in 10). Since then, the estimated lifetime risk increased gradually until the beginning of the new millen-nium, when a slight decrease occurred. One in eight girls (or 12.5%) born in the United States today will be diagnosed with breast cancer at some time in their lives.[3]

Individual differences in age, family history, reproductive history, race or ethnicity, and other factors can dramatically reduce or increase a woman's risk of breast cancer.[3] Individual evaluation and assessment can help practitioners and patients determine individual risk and plan the proper course of action for follow-up.

What Is Risk?

A risk factor is anything that increases the probability of the development of a disease process.[4] In evaluating clinical management strategies, individual risk assessment is more useful for patients than data on the overall population risk.[5] An individual's risk can be expressed in a number of ways: lifetime risk, 5-year risk, absolute risk, and relative risk. Risk assessment can be determined by means of a variety of valid and reliable tools, which are discussed in detail later in this chapter.

Like all medical decisions, the potential benefits of a course of treatment or more intensive screening should be balanced against the risks and costs. Many women have one or more risk factors for breast cancer but do not develop the disease. Most women with breast cancer have no apparent risk factors other than gender and age. Also, most women who have a risk factor and develop breast cancer cannot actually confirm that the risk factor contributed to their diagnosis. Risk factors should not be seen as predictive of breast cancer, and similarly the absence of risk factors should not lead to complacency. Risk assessments can be a guide to help women and their health care providers make informed decisions about the need for earlier, more intensive, or more frequent screenings, genetic counseling, or even prophylactic treatments.

Risk Factors

Gender and age are the two greatest risk factors for breast cancer, which in effect makes every woman "at risk" for breast cancer. Certain specific modifiable and nonmodifiable risk factors put an individual woman at higher than average risk for breast cancer. Modifiable risk factors are those in a woman's control, such as being overweight, drinking alcohol, not exercising, and postmenopausal hormone therapy. Nonmodifiable risk factors—those outside a woman's control—include age, family history, genetics, bone density, and breast density.

Table 4-1 shows the relative risk of many modifiable and nonmodifiable risk factors. Nonmodifiable factors tend to have the greater relative risk (1.1 to 10 times greater risk, excluding "being female" as a risk factor) than modifiable factors (1.1 to 4.0 times greater risk).[6] However, since most women with breast cancer have no identifiable risk factors other than gender and age, it behooves women and their physicians to reduce risk wherever possible by addressing lifestyle changes such as losing weight and increasing exercise. See Chapter 7 for an in-depth discussion of lifestyle changes that may reduce risk.

Gender

The number one risk factor for breast cancer is gender. Less than 1% of all breast cancers are found in men, although the incidence among men has increased 60% since 1990.[7] The mean age at diagnosis for men is 60 to 70 years. Survival rates for men are more or less the same as for women, although recent studies have found that African-American men have a lower survival rate.[8] A family history of male breast cancer is indicative of a possible genetic mutation, and high-risk screening should be considered for others in the family.[9]

Age

Age is a common risk factor for all women. As a woman gets older, she has a greater risk of

Table 4-1. Modifiable versus Nonmodifiable Risks

Risk Factor	Approximate Relative Risk
Modifiable Risk Factors (Range 1.1–4 times greater risk)	
Radiation exposure or frequent x-rays during youth	2.0–4.0
Fist child after age 30	1.4–2.0
Not having children (vs women who give birth at age 35 or younger)	1.5–2.0
Postmenopausal hormone use, estrogen plus progestin (current or recent use for 5 or more years)	1.3–2.0
Overweight/weight gain	1.2–1.5
Drinking alcohol (2–4 drinks/day)	1.4
Current or recent use of birth control pills	1.1–1.3
Lack of exercise	1.2
Not breastfeeding	1.1–1.2
Nonmodifiable Risk Factors (Range 1.1–99 times greater risk)	
Female (vs male)	99.0
Carcinoma in situ (lobular)	7.0–10.0
Confirmed genetic mutations (BRCA1 or BRCA2)	6.0–10.0
Age (risk over age 50 vs risk up to age 50)*	6.0
Family history of breast cancer (2 immediate family members affected)	4.0–6.0
High breast density	3.0–6.0
Personal history of breast cancer	2.0–6.0
Benign breast disease (proliferative): atypical hyperplasia	4.0
High bone density	1.5–3.5
Family history of breast cancer (mother affected before age 60)	2.0–3.0
High levels of estrogen in the blood after menopause	2.0
Menopause at age 55 or older	2.0
Benign breast disease (proliferative): usual hyperplasia	1.5–1.9
High socioeconomic status	1.2–1.8
Family history of breast cancer (mother affected after age 60)	1.4
First period before age 12	1.2–1.3
Being tall	1.2
Ashkenazi Jewish heritage	1.1

Based on Susan G. Komen for the Cure website: Risk Factors and Prevention, Summary Table of Relative Risks. cms.komen.org/komen/AboutBreastCancer/RiskFactorsPrevention/index.htm.
*Data from SEER, 2004.

developing breast cancer (Fig. 4-1). In the United States, 95% of the women diagnosed with breast cancer each year are age 40 or older.[10] A woman today faces a one in eight chance of being diagnosed with breast cancer in her lifetime, and half of that risk is incurred after age 60.[5] From 2005 to 2006, the median age at diagnosis for cancer of the breast was 61.[1] Because rates of breast cancer rise with age, estimates of risk at

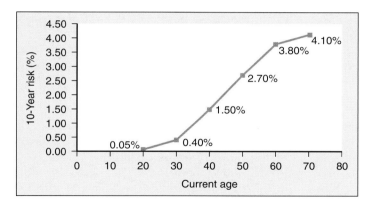

Figure 4-1. A woman's absolute risk of developing breast cancer within the next 10 years.

Table 4-2. Age-Specific Probabilities of Developing Invasive Female Breast Cancer*

If Current Age Is:	The Probability of Developing Breast Cancer in the Next 10 Years Is:†	Or 1 in:
20	0.06%	1760
30	0.44%	229
40	1.44%	69
50	2.39%	42
60	3.40%	29
70	3.73%	27
Lifetime risk	12.08%	8

*Among those free of cancer at beginning of age interval. Based on cases diagnosed 2004–2006. Percentages and "1 in" numbers may not be numerically equivalent due to rounding.
†Probability derived using NCI DevCan Software, Version 6.4.0.
From American Cancer Society, Breast Cancer Facts & Figures 2009–2010. Atlanta: American Cancer Society, Inc., Table 5.

specific ages are more meaningful as a clinical tool than estimates of lifetime risk.[3] Table 4-2 shows the probability of a woman developing breast cancer by age group.[10]

Worldwide, this pattern of late-life or post-menopausal breast cancer is associated with more developed economies or Westernized societies. Premenopausal breast cancer rates are similar throughout the world, suggesting that the disease mechanisms for premenopausal breast cancer are the same worldwide. However, because developed countries see much higher rates of postmenopausal breast cancer,[10] the disease mechanism is thought to be secondary to lifestyle decisions. Within one or two generations, women who move from an undeveloped country to a more developed country exhibit breast cancer rates similar to those of their adopted country, which suggests environmental influences.[10]

Inherited Risk Factors

Family history and genetics affect a woman's risk for breast cancer. Overall, only 5% to 10% of breast cancers are thought to be due to an inherited trait. Women up to age 70 who are *BRCA1* or *BRCA2* mutation carriers have a cumulative risk of 46% and 43%, respectively.[11]

Our understanding of the genetic link to breast cancer and our ability to test for genetic causes is incomplete. Many families have evidence of a genetic risk factor, but no specific mutated gene can be identified. It is important for the health care provider to take a detailed multigenerational family history to identify families with potential genetic risk for breast cancer.[12]

Family History

Because of the high incidence of breast cancer in the general population, it is not uncommon for a woman to report a history of breast cancer in her family. Fully 50% of women diagnosed with breast cancer report a relative of any degree with breast cancer.[2] Yet *BRCA1* and *BRCA2* genes are present in less than 10% of women with breast cancer.[2]

Three factors are important in examining family history: the degree of the relationship between the patient and the relatives who have had breast cancer, the age at diagnosis of the relatives with breast cancer, and the history of other associated genetic cancers, such as ovarian cancer.

Degree of relationship
   First degree (mother, sister, daughter, father)
   Second degree (grandmother, aunt, or niece)
   Beyond (great-grandmother, great-aunt, cousin)

Age at diagnosis of relatives

Genetic cancers are strongly linked to premenopausal incidence[13]

First-degree relative diagnosed *before age 60* is associated with increased risk

Associated genetic factors

Family history of ovarian cancer may indicate increased risk for breast and ovarian cancer

Multigenerational ovarian cancer or premenopausal breast cancer

Family history of Ashkenazi Jewish heritage indicates increased risk of presence of mutated genes

Personal or family history of male breast cancer

A woman with a first-degree relative with breast cancer has a two to three times greater risk for the disease than a woman with no family history. For women with *more than one* immediate female family member with breast cancer, the lifetime excess incidence of disease is 13.3%.[14]

Breast cancer in a close male relative (father, brother, uncle) is rare but should be regarded as a significant risk factor. The paternal family history should also be included in any assessment, since genetic mutations may pass from the father's side without resulting in a male breast cancer (see Chapter 5). A history of prostate cancer may also be an indicator of increased risk or a genetic cause, especially when prostate cancer was found at an early age.[14]

Table 4-3 shows the genes that have been identified as playing a role in breast cancer, along with the frequency of the mutation in the general population, the relative risk both under age 50 and for the decade following age 50, and the absolute lifetime risk. Genetic counseling is important for a woman with a strong family history of breast cancer or related cancers so that she and her family can understand what genetic testing means and, more important, what it *doesn't* mean.

Race and Ethnicity

The incidence of breast cancer in the United States varies by race, as shown in Table 4-4. White women have the highest incidence, followed by African-American women, with an 11% lower incidence. Women of Hispanic or Asian/Pacific Island heritage have an incidence of breast cancer around 33% lower than that of white women.[1]

The causes of these differences are not well understood, although differences in genetics, lifestyle, and access to health care all are likely to play a role. Women born in Asia, for example, have a low risk of developing breast cancer, but their daughters and relatives who are born in North America have a risk profile similar to that of white American women. This seems to indicate that environmental or lifestyle factors are at play. African-American women under age 50 have a higher age-specific incidence of breast cancer than that of white women,[1] and the stage at diagnosis for all African Americans is often more advanced than that for white women. This points to differences in genetics that put African-American women at slightly greater risk for premenopausal breast cancer.

The mortality of breast cancer also differs among different races. As Figure 4-2 demonstrates, African-American women have a lower incidence of breast cancer than white women, but the mortality of breast cancer is greater among African-American women. Incidence and mortality rates have been declining for both

Table 4-3. Breast Cancer: Associated Genes

Gene	Frequency	RR Age < 50	RR Age 50–69	Absolute Risk
BRCA1	0.1%	33	15	~41%
BRCA2	0.13%	12	12	~45
TP53	0.01%	NA	NA	90%
PTEN	<0.01%	NA	NA	30%
ATM	0.5%	5	1.5	15%
CHEK2	0.5%	3	2	10%

RR, relative risk.
From Santen R, Boyd N, Chlebowski R, et al: Critical assessment of new risk factors for breast cancer: considerations for development of an improved risk prediction model. Endocr Rel Cancer 14:169–187, 2007, Fig. 6.

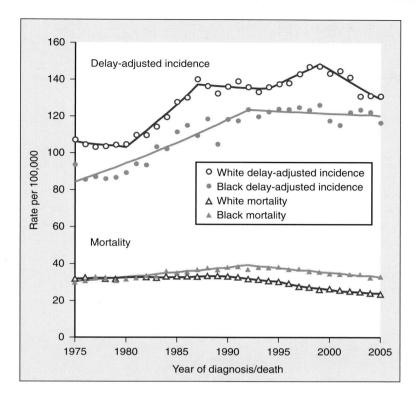

Figure 4-2. Breast cancer delay-adjusted incidence and mortality: white women versus black women, 1975–2005. (From SEER.cancer.gov.)

Table 4-4. Breast Cancer Incidence Rates by Race (U.S. 2002–2006)

Race/Ethnicity	Female
All races	123.8 per 100,000 women
White	127.8 per 100,000 women
Black	117.7 per 100,000 women
Asian/Pacific Islander	89.5 per 100,000 women
American Indian/Alaska Native*	74.4 per 100,000 women
Hispanic†	88.3 per 100,000 women

*Rates are age-adjusted to the 2000 standard population.
†Persons of Hispanic origin may be any race. Data from SEER Stat Fact Sheets: Cancer of the Breast. http://seer.cancer.gov/statfacts/html/breast.html

races since 2000. Current 5-year relative survival rates by race are 89.4% for white women and 85.4% for black women.[1] This decline followed the decrease in use of exogenous hormones in postmenopausal women. Factors associated with improved survival may include increased screening leading to early detection and improved screening technologies.

Behavioral Factors

For women concerned about breast cancer, some lifestyle changes may lead to reduced risk.

For a more in-depth analysis of these lifestyle risk factors, see Chapter 7.

Weight

Postmenopausal women who have gained 25.0 kg or more since age 18 have an increased risk of developing breast cancer.[15] Adipose tissue stores endogenous hormones; therefore, excess weight may be a modifiable risk factor. Before menopause, being slightly overweight decreases a woman's risk of breast cancer. After menopause, however, being overweight increases risk by 30% to 60%.[16] Increased body fat during childhood and adolescence is associated with reduced incidence of premenopausal breast cancer, independent of adult body mass index and menstrual cycle characteristics.[17]

Lack of Exercise

Information on exercise and breast cancer risk has been expanding recently. Some studies confirm that women who are physically active on a regular basis have a lower risk (0.8 relative risk) of developing the disease compared with that of women who are sedentary.[18] In addition, it is suspected that additional mechanisms beyond weight reduction influence the protective effects from physical activity.[19] Because exercise can delay a girl's first menstrual period, facilitate weight control, or reduce the frequency of regular menstrual cycles,[20] regular exercise can help decrease the total amount of estrogen a woman is exposed to over her lifetime.

Alcohol

Alcohol consumption increases breast cancer risk 1.2 to 1.6 times, and the risk rises with increased consumption.[21] The impact of alcohol does not appear to be different in women who are at high risk compared with those of normal risk. Neither the use of concurrent hormone replacement therapy nor the presence of benign breast disease in postmenopausal women who consume greater amounts of alcohol appears to increase risk further.[21]

Radiation Exposure

Studies have shown that treatment of certain diseases such as scoliosis, with radiation doses between 1 and 3 Gy before the age of 40 years increases the risk of breast cancer.[22] Risks are increased with higher total doses of radiation at a young age. Women exposed in childhood or adolescence have the greatest risk, whereas those 50 years or older at the time of exposure experience no added risk. The latent period can be many years, and increased surveillance should begin 8 to 10 years after exposure.[23] Very low doses of radiation, as in mammography, have an insignificant impact on breast cancer risk.

Menstrual and Reproductive Factors

As stated previously, longer-term exposure to estrogen is associated with increased breast cancer risk. This can be related to early menarche, late menopause, or hormone replacement therapy. Other factors, such as a woman's age when she has her first child and extended periods of breastfeeding, may influence breast cancer risk.

Early Menarche/Late Menopause/ Estrogen Levels

Estrogen plays an important role in breast cancer development. The risk of breast cancer is

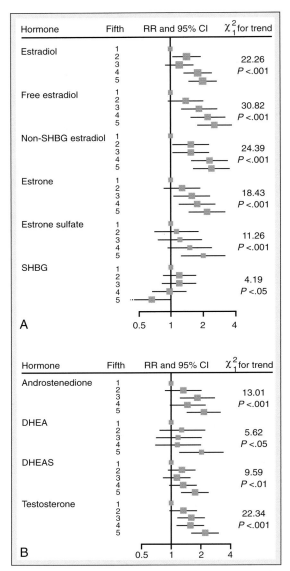

Figure 4-3. Relative risk (RR) of breast cancer by quintile of estrogen concentration (**A**) and androgen concentration (**B**). (From Key T, Appleby P, Barnes I, Reeves G: Endogenous Hormones and Breast Cancer Collaborative Group. Endogenous sex hormones and breast cancer in postmenopausal women: reanalysis of nine prospective studies. J Natl Cancer Inst 94:606–616, 2002, Fig. 1.)

increased 2.0 times among postmenopausal women who have high levels of estradiol circulating in their bloodstream.[24] Figure 4-3 shows the relative risk associated with plasma estrogen and androgen concentrations grouped by quintiles.

Blood estrogen levels are not currently used to assess a woman's risk of breast cancer; however, certain markers can be used to indicate estrogen exposure. These include a woman's age at her first menses, her age at menopause, and her age at first live birth.

It is thought that women who began menses before age 12 have an increased risk compared with women who began after age 15.[24] Studies have shown that women who go through natural menopause after age 55 have a slightly higher risk than that of women who are menopausal before 45 years of age.[25] The average age at menopause in the United States is just over 51 years. Early menopause leads to a lower relative risk of breast cancer, whether menopause is natural or induced (chemically or surgically). In instances of extremely high risk, oophorectomy in premenopausal women may be considered to reduce estrogen exposure and therefore decrease lifetime risk of breast cancer.[24]

Pregnancy and Childbearing

Pregnancy increases breast cancer risk slightly for the first 10 years after birth, but the risk eventually drops to below that of women without children. Overall, therefore, bearing children has a protective effect. The younger a woman is when she has her first child, the sooner the effect of pregnancy becomes protective.[26] Studies suggest that women who are younger than 30 years of age at the first live birth have a lower risk of developing breast cancer than those who have their first child later.[22,26] The number of children a woman has also makes a difference; protection against breast cancer increases as the number of children increases. The effect of in vitro fertilization on breast cancer risk is not yet known and requires further evaluation.[27]

Breastfeeding

Breastfeeding alters menstrual cycles, resulting in some cycles without estrogen peaks and missed menstrual periods. In addition, breastfeeding stimulates the breast tissue to mature into type 4 lobules, and this also decreases cancer risk. The combination of pregnancy and breastfeeding results in an overall reduction in estrogen exposure and thus in decreased breast cancer risk.[28]

The pattern of breastfeeding is an important factor in protection from breast cancer. Women who breastfeed continuously for more than 12 months decrease their risk further. In countries where women breastfeed for extended periods of time (more than 25 months), protection is even greater.[29]

Birth Control

Oral contraceptives are associated with a slight increase in breast cancer risk, but this risk decreases within 10 years after discontinuance.[1] This varies with the type of estrogen/progesterone combination oral contraceptive.

Since most women of reproductive age have a very low risk of breast cancer, even an increase in relative risk means that the absolute risk remains low. As shown in Table 4-2, only 1 in 229 women age 30 will develop breast cancer in the next 10 years, so a 20% increase in relative risk would mean that an additional 2 of every 1145 women of that age would develop breast cancer because of the use of oral contraceptives.[2]

Hormone Replacement Therapy

Over the last few decades, many women have used hormone replacement therapy (HRT) (usually in the form of estrogen plus progestin) to moderate the effects of menopause. Some women have used this therapy as a short-term solution, but others have taken these drugs for many years. Current research shows that the risks of using combination HRT outweigh its benefits.[24] All women, especially women at high risk for breast cancer, are encouraged to avoid long-term (more than 5 years) hormone replacement, if possible.[30] The Women's Health Initiative (WHI), sponsored by the National Institutes of Health (NIH), undertook comprehensive research that has changed the use of postmenopausal hormones. The study was stopped in 2002 because of findings that the risks of taking combined estrogen and progestin were greater than the benefits to postmenopausal women. (Note that women who have had a hysterectomy and were on estrogen replacement therapy only did not have an increased incidence of breast cancer.) As a result of these findings, use of combination hormone replacement therapy (HRT) dropped dramatically in postmenopausal women.[30] Recent studies suggest that the recent drop seen in the incidence of breast cancer (see Fig. 4-2) is due to this drop in the use of HRT.[1,31]

Bone Density

High bone density is an indicator of elevated blood estrogen and may be a surrogate breast cancer risk factor. Early research suggests that women with the highest bone density have about twice the breast cancer risk of those with the lowest bone density.[14] In contrast, height loss may represent a surrogate marker for reduced estrogen exposure, with loss of more than 2.5 cm in height since age 20 resulting in a 20% lower risk of developing breast cancer. Fracture history is another potential surrogate marker for reduced estrogen exposure. Women with a history of fracture within 5 years have a 40% decreased risk of developing breast cancer. Further studies are needed to confirm these findings and to evaluate the accuracy of subjects' recall of height loss or prior fractures.[14]

Breast Density

The WHI found that women taking estrogen and progestin had increased density of breast tissue.[30] The risk of breast cancer increases with increasing breast density and with a greater proportion of breast tissue to adipose tissue. Women with denser breasts as assessed by mammography have a three to six times greater risk of developing breast cancer. Because of the lack of an agreed-upon standard for assessing breast density, health care providers do not yet regularly use breast density to assess breast cancer risk.[31] For women with increased breast density, digital mammography may offer screening benefits over standard mammography (see Chapter 8; Chapter 9, Figs. 9-1 through 9-3).[32]

Breast Health

Breast health can be a good indicator of a woman's overall risk of developing breast cancer. Women who have had benign breast biopsies have subsequently been found to have increased risk of breast cancer. The magnitude of that risk depends on the pathologic changes identified. Nonproliferative breast disease confers no increased risk for the future development of breast cancer, whereas atypical proliferative changes indicate that the breast tissue is changing in a manner that does increase the risk for the future development of breast cancer. For a more complete discussion of the relative risks associated with these benign breast changes, see Chapters 1 and 2.

Personal History of Breast Cancer or Other Cancers

Breast cancer survivors have a greater risk of developing a new and unrelated case of breast cancer than those who have never had breast cancer. A survivor's risk of developing a second breast cancer increases 0.5% to 1.0% per year.[33] The absolute risk of contralateral breast cancer in women with a personal history of breast cancer is estimated to be 6.1% to 12% during the 10 to 20 years after diagnosis.[34] The risk of contralateral breast cancer is decreased by adjuvant therapies such as chemotherapy and hormonal therapy.

Women with a history of certain other cancers also have an increased risk of developing breast cancer. Adolescent Hodgkin's disease represents a particular risk if the patient received radiation treatment as part of her therapy. A woman's exposure to intensive radiation at a young age increases her risk of breast cancer to 39 times the rate of those not exposed.[23]

In addition to Hodgkin's disease, other cancers that have been linked to an increased risk of breast cancer include ovarian, uterine, colon, and thyroid cancers, as well as melanoma. The exact reasons for these links aren't known, although it is likely that there are shared genetic components among the cancers.[33]

Unproven Risk

A number of environmental and lifestyle factors have been proposed as increasing the risk of breast cancer, although at this time studies do not support these proposals. The following have not been shown to result in increased risk of breast cancer: tobacco, environmental pollution, night shift work, antibiotics, high-fat diet, caffeine intake, antiperspirants and deodorants, underwire bras, and breast augmentation or reduction.

Risk Assessment Tools

Several tools are available to health practitioners to evaluate an individual's risk of breast cancer. These include the Gail model, the Claus model, the Tyrer-Cuzick model, and the BRCAPRO model. An accurate and detailed family history is essential in the use of all risk assessment tools. The models provide a snapshot of a woman's risk *today*, using current risk factors. Risk factors can change considerably over time, so it is useful to reassess risk at 2- to 3-year intervals.[34]

Each model has its strengths and weaknesses, with studies showing that different models are more accurate than others in predicting risk for women with particular risk factors. Therefore, it may be beneficial to use several tools to provide a more complete perspective on a patient's overall risk.[34] Table 4-5 compares the characteristics of the available models.

The goal of breast cancer risk assessment is to develop individual breast health management strategies for women. Such strategies may increase early detection and improve survival rates in high-risk women while decreasing cost, complications, and unnecessary anxiety in low-risk women.[14]

Gail Model

The Gail model, which has been well tested for reliability and validity, is the model that is perhaps the most frequently used by practitioners. It is an interactive tool developed by the National Cancer Institute (NCI) and the National Surgical Adjuvant Breast and Bowel Project (NSABP). The tool can be easily accessed by providers and the general public online at www.cancer.gov/bcrisktool/. Figure 4-4 shows the Gail model risk assessments for two different persons.[35] Risk estimates are a composite of risk factors according to the individual's age, age of first menses, age at first live birth, history of biopsies and atypical hyperplasia, first-degree relatives with breast cancer, and race/ethnicity.[3] This tool provides 5-year and lifetime risk estimates for a woman (from 35 years of age to 90 years), with comparison to women of the same age who are at average risk for developing breast cancer. A rather complicated formula (shown in Box 4-1) is used to determine risk in the Gail model; therefore, none of the risk factors used in the Gail model can be easily considered in isolation from the others.[35]

The Gail model should not be used when a woman has a history of breast cancer or carcinoma in situ (CIS). It does not incorporate

Table 4-5. Characteristics of Breast Cancer Risk Assessment Tools

	Gail Model	Claus Model	Tyrer-Cuzick Model	BRCAPRO Model
Use/application	Assessing 5-year and lifetime risks of Caucasian women with no family history, or first-degree relatives with postmenopausal breast cancer	Assessing breast cancer risks of individuals with 0–2 first-degree or second-degree relatives with breast cancer	Includes paternal and maternal second-degree relatives with a history of breast and ovarian cancer	For assessing the probability of a *BRCA1* or *BRCA2* mutation in individuals with a family cancer syndrome
Family history	First-degree relatives with breast cancer	First- and second-degree relatives with breast cancer, with age at onset	First- and second-degree relatives with breast cancer, with age at onset	Multigenerational breast and ovarian cancer, with age at onset
Additional characteristics	Current age Age at menarche Age at first live birth Number of biopsies Atypical hyperplasia Race	Current age		Diagnosis and age in specific family history
Strengths	Incorporates some additional risk factors	Incorporates ovarian cancer and paternal family history	Includes paternal and maternal second-degree relatives with a history of breast and ovarian cancer	Incorporates mutigenerational breast and ovarian cancers and age at onset Evaluates probability of *BRCA1* or *BRCA2* gene mutation

	Biopsies, Family History, Late Childbearing	No Biopsies	No Biopsies, Young Childbearing	Black, No Biopsies	Age 60, No Biopsies
5-Year risk					
This woman	4.4%	1.7%	1.5%	1.7%	2.9%
Average woman, same age and race	1.0%	1.0%	1.0%	0.9%	1.8%
Lifetime risk (to age 90)					
This woman	27.7%	18.5%	17.1%	12.6%	14.3%
Average woman, same age and race	11.9%	11.9%	11.9%	9.1%	9.1%
History of breast cancer, DCIS, or LCIS?	No	No	No	No	No
What is the woman's age?	45	45	45	45	60
What was the woman's age at the time of her first menstrual period?	12–13	12–13	12–13	12–13	12–13
What was the woman's age at the time of her first live birth of a child?	≥30	≥30	<20	≥30	≥30
How many of the woman's first-degree relatives—mother, sisters, and/or daughters—have had breast cancer?	1	1	1	1	1
Has the woman ever had a breast biopsy?	Yes	No	No	No	No
How many breast biopsies (positive or negative) has the woman had?	1	–	–	–	–
Has the woman had at least one breast biopsy with atypical hyperplasia?	No	–	–	–	–
What is the woman's race/ethnicity?	White	White	White	Black	White

Figure 4-4. Gail model risk assessments. DCIS, ductal carcinoma in situ; LCIS, lobular carcinoma in situ. (From www.cancer.gov/bcrisktool.)

Box 4-1. Formula to Determine Risk in the Gail Model

Log odds = –0.74948 + 0.09401 × age menarche
+ 0.52926 × number of biopsies + 0.21863
× age at first live birth
+ 0.95830
× number of relatives with breast cancer
+ 0.01081 × age (<50 versus 50 +)
– 0.28804 × (number of biopsies × age)
– 0.19081 × (age first birth
× number of relatives with breast cancer)

From McTiernan A, Kuniyuki A, Yasui Y, et al: Comparisons of two breast cancer risk estimates in women with a family history of breast cancer. Cancer Epidemiol Biomarkers Prev 10:333–338, 2001.

---

strong family histories of multigenerational breast or ovarian cancer, exposure to radiation therapy to the chest, or lifestyle habits. The model assumes annual breast cancer screening, and it has been modified to improve reliability in all age groups. Validity has not been fully established in minority populations.[35] In the Breast Cancer Prevention Trial, the modified Gail model showed excellent prediction for prospective breast cancer risk, with a ratio of observed to predicted cancers of 1.03 (95% confidence intervals 0.88 to 1.21).[35]

Claus Model

The Claus model, developed by the Cancer and Steroid Hormone (CASH) study, is another commonly used risk assessment tool. Whereas the Gail model considers first-degree relatives, the Claus model incorporates maternal *and* paternal breast cancer history, ovarian cancer history, first- and second-degree relatives, and current age. Estimates derived from the Claus model are based solely on family history, whereas the Gail model also incorporates reproductive variables, atypical hyperplasia, and a history of breast biopsies.[14]

The Gail model and the Claus model are not closely correlated, with discrepancies seen in nulliparity, multiple benign breast biopsies, and paternal history of breast cancer. A positive Claus test (12% or greater risk of breast cancer by age 79) was predictive of a positive Gail test 85.4% of the time, whereas a negative Claus test (less than 12% risk) predicted a negative Gail test only 53.1% of the time[36] (Table 4-6).

Table 4-6. Sensitivity of Claus Model for Predicting Individuals with Above-Average Risk (≥12% Risk to Age 79), Assuming the Gail Model as Gold Standard*

Claus Risk (%)	NSABP-Modified Gail Risk		
	≥12%	<12%	Total
≥12%	146	25	171
<12%	150	170	320
Total	296	195	491

*Sensitivity of Claus for measuring Gail, 146/296 = 49.3%; specificity of Claus for measuring Gail, 170/195 = 87.2%; predictive value of a positive Claus test, 146/171 = 85.4%; predictive value of a negative Claus test, 170/320 = 53.1%.
From McTiernan A, Kuniyuki A, Yasui Y, et al: Comparisons of two breast cancer risk estimates in women with a family history of breast cancer. Cancer Epidemiol Biomarkers Prev 10:333–338, 2001, Table 6.

Tyrer-Cuzick Model

The Tyrer-Cuzick model is a newer, more comprehensive model that includes paternal as well as maternal second-degree relatives with a history of breast and ovarian cancer. This model has not been validated as thoroughly as the Gail and Claus models, but it performed substantially better in one prospective study.[14]

The Family History Evaluation and Screening Programme followed up 1933 women, of whom 52 developed cancer. All models were applied to these women over a mean follow-up of 5.27 years to estimate risk of breast cancer. The ratios (95% confidence intervals) of expected-to-observed numbers of breast cancers were 0.48 (0.20 to 0.64) for Gail, 0.56 (0.43 to 0.75) for Claus, and 0.81 (0.62 to 1.08) for Tyrer-Cuzick. This study concluded that "the Tyrer-Cuzick model is the most consistently accurate model for prediction of breast cancer. The Gail and Claus models seem to underestimate risk."[37]

Studies of the Tyrer-Cuzick model are promising, but further validation is needed, and it is recommended that the model be used in conjunction with other risk assessment tools. A software version of the Tyrer-Cuzick model (IBIS Breast Cancer Risk Evaluation Tool, Risk-FileCalc version 1.0, copyright 2004) is available by contacting IBIS (ibis@cancer.org.uk).

BRCAPRO Model

Models that estimate the probability of detecting a *BRCA1* or *BRCA2* mutation in a given family or individual have been published. There are four widely used probability models, referred to as Couch, Shattuck-Eidens, Frank, and BRCAPRO. Of these, BRCAPRO is the most commonly used model.[14]

BRCAPRO is a mendelian model based on reported family history of breast and ovarian cancer. Accurate information concerning diagnosis and age at diagnosis is essential for this tool to be useful in the estimation of risk. Minor errors in reporting family history can have a significant effect on the probability estimate.

Figure 4-5 demonstrates why the BRCAPRO model must be used carefully.[38] In this example, the choice of the proband (the family member through whom a family's medical history comes to light) significantly affects the results.[38]

The Future

Greater accuracy in risk prediction helps women make accurate and effective choices in medical treatment. Current models are used to support the prophylactic use of tamoxifen or surgery in many high-risk women. Women may forgo treatment if they perceive that the risk of developing breast cancer is not great enough to offset the side effects of therapy. It is imperative that we recognize and study other factors that influence risk and incorporate them into valid and reliable assessment tools.

The Breast Cancer Prevention Collaborative Group (BCPCG) agrees that quantitative breast density, state of the art plasma estrogen and androgen measurements, history of fracture and height loss, body mass index, and waist–hip ratio should be priorities for further testing as factors in future risk models.[14] If found to be good predictors of risk, these parameters could be added to risk assessment tools in the practice setting.

Discussing Risk with Patients

Breast cancer is a devastating and life-changing diagnosis, fraught with emotional, mental, and physical challenges. Because of this, discussing the risk of breast cancer is a sensitive and potentially emotional issue. Discussions should encompass a thorough explanation of what is meant by the term "risk" and how it relates directly to an individual patient's situation. Health care providers should be aware that

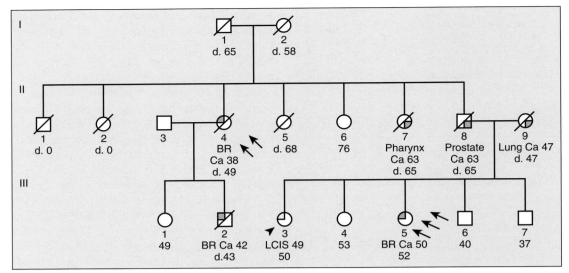

Figure 4-5. Family history of breast cancer in a family of German/Italian ethnicity and the pitfalls of using models to assess genetic risk factors. Women (○); men (□). Age is current or age at death (designated by a diagonal slash). Partial shading of upper left of symbol indicates lobular carcinoma in situ. Shading of lower right indicates a nonbreast, nonovarian primary cancer. Double and triple arrows indicate proband used for BRCAPRO calculation. BR Ca, breast cancer. (From Domchek SM, Eisen A, Calzone K, et al: Application of breast cancer risk prediction models in clinical practice. J Clin Oncol 21:593–601, 2003, Fig. 2.)

patients may enter the discussion with an inaccurate perception of their risk, either overestimating it or underestimating it. The discussions should also center on how the risk evaluation can provide practitioners and patients with a guideline for follow-up evaluations, screening, and prevention.

Perceived Risk

As previously mentioned, women often have inaccurate perceptions of their own risk of breast cancer. In one study, women were asked to estimate the probability that they would develop breast cancer within the next 10 years, and this estimate was then compared with one derived from the Gail model. Researchers "found that the women overestimated their probability of dying of breast cancer by more than 20-fold."[36]

Another study found that women were very inaccurate in estimating their absolute risk of breast cancer but more accurate in estimating relative risk. Even so, the majority of individuals classified as underestimators by one method were classified as overestimators using the other method.[39] Any discussion of risk must recognize that a woman's initial perceived risk of breast

cancer is likely to be inaccurate, usually overestimating the risk.

Risk Interpretation

There are several ways of expressing a person's risk: lifetime risk versus 3-year, 5-year, or 10-year risk, and absolute versus relative risk. (See the section. "What Is Risk?" at the beginning of the chapter.) Using all four approaches together can be useful in providing a patient with an overall perspective on her risk.[6] For example:

- A woman in her mid 30s might have a higher relative risk compared with that of other women of the same age, but her absolute risk of breast cancer remains low.
- A woman in her 60s might have a lower relative risk of breast cancer compared with that of women of the same age, but her absolute risk is high.
- A woman might have a high lifetime risk of breast cancer, but her 5-year risk might be low.

These near-term, long-term, relative, and absolute risks can help a woman and her family make effective decisions on the course of action for surveillance, follow-up, and treatment. Greater risk, however, is not necessarily predictive of breast cancer in a particular individual. Rather, the risk numbers express the expected rate of occurrence among a larger pool of women.[6]

What constitutes "high risk" is a matter of personal discussion between a woman and her physician. To some, a relative risk factor of two times the normal risk factor (two times the normal expected risk *for a woman of a given age*) might be considered high risk. To others, because breast cancer is the most common type of non-skin cancer diagnosed in women, even a risk factor of 1% seems high risk. The NCCN Clinical Practice Guidelines in Oncology suggests that a 5-year Gail model absolute risk of 1.67% or greater is considered high risk.[6]

Management Strategies for High-Risk Patients

Once a woman has been identified as being at high risk, specific strategies can be taken to reduce the risk and improve the chances for early detection.[5] Risk reduction options may be used in combination or sequentially and may change as she progresses through the life cycle.

Management options for women at high risk are discussed in Chapter 9, Screening of High-Risk Patients. Research on breast cancer prevention among high-risk populations continues.

Risk Assessment Clinics

As information about breast cancer risk and early detection is better disseminated, individuals are looking for resources to help them evaluate personal risks and implement a plan of care for prevention and early detection. Risk assessment clinics can provide an organized and consistent approach to risk evaluation and management, and they often combine multiple disciplines to address the unique needs of individuals throughout the risk spectrum. Program goals usually focus on the needs of individuals at risk for breast cancer, but they may also include research and education of health care providers. The NCCN Clinical Practice Guidelines in Oncology, Breast Cancer Risk Assessment and Breast Cancer Risk Reduction v.1.2007 are available online at www.NCCN.org and provide detailed mapping of interventions. Table 4-7 summarizes recommended NCCN management strategies for the prevention of breast cancer.[6]

Table 4-7. Algorithm for Breast Cancer Screening and Prevention

Average Risk	
5-year Gail model risk <1.67%	Annual physical exam
	Annual screening mammogram beginning at age 40
	Encourage breast self-exam (BSE)
	Reassess risk every 2–3 years
High Risk	
5-year Gail model risk ≥1.67%	Physical exam every 6–12 months
	Annual mammogram, begin age 40
	Encourage BSE
	Consider tamoxifen or prevention trial
Prior thoracic radiation	Physical exam every 6–12 months
	Annual mammogram at 10 years after treatment, no later than age 40
	Encourage BSE
	Consider tamoxifen or prevention trial
Lobular carcinoma in situ or atypical hyperplasia	Physical exam every 6–12 months
	Annual mammogram
	Encourage BSE
	Consider tamoxifen or prevention trial
Strong family history of genetic predisposition	Physical exam every 6–12 months
	Annual mammogram (at 25, or 10 years before earliest index case)
	Encourage BSE
	Consider tamoxifen or prevention trial
	Consider prophylactic mastectomy
	Consider prophylactic oophorectomy

Adapted from NCCN Clinical Practice Guidelines in Oncology, 2007.

The core component of these programs is the multidisciplinary team. Often headed by board-certified medical or surgical oncologists, the team may include genetic counselors, advanced practice nurses, social workers, and support staff with training and experience in genetics and oncology. Services vary depending on the resources available. Consultants in imaging, pathology, nutrition, reconstructive surgery, and gynecology are examples of additional essential resources.[12]

Conclusion

Although the lifetime risk of breast cancer in the United States is 12.7% (1 woman of 8),[2] individual differences in age, family history, reproductive history, and other factors dramatically reduce or increase a woman's risk of breast cancer. Gender, age, and family history are the three most important risk factors for women in relation to breast cancer. In the United States, approximately 5% to 10% of all breast cancers are related to *BRCA1* or *BRCA2* mutations.[12] Prevention, early detection, and intervention are steadily improving as a result of advances in research, technology, and patient education. Individualized breast cancer risk assessment is paramount to ensure and promote breast health.

References

1. SEER Stat Fact Sheet. http://seer.cancer.gov/statfacts/html/breast.html. Accessed 2/19/2010.
2. American Cancer Society: Cancer Facts and Figures 2008. www.cancer.org/downloads/STT/2008CAFFfinalsecured.pdf. Accessed 12/22/2008.
3. American Cancer Society: Detailed guide: breast cancer (2009). http://www.cancer.org/docroot/CRI/content/CRI_2_4_1X_What_are_the_key_statistics_for_breast_cancer_5.asp?sitearea=. Accessed 2/19/2010.
4. National Cancer Institute Fact Sheet: Probability of Breast Cancer in American Women. www.cancer.gov/cancertopics/factsheet/Detection/probability-breast-cancer. Accessed 12/22/2008.
5. Abeloff MD, Wolff AC, Wood WC, et al: Cancer of the breast. In Abeloff MD, Armitage JO, Niederhuber JE, et al (eds): Clinical Oncology, 3rd ed. Philadelphia: Churchill Livingstone, 2004, pp 2379–2385.
6. NCCN Clinical Practice Guidelines in Oncology. (2008). www.nccn.org. Accessed 12/22/2008.
7. Susan G. Komen for the Cure website: Risk Factors & Prevention, Summary Table of Relative Risks. http://ww5.komen.org/BreastCancer/RiskFactorsSummaryTable.html?terms=relative=risks. Accessed 1/26/2009.
8. National Cancer Institute: Male breast cancer treatment. www.cancer.gov/cancertopics/pdq/treatment/malebreast/healthprofessional. Accessed 12/22/2008.
9. American Society of Clinical Oncology: Racial disparities seen in male breast cancer survival. Science Daily March 18, 2007. www.sciencedaily.com/releases/2007/03/070317125448.htm. Retrieved 10/29/07.
10. American Cancer Society: Breast Cancer Facts & Figures 2009–2010, www.acsevents.org/downloads/STT/F861009_final%209-08-09.pdf. Accessed 3/10/2010.
11. Jatoi I, Anderson W: Management of women who have a genetic predisposition for breast cancer. Surg Clin North Am 88: 845–861, 2008.
12. Vogel V, Bevers T: Handbook of Breast Cancer Risk-Assessment. Boston: Jones and Bartlett Publishers, 2003, p 3.
13. Bell D, Kim S, Godwin A, et al: Genetic and functional analysis of CHEK2 (CHK2) variants in multiethnic cohorts. Int J Cancer 121:2661–2667, 2007.
14. Santen R, Boyd N, Chlebowski R, et al: Critical assessment of new risk factors for breast cancer: considerations for development of an improved risk prediction model. Endocr Rel Cancer 14:169–187, 2007.
15. Eliassen H, Colditz G, Colditz B, et al: Adult weight change and risk of postmenopausal breast cancer. JAMA 296(2):193–201, 2006.
16. van den Brandt PA, Spiegelman D, Yaun S, et al: Pooled analysis of prospective cohort on height, weight, and breast cancer risk. Am J Epidemiol 152:514–527, 2000.
17. Baer H, Colditz G, Rosner B, et al: Body fatness during childhood and adolescence and incidence of breast cancer in premenopausal women: a prospective cohort study. Breast Cancer Res 7(3):R314–R325, 2005.
18. Kruk J: Lifetime physical activity and the risk of breast cancer: a case-control study. Cancer Detect Prev 31(1):18–28, 2007.
19. Bernstein L, Patel A, Ursin G, et al: Lifetime recreational exercise activity and breast cancer risk among black women and white women. J Natl Cancer Inst 97(22):1671–1679, 2005.
20. Willett W, Rockhill B, Hankinson S, et al: Nongenetic factors in the causation of breast cancer. In Harris JR, Lippman ME, Morrow M, Osborne CK: Diseases of the Breast, 3rd ed. Philadelphia: Lippincott Williams & Wilkins, 2004, Chap. 16.
21. Horn-Ross PL: Patterns of alcohol consumption and breast cancer risk in the California Teachers Study cohort. Cancer Epidemiol Biomark Prev 13(3):405–411, 2004.
22. Preston D, Mattsson A, Holmberg E, et al: Radiation effects on breast cancer risk: a pooled analysis of eight cohorts. Radiat Res 158:220–235, 2002.
23. Travis L, Hill D, Dores G, et al: Breast cancer following radiotherapy and chemotherapy among young women with Hodgkin disease. JAMA 290(4):465–475, 2003.
24. The Endogenous Hormones and Breast Cancer Collaborative Group: Endogenous sex hormones and breast cancer in postmenopausal women: reanalysis of nine prospective studies. J Natl Cancer Inst 94:606–616. 2002.
25. Butler L, Potischman N, Newman B, et al: Menstrual risk factors and early-onset breast cancer. Cancer Causes Control 11(5): 451–458, 2000.
26. Russo J, Moral R, Balogh G, et al: The protective role of pregnancy in breast cancer. Breast Cancer Res 7(3):131–142, 2005.
27. Salhab M, Al Sarakbi W, Mokbel K: In vitro fertilization and breast cancer risk: a review. Int J Fertil Womens Med 50(6): 259–266, 2005.
28. National Cancer Institute: Breast Cancer Prevention Institute Online Booklet. www.bcpinstitute.org/booklet4.htm. Accessed 1/12/2007.
29. Chang-Claude J, Eby N, Kiechle M, et al: Breastfeeding and breast cancer risk by age 50 among women in Germany. Cancer Causes Control 11(8):687–695, 2000.
30. National Institutes of Health: Menopausal hormone therapy. September 2006. www.nih.gov/phtindex.htm. Accessed 1/15/07.
31. Barlow W, White E, Ballard-Barbash R, et al: Prospective breast cancer risk prediction model for women undergoing screening mammography. J Natl Cancer Inst 98:1204–1214, 2006.
32. Yaffe M, Mainprize J, Jong R: Technical developments in mammography. Health Phys 95(5):599–611, 2008.
33. Nissen M, Lazovich D, Jolitz G: Breast carcinoma after cancer at another site: method of detection, tumor characteristics, and surgical treatment. Cancer 89:1999–2005, 2000.
34. Hollingsworth A, Singletary E, Morrow M: Current comprehensive assessment and management of women at increased risk for breast cancer. Am J Surg 187:349–362, 2004.

35. National Cancer Institute: Breast Cancer Risk Assessment Tool: an interactive tool for measuring the risk of invasive breast cancer. www.cancer.gov/bcrisktool/ Accessed 2/2/2009.

36. McTiernan A, Kuniyuki A, Yasui Y, et al: Comparisons of two breast cancer risk estimates in women with a family history of breast cancer. Cancer Epidemiol Biomark Prev 10:333–338, 2001.

37. Amir E, Evans D, Shenton A, et al: Evaluation of breast cancer risk assessment packages in the family history evaluation and screening programme. J Med Genet 40:807–814, 2003.

38. Domchek S, Eisen A, Calzone K, et al: Application of breast cancer risk prediction models in clinical practice. J Clin Oncol 21:593–601, 2003.

39. Bottorff J, Richardson C, Balneaves L, et al: Unraveling women's perceptions of risk for breast cancer. Health Ed Res 19:469–475, 2004.

Genetics

5

Jennifer E. Axilbund, Amy L. Gross, and Kala Visvanathan

KEY POINTS

- Most hereditary cancer predisposition syndromes are inherited in an autosomal dominant pattern.
- In approximately 50% of families suggestive of hereditary breast cancer, the cancer is due to hereditary breast and ovarian cancer (HBOC) syndrome.
- Features suggestive of HBOC include premenopausal breast cancer, ovarian cancer, and male breast cancer.
- Two genes responsible for HBOC are *BRCA1* and *BRCA2*, which appear to function as tumor suppressor genes and are involved in DNA repair.
- Mutations in *BRCA1* and *BRCA2* have a high penetrance, conferring a lifetime risk of ovarian cancer between 20% and 65%. *BRCA1* mutations are associated with a higher risk of ovarian and primary peritoneal cancer compared with *BRCA2* mutations and also are associated with earlier age of onset of cancer.
- The precise factors dictating whether an individual with a specific *BRCA1* or *BRCA2* mutation will develop breast cancer are thought to depend on other genetic and environmental risk modifiers.
- Genetic testing for *BRCA1* and *BRCA2* is clinically available, and for most families involves full sequencing of both genes.
- A very small proportion of hereditary breast cancer is due to rare syndromes, including Li-Fraumeni syndrome, Cowden syndrome, Peutz-Jeghers syndrome, and hereditary diffuse gastric cancer.
- Low-penetrance genes associated with breast cancer risk have been identified; however, their clinical implication is still being elucidated.
- If a patient's personal or family history is suggestive of hereditary breast cancer, she should be referred for genetic counseling and discussion of screening and preventive strategies.
- Interventions for women with a hereditary breast cancer syndrome include intensive cancer screening, chemoprevention, and prophylactic surgery.
- DNA banking for the future by women with breast cancer that is not explained by current genetic technology is also an option that should be discussed with and undertaken by some families.

Introduction

Most breast cancers are sporadic and likely due to a combination of genetic and environmental factors, but an estimated 5% to 10% of breast cancers are "hereditary," meaning attributable primarily to mutations in a specific gene. About 50% of hereditary breast cancers are believed to be due to the hereditary breast and ovarian cancer syndrome (HBOC).[1,2] With only 1% of breast cancers being attributable to a handful of very rare syndromes (discussed in the text that follows), this leaves 50% that are due to yet undiscovered genetic factors.

Recognizing hereditary breast cancer is an academic exercise, but it can also be helpful to families for several reasons. For a woman with breast cancer, the identification of a mutation can help to explain her cancer as well as predict her risk of developing other related cancers. For a woman with no personal history of cancer, but with a strong family history of breast cancer, it can help to better define her risk of breast and other related cancers, enabling consideration of more specific screening and risk reduction options. In both cases, such genetic information can also be useful when assessing risk to family members, particularly children, siblings, and parents. Such information may also decrease anxiety, since studies have shown that women with a family history on average have a higher perceived risk of developing breast cancer than their actual risk.[3]

The overall goal of cancer risk assessment is twofold: (1) to target high-risk groups with more aggressive screening and risk-reduction strategies so as to favorably impact overall survival, and (2) to minimize overtreatment and its associated complications such as increased false-positive tests in low-risk groups.

Genetics Review: Autosomal Dominant Inheritance

Most hereditary cancer predisposition syndromes are inherited in an autosomal dominant pattern. Humans have 46 chromosomes, arranged into 23 pairs. The first 22 pairs are called autosomes and are present in both males and females. The 23rd pair constitutes the sex chromosomes, with females having two X chromosomes and males having one X and one Y chromosome. The genes for most currently recognized hereditary cancer syndromes are located on the autosomes, meaning that rather than being sex-linked, they can be inherited and transmitted by both males and females. For this reason, it is important to consider both maternal and paternal family history when assessing cancer risk.

When a parent has a mutation in a hereditary cancer gene, he or she has one copy of the gene with the mutation and one copy without it. Each offspring of that individual inherits one copy of the parent's gene. Thus, there is a 50% chance that it is the copy with the mutation and a 50% chance that it is the copy without the mutation. If a child of a mutation carrier inherits the mutation, he or she can pass it on to future children. However, members of a family who are shown not to have a mutation previously identified in another relative cannot pass it to their own offspring.

Hereditary Breast and Ovarian Cancer Syndrome (HBOC)

Features and Cancer Risks

The two genes BRCA1 and BRCA2 were initially discovered by studies of families strongly suggestive of hereditary breast cancer. Thus, they are named breast cancer susceptibility gene 1 (BRCA1) and breast cancer susceptibility gene 2 (BRCA2). Several hundred mutations have been reported in BRCA1 and BRCA2 since their identification, some of which are associated with an increased cancer risk.[4]

Functions of BRCA Genes

The BRCA1 and BRCA2 genes are known to be involved, both separately and coordinately, in DNA double-stranded break repair. These breaks can occur in response to ionizing radiation or DNA cross-linking agents such as the chemotherapeutic agent, cisplatin. Repair occurs through homologous recombination, by which homologous, undamaged DNA strands are invaded by a damaged single-stranded DNA. Homologous sequences are then paired, resulting in an undamaged double-stranded DNA molecule. The double-stranded break repair pathway is complex and involves numerous other genes in addition to BRCA1 and BRCA2. Impairment in DNA repair has been associated with increased cancer risk.

BRCA genes are considered to act as tumor suppressor genes, because an inherited deleterious mutation in one allele represents the first "hit" in Knudsen's two-hit hypothesis of tumorigenesis. If the second allele loses its function within a cell (through accumulation of damage), cancer can develop as a result of the cell's inability to repair acquired abnormalities. Precisely why the BRCA1 and BRCA2 genes predispose specifically to breast and ovarian cancer is still unclear.

The involvement of the BRCA1/2 genes in DNA repair is also thought to explain why women with BRCA1/2-related breast cancer have a better response to cisplatin-based regimens than those with sporadic breast cancer.[5] Cisplatin generates a highly reactive species after intracellular aquation. This species binds to DNA, causing intra-strand cross-links primarily between adjacent guanines in the DNA helix major groove. Among other cytotoxic effects, it is believed that the cisplatin-induced adducts may induce the mismatch repair (MMR) complex to produce single-stranded DNA breaks, resulting in cytotoxicity and cell death.[6]

Poly(ADP) ribose polymerase (PARP) inhibitors represent a novel investigational treatment for BRCA1/2-related cancers. PARP inhibitors decrease cells' ability to repair single-stranded breaks in DNA. BRCA-deficient tumor cells are sensitive to these agents, because increases in single-stranded breaks increase rates of double-stranded breaks, which can lead to increased death for these cells. PARP inhibitors therefore may act as selective BRCA-deficient tumor cell killers and are currently in clinical development and phase I and II trials for this use.

Prevalence and Penetrance of *BRCA1/2* Mutations

For genetic testing of *BRCA1* and *BRCA2* to be useful to families at high risk for a mutation in these genes, it is necessary to have accurate assessments of their prevalence (how common the mutations are in a particular population) and penetrance (the likelihood of mutation carriers developing cancer). Although thought to be responsible for one half of hereditary breast cancers,[2] mutations in these two genes are generally rare. Estimations of mutation prevalence in the U.S population range from approximately 0.1% to 0.76% (1 in 1000 to 1 in 132).[7–9] However, in women of Ashkenazi Jewish (Eastern European) descent, approximately 2.5% (1 in 40) are believed to be mutation carriers.[10]

BRCA1 and *BRCA2* mutations have a high penetrance. The lifetime risk of invasive breast cancer with a *BRCA1* or *BRCA2* mutation ranges from 36% to 85%, depending on the study methodology.[11–14] Original data were based primarily on highly selected families such as those used for positional cloning of the genes. In these families, the estimated lifetime risk of breast cancer was over 80%; in *BRCA1* carriers, the lifetime risk for ovarian cancer was between 40% and 65%, and for *BRCA2* carriers, it was 20%.[15,16] Later studies have used case-based ascertainment and, to a lesser extent, population-based data. Population-based designs to ascertain penetrance are usually performed on specific subpopulations (e.g., Ashkenazi Jews) known to harbor a high incidence of founder mutations to obtain an adequate number of carriers. One study of the Ashkenazim showed a 56% lifetime risk (to age 70 years) for breast cancer and a 16% lifetime risk of ovarian cancer but did not distinguish between *BRCA1* and *BRCA2*.[10] By comparison, case-based ascertainment usually yields higher penetrance estimates, with 69% and 74% lifetime risk of breast cancer, and 54% and 23% risk of ovarian cancer in Ashkenazi Jews with mutations in *BRCA1* and *BRCA2*, respectively.[12] A meta-analysis of case-based studies showed a 65% lifetime risk for breast cancer and 39% risk for ovarian cancer in all-comers with mutations in *BRCA1*; corresponding values for *BRCA2* were 45% and 11%.[14] A recent meta-analysis (including both Ashkenazi and non-Ashkenazi Jewish popula-

tions) estimated the lifetime risk of breast cancer as 55% in *BRCA1* carriers and 47% in *BRCA2* carriers; ovarian cancer risk was estimated as 39% in *BRCA1* carriers and 17% in *BRCA2* carriers.[17]

Penetrance estimates may also vary, based not only on the populations studied, but also on other risk factors such as oral contraceptive use, parity, and oophorectomy,[18] and on the specific location of the mutation within the gene. Analysis of *BRCA1* cancer families has revealed a correlation between the mutation site and the relative risk of breast versus ovarian cancer. 3′ Mutations, which cause truncation of the C-terminal region, are associated with a higher proportion of breast than ovarian cancers, whereas 5′ mutations, which delete a large segment of the BRCA1 protein, are associated with a mixture of breast and ovarian cancers.[19] Mutations in the central region of *BRCA2* (referred to as the "ovarian cancer cluster region") have been shown to be associated with a decreased risk of breast cancer relative to ovarian cancer risk.[20]

Features of *BRCA1*- and *BRCA2*-Related Cancers

Compared with that of the general population, *BRCA1* and *BRCA2* mutation carriers have an increased risk of developing breast cancer. The lifetime risk of invasive breast cancer conferred by a *BRCA1* or *BRCA2* mutation is estimated to be between 36% and 85%. *BRCA1*- and *BRCA2*-associated breast cancers are diagnosed at a younger age, often premenopausally.[21] This is particularly true for *BRCA1* carriers, approximately 20% of whom develop breast cancer before age 40, with 50% by age 50.[22] A recent retrospective cohort study indicated that ductal carcinoma in situ (DCIS), with or without invasive cancer, is just as prevalent in mutation carriers (37%) as in high-risk noncarriers (34%) but that it may develop at an earlier age.[23] A population-based case-control study looked at the prevalence of *BRCA1* and *BRCA2* mutations in women diagnosed with DCIS. It was found that mutation prevalence rates in this group were similar to those found in women with invasive breast cancer, suggesting that the criteria used to assess eligibility for screening and risk for positive mutation-carrier status should include diagnoses of DCIS.[24] In another cohort study of mutation carriers with stage I or II breast cancer, it was found that the risk of a second primary breast cancer in the contralateral breast was approximately 30% over 10 years, and even higher in women who did not use chemoprevention or undergo oophorectomy.[25]

In addition to a lower age of onset, *BRCA1*-related breast cancers typically have features associated with a poorer prognosis, including numerous mitoses and substantial pleomorphism.[26] Compared with sporadic and *BRCA2*-related cancers, *BRCA1*-type breast cancers characteristically exhibit higher frequency of grade 3 tumors and lower frequency of both estrogen receptors (ER) and progesterone receptors (PR), and they are rarely *HER2/neu*-positive.[27] Approximately 75% of *BRCA2*-associated breast cancers are hormone receptor–positive, whereas a similar percentage of *BRCA1*-associated breast cancers are not positive.[27] The lack of estrogen, progesterone, and *HER2* receptor expression constitutes the "triple-negative" or basal phenotype, which has been identified as having a poorer prognosis than other tumors because of the limited number of therapies that can specifically target these cells.

Compared with the general population, *BRCA1* and *BRCA2* mutation carriers also have an increased risk of ovarian cancer. The lifetime risk of ovarian cancer in the general population is approximately 1.3%, whereas the lifetime risk of *BRCA* mutation carriers is estimated to be 10% to 60%. *BRCA1* mutations confer a higher risk of ovarian and primary peritoneal cancer compared with risk from *BRCA2* mutations, and they are associated with earlier age at onset. Fallopian tube cancers, though much rarer than ovarian cancer, are also higher in carriers than in noncarriers,[28] and again this risk is increased in *BRCA1* carriers than in *BRCA2* carriers. *BRCA1*- and *BRCA2*-associated ovarian cancers are pathologically and histologically indistinguishable from one another. However, they are generally of serous histology, with endometrioid being the next most common. Mucinous tumors are unlikely to be associated with *BRCA1* or *BRCA2* mutations, whereas rarer forms such as clear cell tumors are not common enough for an association (or lack thereof) to be determined to date. In addition, borderline and low-malignant-potential tumors of the ovary are not believed to be associated with *BRCA1* or *BRCA2* mutations.[20]

Males with *BRCA1* and *BRCA2* mutations also have an increased risk of developing cancer. Although the risk of male breast cancer is known to be increased with *BRCA1* mutations, it is higher with *BRCA2* mutations, with a lifetime risk estimate of approximately 5% to 6% compared with approximately 0.1% in men who are noncarriers. The lifetime risk of prostate cancer is also increased, but has not been reliably quantified. Although there is a trend toward younger-onset prostate cancer, it is not strikingly young, as is often seen with the breast cancer in females.

The association of other cancers with *BRCA1* and *BRCA2* mutations has been studied in a number of cohorts. In particular, *BRCA2* mutations are associated with an increased risk of pancreatic cancer and melanoma.[10,29] Unfortunately, the lifetime risk of developing these malignancies has not been reliably quantified. A kin-cohort study of unselected patients newly diagnosed with ovarian cancer looked at cancer incidence in first-degree relatives of confirmed *BRCA1* and *BRCA2* mutation carriers. A higher risk ratio was associated with ovarian, female breast, and testicular cancer in *BRCA1* carriers, with higher risk for ovarian, female and male breast, and pancreatic cancers in *BRCA2* carriers.[8]

The precise factors that determine which mutation-positive women will, and will not, develop cancer are unknown. Variation in penetrance of *BRCA1* and *BRCA2* has resulted in the identification of possible cancer risk modifiers in carriers. Both hormonal and genetic influences have been examined. The use of oral contraceptives, for example, has been reported to protect against ovarian cancer in noncarriers.[30] Studies in carriers present differential risk in regard to breast or ovarian cancer, showing a protective effect of oral contraceptives against ovarian cancer[31] or no reduction in risk.[32] However, a clinical dilemma is presented by data suggesting that the use of oral contraceptives in *BRCA1* carriers may also significantly increase breast cancer risk.[18] At present, oral contraceptive use is not actively recommended for ovarian cancer prevention, but short-term use for contraceptive needs is not contraindicated.

The relation between endogenous hormonal factors to breast and ovarian cancer risk has also been assessed in *BRCA1* and *BRCA2* carriers.

In a study of the reproductive histories of *BRCA1* carriers, the risk of breast cancer was increased in those who experienced menarche before age 12, and in those with parity of less than three.[31] It is interesting to note that the risk of ovarian cancer in *BRCA1* carriers has been found to be lower with greater parity, in contrast to *BRCA2* carriers, in whom parity was associated with a significant increase in ovarian cancer risk.[33] Further studies to address these gene-environment and gene-gene interactions are ongoing. These studies are needed to potentially make it possible to provide more personalized risk estimates for the individual woman.

Genetic Testing

Family history features suggestive of a *BRCA1* or *BRCA2* mutation include premenopausal breast cancer, ovarian cancer, and male breast cancer. A referral for genetic counseling is indicated if the medical or family history is consistent with hereditary breast and ovarian cancer (Box 5-1).

Because of autosomal dominant inheritance, it is most informative to begin genetic testing in a family member who has had the cancer of concern. This is because one goal of genetic testing is to first identify the mutation in a relative with cancer in the family and then determine which other relatives did, and did not, inherit it. Those who did inherit the mutation have an increased risk of developing specific malignancies, whereas the risk of cancer for those who did not inherit it is much lower and based on other cancer-specific risk factors, such

as age at menarche, age at menopause, body mass index (BMI), and hormone replacement therapy (HRT).

Consider the following scenario, which is illustrated in Figure 5-1. Mary is concerned about her risk of developing breast cancer, since her mother (Susan) was recently diagnosed with the disease. Mary's maternal aunt (Jane) is deceased as a result of breast cancer, suggesting a hereditary component to the family history. If Mary chooses to undergo genetic testing and no mutations are detected (i.e., a negative result), there are two possible explanations for this result. First, Susan's and Jane's breast cancers may be due to a mutation in the gene for which Mary was tested. However, because of autosomal dominant inheritance, Mary did not inherit the mutation from Susan. Thus, Mary's risk of developing breast cancer is likely closer to that of the general population and is based on her own risk factors, since her family history of breast cancer is attributable to a genetic mutation that Mary does not have. However, the second possibility is that Susan's and Jane's cancers are due to a mutation in a gene that was not tested or that has not yet been discovered. Therefore, it is not possible to determine whether Mary has the same mutation. In this scenario, Mary remains at an increased risk for breast cancer based on her genetically unexplained family history. It is not possible to distinguish between these two possible explanations without genetically testing Susan.

Box 5-1. Features Indicating a Need for Referral for Cancer Genetic Counseling

---

Breast cancer diagnosed before menopause (typically before age 50)

Member of a family with a known *BRCA1* or *BRCA2* mutation

Two breast primaries in a single individual, particularly when one was diagnosed premenopausally

Breast and ovarian cancer in a single individual

Personal or family history of male breast cancer

Two breast cancers or ovarian cancers in close relative(s) from the same side of family (maternal or paternal)

Breast or ovarian cancer in a member of a high-risk population (i.e., Ashkenazim)

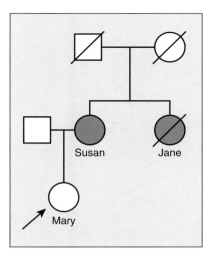

Figure 5-1. Mary is concerned about her risk for breast cancer because her mother Susan and her maternal aunt Jane both had breast cancer. Genetic testing is most informative if it begins with Susan.

By contrast, if genetic testing were performed on Susan and a mutation were detected, one could reasonably attribute her breast cancer to the identified mutation. Determining whether Mary has this same mutation would then indicate whether she, too, has an increased risk of breast cancer. It can also determine whether Mary's offspring would have an increased risk of breast cancer.

Genetic analysis of the *BRCA1* and *BRCA2* genes is clinically available. For most families, full sequencing of both genes is required and is considered the most reliable method of gene analysis. However, an estimated 12% of deleterious mutations are large genomic deletions or duplications, which are not detectable with sequencing.[34] Therefore, additional testing technology, such as Southern blot analysis, may be necessary in families with a cancer pattern strongly suggestive of a hereditary component. If a woman with breast cancer undergoes full analysis of both genes and a mutation is identified, the mutation likely explains the most significant genetic component of her cancer. It also indicates that she has an increased risk of ovarian cancer, and intensive screening or consideration of ovarian cancer risk-reducing options is indicated. In addition, it is possible to offer predictive genetic testing to other interested family members to identify those who also have an increased risk of developing breast and ovarian cancer.

If no mutations are identified, the woman's breast cancer is genetically unexplained. Possible explanations are that (1) there is a *BRCA1* or *BRCA2* mutation that is not identifiable using current technology, (2) the family history is due to a rare breast cancer syndrome (discussed later in text), (3) there is a mutation in an undiscovered gene, or (4) the breast cancer is due to a combination of many genetic and environmental factors. The woman's risk for a future malignancy, and cancer risk for her relatives, is based on her family history.

A third possible result of genetic analysis is a variant of uncertain significance, which is a change in the DNA sequence whose role in cancer development is not known. Through research, some variants are ultimately determined to be polymorphisms (normal genetic variation between individuals and populations), whereas others are ultimately classified as deleterious (cancer-causing). Until the significance of the variant is determined, genetic testing is generally not offered to unaffected relatives. Uncertain variants are detected in approximately 10% of samples tested from Caucasian individuals. In non-Caucasian populations, such as African Americans, the chance of an uncertain variant increases owing to less available genetic data in minority ethnicities.

In persons of Ashkenazi Jewish descent, genetic testing usually begins with analysis of three founder mutations. The 187delAG and 5385insC mutations in the *BRCA1* gene and the 6174delT mutation in the *BRCA2* gene account for approximately 90% of *BRCA1* and *BRCA2* mutations detected in the Ashkenazim. Because of the high detection rate with this three-mutation panel, full sequencing is generally considered only in Ashkenazi Jewish persons with a high pre-test probability of a deleterious mutation and whose test results are negative for the three founder mutations. Other populations known to have founder mutations include Icelanders (999del5 in *BRCA2*) and those from Finland, France, Russia, Denmark, Sweden, Belgium, and the Netherlands.[35]

Once a mutation has been identified in a family, other relatives have the option of undergoing testing for that specific mutation. This is due to the rarity of *BRCA1* and *BRCA2* mutations, such that one seldom sees a family with more than one mutation. However, because these mutations are more common among Ashkenazi Jews and there are a significant number of Ashkenazi families with more than one mutation, testing for the entire founder mutation panel is generally recommended even when only one founder mutation has been identified in the family.

Because of patent and licensing constraints, sequencing of *BRCA1* and *BRCA2* is clinically available only through Myriad Genetic Laboratories (Salt Lake City, Utah). Peripheral blood is the preferred specimen, and turn-around time for the analysis is generally 3 to 4 weeks. Full sequencing costs more than $3000, whereas the Ashkenazi Jewish founder mutation panel is around $500 and mutation-specific testing is approximately $400. Most insurance companies cover a portion, if not all, of the cost for patients whose medical or family history is suggestive of an underlying mutation. Because of the expense, however, the laboratory offers insurance preauthorization services. These costs may change in the future.

Management: Screening and Risk Reduction Options

Breast Cancer

Screening and risk reduction strategies for the breast in female BRCA1 and BRCA2 mutation carriers fall into three general categories: intensive cancer screening, chemoprevention, and prophylactic surgery. According to recommendations of the National Comprehensive Cancer Network (NCCN), women with BRCA1 or BRCA2 mutations should have a clinical breast examination by a healthcare provider at least every 6 months, beginning at age 25 years (www.nccn.org). Mammograms generally begin at age 25 years, but can be adjusted based on the cancer pattern in the family, since there is also the issue of radiation risk. Adjuvant ultrasound is also a consideration for women with dense breast tissue; studies are ongoing to determine its effectiveness.

Recently, magnetic resonance imaging (MRI) has become a more routine part of breast screening for mutation carriers. The American Cancer Society recommends that women with a high risk of developing breast cancer (greater than 20% lifetime risk) should get an MRI and a mammogram every year. The optimal interval for MRIs has not yet been established.[36] A review of the effectiveness of MRI as an addition to mammography and ultrasound in screening high-risk young women found consistent evidence that MRI as a screening strategy provides high sensitivity compared with that of mammography alone or mammography and ultrasound with or without clinical breast exam.[37] Whether this higher sensitivity translates into a reduction in patient mortality compared with that with mammography alone is presently unclear. This is an evolving field.

Risk reduction options include chemoprevention or prophylactic bilateral mastectomy. Data on the effectiveness of chemoprevention with tamoxifen in BRCA1 and BRCA2 carriers have been extrapolated from large trials within the general population. The National Surgical Adjuvant Breast and Bowel Project (NSABP) prevention trials showed a 62% decrease in the risk of breast cancer in BRCA2-positive women who received tamoxifen for 5 years versus no reduction in breast cancer incidence among BRCA1-positive women.[38] However, another study examined the effects of tamoxifen on prevention of contralateral breast cancer in mutation carriers and found that the drug did provide protection overall, but the protection reached significance only in BRCA1 mutation carriers.[39] This is an interesting finding in light of the lack of hormone receptor expression seen in BRCA1 relative to BRCA2 cancers and is yet to be replicated.

Another risk-reduction option is prophylactic bilateral mastectomy, which reduces the risk of breast cancer by at least 90% in unaffected mutation carriers.[21,40] For women with breast cancer who opt for contralateral prophylactic mastectomy, the rate of a contralateral malignancy is also reduced by 90%.[41] However, therapeutic and/or contralateral mastectomy does not reduce the risk of chest wall or distant recurrence. Furthermore, although such surgery results in the greatest reduction in breast cancer risk, it is often an emotionally difficult choice for women. Although expected to decrease mortality, the efficacy of bilateral prophylactic mastectomy in prolonging survival has not yet been shown in prospective studies.

Ovarian Cancer

Although there is no evidence that ovarian cancer screening is efficacious in BRCA1 and BRCA2 mutation carriers or the general population, at present mutation-positive women who have not completed their family are recommended to have pelvic examination, transvaginal ultrasound, and serum CA-125 testing every 6 to 12 months. Studies examining the ability of this surveillance to detect early-stage ovarian cancers have had mixed results, with one group finding four of five cancers detected at stage I or II[42] and a review of other studies finding 63% of screen-detected ovarian cancers at stage IIC or greater.[43] The authors of the latter study suggest that the features of BRCA-related ovarian tumors—primarily high-grade serous and endometrioid—progress relatively rapidly to an advanced stage, making early detection difficult. The use of oral contraceptives as chemoprevention for ovarian cancer in BRCA mutation carriers has been suggested by studies showing significant reduction of risk. However, their use is not routinely recommended owing to the possibility of increased breast cancer risk.

For those who have completed childbearing, prophylactic bilateral salpingo-oophorectomy is the standard of care. Such surgery, when compared with increased surveillance, reduces the risk of ovarian cancer by 80% to 90%.[44,45] The majority of the remaining risk is attributed to primary peritoneal cancer, although a small proportion may arise in the remnant of the fallopian tube remaining in the uterus. There is also some suggestion of an association between uterine papillary serous carcinoma and *BRCA1* mutations, although this is primarily based on case reports in the literature rather than on large numbers of patients. However, for these reasons, some women also consider concurrent hysterectomy, but this is not a standard recommendation for all mutation-positive women. In addition, up to 4% of mutation-positive women undergoing prophylactic oophorectomy will have an occult cancer identified.[46] For this reason, it is generally recommended that a gynecologic oncologist either perform the surgery or be available for staging, if necessary. So far, a survival benefit has been shown in the short term but not in the long term.[47]

Timing of prophylactic oophorectomy post-childbearing may differ depending on the underlying gene mutation and the family history. It is typically recommended that *BRCA1/2* mutation-positive women pursue surgery in their mid to late 30s or early 40s. An added benefit of bilateral oophorectomy, particularly when it occurs before menopause, is a reduction in breast cancer risk of up to 50%.[44] What is unknown at this time is whether the reduction in breast cancer risk conferred by prophylactic bilateral salpingo-oophorectomy is of the same magnitude in *BRCA1* carriers as in *BRCA2* carriers. Recently, it was reported that bilateral salpingo-oophorectomy resulted in a 72% reduction in breast cancer risk in *BRCA2* mutations carriers, with only a 45% risk reduction in *BRCA1* mutation carriers.[48] This suggests an age-dependent benefit.[49] Ultimately, timing of the surgery depends on a combination of factors, including the gene involved and the woman's own medical and psychosocial history.

Hormone replacement therapy (HRT) is often an issue of concern for mutation-positive women, since they are usually premenopausal at the time of prophylactic oophorectomy. Thus, entry into menopause is sudden, and severity of symptoms varies. Short-term HRT for severe menopausal side effects (e.g., vasomotor symptoms and insomnia) is an option to provide improvement in quality of life, particularly estrogen, if only the uterus has been removed.

Current views on HRT in this high-risk population vary considerably, ranging from no HRT to HRT until the age at which menopause would have naturally occurred. Data on HRT in *BRCA1* and *BRCA2* carriers has been extrapolated from data from the general population, and there is a need to evaluate its use in this population prospectively. Long-term HRT is not uniformly recommended because of the already greatly increased risk of breast cancer due to mutation status, but further studies on the long-term effects of ovarian removal on the brain, bone, and cardiovascular system are needed.

Rare Hereditary Breast Cancer Syndromes

The following syndromes (summarized in Table 5-1) each account for less than 1% of hereditary breast cancer. All are inherited in an autosomal dominant pattern, as with *BRCA1* and *BRCA2*. Recognition of these syndromes is important because each is associated with appreciable cancer risk as well as other potential health complications. Identification of these rare syndromes can make a direct impact on management of affected patients and their family members.

Li-Fraumeni Syndrome

Li-Fraumeni (LFS) syndrome was originally named "SBLA syndrome" because of the six cardinal cancers used to define the syndrome: *s*arcomas of the bone, soft tissue *s*arcomas, *b*reast cancer, *b*rain tumors, acute *l*eukemias, and *a*drenocortical cancer. Although these cancers are the main components of LFS and are integral to the diagnostic criteria (Box 5-2), at least 25% of cancers identified in LFS families are non-cardinal cancers. Other cancers suggested to be part of the LFS spectrum are lung cancer, gastric cancer, pancreatic cancer, Wilms' tumor, malignant phyllodes tumors, colorectal cancer, and choroid plexus carcinoma.[52-55] It is interesting that Birch and associates[52] did not find a significant excess of leukemia in the LFS families that they studied. However, because of ascertainment issues, syndrome rarity, and the presence of presumably nonsyndromic cancers within syndromic families, the full spectrum of associated cancers is unknown, thus complicating screening recommendations.

The lifetime risk of cancer associated with LFS is very high. Chompret and associates[56] cal-

Table 5-1. Hereditary Syndromes Conferring a Substantially Increased Risk for Breast Cancer

Syndrome	Gene	Breast Cancer Risk	Associated Non-Breast Cancers	Nonmaligant Features
Hereditary breast and ovarian cancer syndrome (HBOC)	BRCA1 BRCA2	36–85%	Ovarian, pancreatic, prostate, melanoma	None reported
Li-Fraumeni syndrome (LFS)	p53	80–90% (extrapolated based on overall lifetime cancer risk estimates)	Sarcomas, acute leukemias, adrenocortical, brain, lung, gastric, pancreatic, colorectal, Wilms' tumor, malignant phyllodes, choroid plexus carcinoma	None reported
Cowden syndrome (CS)	PTEN	20–50%	Thyroid, endometrial	Mucocutaneous lesions, benign thyroid conditions, benign breast disease, genitourinary abnormalities, uterine fibroids
Peutz-Jeghers syndrome (PJS)	STK11/ LKB1	32–54%	Gastrointestinal (stomach, small intestine, colon), pancreatic, ovarian, testicular, lung	Mucocutaneous melanin pigmentation, gastrointestinal hamartomas
Hereditary diffuse gastric cancer (HDGC)	CDH1	39–52%	Gastric	None reported

Box 5-2. Criteria for Classic Li-Fraumeni syndrome (LFS) and Li-Fraumeni-like syndrome (LFL)

Classic Li-Fraumeni syndrome[50]
A proband with a sarcoma diagnosed before age 45 and
A first-degree relative diagnosed before age 45 with any cancer and
A first- or second-degree relative diagnosed before age 45 with any cancer or with a sarcoma at any age

Li-Fraumeni-like syndrome[51]
A proband with any childhood cancer or sarcoma, brain tumor, or adrenocortical tumor diagnosed before age 45 and
A first- or second-degree relative diagnosed at any age with a typical LFS cancer (sarcoma, breast cancer, brain tumor, adrenocortical tumor or leukemia) and
A first- or second-degree relative diagnosed before age 60 with any cancer

culated a lifetime cancer risk of 73% for males and 100% for females, attributing the excess risk for females to the high risk of breast cancer. Age-related risks have also been calculated, with a 15% cancer risk by age 15 years, 54% by age 16 to 45 years, and 68% for those over 45 years.[56] However, median ages at diagnosis vary by cancer type, with 3 years as the median age at diagnosis for adrenocortical cancer, 14 to 15 years for sarcomas, 16 years for brain tumors, 27 years for leukemia, and 33 years for breast cancer.[57] A sample LFS pedigree is seen in Figure 5-2.

A significant issue with LFS is the risk for subsequent primary cancers. In a study of 24 LFS kindreds, Hisada and associates[56] showed that the cumulative probability of a second primary cancer was 57% at 30 years of follow-up, and the risk was higher (67% at 20 years of follow-up; 100% at 30 years of follow-up) when the first primary cancer was a soft tissue sarcoma. There was also a higher risk when the first cancer occurred before age 20 years (83-fold), but no excess risk was noted when the first cancer occurred after age 45 years. Second primary cancers occurred at a median of 6 years after the first cancer, with a range of 1 to 27 years. The cumulative probability of a third primary cancer was 38% at 10 years of follow-up after the second primary cancer. Of note, aside from the soft tissue sarcoma association, the second primary risk did not differ between cardinal LFS cancers and rarer LFS cancers.

After radiation, second primary cancers have also been evaluated. In the study by Hisada and associates,[58] 9 of the 30 patients who developed a second primary cancer had received radiation treatment for their first cancer. Six of the nine patients developed a total of eight cancers within the treatment field, at a median of 11 years after

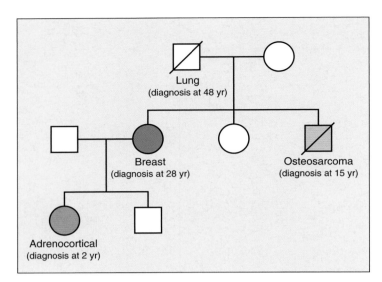

Figure 5-2. Typical pedigree from a family with associated cancers of Li-Fraumeni syndrome.

radiation. The subsequent primary cancers were mostly sarcomas, although one was a breast cancer in a woman previously treated for osteosarcoma, soft tissue sarcoma, and a prior breast cancer. Development of second primary cancers has also been reported specifically in LFS women who received radiation for treatment of breast cancer.[59,60] This has led to postulation that mastectomy may be preferable to breast conservation in women with LFS-related breast cancer. At the least, detailed discussion of the risks is warranted before making final treatment decisions.

Li-Fraumeni syndrome is associated with germline mutations in the *p53* gene. David Lane[61] dubbed *p53* "The Guardian of the Genome," because of its biologic function as a G1 checkpoint control for DNA damage. *p53* is somatically mutated in about half of all human cancers, although mutation prevalence varies by tissue type. The p53 protein directs p21 to interact with cdk2, regulating cell division. Absent *p53* function results in lack of p21 production, causing uncontrolled cell division and tumorigenesis. Approximately 80% of families who meet the strictest criteria for LFS have a detectable *p53* mutation. However, the likelihood of mutation detection is lower for families meeting the LFS-like (LFL) criteria (see Box 5-2). De novo mutations have been reported, with a possible de novo rate as high as 24%.[56] Salmon and associates[60] postulated that the number of de novo mutations may actually be underestimated owing to selection bias, since mutation studies are usually conducted in those with the strongest family histories. Alternatively, de novo mutations may represent

the most severe cases, resulting in decreased life expectancy and failure to reproduce.

Management of LFS is complicated. Given the dramatic risk for young-onset breast cancer, increased breast surveillance is recommended, and the approach is routinely updated by the NCCN (www.nccn.org). However, potential risks of mammography-related radiation have been questioned, leading to a potentially more prominent role for MRI. Prophylactic mastectomy is assumed to substantially lower breast cancer risk based on *BRCA1* and *BRCA2* data, although LFS-specific studies have not been performed. Recommended screening also includes annual urinalysis, complete blood cell count, abdominal ultrasound, and organ-targeted surveillance based on family history beginning in childhood; however, effect on mortality has not been studied. Generally, affected families are strongly encouraged to pay attention to concerning, lingering symptoms, and seek prompt medical attention.

Cowden Syndrome

Cowden syndrome (CS) is part of the *PTEN* hamartoma tumor syndrome (PHTS), which also includes Bannayan-Riley-Ruvalcaba syndrome, Proteus syndrome, and Proteus-like syndrome. These syndromes are allelic, meaning that they all are associated with mutations in *PTEN*, but with differing features. CS is associated with both malignant and nonmalignant neoplasms. Female breast cancer is the most common CS-associated malignancy, with a lifetime risk of 25% to 50% and an average age at diagnosis of 38 to 46 years.[62] Male breast cancer has been reported in patients with CS.[63] The risk of developing contralateral primary breast cancer in women is not known. Other CS-associated malignancies include a 10% lifetime risk of thyroid cancer (predominantly follicular, although papillary has been reported) and a 5% to 10% lifetime risk of endometrial cancer. Renal carcinoma, melanomas, and glial tumors have also been reported in CS, but the lifetime risks have not been quantified.[64]

Cowden syndrome is also associated with nonmalignant features, of which the most prominent are mucocutaneous findings (Fig. 5-3). Trichilemmomas and papillomatous papules are around 99% penetrant by the time a person is in the 20s; trichilemmomas are most often found at the hairline, whereas papillomatous papules usually occur on the face, hands, and feet (pressure points) or oral mucosa (as reviewed in Gustafson and associates[65]). A detailed list of nonmalignant features is given in Box 5-3.

Cowden syndrome is due to mutations in the *PTEN* (*p*hosphatase and *ten*sin homologue deleted on chromosome ten) gene. Approximately 80% to 90% of persons who meet CS diagnostic criteria have an identifiable *PTEN* mutation, some of which are found in the promoter region. PTEN is a protein phosphatase and inhibits cell migration and cell spreading (reviewed in Eng[66]). It also mediates cell cycle arrest at G1 and influences apoptosis and has both nuclear and cytoplasmic localization. This dual localization likely contributes to *PTEN's* role in carcinogenesis.

The mucocutaneous symptoms of CS rarely require intervention, unless they are irritating or disfiguring. If CS is symptomatic, treatment ranges from topical agents to surgical excision. Treatment of associated cancers does not differ from the sporadic counterparts, although attention should be paid to the possibility of secondary malignancies. The NCCN updates CS surveillance recommendations annually, but generally recommends consideration of thyroid surveillance with annual thyroid ultrasound beginning at age 18 years. Endometrial screening has also been proposed, but efficacy is unproven. Breast surveillance is similar to that recommended for *BRCA1* and *BRCA2* mutation carriers, including semiannual clinical breast exams beginning at age 25 years, annual mammography, and breast MRI beginning at age 30 to 35 years or earlier, depending on family history.

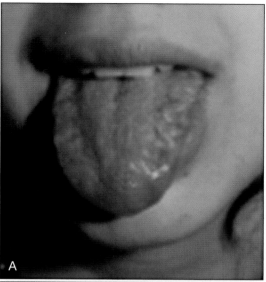

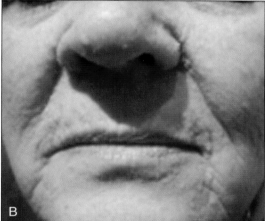

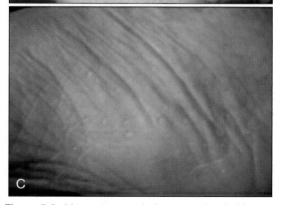

Figure 5-3. Mucocutaneous lesions associated with Cowden syndrome. (A, From http://www.uveitis.org/medical/articles/case/Cowden_sy.html. B, C, From Kovich O, Cohen D: Cowden's syndrome. Dermatol Online J 10(3):3, Figs. 1 and 2.)

Box 5-3. Operational Diagnostic Criteria for Cowden Syndrome

Diagnostic criteria of an individual

Mucocutaneous lesions, alone, if:
  Six or more facula papules (at least three trichilemmomas) *or*
  Cutaneous facial papules and oral mucosal papillomatosis *or*
  Oral mucosal papillomatosis and acral keratoses *or*
  Six or more palmoplantar keratoses
Two or more major criteria *or*
One major and three or more minor criteria *or*
Four or more minor criteria

Diagnostic criteria in a family with an individual who is diagnostic for Cowden syndrome

Pathognomonic criteria *or*
One major criteria *or*
Two minor criteria *or*
History of Bannayan-Riley-Ruvalcaba syndrome (BRRS)

Pathognomonic criteria

Adult Lhermitte-Duclos disease (LDD)
Mucocutaneous lesions
  Trichilemmomas (facial)
  Papillomatous papules
  Acral keratoses

Major criteria

Breast cancer
Thyroid cancer (especially follicular)
Macrocephaly (>97th percentile)
Endometrial cancer

Minor criteria

Benign thyroid lesions (e.g., multinodular goiter, adenoma)
Mental retardation (IQ < 75)
Gastrointestinal hamartomas
Fibrocystic breast disease
Lipomas
Fibromas
Genitourinary tumors (especially renal cell carcinoma)
Genitourinary structural manifestations
Uterine fibroids

Adapted from National Comprehensive Cancer Network Practice Guidelines in Oncology v.1.2010: NCCN Guidelines for Detection, Prevention, and Risk Reduction: Genetic/Familial High-Risk Assessment: Breast and Ovarian (www.nccn.org).

Prophylactic mastectomy is assumed to substantially lower breast cancer risk based on *BRCA1* and *BRCA2* data, although CS-specific studies have not been performed.

Peutz-Jeghers Syndrome

Peutz-Jeghers syndrome (PJS) is defined by the presence of gastrointestinal polyposis and mucocutaneous pigmentation. The polyps are Peutz-

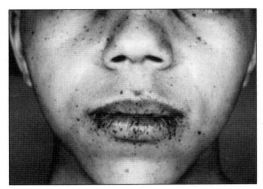

Figure 5-4. Mucocutaneous melanin pigmentation characteristic of Peutz-Jeghers syndrome. (From Division of Gastroenterology, The Johns Hopkins Hospital, 1999, www.hopkins-gi.org)

Jeghers–specific hamartomas that histologically have mucosa interdigitated with smooth muscle in a branched pattern. They can occur throughout the gastrointestinal tract, but are most prevalent in the small bowel. The average age at diagnosis of PJS is 23 years in men and 26 years in women, owing in large part to small bowel intussusception or other gastrointestinal symptoms. One study showed that laparotomy for bowel obstruction occurred in 30% of affected persons by age 10 years, increasing to 68% by age 18 years.[67]

Peutz-Jeghers syndrome's mucocutaneous pigmentation usually occurs in infancy or early childhood, but fades with age, often becoming unnoticeable by one's 20s. The spots are usually dark brown or dark blue and range from 1 to 5 mm (Fig. 5-4). Most commonly, the spots are located on the lips, buccal mucosa, hands, and feet.

Peutz-Jeghers syndrome is associated with dramatically increased risk for a variety of malignancies, with a lifetime relative risk of developing any cancer ranging from 9.9-fold to 15.2-fold (37% to 93%).[68–70] Increased risk for malignancy with PJS includes cancers of the breast, colon, small intestine, stomach, esophagus, pancreas, lung, testes, uterus, ovaries, and cervix. Specifically, females are at risk for bilateral ovarian sex cord tumors with annular tubules (SCTAT) that are multifocal and usually benign.[71] Males have been shown to develop calcifying Sertoli cell tumors of the testes that can cause gynecomastia due to secreted estrogen.[72] In a review of 419 patients with PJS, the lifetime risk (to age 70 years) was 57% for developing gastrointestinal cancer, 18% for gynecologic cancer, 17% for lung cancer, and 11% for pancreatic cancer.[73]

Breast cancer is one of the most significant malignancies associated with PJS, with lifetime risk estimates ranging from 32% to 54%.[70,74] Age-related risk is 8% by age 40 years, 13% by 50 years, 31% by 60 years, and 45% by 70 years,[73] although Giardiello and associates[70] reported a mean age at diagnosis of 37 years. Male breast cancer and bilateral breast cancer have also been reported.[73,75,76]

Peutz-Jeghers syndrome is due to mutations in the *STK11* (LKB1) gene. The LKB1 protein physically associates with *p53* and regulates specific *p53*-dependent apoptotic pathways. Thus, LKB1 loss of function leads to deficient apoptosis of intestinal epithelial cells.[77] Genetic testing is recommended for people meeting diagnostic criteria (Box 5-4), and almost half of detected mutations are large rearrangements.[78] In addition, the mutation detection rate is higher for patients with a positive family history than for those with apparently de novo mutations.

Management for persons with PJS is complex, with surveillance beginning at birth for some neoplasms.[79] Upper endoscopy and small bowel series begin at age 8 years, with the addition of colonoscopy at age 18 years. Gynecologic screening begins at age 21 years, with consideration of pancreatic surveillance at age 25 years. Breast-specific screening has been extrapolated from that recommended for *BRCA1* and *BRCA2* mutation carriers and includes semiannual clinical breast exams and annual mammograms and breast MRI beginning at age 25 years. As with most rare syndromes, syndrome-specific screening studies have not been performed, but management recommendations are based on expert opinion.

Hereditary Diffuse Gastric Cancer

Hereditary diffuse gastric cancer (HDGC) syndrome was first recognized in three Maori kindreds[80] and has since been found in varying ethnicities. The predominant feature is diffuse gastric cancer, also referred to as linitis plastica, which spreads submucosally. The risk of gastric cancer by age 80 years was calculated to be 67% for males and 83% for females, with an average age at diagnosis of 38 years. The risk of lobular breast cancer was also increased in affected families, with a lifetime risk of 39% and an average age at diagnosis of 53 years. However, it is important to note that these risks were derived from 11 families ascertained through strict criteria (at least three cases of diffuse gastric cancer).[81] Evaluation of four families with a specific founder mutation showed a breast cancer risk of 52%.[82] Penetrance data for less highly-selected families are lacking.

Hereditary diffuse gastric cancer is due to mutations in the *E-cadherin* (*CDH1*) gene, which is a calcium-dependent cell-cell adhesion glycoprotein integral to adhesive properties between epithelial cells. Approximately 50% of families suggestive of HDGC have a detectable *CDH1* mutation, suggesting genetic heterogeneity.

Note that loss of *E-cadherin* is present in more than 90% of sporadic lobular breast cancers, but in only 5% to 10% of ductal breast cancers.[83] Initial criteria for consideration of *CDH1* testing were developed by the International Gastric Cancer Linkage Consortium and required two or more documented cases of diffuse gastric cancer in first- or second-degree relatives, with at least one diagnosed before age 50 years, or three or more first- or second-degree relatives with diffuse gastric cancer at any age. Brooks-Wilson and associates[84] proposed revised criteria (Box 5-5), which are now used in Western populations. However, the criteria may be too broad for use in countries with a high incidence of gastric cancer, such as Japan and Korea. The contribution of *CDH1* mutations to hereditary breast cancer is unknown.

Twenty-three *BRCA1/2*-negative families with hereditary (defined as no family history of gastric cancer *and* two or more cases of breast cancer of specified degree of relativity *or* a

Box 5-5. Criteria for Consideration of CDH1 Molecular Genetic Testing in Individuals with Gastric Cancer

Two or more cases of gastric cancer in a family, with at least one diffuse gastric cancer diagnosed before age 50

Three or more cases of gastric cancer in a family, diagnosed at any age, with at least one documented case of diffuse gastric cancer

An individual diagnosed with diffuse gastric cancer before age 45*

An individual diagnosed with both diffuse gastric cancer and lobular breast cancer

One family member diagnosed with diffuse gastric cancer and another with lobular breast cancer

One family member diagnosed with diffuse gastric cancer and another with signet ring colon cancer

*Lowering the cutoff age to before age 40 has been proposed.
Data from Brooks-Wilson AR, Kaurah P, Suriano G, et al: Germline E-cadherin mutations in hereditary diffuse gastric cancer: assessment of 42 new families and review of genetic screening criteria. J Med Genet 41(7):508–517, 2004.

proband with breast cancer diagnosed before age 45 years) lobular or mixed ductal and lobular breast cancer were screened for *CDH1* mutations.[85] One person was found to have a *CDH1* mutation. This patient was diagnosed with lobular breast cancer at age 42 years, and her mother was diagnosed with lobular breast cancer at age 28 years, but she had no other family history of gastric or breast cancer. If larger studies of familial lobular breast cancer kindreds confirm these findings, *CDH1* may be a consideration for breast-specific hereditary cancer families, even in the absence of a gastric cancer.

Surveillance for breast cancer includes semiannual clinical breast exams and annual mammograms. However, MRI appears to be better than mammography at detecting lobular cancers, indicating a role for MRI as a regular component of screening.[86] Screening for gastric cancer is less straightforward, since the cancer usually develops submucosally. Chromoendoscopy and endoscopic ultrasound have been proposed, but not proved reliable for detecting gastric carcinoma prior to metastasis. Therefore, strong consideration must be given to prophylactic gastrectomy after thorough discussion of the associated morbidity.

Low-Penetrance Genes

Low-penetrance genes may ultimately account for a significant proportion of breast cancer seen

in excess of the general population risk for this malignancy. However, their precise role in cancer development is not yet well understood. Therefore, testing for these alterations is not routinely recommended at this time. Despite this, it is important to be aware of their existence, since they are active areas of genetic research.

Ataxia-telangiectasia (AT) is an autosomal recessive syndrome characterized by progressive cerebellar ataxia, ocular telangiectasias, and increased risk for malignancy. Heterozygotes (unaffected carriers) are thought to have a twofold increased risk of breast cancer (as reviewed in Ahmed and Rahman[87] and Prokopcova and associates[88]). This is of particular importance to mothers, sisters, and daughters of individuals with AT. However, approximately 1% of the general population has a mutation in the *ATM* gene, which is associated with AT. Furthermore, studies looking at series of breast cancer cases have failed to clarify the contribution of *ATM* mutations to breast cancer as a whole. Therefore, at this time, increased breast cancer screening is reasonable for known carriers ascertained through a family member known to have AT, but screening of the general population and/or breast cancer population for *ATM* mutations is not recommended.

The *CHEK2* gene (cell cycle checkpoint kinase 2) has been suggested as a potential contributor to familial breast cancer. Originally, *CHEK2*, including the common *1100*C mutation, was thought to be a second LFS-associated gene; however, more recent data do not support this.[89] Most recently, Weischer and associates[90] performed a meta-analysis showing aggregated odds ratios of 2.7 for unselected breast cancer, 2.6 for early-onset breast cancer, and 4.8 for familial breast cancer, and they calculated a cumulative breast cancer risk of 37% by age 70 years for individuals with the *CHEK2*1100*C mutation. However, a thoughtful commentary by Offit and Garber[91] cited ascertainment issues in the studies included within the meta-analysis, population heterogeneity, and prevalence of phenocopies (mutation-negative individuals who still develop breast cancer) within *CHEK2* families; they concluded that currently available data do not support routine clinical testing for *CHEK2*.

Genetic Assessment

Women with a personal or family history suggestive of hereditary breast cancer should be referred for genetic counseling and discussion of screening and risk reduction options. Although it varies from clinic to clinic, patients referred for genetic counseling typically meet with a genetic counselor and a physician with expertise in cancer genetics.

Genetic Counseling Process

During the cancer genetics consultation, the patient's medical history is reviewed. If the patient has had cancer, particular attention is paid to the age at diagnosis and any other prior or synchronous malignancies. Menopausal status is noted for women with breast cancer; for those with ovarian cancer in particular, pathology is important.

The family history is also collected, including health history for all first- and second-degree relatives, living or deceased. Maternal family history and paternal family history are equally important because of autosomal dominant inheritance. Ages at cancer diagnosis are recorded, and, if possible, pathology reports are obtained to verify accuracy of patient report. This information is then used to construct a pedigree, which is a visual representation of the family history that makes a cancer pattern more easily identifiable (Fig. 5-5). The pedigree is the most valuable tool for cancer genetics risk assessment.

The genetics provider reviews the medical and family history with the patient and discusses the presence or absence of features suggestive of a hereditary cancer syndrome. In addition to an overall impression, it is sometimes possible to use one of several statistical models to predict the likelihood of detecting a mutation in one of the currently known cancer predisposition genes. The genetics provider also discusses modification of cancer risk based on the outcome of genetic testing and discusses how the results influence the risk for a future malignancy. Basic genetics is also overviewed, along with a discussion of how the patient's results are expected to affect other family members, both medically and emotionally. Finally, the psychosocial aspects of genetic testing are reviewed, including potential risks as depression, fear, anxiety, and stigma, as well as guilt, particularly when the patient is a parent. The genetics provider then discusses how various test results will affect medical management, including increased screening versus risk reduction, and the patient is familiarized with how the options are influenced by the various possible test results. Provision of this information assists the patient in assessing the personal usefulness of genetic testing, in weighing the risks and benefits, and in making a personally informed choice.

If the patient chooses to undergo genetic testing, written informed consent is obtained. When the results are available, they are communicated to the patient either in person at a scheduled follow-up visit, or over the telephone,

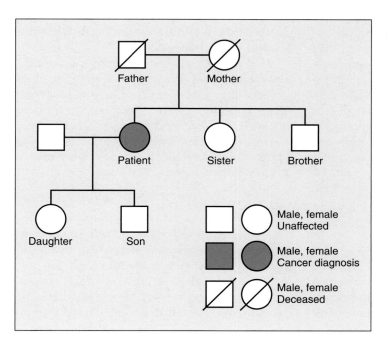

Figure 5-5. A pedigree provides a visual representation of a family history.

depending on clinic and provider preference. For patients with an identified mutation who receive a phone disclosure, a return visit is strongly recommended to finalize the management discussion, whereas those without a detectable mutation are given the option of a return visit. Patients, regardless of the result, are also encouraged to maintain periodic contact with the cancer genetics service, since it is a rapidly advancing field.

Special Considerations

Genetic Discrimination

Some patients are concerned about the potential for genetic discrimination, which is the theory that insurance companies could use genetic information to increase premiums or discontinue coverage. Federal HIPAA (The Health Insurance Portability and Accountability Act) legislation protects patients with group health insurance coverage so that individuals within the group cannot be dropped from the plan and individual rates within the group cannot be increased. However, premiums for the entire group can be increased, but this is less likely to happen with large groups. The federal legislation does not protect individually obtained health plans, however, such as those often held by people who are self-employed. Depending on the state in which a patient lives, there may be state-level protection that extends to individual policies. In addition, the Genetic Information Nondiscrimination Act (GINA) has been proposed, which is federal legislation that extends to individual health plans. Life, disability, and long-term care insurance have no protection from discrimination on the federal level or in many states. An important consideration, though, is that a patient's prior diagnosis of cancer is expected to have a greater impact on insurability than any subsequent genetic information about cancer risk. Therefore, genetic discrimination is often a greater concern for family members who have not been diagnosed with cancer.

Testing of Minors

The American College of Medical Genetics advises that genetic testing should be performed on minors only when the results will have an impact on medical management in childhood or adolescence. Although there are certainly exceptions, cancer is generally an adult-onset disease, even when associated with hereditary predisposition. With hereditary breast and ovarian cancer and Cowden syndrome, for example, screening is usually initiated between ages 25 and 35 years. Thus, for these syndromes, it is recommended that genetic testing be deferred until the age at which intensive screening is to begin so that the individual can decide for him- or herself whether the information is desired. With a notably early-onset cancer in a family, predictive genetic testing may be considered earlier than age 18 years, but is generally discouraged. By comparison, Peutz-Jeghers syndrome and Li-Fraumeni syndrome can cause childhood complications or malignancy, warranting consideration of genetic testing before the age of majority.

DNA Banking

Only 50% of hereditary breast cancer is explained by current genetic technology. Therefore, many of the women who undergo genetic testing will not have a detectable mutation, but whose testing may still be suspicious for a hereditary form of cancer. Because the genetic test results can be of great importance to family members, women with advanced breast cancer suggestive of a hereditary syndrome should be encouraged to consider DNA banking. DNA banking allows for storage of a DNA sample, making it accessible to family members in the future when more genes are identified. DNA banking is of particular consideration for women with advanced disease and a poor prognosis.

How to make a referral for genetic assessment or to a high-risk clinic: Most university medical centers offer cancer genetics services. Directories of cancer genetics professionals can be accessed through the National Society of Genetic Counselors (http://www.nsgc.org), GeneClinics (http://www.geneclinics.org), and the National Cancer Institute (http://www.cancer.gov).

Conclusion

The last 20 years have yielded substantial progress in the understanding of the basic science of hereditary breast cancer syndromes, the *BRCA1*, *BRCA2*, and rarer genes, and their role in hereditary cancer susceptibility. Developments in the translation of these findings into clinical applications are emerging, but important questions remain. Research is needed to better define not only the environmental and genetic factors dictating which mutation carriers will develop cancer, but also the efficacy of preventive interventions in this specific population.

Information on high-risk cancer genetics clinics is available on the websites of most National Cancer Institute (NCI)-designated comprehensive cancer centers. These facilities can provide a more detailed risk assessment as well as genetic counseling and testing, breast screening, and risk-reduction strategies for women at increased risk.

References

1. Ford D, Easton DF, Stratton M, et al: Genetic heterogeneity and penetrance analysis of the BRCA1 and BRCA2 genes in breast cancer families. The Breast Cancer Linkage Consortium. Am J Hum Genet 62(3):676–689, 1998.
2. Martin AM, Blackwood MA, Antin-Ozerkis D, et al: Germline mutations in BRCA1 and BRCA2 in breast-ovarian families from a breast cancer risk evaluation clinic. J Clin Oncol 19(8):2247–2253, 2001.
3. Garber JE: Validation of family history of breast cancer and identification of the BRCA1 and other syndromes using a population-based cancer registry. J Womens Health 6(3):349–351, 1997.
4. Brody LC, Biesecker BB: Breast cancer susceptibility genes. BRCA1 and BRCA2. Medicine 77(3):208–226, 1998.
5. Cass I, Baldwin RL, Varkey T, et al: Improved survival in women with BRCA-associated ovarian carcinoma. Cancer 97(9):2187–2195, 2003.
6. Camidge DR, Jodrell DI: Chemotherapy. In Knowles MA, Selby PJ (ed): Introduction to the Cellular and Molecular Biology of Cancer, 4th ed. New York: Oxford University Press, 2005, pp 399–413.
7. Ford D, Easton DF, Peto J: Estimates of the gene frequency of BRCA1 and its contribution to breast and ovarian cancer incidence. Am J Human Genet 57(6):1457–1462, 1995.
8. Risch HA, McLaughlin JR, Cole DE, et al: Population BRCA1 and BRCA2 mutation frequencies and cancer penetrances: a kin-cohort study in Ontario, Canada. J Natl Cancer Inst 98(23):1694–1706, 2006.
9. McClain MR, Palomaki GE, Nathanson KL, Haddow JE: Adjusting the estimated proportion of breast cancer cases associated with BRCA1 and BRCA2 mutations: public health implications. Genet Med 7(1):28–33, 2005.
10. Struewing JP, Hartge P, Wacholder S, et al: The risk of cancer associated with specific mutations of BRCA1 and BRCA2 among Ashkenazi Jews. N Engl J Med 336(20):1401–1408, 1997.
11. Hopper JL, Southey MC, Dite GS, et al: Population-based estimate of the average age-specific cumulative risk of breast cancer for a defined set of protein-truncating mutations in BRCA1 and BRCA2. Australian Breast Cancer Family Study. Cancer Epidemiol Biomarkers Prev 8(9):741–747, 1999.
12. King MC, Marks JH, Mandell JB, New York Breast Cancer Study G: Breast and ovarian cancer risks due to inherited mutations in BRCA1 and BRCA2. Science 302(5645):643–646, 2003.
13. Satagopan JM, Offit K, Foulkes W, et al: The lifetime risks of breast cancer in Ashkenazi Jewish carriers of BRCA1 and BRCA2 mutations. Cancer Epidemiol Biomarkers Prev 10(5):467–473, 2001.
14. Antoniou A, Pharoah PD, Narod S, et al: Average risks of breast and ovarian cancer associated with BRCA1 or BRCA2 mutations detected in case series unselected for family history: a combined analysis of 22 studies. Am J Hum Genet 72(5):1117–1130, 2003.
15. Ford D, Easton DF, Bishop DT, et al: Risks of cancer in BRCA1-mutation carriers. Breast Cancer Linkage Consortium. Lancet 343(8899):692–695, 1994.
16. Easton DF, Ford D, Bishop DT: Breast and ovarian cancer incidence in BRCA1-mutation carriers. Breast Cancer Linkage Consortium. Am J Hum Genet 56(1):265–271, 1995.
17. Chen S, Parmigiani G: Meta-analysis of BRCA1 and BRCA2 penetrance. J Clin Oncol 25(11):1329–1333, 2007.
18. Narod SA, Dube MP, Klijn J, et al: Oral contraceptives and the risk of breast cancer in BRCA1 and BRCA2 mutation carriers. J Natl Cancer Inst 94(23):1773–1779, 2002.
19. Gayther SA, Warren W, Mazoyer S, et al: Germline mutations of the BRCA1 gene in breast and ovarian cancer families provide evidence for a genotype-phenotype correlation. Nat Genet 1995;11(4):428–433, 1995.
20. Risch HA, McLaughlin JR, Cole DE, et al: Prevalence and penetrance of germline BRCA1 and BRCA2 mutations in a population series of 649 women with ovarian cancer. Am J Hum Genet 68(3):700–710, 2001.
21. Meijers-Heijboer EJ, Verhoog LC, Brekelmans CT, et al: Presymptomatic DNA testing and prophylactic surgery in families with a BRCA1 or BRCA2 mutation. Lancet 355(9220):2015–2020, 2000.
22. Claus EB, Schildkraut JM, Thompson WD, Risch NJ: The genetic attributable risk of breast and ovarian cancer. Cancer 77(11):2318–2324, 1996.
23. Hwang ES, McLennan JL, Moore DH, et al: Ductal carcinoma in situ in BRCA mutation carriers. J Clin Oncol 25(6):642–647, 2007.
24. Claus EB, Petruzella S, Matloff E, Carter D: Prevalence of BRCA1 and BRCA2 mutations in women diagnosed with ductal carcinoma in situ. JAMA 293(8):964–969, 2005.
25. Metcalfe K, Lynch HT, Ghadirian P, et al: Contralateral breast cancer in BRCA1 and BRCA2 mutation carriers. J Clin Oncol 22(12):2328–2335, 2004.
26. Pathology of familial breast cancer: differences between breast cancers in carriers of BRCA1 or BRCA2 mutations and sporadic cases. Breast Cancer Linkage Consortium. Lancet 349(9064):1505–1510, 1997.
27. Weber F, Shen L, Fukino K, et al: Total-genome analysis of BRCA1/2-related invasive carcinomas of the breast identifies tumor stroma as potential landscaper for neoplastic initiation. Am J Hum Genet 78(6):961–972, 2006.
28. Aziz S, Kuperstein G, Rosen B, et al: A genetic epidemiological study of carcinoma of the fallopian tube. Gynecol Oncol 80(3):341–345, 2001.
29. Cancer risks in BRCA2 mutation carriers. The Breast Cancer Linkage Consortium. J Natl Cancer Inst 91(15):1310–1316, 1999.
30. Risch HA, Weiss NS, Lyon JL, et al: Events of reproductive life and the incidence of epithelial ovarian cancer. Am J Epidemiol 117(2):128–139, 1983.
31. Narod SA, Risch H, Moslehi R, et al: Oral contraceptives and the risk of hereditary ovarian cancer. Hereditary Ovarian Cancer Clinical Study Group. N Engl J Med 339(7):424–428, 1998.
32. Modan B, Hartge P, Hirsh-Yechezkel G, et al: Parity, oral contraceptives, and the risk of ovarian cancer among carriers and noncarriers of a BRCA1 or BRCA2 mutation. N Engl J Med 345(4):235–240, 2001.
33. McLaughlin JR, Risch HA, Lubinski J, et al: Reproductive risk factors for ovarian cancer in carriers of BRCA1 or BRCA2 mutations: a case-control study. Lancet Oncol 8(1):26–34, 2007.
34. Walsh T, Casadei S, Coats KH, et al: Spectrum of mutations in BRCA1, BRCA2, CHEK2, and TP53 in families at high risk of breast cancer. JAMA 295(12):1379–1388, 2006.
35. Szabo CI, King MC: Population genetics of BRCA1 and BRCA2. Am J Hum Genet 60(5):1013–1020, 1997.
36. Saslow D, Boetes C, Burke W, et al: American Cancer Society Guidelines for Breast Screening with MRI as an Adjunct to Mammography. CA Cancer J Clin 57(2):75–89, 2007.
37. Lord SJ, Lei W, Craft P, et al: A systematic review of the effectiveness of magnetic resonance imaging (MRI) as an addition to mammography and ultrasound in screening young women at high risk of breast cancer. Eur J Cancer 43(13):1905–1917, 2007.
38. King MC, Wieand S, Hale K, et al: Tamoxifen and breast cancer incidence among women with inherited mutations in BRCA1 and BRCA2: National Surgical Adjuvant Breast and Bowel Project (NSABP-P1) Breast Cancer Prevention Trial. JAMA 286(18):2251–2256, 2001.
39. Narod SA, Brunet JS, Ghadirian P, et al: Tamoxifen and risk of contralateral breast cancer in BRCA1 and BRCA2 mutation car-

riers: a case-control study. Hereditary Breast Cancer Clinical Study Group. Lancet 356(9245):1876–1881, 2000.

40. Rebbeck TR, Friebel T, Lynch HT, et al: Bilateral prophylactic mastectomy reduces breast cancer risk in BRCA1 and BRCA2 mutation carriers: the PROSE Study Group. J Clin Oncol 22(6):1055–1062, 2004.
41. van Sprundel TC, Schmidt MK, Rookus MA, et al: Risk reduction of contralateral breast cancer and survival after contralateral prophylactic mastectomy in BRCA1 or BRCA2 mutation carriers. Br J Cancer 93(3):287–292, 2005.
42. Scheuer L, Kauff N, Robson M, et al: Outcome of preventive surgery and screening for breast and ovarian cancer in BRCA mutation carriers. J Clin Oncol 20(5):1260–1268, 2002.
43. Hogg R, Friedlander M: Biology of epithelial ovarian cancer: implications for screening women at high genetic risk. J Clin Oncol 22(7):1315–1327, 2004.
44. Rebbeck TR, Lynch HT, Neuhausen SL, et al: Prophylactic oophorectomy in carriers of BRCA1 or BRCA2 mutations. N Engl J Med 346(21):1616–1622, 2002.
45. Kauff ND, Satagopan JM, Robson ME, et al: Risk-reducing salpingo-oophorectomy in women with a BRCA1 or BRCA2 mutation. N Engl J Med 346(21):1609–1615, 2002.
46. Laki F, Kirova YM, This P, et al: Prophylactic salpingo-oophorectomy in a series of 89 women carrying a BRCA1 or a BRCA2 mutation. Cancer 109(9):1784–1790, 2007.
47. Domchek SM, Friebel TM, Neuhausen SL, et al: Mortality after bilateral salpingo-oophorectomy in BRCA1 and BRCA2 mutation carriers: a prospective cohort study. Lancet Oncol 7(3):223–229, 2006.
48. Kauff ND, Domchek SM, Friebel TM, et al: Multi-center prospective analysis of risk-reducing salpingo-oophorectomy to prevent BRCA-associated breast and ovarian cancer. J Clin Oncol 24:49s, 2006.
49. Chen S, Iversen ES, Friebel T, et al: Characterization of BRCA1 and BRCA2 mutations in a large United States sample. J Clin Oncol 24(6):863–871, 2006.
50. Li FP, Fraumeni JF Jr.: Soft-tissue sarcomas, breast cancer, and other neoplasms. A familial syndrome? Ann Intern Med 71(4):747–752, 1969.
51. Birch JM, Hartley AL, Tricker KJ, et al: Prevalence and diversity of constitutional mutations in the p53 gene among 21 Li-Fraumeni families. Cancer Res 54(5):1298–1304, 1994.
52. Birch JM, Alston RD, McNally RJ, et al: Relative frequency and morphology of cancers in carriers of germline TP53 mutations. Oncogene 20(34):4621–4628, 2001.
53. Nichols KE, Malkin D, Garber JE, et al: Germ-line p53 mutations predispose to a wide spectrum of early-onset cancers. Cancer Epidemiol Biomarkers Prev 10(2):83–87, 2001.
54. Wong P, Verselis SJ, Garber JE, et al: Prevalence of early onset colorectal cancer in 397 patients with classic Li-Fraumeni syndrome. Gastroenterology 130(1):73–79, 2006.
55. Krutilkova V, Trkova M, Fleitz J, et al: Identification of five new families strengthens the link between childhood choroid plexus carcinoma and germline TP53 mutations. Eur J Cancer 41(11):1597–1603, 2005.
56. Chompret A, Brugieres L, Ronsin M, et al: P53 germline mutations in childhood cancers and cancer risk for carrier individuals. Br J Cancer 82(12):1932–1937, 2000.
57. Olivier M, Goldgar DE, Sodha N, et al: Li-Fraumeni and related syndromes: correlation between tumor type, family structure, and TP53 genotype. Cancer Res 63(20):6643–6650, 2003.
58. Hisada M, Garber JE, Fung CY, et al: Multiple primary cancers in families with Li-Fraumeni syndrome. J Natl Cancer Inst 90(8):606–611, 1998.
59. Limacher JM, Frebourg T, Natarajan-Ame S, Bergerat JP: Two metachronous tumors in the radiotherapy fields of a patient with Li-Fraumeni syndrome. Int J Cancer 96(4):238–242, 2001.
60. Salmon A, Amikam D, Sodha N, et al: Rapid development of post-radiotherapy sarcoma and breast cancer in a patient with a novel germline 'de-novo' TP53 mutation. Clin Oncol 19(7):490–493, 2007.
61. Lane DP: Cancer. p53, guardian of the genome. Nature 358(6381):15–16, 1992.
62. Eng C: Cowden syndrome. J Genet Couns 6(2):181–192, 1997.
63. Fackenthal JD, Marsh DJ, Richardson AL, et al: Male breast cancer in Cowden syndrome patients with germline PTEN mutations. J Med Genet 38(3):159–164, 2001.
64. Eng C: Will the real Cowden syndrome please stand up: revised diagnostic criteria. J Med Genet 37(11):828–830, 2000.

65. Gustafson S, Zbuk KM, Scacheri C, Eng C: Cowden syndrome. Semin Oncol 34(5):428–434, 2007.
66. Eng C: PTEN: one gene, many syndromes. Hum Mutat 22(3):183–198, 2003.
67. Hinds R, Philp C, Hyer W, Fell JM: Complications of childhood Peutz-Jeghers syndrome: implications for pediatric screening. J Pediatr Gastroenterol Nutr 39(2):219–220, 2004.
68. Boardman LA, Thibodeau SN, Schaid DJ, et al: Increased risk for cancer in patients with the Peutz-Jeghers syndrome. Ann Intern Med 128(11):896–899, 1998.
69. Lim W, Hearle N, Shah B, et al: Further observations on LKB1/STK11 status and cancer risk in Peutz-Jeghers syndrome. Br J Cancer 89(2):308–313, 2003.
70. Giardiello FM, Brensinger JD, Tersmette AC, et al: Very high risk of cancer in familial Peutz-Jeghers syndrome. Gastroenterology 119(6):1447–1453, 2000.
71. Young RH: Sex cord-stromal tumors of the ovary and testis: their similarities and differences with consideration of selected problems. Mod Pathol 18(Suppl 2):S81–S98, 2005.
72. Young S, Gooneratne S, Straus FH II, et al: Feminizing Sertoli cell tumors in boys with Peutz-Jeghers syndrome. Am J Surg Pathol 19(1):50–58, 1995.
73. Hearle N, Schumacher V, Menko FH, et al: Frequency and spectrum of cancers in the Peutz-Jeghers syndrome. Clin Cancer Res 12(10):3209–3215, 2006.
74. Lim W, Olschwang S, Keller JJ, et al: Relative frequency and morphology of cancers in STK11 mutation carriers. Gastroenterology 126(7):1788–1794, 2004.
75. Riley E, Swift M: A family with Peutz-Jeghers syndrome and bilateral breast cancer. Cancer 46(4):815–817, 1980.
76. Conneely JB, Kell MR, Boran S, et al: A case of bilateral breast cancer with Peutz-Jeghers syndrome. Eur J Surg Oncol 32(1):121–122, 2006.
77. Karuman P, Gozani O, Odze RD, et al: The Peutz-Jeghers gene product LKB1 is a mediator of p53-dependent cell death. Mol Cells 7(6):1307–1319, 2001.
78. Aretz S, Stienen D, Uhlhaas S, et al: High proportion of large genomic STK11 deletions in Peutz-Jeghers syndrome. Hum Mutat 26(6):513–519, 2005.
79. Giardiello FM, Trimbath JD: Peutz-Jeghers syndrome and management recommendations. Clin Gastroenterol Hepatol 4(4):408–415, 2006.
80. Guilford P, Hopkins J, Harraway J, et al: E-cadherin germline mutations in familial gastric cancer. Nature 392(6674):402–405, 1998.
81. Pharoah PD, Guilford P, Caldas C: Incidence of gastric cancer and breast cancer in CDH1 (E-cadherin) mutation carriers from hereditary diffuse gastric cancer families. Gastroenterology 121(6):1348–1353, 2001.
82. Kaurah P, MacMillan A, Boyd N, et al: Founder and recurrent CDH1 mutations in families with hereditary diffuse gastric cancer. JAMA 297(21):2360–2372, 2007.
83. Qureshi HS, Linden MD, Divine G, Raju UB: E-cadherin status in breast cancer correlates with histologic type but does not correlate with established prognostic parameters. Am J Clin Pathol 125(3):377–385, 2006.
84. Brooks-Wilson AR, Kaurah P, Suriano G, et al: Germline E-cadherin mutations in hereditary diffuse gastric cancer: assessment of 42 new families and review of genetic screening criteria. J Med Genet 41(7):508–517, 2004.
85. Masciari S, Larsson N, Senz J, et al: Germline E-cadherin mutations in familial lobular breast cancer. J Med Genet 44(11):726–731, 2007.
86. Schelfout K, Van Goethem M, Kersschot E, et al: Preoperative breast MRI in patients with invasive lobular breast cancer. Eur Radiol 14(7):1209–1216, 2004.
87. Ahmed M, Rahman N: ATM and breast cancer susceptibility. Oncogene 25(43):5906–5911, 2006.
88. Prokopcova J, Kleibl Z, Banwell CM, Pohlreich P: The role of ATM in breast cancer development. Breast Cancer Res Treat 104(2):121–128, 2007.
89. Evans DG, Birch JM, Narod SA: Is CHEK2 a cause of the Li-Fraumeni syndrome? J Med Genet 45(1):63–64, 2008.
90. Weischer M, Bojesen SE, Ellervik C, et al: CHEK2*1100delC genotyping for clinical assessment of breast cancer risk: meta-analyses of 26,000 patient cases and 27,000 controls. J Clin Oncol 26(4):542–548, 2008.
91. Offit K, Garber JE: Time to check CHEK2 in families with breast cancer? J Clin Oncol 26(4):519–520, 2008.

6

Strategies for Risk Reduction

Anna Voltura and Lisa Jacobs

KEY POINTS

- Chemoprevention is the use of chemotherapeutics to stabilize, suppress, or reverse the mechanisms whereby a precancerous lesion becomes a cancerous lesion.
- The 1992 National Surgical Adjutant Breast and Bowel Project 1 (NSABP) launched the Breast Cancer Prevention Trial P-1 (BCPT P-1) to evaluate the potential of tamoxifen as a chemopreventive drug for breast cancer in high-risk women (i.e., age 60 years or older and women 35 to 59 with a Gail model risk of 1.66 or a history of lobular carcinoma in situ [LCIS]) and found that tamoxifen reduced the risk of invasive cancer by 49% and ductal carcinoma in situ (DCIS) by 50%. In women with atypical ductal hyperplasia (ADH), the risk was reduced by 56% and in those with LCIS by 86%. Women with a *BRCA2* mutation had a reduction of 62%.
- The Study of Tamoxifen and Raloxifene (STAR/P2) trial proved that raloxifene (Evista) was equivalent to tamoxifen in risk reduction for invasive cancer but not for DCIS.
- Both tamoxifen and raloxifene increase the risk of endometrial cancer, thromboembolic events, cataracts, and stroke.
- Tamoxifen and raloxifene have both been approved by the Food and Drug Administration (FDA) for use in chemoprevention of breast cancer in high-risk women.
- European studies have confirmed tamoxifen for use in high-risk women to reduce the occurrence of breast cancer.
- Aromatase inhibitors are under study as chemopreventive agents in breast cancer.
- Soy has not proved to be chemopreventive in breast cancer but is thought to have a protective effect.
- Genetic counseling is imperative in determining those women who have an increased risk of breast cancer and may benefit from tamoxifen or raloxifene.
- Physicians who dispense tamoxifen and raloxifene for chemoprevention of breast cancer must be skilled at risk determination of breast cancer, risk of tamoxifen and raloxifene use, and counseling.
- Bilateral prophylactic mastectomy is considered for patients who do not have a breast cancer diagnosis but are at high risk for developing the disease.
- Contralateral prophylactic mastectomy is considered for patients who have a current or previous diagnosis of breast cancer.
- High-risk patients are those with *BRCA* mutations, a strong family history of breast cancer, or histologic risk factors.
- Other reasons for prophylactic mastectomy include conditions that make surveillance difficult and reconstructive issues.
- A multidisciplinary team approach to patient selection is necessary when discussing prophylactic mastectomy with a patient.
- Counseling on the risks and benefits of prophylactic mastectomy and on reconstruction and psychosocial issues of the procedure is essential.

For those women at increased risk of developing breast cancer, improved methods of risk and genetic assessment have occurred simultaneously with improved methods of risk reduction. Women identified as having an increased risk for development of breast cancer can be offered a variety of increased surveillance strategies or risk-reducing interventions. Chemoprevention combined with increased surveillance is one option. A second option is surgical risk reduction with prophylactic mastectomy.

The selection of women who should be counseled regarding risk-reduction strategies is dependent on reliable and thorough risk assessment (see Chapters 4 and 5). After a woman has been identified as having increased risk of developing breast cancer, a variety of options are available to her, ranging from increased surveillance to chemoprevention to surgical intervention. Multidisciplinary evaluation and management, including overall health of the woman, comorbid conditions, possible risks and benefits of each method, psychological impact of the intervention, and long-term consequences must be considered before a management strategy is implemented.

CHEMOPREVENTION

Concepts of Chemoprevention

The concept of chemoprevention was eloquently presented by Michael Sporn[1] in 1975 while discussing the use of retinoids in prevention of epithelial cancers. The discussion centered on the idea that cancer prevention should be studied and implemented in the fight against cancer. The process of a normal cell becoming a cancerous cell is one that occurs over time, and if we can stop the advancement of that process we can actually prevent the cancer from occurring. Chemoprevention is the use of chemotherapies to stabilize, suppress, or reverse the mechanisms by which a precancerous lesion becomes a cancerous lesion. Breast cancer research has led the way in analyzing and implementing models of chemoprevention.

Chemoprevention for breast cancer evolved from the treatment of breast cancer. Tamoxifen, a first-generation selective estrogen receptor modulator (SERM) has been extensively used in the treatment of breast cancer. Many studies of tamoxifen use in breast cancer treatment have shown a secondary effect of reducing primary breast cancer in the contralateral breast by 40% to 50%.[2-4] This finding elucidated tamoxifen as a chemopreventive agent for breast cancer and launched the first prospective randomized phase III trial of the efficacy of any chemopreventive agent—this one specifically for preventing breast cancer in high-risk women.[5] Figure 6-1 shows the decision points that a SERM must pass to modulate estrogen-like actions in a target tissue.

Tamoxifen Chemoprevention Studies

In 1992, the National Adjuvant Breast and Bowel Project (NSABP) started the Breast Cancer Prevention Trial P-1 (BCPT P-1) to evaluate the potential of tamoxifen in preventing breast cancer in high-risk women.[6] In this study, 13,388 women 35 years and older with

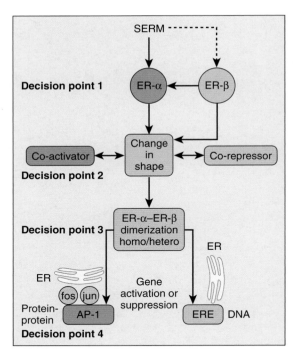

Figure 6-1. Decision points that a selective estrogen receptor modulator (SERM) must pass to modulate estrogen-like actions in a target tissue. A SERM can bind to either ER-α or ER-β, and the complexes can then recruit co-activators or co-repressors. The complexes might homo- or heterodimerize and modulate genes by either a nontraditional pathway of protein-protein interactions (AP-1) or a traditional pathway (ER-DNA). (From Park WC, Jordan VC: Selective estrogen receptor modulators (SERMS) and their roles in breast cancer. Trends Mol Med 8(2):82–88, 2002.)

an increased risk of breast cancer according to the Gail model risk factors were randomized to tamoxifen 20 mg a day or placebo for 5 years (Table 6-1). The Gail model is based on age, number of first-degree relatives with breast cancer, nulliparity or age at first live birth, number of breast biopsies, presence of atypical hyperplasia, and age at menarche.[7] The three high-risk groups included women 60 years of age and older (baseline risk 1.66), women 35 to 59 years who had a predicted 5-year risk of breast cancer development of at least 1.66, and women who had a history of lobular carcinoma in situ (LCIS).[8] In the final analysis (Table 6-2), the cohort's 5-year predicted breast cancer risk ratio was an average of 2.33, whereas 70% of the women were younger than 60 years.

The results of the BCPT P-1 trial were overwhelmingly positive, and the trial was unblinded in 1998. Among women with increased risk of

Table 6-1. Cohort Characteristics of the BCPT P-1 Trial

Age (years)	
35–39	2.6%
40–49	36.7%
50–59	30.8%
60–69	24.0%
>70	6.0%
Ethnicity/race	
White	96.4%
Black	1.7%
Other races	1.9%
Risk assessment	
History of lobular carcinoma in situ	6.3%
History of atypical ductal hyperplasia	9.1%
No first-degree relative with breast cancer	23.8%
One first-degree relative with breast cancer	56.8%
Two first-degree relatives with breast cancer	16.4%
Three or more first-degree relatives with breast cancer	3.0%
Prior surgery	
Women with hysterectomy	37.1%

Data from Fisher B, Costantino JP, Wickerham L, et al: Tamoxifen for prevention of breast cancer: report of the National Surgical Adjuvant Breast and Bowel Project P-1 Study. J Natl Cancer Inst 90(18):1371–1388, 1998, Table 2.

Table 6-2. BCPT P-1: Percentage of Women per Risk Ratio

Risk Ratio	Percentage of Women
≤2.00	25.0
2.01–3.00	31.0
3.01–5.00	26.6
≥5.01	17.4

Data from Fisher B, Costantino JP, Wickerham L, et al: Tamoxifen for prevention of breast cancer: report of the National Surgical Adjuvant Breast and Bowel Project P-1 Study. J Natl Cancer Inst 90(18):1371–1388, 1998, Table 2.

Table 6-3. BCPT P-1: Percentage of Invasive Breast Cancer Reduced

Total group	49
Women < 49 yr	44
Women 50–59 yr	51
Women > 60 yr	55
Women with LCIS	56
Women with ADH	86

LCIS, lobular carcinoma in situ; ADH, atypical ductal hyperplasia.
Data from Fisher B, Costantino JP, Wickerham L, et al: Tamoxifen for prevention of breast cancer: report of the National Surgical Adjuvant Breast and Bowel Project P-1 Study. J Natl Cancer Inst 90(18):1371–1388, 1998, Table 2.

gen receptor. How then does tamoxifen affect tumors of women with mutations in *BRCA1* and *BRCA2*? *BRCA1* tumors tend to be ER negative, whereas *BRCA2* tumors tend to be ER positive. Blood samples were obtained from BCPT participants at entry into the initial study. Genomic analysis of *BRCA1* and *BRCA2* for 288 women who developed breast cancer after entry into the BCPT was undertaken.[9] Tamoxifen reduced breast cancer incidence in *BRCA2* carriers by 62%, whereas it did not reduce the incidence in *BRCA1* carriers who tend toward ER-negative tumors.[9] In 2005, an update of the initial findings from the BCPT P-1 trial was presented. After 7 years' follow-up, the data still support the conclusive results.[8]

Tamoxifen Risks and Complications

We cannot speak of the benefits of tamoxifen without speaking of the possible risks and complications. Women who received tamoxifen in the BCPT P-1 trial had a 2.53 greater risk of endometrial cancer. The absolute risk of developing endometrial cancer was 0.79% in the tamoxifen group compared with 0.37% in the control group. The risk was higher in women over 50 years old, who demonstrated a risk ratio of 4.01 in developing endometrial cancer while taking tamoxifen.[6] Although the development of endometrial cancer has long been thought to be the major disadvantage of taking tamoxifen, all the endometrial tumors found in women in the trial were early-stage and readily treated. No deaths from endometrial cancer occurred. There was an increase in cataract development and consequent surgery for cataracts in women taking tamoxifen, with a risk ratio average of 1.35, indicating only a very slight significance.[6]

breast cancer, tamoxifen reduced the risk of invasive breast cancer by 49% and the risk of noninvasive breast cancer (ductal carcinoma in situ [DCIS]) by 50%.[6] The amount of risk reduction varied with age and with diagnosis of LCIS and atypical ductal hyperplasia (ADH) (Table 6-3). Although women of all ages saw a benefit from tamoxifen, the greatest effect was seen in women with ADH and LCIS, with a decrease of 56% and 86%, respectively, in the incidence of breast cancer. Tamoxifen reduced the incidence of estrogen-receptor (ER) positive tumors but had no effect on ER-negative tumors. This is logical since tamoxifen targets the estro-

A 19.5% decrease in fractures was also seen in the group of women taking tamoxifen. However, this did not reach statistical significance.[6]

Thromboembolic events were seen at an impressively high rate and proved to be a more worrisome complication in those taking tamoxifen. Pulmonary embolus was increased by a risk ratio of 3.01.[6] Pulmonary emboli were seen predominantly in women 50 years and over by a risk ratio of 3.19 compared with women 49 years and younger, who had a risk ratio of 2.03. Deep venous thrombosis was also seen more often in women who took tamoxifen compared with that seen in the control group. Again, the incidence occurred more often in women 50 years and older with a risk ratio of 1.71, compared with 1.39 in women 49 years and younger. Stroke incidence was only slightly increased in the tamoxifen group with a risk ratio of 1.59, which was not statistically significant. It is interesting that the incidence of heart disease was the same in both groups, indicating no protection from heart disease with tamoxifen.

Raloxifene Chemoprevention Studies

In an effort to continue to search for a drug with a high-benefit, low-risk ratio for use in the prevention of breast cancer, the NSABP initiated another study. The Study of Tamoxifen and Raloxifene (STAR) P-2 trial began on July 1, 1999, and closed on December 31, 2005.[10] The study group consisted of 19,747 postmenopausal women of mean age 58.5 years with a mean risk ratio of 4.03 for developing breast cancer in 5 years (Table 6-4). The STAR trial disseminated from the Multiple Outcomes of Raloxifene Evaluation (MORE) trial and the subsequent

4-year follow-up trial, Continuing Outcomes Relevant to Evista (CORE) trial.[11] These studies were undertaken to assess raloxifene in preventing fractures in postmenopausal women. A secondary outcome from the MORE and CORE trials was that raloxifene was noted to reduce the risk of breast cancer compared with tamoxifen, whereas it may have a decreased risk of endometrial cancer compared with tamoxifen.[11] A subsequent study looking at the breakdown of subgroups in the MORE and CORE trials published in 2006 showed that raloxifene reduced the risk of breast cancer in postmenopausal women regardless of risk factors. However, the effect was greater in women with increased risk of developing breast cancer, varying from 33% to 89% decreases in breast cancer occurrence congruent with the estimated risk.[12] This proved that the effect of raloxifene was greater in higher-risk women. Other examinations of the MORE study data have shown that the reduction of breast cancer risk seen in the use of raloxifene is dependent on the level of endogenous estrogen (Fig. 6-2).

The STAR P-2 trial results were published in 2006 and established that raloxifene was as effective in reducing the risk of invasive breast cancer; however, it did not reduce the risk of DCIS.[10] The raloxifene group had fewer thromboembolic events and cataracts but the same

Table 6-4. Risk Ratio According to Percentage of Women in STAR P-2 Trial	
Risk Ratio	**Percentage of Women**
≤2.00	11.0
2.01–3.00	30.3
3.01–5.00	31.4
≥5.01	27.3

Data from Vogel VG, Costantino JP, Wickerham L, et al: Effects of tamoxifen vs raloxifene on the risk of developing invasive breast cancer and other disease outcomes: The NSABP Study of Tamoxifen and Raloxifene (STAR) P-2 Trial. JAMA 295(23):2727–2926, 2006, Table 1.

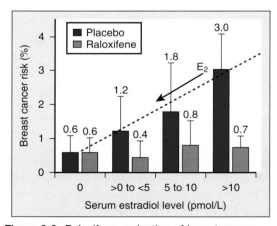

Figure 6-2. Raloxifene, reduction of breast cancer risk, and endogenous estrogen levels. In the MORE study, the reduction of breast cancer seen in the use of raloxifene is dependent on the endogenous estrogen level. E_2, estradiol. (From Cummings SR, Duong T, Kenyon E, et al: Serum estradiol level and risk of breast cancer during treatment with raloxifene. JAMA 287:216–220, 2002.)

risk of endometrial cancer.[10] It should be noted that the rate of risk of endometrial cancer in the raloxifene group was 38% lower than in the tamoxifen group; however, it was not statistically significant. Even more importantly, the risk of thromboembolic events was decreased by 30% in the raloxifene group compared with the tamoxifen group, which was significantly different. This should be emphasized, especially considering that the group experiencing thromboembolic events more often were the women who were over 50 years and who had greater representation in the STAR study (Table 6-5). Therefore, the STAR trial gave us another useful chemopreventive agent in the fight against breast cancer, though in a different group of women. Raloxifene is an alternative for lowering the risk of breast cancer in postmenopausal women with moderate to high Gail model risk scores and in those with LCIS.[10] Raloxifene has recently been approved by the Food and Drug Administration (FDA) for use in breast cancer prevention in high-risk women.

Table 6-5. Cohort Characteristics in STAR P-2 Trial

Characteristic	Percentage of Women
Age (years)	
<49	9.0
50–59	49.8
60–69	32.4
>70	8.7
Race/ethnicity	
White	93.5
African American	2.4
Hispanic	2.0
Other	2.1
Risk assessment	
No first-degree relatives with breast cancer	28.8
One first-degree relative with breast cancer	52.2
Two first-degree relatives with breast cancer	15.9
Three or more first-degree relatives with breast cancer	3.0
History of lobular carcinoma in situ	9.2
History of atypical ductal hyperplasia	22.8
Hysterectomy	51.4

Data from Vogel VG, Costantino JP, Wickerham L, et al: Effects of tamoxifen vs raloxifene on the risk of developing invasive breast cancer and other disease outcomes: The NSABP Study of Tamoxifen and Raloxifene (STAR) P-2 Trial. JAMA 295(23):2727–2926, 2006, Table 1.

International Chemoprevention Studies

Another trial, International Breast Cancer Intervention Study (IBIS-1), enrolled 7154 women between 1992 and 2001.[13] This was a double-blind study in which women took either tamoxifen or placebo for 5 years with a median follow-up of 8 years. The primary outcome was the occurrence of invasive breast cancer or DCIS. These women were between 35 and 70 years old and were eligible on the following criteria: at least a 2.0 relative risk of breast cancer development for ages 45 to 70, a 4.0 relative risk for ages 40 to 44, and a 10.0 relative risk for ages 35 to 39. This study was conducted in Australia, New Zealand, and the United Kingdom. Obviously, these women had a much higher cumulative risk than those in the BCPT P-1 and P-2 trials. Initial results released in 2002 indicated a risk reduction of 32%, which was not statistically significant. There was no significant increase in endometrial cancer; however, there was a significant increase in thromboembolic events.[13] Of note is that nearly 50% of the thromboembolic events occurred within 3 months of major surgery or prolonged immobilization. The initial interpretation was that there was not enough evidence to support a positive benefit-to-risk ratio. In 2007, after a median follow-up of 96 months, the results subsequently confirmed that tamoxifen reduces the risk of ER-positive breast cancer in women who have a significantly increased risk for developing breast cancer.[14] Note that this study indicates that the effects of tamoxifen last for at least 10 years after follow-up, whereas the major adverse effects do not continue after the 5-year treatment period.[14]

Two large European studies have also looked at tamoxifen in the prevention of breast cancer: the Royal Marsden Tamoxifen Breast Cancer Prevention Trial (Marsden) from Great Britain and the Italian Randomized Tamoxifen Prevention Trial Among Women with Hysterectomy (Italian). Early results from these trials showed minimal protective effect from tamoxifen, possibly because of the small number of women enrolled (Fig. 6-3). However, both studies have recently reported significant positive results with tamoxifen in the prevention of breast cancer in high-risk women.[15,16] The Marsden trial enrolled a total number of 2471, with a median 13.2-year follow-up. The women were randomly assigned

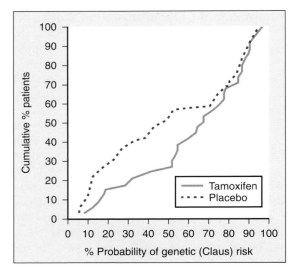

Figure 6-3. Analysis of the Marsden Tamoxifen Trial. Seventy patients developed breast cancer during the Marsden trial. There was a reduced incidence of breast cancer in women on tamoxifen who had a lower risk on the Claus model, but the difference was not statistically significant (*P* = .06). (From Kote-Jarai Z, Powles TJ, Mitchell G, et al: BRCA1/BRCA2 mutation status and analysis of cancer family history in participants of the Royal Marsden Hospital Tamoxifen Chemoprevention Trial. Cancer Lett 247:259–265, 2007.)

to take tamoxifen daily or placebo for 8 years. The primary outcome was the occurrence of invasive breast cancer. The results showed a 39% decrease in the incidence of breast cancer in ER-positive tumors.[15] This was seen after the 8-year treatment period compared with during the treatment period. This seemed to indicate a long-term preventive effect rather than a treatment effect of tamoxifen.[15] In this trial, participants were younger and had a higher relative risk that was based on their family history of breast cancer. The difference in patient characteristics and the sample size studied may account for the differences in initial findings (Table 6-6).

The Italian study, which also initially demonstrated no reduction in risk of breast cancer, recently reported its findings after 11 years of

follow-up.[16] The study ran from October 1, 1992, until December 31, 1997. Women who had undergone hysterectomy (*n* = 5408) were enrolled and were given tamoxifen (20 mg/day) for 5 years or placebo. Fifty percent of the women had also undergone bilateral oophorectomy and were therefore considered low risk for developing breast cancer. The results indicate that tamoxifen decreases the risk of breast cancer in high-risk women. Women who had bilateral oophorectomy or were otherwise at low risk for developing breast cancer did not see a decrease in breast cancer incidence with tamoxifen.[16] It is interesting to note that the women who were taking hormonal replacement therapy (HRT) at the time of the study did not stop HRT. The study did reveal a 50% to 60% decreased incidence of breast cancer in women taking HRT in the tamoxifen arm versus those taking placebo.[16]

Impact of Chemoprevention on Benign Breast Disease

The plethora of data obtained from the BCPT P-1 trial has many uses for various types of analysis. One interesting substudy was concerned with how tamoxifen affects benign breast disease. This was published in 2003 and concludes that women who received tamoxifen, especially those younger than 50 years, had a reduced incidence of clinically detected benign breast disease and therefore obtained fewer breast biopsies.[17] The types of benign breast disease evaluated are listed in Box 6-1. Of these, the decrease in incidence was more often seen in hyperplasia and metaplasia.[17] Biopsies required for hyperplasia and metaplasia were significantly reduced by 41% in premenopausal women. This could potentially decrease the morbidity and costs of continual radiographic and surgical diagnosis and treatment associated with benign breast disease. Does this outweigh the risk of taking tamoxifen? The study did not advocate

Table 6-6. Cohort Characteristics in International Trials			
Trial	**Size of Cohort**	**Mean Age (years)**	**Mean Risk Ratio**
International Breast Cancer Intervention Study-1	7152	35–70	2.0–10.0
Royal Marsden Tamoxifen Breast Cancer Prevention Trial	2471	47	Family history
Italian Randomized Tamoxifen Prevention Trial	5408	30–70	Not reported

Box 6-1. Types of Benign Breast Disease Assessed	
Adenosis	Fibroadenoma
Cyst	Fibrosis
Duct ectasia	Hyperplasia
Fibrocystic disease	Metaplasia

the use of tamoxifen in cases of established benign breast disease, but rather it emphasized the effects of tamoxifen on tumor genesis at an earlier stage than was previously thought.[17]

Aromatase Inhibitor Chemoprevention Studies

Aromatase inhibitors are now being tested in breast cancer prevention trials.[18] They are the most frequently used antihormonal treatment for ER breast cancer in postmenopausal women. Aromatase inhibitors suppress aromatase enzyme activity, thus decreasing the production of estrogen. Adverse effects are therefore from the overall depletion of estrogen. There is no increase in endometrial cancer or thromboembolic events, as seen with tamoxifen. However, aromatase inhibitors are associated with an increase in bone fractures, vaginal dryness, loss of libido, and musculoskeletal symptoms.[18] The ongoing trials testing aromatose inhibitors for prevention are International Breast Cancer Intervention Study II, Aromasin Prevention Study, and the National Cancer Institute of Canada Clinical Trials Group MAP.3 Breast Cancer Prevention Trial.[18] The results of these studies will be interesting and may very well change how we practice chemoprevention for breast cancer.

Phytoestrogens as Chemopreventive Agents

Other areas of study for chemoprevention have focused on phytoestrogens or soy products. Initially, it was thought that phytoestrogens may be protective against breast cancer because of the low incidence of breast cancer in Asian women, who have high phytoestrogen consumption. It has been further noted that when Asian women adopt a Western diet and lifestyle, the rate of breast cancer increases. This association has recently been disproved by a prospective longitudinal study, the Japan Collaborative

Cohort (JACC) Study.[19] The study ran from 1988 to 1990 and included 30,454 women ages 40 to 79, with a mean follow-up of 7.6 years. The women completed a questionnaire on diet and other lifestyle features, and hazard ratios were then calculated to assess the association between soy intake and the risk of breast cancer. This longitudinal study demonstrated that there was no significant association between the risk of breast cancer and the consumption of phytoestrogens.[19-21] The JACC also looked at fat and fatty acids in this same cohort and found that there was no increased risk of breast cancer associated with total or saturated fat intake.[20] However, it did suggest a protective effect of long-chain omega-3 fatty acids abundantly found in fish.[19,20] These same studies have indicated that the importance of phytoestrogen consumption may be ingestion during puberty or possibly when in utero through the placenta.

Strategies for Preventing Estrogen Receptor-Negative Tumors

As previously discussed, tamoxifen reduces the incidence of ER-positive tumors but has no effect on ER-negative tumors. Strategies to prevent ER-negative tumors are actively being sought, with phase I and II chemoprevention trials of novel agents targeting alternative important molecular pathways (Fig. 6-4). A number of trials with new potential chemopreventive agents are being planned in women with an increased risk for ER-negative breast cancer. These include tyrosine kinase inhibitors, cyclin-dependent kinase inhibitors, ligands for peroxisome proliferator-activated receptor c (PPAR ligands, glitazones), RXR selective ligands (rexinoids), COX (cyclooxygenase)-2 selective inhibitors, demethylating agents, histone deacetilase inhibitors, and vitamin D_3 derivatives.[22]

Translation of Studies into Clinical Use of Tamoxifen

The BCPT P-1 is a landmark trial that has brought chemoprevention to the threshold of being the standard of care. Shortly after presentation of the data from the BCPT P-1, the FDA approved tamoxifen for use as a chemopreventive agent in high-risk women. Raloxifene was initially FDA approved for use in the prevention and treatment of osteoporosis in postmeno-

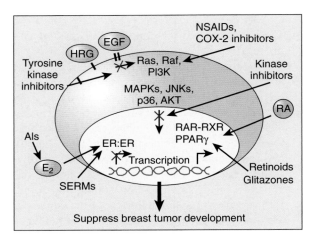

Figure 6-4. Novel targets for the prevention of breast cancer. Strategies to prevent estrogen receptor (ER)-negative tumors are actively being sought. Potential chemopreventive agents include tyrosine kinase inhibitors, cyclin-dependent kinase inhibitors, ligands for peroxisome. E_2, estradiol; NSAIDS, nonsteroidal noninflammatory drugs; SERMs, selective estrogen receptor modulators. (From Gasco M, Argusti, A, Bonanni B, Decensi A: SERMs in chemoprevention of breast cancer. Eur J Cancer 41:1980–1989, 2005.)

pausal women and only recently was approved for chemoprevention for postmenopausal women at high risk for breast cancer. More than 500,000 women in the United States are taking raloxifene for osteoporosis.[10] Some of these women are also getting the benefit of decreased breast cancer incidence, which may be part of the reason their physicians chose raloxifene to treat their osteoporosis. The update of the BCPT P-1 trial presented in 2005 claims that 2.5 million women could have a net benefit from the use of tamoxifen.[8] Why then do we not see tamoxifen used more often in the setting of chemoprevention?

All these data support tamoxifen for prevention of breast cancer. The next step is to translate these findings into clinical practice. The risk of developing breast cancer is the primary determining factor of the net benefit of tamoxifen as a chemopreventive agent. The higher the risk of breast cancer, the greater the net benefit. The absolute risks from tamoxifen of endometrial cancer, stroke, pulmonary embolus, and deep venous thrombosis increase with age and differ between black and white women.[23] Therefore, tamoxifen is most beneficial for younger women who have an elevated risk of breast cancer.[23] Tamoxifen appears to reduce the risk of developing ER-positive breast cancer for at least 10 to 15 years after treatment ends.[13,15,24]

Translation of the prevention trials into clinical use must first be approached by calculating the risk of developing breast cancer. The method of calculating the 5-year risk was based on the model of Gail and colleagues.[7,23] A computer program designed to help health care practitioners estimate the risk of invasive breast cancer for a given patient can be obtained from the National Cancer Institute.[23] Other strong risk factors include women with LCIS who have a risk ratio of 6.47 and women with DCIS who have a risk ratio of 14.7.[23] Women who carry the mutations in *BRCA1* and *BRCA2* are thought to have a cumulative breast cancer risk of 37% to 85%.[23] Thus, when counseling a patient on the use of tamoxifen in prevention of breast cancer, the patient's risk needs to be adequately estimated.

Genetic Counseling

Genetic counseling is imperative in helping to determine which women are at high risk for breast cancer and may therefore benefit from taking tamoxifen. A well-trained genetic counselor can calculate the relative risk for the patient and then discuss possible options for prevention. Physicians who counsel patients on the use of tamoxifen for prevention of breast cancer need to be adequately trained in counseling patients based on benefit:risk ratio. Counseling includes involving the patient in the decision-making process. Analyzing the patient's quantitative risk of developing breast cancer is essential. Evaluating the patient's risk of incurring potential side effects cannot be understated. Weighing the patient's perceived risk of breast cancer is also important.[23,25] Risk perception has been shown to be associated with health behavior.[25] Accurately analyzing a patient's risk and subsequently educating this patient on her risk can alleviate false risk perception (either high or low). If a patient understands her true risk, she can then monitor her health behavior appropriately.[25]

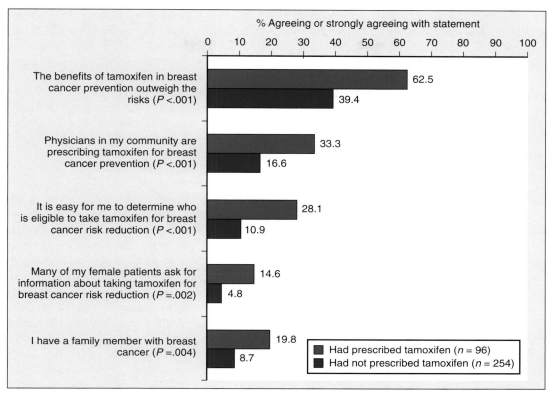

Figure 6-5. Prescription of tamoxifen for breast cancer prevention by primary care physicians. A survey of 350 physicians showed that relatively few (27.4%) had prescribed tamoxifen for breast cancer prevention. Certain attitudes were also strongly associated with a willingness to prescribe tamoxifen for breast cancer prevention. (From Armstrong K, Quistbert DA, Mico E, et al: Prescription of tamoxifen for breast cancer prevention by primary care physicians. Arch Intern Med 166:2260–2265, 2006.)

Tamoxifen is well known to oncologists, who have used it for years in the treatment of breast cancer. To other types of physicians, tamoxifen is viewed as a cancer drug and thus characterized as toxic. It is felt that primary care physicians, who are the most involved in preventive care, view tamoxifen as too toxic.[26] In contrast, primary care physicians are familiar with raloxifene, which is widely prescribed for the prevention and treatment of osteoporosis in postmenopausal women. In a recent study, it was found that primary care physicians who prescribed tamoxifen for breast cancer prevention were older and less likely to be women and saw more than 100 patients per week.[26] They were also more likely to have a family member with breast cancer[26] (Fig. 6-5). Overall, the factor most commonly associated with a prescription of tamoxifen was the patient's request for information about tamoxifen. Therefore, familiarity with tamoxifen, knowledge of the conclusive studies, and the ability to calculate a patient's

risk are important factors in prescribing tamoxifen for breast cancer prevention.

Cost-Effectiveness of Tamoxifen and Chemoprevention

It is interesting to look at the cost-effectiveness of tamoxifen in the prevention of breast cancer. Obviously, many women who have an increased risk of breast cancer will never develop breast cancer. For women with a 5-year risk of 1.66 of developing breast cancer, one would have to treat 120 women to save 1 from getting breast cancer. For women with an increased risk ratio of 2.3, one would have to treat 87 women to prevent 1 from getting breast cancer. Tamoxifen is felt to be cost-effective as a primary breast cancer prevention in women with prior ADH, LCIS, or a 5-year Gail model risk score of 5 or greater.[24] In this group of women, one would have to treat 40 to save 1 from getting breast cancer. The cost-effectiveness of tamoxifen use in breast cancer prevention is significant. The incremental cost-effectiveness of tamoxifen is $41,372 per life-year gained for women 35 to 49 years; for women 50 to 59 years and older than 60 cost-effectiveness is $68,349 and $74,981, respectively.[27,28] These figures were based on the economy of 1999. Adjusting for inflation, the current cost-effectiveness of tamoxifen is $50,063.60 per life-year gained for women 35 to 49 years, $82,702.03 for women 50 to 59 years, and $90,733.31 for women 60 years and older.

PROPHYLACTIC MASTECTOMY

Research in chemoprevention has produced strong evidence that the incidence of breast cancer can be reduced in a high-risk population. However, the degree of risk reduction, coupled with the side effects of the medication and the length of treatment, have prompted many women to decline chemoprevention. Another method of risk reduction is prophylactic mastectomy (PM). Compared to chemoprevention, this method has the advantages of being accomplished over a shorter period of time and resulting in greater risk reduction. This option is particularly attractive to patients who carry gene mutations that increase their risk of developing breast cancer. However, the psychological and physiologic impact of this intervention is more intense. Fortunately, the emotional impact of prophylactic mastectomy has been somewhat diminished by reconstruction options currently available. The surgical interventions, though, have significant operative risk that must be considered.

Overview of Prophylactic Mastectomy

Prophylactic mastectomy (PM) is the surgical removal of the breast for reasons other than that the breast contains cancer. PM is a procedure that the patient chooses to have performed.[29] Bilateral prophylactic mastectomy (BPM) is usually performed on women who have a high risk of developing breast cancer but no personal history of breast cancer. High-risk women include those who carry the BRCA gene mutation, those with a strong family history of breast cancer or a combination of breast and ovarian cancer, and those with a histologically proven proliferative breast disease. In addition, women with breast cancer in one breast may choose to have the opposite (contralateral) breast removed in order to reduce the risk for developing cancer in this breast or to achieve symmetry. The use of contralateral prophylactic mastectomy (CPM) has doubled in the past six years.[30] It must be noted that PM to reduce the risk of breast cancer remains controversial because there are no prospective studies to support the benefits and outline the risks.

Other benign breast conditions that may lead patients to consider PM include difficulty in examining the breasts due to fibrocystic mastopathy, the presence of dense breast tissue that makes the interpretation of mammograms difficult, a history of multiple previous negative breast biopsies, severe and incapacitating mastodynia, chronic mastitis, and failed cosmetic procedures. For these conditions PM is by no means conventional therapy and should be considered only for those conditions refractory to medical therapy.

Patient Selection

Who then do we select for PM? It is important to remember that it is the women's choice whether or not to have this treatment. Certainly, some patients have a higher risk of developing breast cancer than others and are therefore good candidates for PM; however, there are no prospective studies indicating overall survival benefit in patients undergoing PM for cancer prevention as compared to patients with similar risk who do not have PM. Studies do show that BPM reduces the risk of breast cancer development in women with BRCA1 and BRCA2 mutations by 90%.[31] In women with a family history of breast cancer and unknown BRCA status, risk reduction of developing breast cancer was as high 94%.[32] Similarly, studies have shown that CPM will reduce the risk of developing breast cancer, but no survival benefit has been shown.[29,30] Clearly, it is important for those who may test positive for the BRCA gene mutation to be tested so that an accurate assessment of risk can be made. Such assessment should include consultation with a genetic counselor, and only after the patient's risk has been determined is the patient able to weigh the potential risks and benefits of PM.

To date, the strongest predictor of a woman's risk of developing breast cancer is the presence of the *BRCA1* or *BRCA2* gene mutation. Those patients who test positive for the gene will see the greatest reduction in risk with PM. Several retrospective studies show the risk reduction for breast cancer development of BPM in *BRCA* carriers to be 90% to 95%.[31,32] One prospective study confirms up to 100% risk reduction if bilateral prophylactic salpingo-oophorectomy (PSO) is also performed.[33] Interestingly, two studies using a theoretical mathematical analysis of survival gains showed that BPM may actually improve survival in women who are carriers of the *BRCA* mutation.[34,35] Among women with a positive family history of breast cancer, BPM reduced their risk of developing breast cancer from 90% to 94%, and disease-specific mortality was reduced 81% to 100%.[32] Despite these impressive statistics, women must clearly understand that there is still a lifelong possibility of developing breast cancer even after PM.

For women with a primary breast cancer who choose to have CPM for risk reduction, many studies indicate significant reduction of risk of a secondary breast cancer in the contralateral breast. Of course, the benefit of risk reduction is greatest in those women with the highest risk of contralateral breast cancer. There is a potential 91% risk reduction in women with a *BRCA* mutation and 94% to 96% risk reduction in women with a family history of breast cancer.[29,30] However, demonstrating an overall survival benefit is more difficult because these patients already have a primary breast cancer. The risk of death from the primary cancer is usually higher than the risk of death from a possible secondary contralateral cancer.[36] Similarly, studies assessing overall survival in *BRCA* mutation carriers who developed a primary breast cancer and subsequently choose CPM showed no survival benefit.[37,38,39] However, two of these studies evaluated whether CPM improved survival in relation to the stage of the primary breast cancer and found that survival was slightly improved for stage 1 and stage 2 breast cancer.[38,39]

Patients with a lobular neoplasia have a very specific risk of breast cancer. As indicated above, lobular carcinoma in situ (LCIS) is a significant marker for breast cancer rather than a premalignant lesion.[40,41,42] This is because of the incidence of bilaterality of the breast cancer risk even when the LCIS is found in only one breast. Within 25 years of diagnosis of LCIS in one breast, patients have a 25% chance of developing breast cancer of either the ductal or lobular type in either breast.[40,41] Patients with both LCIS and an invasive carcinoma have a bilaterality rate as high as 57%.[43] Therefore, women with unilateral invasive breast cancer and a coexisting LCIS lesion may benefit more from CPM than those without coexisting LCIS.

The Society of Surgical Oncology (SSO) position statement on prophylactic mastectomy from January 2007 outlines criteria for surgeons to consider when advising patients on either CPM or BPM.[44] The SSO statement suggests that potential indications for BPM for patients without a breast cancer diagnosis include the presence of *BRCA* mutations, a strong family history of breast cancer, and histologic risk factors (atypical ductal or lobular hyperplasia and LCIS). A strong family history is one in which breast cancer has occurred in multiple first-degree relatives or multiple successive generations of family members with breast or ovarian cancer. High-risk pathology is of special concern when present with a strong family history. BPM can be considered in extreme situations such as mammographically dense breast tissue that is difficult to evaluate, several prior breast biopsies for mammographic abnormalities, and a patient's strong concern about breast cancer. When discussing BPM for *BRCA* mutations with a patient, prophylactic oophorectomy should also be considered.

In patients with a current or previous breast cancer, the SSO criterion for CPM includes risk reduction, difficult surveillance, and reconstructive issues concerning symmetry and balance. Many women with breast cancer overestimate their risk for developing a contralateral breast cancer and need to be clearly advised on their individual risk.[2] Factors associated with increased risk for contralateral breast cancer are young patient age, strong family history, *BRCA* mutations, associated LCIS, multicentric cancer, and previous chest wall radiation. Difficult surveillance includes those patients with mammographically dense breasts that are difficult to evaluate, or diffuse indeterminate microcalcifications in the unaffected breast. Women with large and/or ptotic breasts may need to undergo CPM for symmetry or balance. Mastopexy and reduction mammoplasty should also be considered. In women who choose to not have reconstruction, CPM may need to be done to preserve balance. Whether considering BPM or CPM, all patients should be counseled by a multidisciplinary group including the surgical oncologist, medical oncologist, radiologist, pathologist, plastic reconstructive surgeon, and a genetic counselor. Patients should also be advised of alternative risk-reducing measures such as chemoprevention, close surveillance, hormonal therapy, and prophylactic oophorectomy in premenopausal women.

Quality of Life after Prophylactic Mastectomy

As with any surgical procedure, the risks and benefits of PM must be discussed with the patient in order for her to give informed consent to the procedure. Possible complications following PM include sensory loss, bleeding, infection, hematoma, seroma, nonhealing wounds, flap necrosis, and postmastectomy pain syndrome. Complications of reconstruction include implant failure, capsular formation, asymmetry, poor cosmetic outcome, and reconstructive failure. Following PM, 27% to 49.6% of women will experience complications.[45,46] Not all women will choose reconstruction after mastectomy, but all should have the opportunity to consider this step. Reviewed literature shows that between 69% and 84% of women undergoing PM choose reconstruction.[45,46,47] Women who do choose reconstruction need to be appropriately advised of all the possible complications and subsequent need for follow-up surgical procedures to exchange expanders for implants or autologous reconstruction, construct the nipple areolar complex, repair asymmetry, or address complications. Optimal cosmetic outcome usually takes more than one surgical intervention. Patient satisfaction has been negatively correlated with perceived lack of information about reconstruction and possible complications.[48]

Several investigators have assessed quality of life, satisfaction, and body image after mastectomy, including PM. The psychosocial issues of losing one or both breasts are important and must be addressed preoperatively. Many studies confirm that the type of surgery a woman undergoes for her breast cancer or for risk reduction of breast cancer is important for body image and feelings of attractiveness.[49,50] Mastectomy can be perceived as a loss of body part that connotes femininity and womanhood.[51] Many studies indicate that mastectomy with reconstruction can yield high contentment with quality of life and self-esteem.[45,47,52,53] However, many studies conclude that PM may have a negative effect on sexuality and body image.[45,47,48,53] Interestingly, during a long-term follow-up of two years after surgery, women experienced improvements in psychosocial adjustment, returning to presurgical levels.[54] Still, all of these issues must be raised before PM as part of the risks and benefits discussion in order to achieve informed consent.

Summary

The BCPT P-1 study, the MORE/CORE study, and finally the STAR P-2 study all have proved the principle that chemoprevention can reduce the incidence of cancer in women with an increased risk of developing breast cancer. These studies have demonstrated that tamoxifen and raloxifene can be classified as chemopreventive drugs such that they decrease the incidence of breast cancer in women at high risk. The IBIS-1 study showed that tamoxifen reduced the risk of breast cancer in very-high-risk women and further concluded that the effects from tamoxifen last at least 10 years, whereas the potential side effects do not last beyond the time that tamoxifen is taken. The Royal Marsden trial confirms a long-term preventive effect on ER-positive breast cancer with tamoxifen use. The Italian study showed that tamoxifen decreased breast cancer incidence in high-risk women but not in low-risk women. Subsequent studies using the data from the BCPT P-1 trial also indicate a benefit from tamoxifen in benign breast disease and a significant advantage in women positive for the *BRCA2* mutation (Tables 6-7 and 6-8).

The risks associated with tamoxifen use greatly depend on the age of the woman and her ethnicity, since some risks seem to be greater in African American women.[6] Obviously, any woman who is encouraged to take tamoxifen for chemoprevention should have a net benefit of cancer reduction. The net benefit of chemoprevention is highly positive for women younger than 50 years whose predicted breast cancer risk ratio is at least 2.5 over 5 years. It is also highly

Table 6-7. Summary of Randomized Clinical Trials of Chemoprevention for Breast Cancer

Trial	No. of Patients	Cohort	Intervention	Risk Reduction
NSABP BCPT P-1	13,388	Age > 60 yr or 35–59 with 5-year risk >1.66% or ADH or LCIS	Tamoxifen or placebo 5 yr	49% invasive cancer, 50% DCIS
STAR P-2	19,747	Postmenopausal Mean age 58.5 Mean risk 4.03	Tamoxifen or raloxifene 5 yr	Both equally reduced invasive by 49% Raloxifene had no effect on DCIS
MORE and CORE	7,705	Mean age 66.5 with osteoporosis Risk > 1.67	Raloxifene 120 mg vs 60 mg vs placebo 5 yr	76% invasive cancer (89% in those with family history of cancer vs 58% no family history of cancer)
Royal Marsden/UK BCPT	2,471	Mean age 47, higher relative risk based on family history	Tamoxifen vs placebo	35% invasive cancer during 8 year tamoxifen period (nonsignificant) 51% invasive cancer post-tamoxifen period (significant)
Italian Tamoxifen Prevention Trial among women with hysterectomy	5,408	Age 30–70 after TAH, 50% Oophorectomy	Tamoxifen vs placebo	82% in high-risk group and 3% in low-risk group
International Breast Cancer Intervention Study (IBIS-I)	7,152	Age 35–70 with family history, LCIS, ADH	Tamoxifen vs placebo	34% in high-risk group

ADH, atypical ductal hyperplasia; DCIS, ductal carcinoma in situ; LCIS, lobular carcinoma in situ; TAH, total abdominal hysterectomy.

Table 6-8. Risk Ratio for Adverse Outcomes in Each Prevention Trial*

Trial	Endometrial Cancer	Pulmonary Embolus (PE)	Deep Venous Thrombosis	Stroke	Cataracts
BCPT P-1	2.53 <49 yr 1.21 >50 yr 4.01	3.01 <49 yr 2.03 >50 yr 3.19	1.60 <49 yr 1.39 >50 yr 1.71	1.59 <49 yr 0.76 >50 yr 1.75	1.14 Not broken down by age
STAR P-2	0.62 Basically equal in both groups	Tamoxifen 3.01 Raloxifene 3.00	Tamoxifen 1.60 Raloxifene 1.60	Tamoxifen 1.39 Raloxifene 1.33	Tamoxifen 0.92 Raloxifene 0.68
MORE/CORE (raloxifene only)	0.8	3.10	Combined with PE	Not reported	Not reported
Royal Marsden	Tamoxifen total no. of women: 13 Placebo total no. of women: 5	Tamoxifen total no. of women: 8 Placebo total no. of women: 3	Combined with PE	Tamoxifen total no. of women: 7 Placebo total no. of women: 9	Tamoxifen total no. of women: 9 Placebo total no. of women: 1
Italian	Not reported	1.66 for all thromboembolic events	Combined with PE	Not reported	Not reported
IBIS-1	Tamoxifen total no. of women: 11 Placebo total no. of women: 5	Tamoxifen total no. of women: 13 Placebo total no. of women: 10	Tamoxifen total no. of women: 24 Placebo total no. of women: 5	Tamoxifen total no. of women: 13 Placebo total no. of women: 11	Tamoxifen total no. of women: 38 Placebo total no. of women: 37

*Some reported as total number of women in whom adverse outcomes occurred.

positive for Caucasian women younger than 60 whose 5-year predicted rate of developing breast cancer is 4.5.[6,23] Another group of women who should strongly consider taking tamoxifen for prevention are women with LCIS or ADH.[6,23] For these women the 5-year rates of developing breast cancer are 6.5 and 5.0, respectively. Clearly, any woman who is directed to take tamoxifen for chemoprevention of breast cancer must have a positive benefit:risk ratio.[8,23]

For those patients who choose not to pursue chemoprevention but desire risk reduction, prophylactic mastectomy may be an option. Prophylactic mastectomy is performed primarily for risk reduction of breast cancer, and those women at highest risk for developing breast cancer are potential candidates. Risk assessment and appropriate counseling are essential when discussing PM with a patient. Whether the patient is seeking advice for a bilateral prophylactic mastectomy (no evidence of breast cancer) or contralateral prophylactic mastectomy (personal history of breast cancer), indications for consideration should be evaluated by a multidisciplinary team including the surgical oncologist, medical oncologist, pathologist, reconstructive plastic surgeon, and a genetic counselor. The discussion must include the potential risks and benefits of immediate reconstruction, the possible psychosocial implications, and alternative risk-reducing strategies. Importantly, the patient must understand that PM does not provide 100% protection against the development of breast cancer.

References

1. Sporn MB: Approaches to prevention of epithelial cancer during the preneoplastic period. Cancer Res 36:2699–2702, 1976.
2. EBCTCG Collaborators: Early Breast Cancer Trialists Collaborative Group. Tamoxifen for early breast cancer—an over view of the randomized trials. Lancet 351:1451–1467, 1998.
3. Margreiter R, Weigele J: Tamoxifen for premenopausal patients with advanced breast cancer. Breast Cancer Res Treat 4:45–48, 1984.
4. Fisher B, Costantino JP, et al: A randomized clinical trial evaluating tamoxifen in the treatment of patients with node negative breast cancer who have estrogen-receptor positive tumors. N Engl J Med 320:479–484, 1989.
5. Fisher B, Redmond C: New perspective on cancer of the contralateral breast: a marker for assessing tamoxifen as a preventive agent. J Natl Cancer Inst 83:1278–1280, 1991.
6. Fisher B, Costantino JP, Wickerham L, et al: Tamoxifen for prevention of breast cancer: report of the National Surgical Adjuvant Breast and Bowel Project P-1 Study. J Natl Cancer Inst 90(18):1371–1388, 1998.
7. Gail MH, Brintan LA, Byar BP, et al: Projecting individualized probabilities of developing breast cancer for white females who are being examined annually. J Natl Cancer Inst 81:1879–1886, 1989.
8. Fisher B, Costantino JP, Wickerham L, et al: Tamoxifen for the prevention of breast cancer: current status of the National Surgical Adjuvant Breast and Bowel Project P-1 Study. J Natl Cancer Inst 97(22):1652–1662, 2005.
9. King MC, Wieand S, Hale K, et al: Tamoxifen and breast cancer incidence among women with inherited mutations in BRCA1 and BRCA2. JAMA 286(18):2251–2256, 2001.
10. Vogel VG, Costantino JP, Wickerham L, et al: Effects of tamoxifen vs raloxifene on the risk of developing invasive breast cancer and other disease outcomes: The NSABP Study of Tamoxifen and Raloxifene (STAR) P-2 Trial. JAMA 295(23):2727–2926, 2006.
11. Cummings SR, Eckert S, Krueger KA, et al: The effect of raloxifene on risk of breast cancer in postmenopausal women. Results from the MORE randomized trial. JAMA 281(23): 2189–2197, 1999.
12. Lippman ME, Cummings SR, Disch DP, et al: Effect of raloxifene on the incidence of invasive breast cancer in postmenopausal women with osteoporosis categorized by breast cancer risk. Clin Cancer Res 12(17):5242–5247, 2006.
13. Cuzick J, Forbes J, Edwards R, et al: First results from the International Breast Cancer Intervention Study (IBIS-1): a randomized prevention trial. Lancet 360:817–824, 2002.
14. Cuzick J, Forbes J, Sestal I, et al: Long-term results of tamoxifen prophylaxis for breast cancer—96 month follow-up of the randomized IBIS-1 Trial. J Natl Cancer Inst 99(4):272–282, 2007.
15. Powles TJ, Ashley S, Tidy A, et al: Twenty-year follow-up of the Royal Marsden Randomized, Double-Blinded Tamoxifen Breast Cancer Prevention Trial. J Natl Cancer Inst 99(4): 283–290, 2007.
16. Veronesi U, Maisonneuve P, Rotmensz N, et al: Tamoxifen for the prevention of breast cancer: late results of the Italian Randomized Tamoxifen Prevention Trial Among Women with Hysterectomy. J Natl Cancer Inst 99(9):727–737, 2007.
17. Tan-Chiu E, Wang J, Costantino JP, et al: Effects of tamoxifen on benign breast disease in women at high risk for breast cancer. J Natl Cancer Inst 95(2):302–307, 2003.
18. Fabian CJ: The what, why, and how of aromatase inhibitors: hormonal agents for treatment and prevention of breast cancer. Int J Clin Pract 61(12):2051–2063, 2007.
19. Nishio K, Niwa Y, Toyoshima H, et al: Consumption of soy foods and the risk of breast cancer: findings from the Japan Collaborative Cohort (JACC) Study. Cancer Causes Control 18:801–808, 2007 [Abstract].
20. Wakai K, Tamakosi K, Date C, et al: Dietary intakes of fat and fatty acids and risk of breast cancer: a prospective study in Japan. Cancer Sci 96(9):590–599, 2005.
21. Duffy C, Perez K, Partridge A: Implications of phytoestrogen intake for breast cancer. CA Cancer J Clin 57(5):260–277, 2007.
22. Gasco M, Argusti A, Bonanni B, Decensi A: SERMs in chemoprevention of breast cancer. Eur J Cancer 41:1980–1989, 2005.
23. Gail MH, Costantino JP, Bryant J, et al: Weighing the risks and benefits of tamoxifen treatment for preventing breast cancer. J Natl Cancer Inst 91(21):1829–1846, 1999.
24. Fabian CJ, Kimler BF: Selective estrogen-receptor modulators for primary prevention of breast cancer. J Clin Oncol 23(8): 1644–1655, 2005.
25. Levy AG, Shea J, Williams SV, et al: Measuring perceptions of breast cancer risk. Cancer Epidemiol Biomarkers Prev 15(10): 1893–1898, 2006.
26. Armstrong K, Quistberg BA, Micco BA, et al: Prescription of tamoxifen for breast cancer prevention by primary care physicians. Arch Intern Med 166:2260–2265, 2006.
27. Imai H, Kuroi K, Ohsumi S, et al: Economic evaluation of the prevention and treatment of breast cancer: present status and open issues. Breast Cancer 14:81–87, 2007.
28. Noe LL, Becker RV, Gradishar WJ, et al: The cost effectiveness of tamoxifen in the prevention of breast cancer. Am J Managed Care 5(6 Suppl):S389–S406, 1999.
29. Zakaria S, Degnim AC: Prophylactic mastectomy. Surg Clin N Am 87:317–331, 2007.
30. Tuttle TM, Habermann EB, Grund EH, et al: Increasing use of contralateral prophylactic mastectomy for breast cancer patients: a trend toward more aggressive surgical treatment. J Clin Oncol 25(33):1–6, 2007.
31. Rebbeck TR, Friebel T, Lynch HT, et al: Bilateral prophylactic mastectomy reduces breast cancer risk in BRCA1 and BRCA2 mutation carriers: the PROSE study group. J Clin Oncol 22(6):1055–1062, 2004.

32. Hartmann LC, Schaid DJ, Woods JE, et al: Efficacy of bilateral prophylactic mastectomy in women with a family history of breast cancer. N Engl J Med 340(2):77–78, 1999.

33. Meijers-Heijboer H, van Geel B, van Putten WL, et al: Breast cancer after bilateral prophylactic mastectomy in women with a BRCA1 or BRCA2 mutation. N Engl J Med 345(3):159–164, 2001.

34. Schrag D, Kuntz KM, Garber JE, et al: Decision analysis: effects of prophylactic mastectomy and oophorectomy on life expectancy among women with BRCA1 or BRCA2 mutations. N Engl J Med 336(20):1465–1471, 1997.

35. Grann VR, Jacobson JS, Thomason D, et al: Effect of prevention strategies on survival and quality adjusted survival of women with BRCA1/2 mutations: an updated decision analysis. J Clin Oncol 20(10):2520–2529, 2002.

36. Rosen PP, Groshen S, Kinne DW, et al: Contralateral breast carcinoma: an assessment of risk and prognosis in stage 1 and stage 2 patients with 20-year follow-up. Surgery 196(5):904–910, 1989.

37. Brekelmans CT, Seynaeve C, Menke-Plumers M, et al: Survival and prognostic factors in BRCA1-associated breast cancer. Ann Oncol 17(3):391–400, 2006.

38. Peralta EA, Ellenhorn JDI, Wagman LD, et al: Contralateral prophylactic mastectomy improves the outcome of selected patients undergoing mastectomy for breast cancer. Am J Surg 180(6):439–445, 2000.

39. Herrington LJ, Barlow WE, Yu O, et al: Efficacy of prophylactic mastectomy in women with unilateral breast cancer: a cancer research network project. J Clin Oncol 23(19):4275–4286, 2005.

40. Haagensen CD, Lane N, Lattes R, et al: Lobular neoplasia (so-called lobular carcinoma in situ) of the breast. Cancer 42:737–769, 1978.

41. Rosen PP, Kosloff C, Lieberman PH, et al: Lobular carcinoma in situ of the breast. Detailed analysis of 99 patients with average follow-up of 24 years. Am J Surg Pathol 2:225–251, 1978.

42. Andersen JA: Lobular carcinoma in situ of the breast. An approach to rational treatment. Cancer 39:2597–2602, 1977.

43. Lesser MI, Rosen PP, Kinne DW, et al: Multicentricity and bilaterality in invasive breast cancer. Surgery 91:234–240, 1982.

44. Society of Surgical Oncology: Position statement on prophylactic masytectomy. http://www.surgonc.org/default.aspx?id=179&fragment

45. Frost MH, Slezak JM, Tran NV, et al: Satisfaction after contralateral prophylactic mastectomy: the significance of mastectomy type, reconstructive complications, and body appearance. J Clin Oncol 23(31):7849–7856, 2005.

46. Heemskerk-Gerritsen BAM, Brekelmans CTM, Menke-Pluymers MBE, et al: Prophylactic mastectomy in BRCA1/2 mutation carriers and women at risk of hereditary breast cancer: long-term experiences at the Rotterdam family cancer clinic. Ann Surg Oncol 14(12):3335–3344, 2007.

47. Geiger AM, Nekhlyudov L, Herrinton LJ, et al: Quality of life after bilateral prophylactic mastectomy. Ann Surg Oncol 14(2):686–694, 2006.

48. Bresser PJ, Seynaeve C, Van Gool AR, et al: Satisfaction with prophylactic mastectomy and breast reconstruction in genetically predisposed women. Plast Reconstr Surg 117(6):1675–1682, 2006.

49. Rowland JH, Desmond KA, Meyerowitz BE, et al: Role of breast reconstructive surgery in physical and emotional outcomes among breast cancer survivors. J Natl Cancer Inst 92(17):1422–1429, 2000.

50. Pelusi J: Sexuality and body image. Am J Nurs 106(3)(Suppl):32–38, 2006.

51. Wilmoth MC: The aftermath of breast cancer: an altered sexual self. Cancer Nurs 24(4):278–286, 2001.

52. Cocquyt VF, Blondeel PN, Depypere HT, et al: Better cosmetic results and comparable quality of life after skin-sparing mastectomy and immediate autologous breast reconstruction compared to breast conservative treatment. Br J Plast Surg 56:462–470, 2003.

53. Brandberg Y, Sandelin K, Erikson S, et al: Psychological reactions, quality of life, and body image after bilateral prophylactic mastectomy in women at high risk for breast cancer: a prospective 1-year follow-up study. J Clin Oncol 26(24):3943–3949, 2008.

54. Parker PA, Youssef A, Walker S, et al: Short-term and long-term psychosocial adjustment and quality of life in women undergoing different surgical procedures for breast cancer. Ann Surg Oncol 14(11):3078–3089, 2007.

7

Nutrition and Lifestyle

Lisa Ware Corbin

KEY POINTS

- Known breast cancer risk factors (e.g., age at menarche, parity, and heredity) are thought to explain only 25% to 47% of breast cancer risks in the United States, with up to 60% of risks felt to be due to environmental factors.
- The World Cancer Research Fund estimates that about one third of breast cancer risk can be explained by obesity and sedentary lifestyle and 2% to 4% by alcohol consumption—all potentially modifiable risk factors.
- In many cases, when a link between breast cancer and nutrition or lifestyle is thought to be present, retrospective case-control studies have initially found a link, but later prospective cohort studies have found no association or a less dramatic association. Randomized, controlled trials of lifestyle and nutrition interventions to prevent breast cancer are few.
- Achieving or maintaining a healthy weight and participating in regular aerobic exercise both lower a woman's risk for primary and secondary breast cancer.
- A diet high in fruits and vegetables and low in saturated fats is associated with decreased risk of breast cancer; consumption of low-fat dairy products may also be protective.
- Exposure to ionizing radiation to treat childhood cancer increases the risk of breast cancer; exposure to lower levels of radiation does not.
- Supplemental vitamins, minerals, and other compounds probably do not do much to lower a woman's risk of developing breast cancer.

Introduction

"Why me" is a phrase often heard by physicians caring for patients with newly diagnosed breast cancer. "I did everything right—I exercised, I ate well, I took supplements, I tried to minimize stress, I went to church. Why did I get breast cancer?"

Why did she develop breast cancer? What is the evidence that doing things "right" prevents breast cancer? This chapter explores two areas, nutrition and lifestyle, in which a patient's choices may or may not affect her risk of being diagnosed with breast cancer.

In an interesting study published in 2005, patients with cancer (including over 450 patients with breast cancer) were asked why they thought they had developed cancer.[1] Researchers concluded that respondents typically underestimated the importance of behavioral factors that are known to be associated with increased cancer risk, such as obesity and physical inactivity, while overestimating the importance of stress and environmental pollution. The authors stressed that patient education, particularly regarding modifiable risk factors, is paramount. This chapter aims to educate the clinician to be able to educate the patient about which potentially modifiable nutrition and lifestyle factors do or do not place her at increased risk of breast cancer.

Over the last two decades, possible associations among nutrition, lifestyle, and cancer risk have garnered more public attention and press. In 2007, an international committee of experts (World Cancer Research Fund/American Institute for Cancer Research [WCRF/AICR]) provided a summary of scientific evidence on the effect of nutrition on cancer up to the mid-1980s. The report estimated that up to one third of cancer incidence worldwide was preventable by healthy eating, weight control, and appropriate physical activity.[2] Studies of families in Scandinavian countries have suggested that environmental factors may be responsible for up to 80% of breast cancer risk.[3] Also supporting the association between environmental factors and risk of cancer is the fact that rates of breast cancer vary tremendously from country to country, and areas with similar lifestyles (e.g., North America and Western Europe) tend to have similar rates of breast cancer. Furthermore, when women emigrate from a country with a low rate of breast cancer to a country with higher breast cancer incidence, the immigrant's risk of breast cancer rises to mirror that of her adopted country.[4] Moreover, risk continues to rise for second and later generations of immigrants.

Choosing which areas to investigate often begins with thoughts of plausibility, with a focus on areas in which lifestyle choices and nutrition may affect factors known or theorized to be associated with breast cancer, such as exposure to estrogens, exposure to carcinogens, and oxidative stress. Investigation of the possible relation of nutrition, lifestyle, and disease often begins with retrospective epidemiologic searches from which associations—but not conclusions—can be made. If associations are found, prospective observational studies provide more scientifically sound evidence. Finally, prospective, randomized, controlled trials of nutrition and lifestyle interventions may be carried out to solidify the association. These studies usually have much less dramatic results than the epidemiologic studies, but stronger conclusions can be drawn from these less common difficult-to-carry-out trials.

The results of epidemiologic studies can be viewed as a compass, pointing in a general direction, and may constitute all the "evidence" that is available for a certain nutrition/lifestyle suggestion. It may take years or decades of "exposure" (lifestyle choice) to make a difference, and decades-long trials with large enough numbers of participants to show statistical significance may be impractical. If done, however, such trials provide finer tuning for the compass direction suggested by epidemiologic investigation. This chapter presents data from both epidemiologic studies and prospective trials that explore the role of nutrition and lifestyle for primary and secondary prevention of breast cancer.

NUTRITION

Nutrition has been explored as a risk for cancer development, progression, and recurrence. Women's interests have been piqued, as diet and dietary supplements are potentially modifiable and thus give women a sense of control over the disease. Which nutrition factors have links to breast cancer and what can be done about them to lower risk?

Diet

Fruit and Vegetable Intake

Based on a review of data published through the mid-1980s, the 2007 WCRF/AICR report[2] concluded that a high consumption of fruits and vegetables probably decreases the risk of breast cancer. Studies analyzed since that time have not been as definitive, however.[5] In general, retrospective studies are more likely to show an association, whereas prospective studies are not likely to show such an association. For example, in 2001, Smith-Warner and associates[6] pooled data from eight prospective cohort studies and found no evidence of a protective effect for fruit and vegetable intake. The study group chose to analyze cohort studies rather than case-control studies to minimize effects of recall bias and included only studies with at least 200 cases as well as excellent dietary recording/analysis techniques. Studies included not only overall fruit and vegetable intake but also specific groups of fruits and vegetables and individual food items. The pooled studies included 7377 incident invasive breast cancer cases occurring among 351,825 women whose diets were analyzed at baseline. In addition to not finding associations between overall fruit and vegetable intake and breast cancer, subanalysis did not find such associations for green leafy vegetables, 8 botanical groups, or 17 specific fruits and vegetables.

Highlighting the idea that case-control studies likely overestimate associations owing to recall bias, a meta-analysis published in 2003 found a slight protective effect of fruit and vegetable intake in 15 case-control studies but no association in 10 prospective cohort studies.[7]

A large prospective study, the European Prospective Investigation into Cancer and Nutrition (EPIC), followed up 285,526 women between ages 25 and 70 years who were recruited from eight European countries. Participants completed a dietary questionnaire at enrollment (1992–1998) and were followed up for development of cancer until 2002 (mean follow-up 5.4 years). The authors acknowledge that the study period thus far is short, but so far associations between fruit or vegetable intake and breast cancer risk have not been seen.[8] Nevertheless, maintaining a healthy lifestyle includes eating a good balance of various foods each day. Sample recommended diets are shown in Table 7-1.

Glycemic Load

The glycemic index is a value given to specific foods to enable comparison of the relative impact that ingesting each food will have on blood glucose level. Foods with a high glycemic index raise the blood glucose proportionally higher than foods with a lower glycemic index (Table 7-2). It has been theorized that high consumption of foods with a high glycemic index may predispose to the development of cancer because cells with a high metabolic activity are preferential users of glucose. Also, foods with a high glycemic index may contribute to higher insulin levels; insulin has been shown to act as a growth factor and perhaps promotes tumor growth. Epidemiologic studies have shown a very small but statistically significant link between diabetes and risk of breast cancer; patients with type 2 diabetes show elevated blood glucose and insulin levels.[9]

One relatively large cohort study compared women with breast cancer with age-matched women without breast cancer and interviewed all subjects about intake of foods with a high glycemic index. The study enrolled 2569 women with breast cancer; controls were 2588 hospitalized women with unrelated conditions. Compared with women with the lowest intake and adjusting for other risk factors (age, body mass index [BMI], total calorie intake), women with the highest intake of desserts or sugars had multivariate odds ratio [OR] of 1.19 (95% confidence interval [CI] 1.02–1.39).[10]

Saturated Fat

Animal studies have shown saturated fat to be a promoter of mammary carcinogenesis, controlling for total caloric intake. In addition, in many studies high dietary fat intake has been linked to higher serum levels of estradiol.[11]

Some epidemiologic studies have linked fat intake to an increased incidence of breast cancer, but again case-control and prospective cohort studies have yielded conflicting results. In 2003, Boyd and associates[4] combined case-control with cohort studies examining this relationship and estimated a 19% overall increased risk of breast cancer for the highest versus the lowest levels of saturated fat intake. However, when these studies were separated and analyzed according to study types, neither an analysis of the case-control studies nor an analysis of the cohort studies was able to show a significant correlation.[4]

The Women's Health Initiative study, best known for concluding that routine use of postmenopausal hormonal replacement therapy is unwarranted, also investigated the intervention of a low-fat diet on the risk of development of breast cancer.[12] Over 48,800 women ages 50 to 79 at the start of the trial were put on a low-fat diet (with an aim of 20% of calories from fat) or were asked to continue their regular diet. The group assigned to the low-fat diet lowered their fat intake to 24% by the end of the first year, but this number rose to 29% by the end of the sixth year. Still, this was much less than the approximately 37% fat diet that both groups began with and that the normal diet group continued with. There was no statistically significant difference in development of breast cancer between the two groups, although there was a trend toward benefit. A 9% decrease in risk of breast cancer was seen for the low-fat group, but it was not statistically significant. It is interesting that there was a suggestion of a dose-response relationship, since women who had the highest fat intake at the start of the study and who reduced fat intake the most saw the greatest reduction in risk.

One criticism of the study was that no differentiation was made between "good fats" (mono-unsaturated and polyunsaturated) and "bad fats" (saturated fats and trans-fats). Other critics note that the effects of diet may require longer follow-up to be seen (study participants were followed up for an average of 8.1 years). Although this study does not provide conclusive evidence that a low-fat diet reduces the risk of breast cancer, for general and cardiac health reasons, the U.S. Dietary Guidelines for Americans still recommend that adults keep total fat intake to 20% to 35% of calories, with saturated fats making up less than 10% of total caloric intake.

Decreasing dietary fat intake may have more of a benefit in prevention of secondary breast cancer. The Women's Intervention Nutrition Study randomized 2437 women with early-stage, treated breast cancer in a prospective manner to a dietary intervention group ($n = 975$)

Table 7-1. Sample USDA Food Guide and the DASH Eating Plan at the 2000-Calorie Level*
(Amounts of various food groups that are recommended each day or each week in the USDA Food Guide and in the DASH Eating Plan (amounts are daily unless otherwise specified) at the 2000-calorie level. Also identified are equivalent amounts for different food choices in each group. To follow either eating pattern, food choices over time should provide these amounts of food from each group on average.)

Food Groups and Subgroups	USDA Food Guide Amount[†]	DASH Eating Plan Amount	Equivalent Amounts
Fruit Group	2 cups (4 servings)	2 to 2.5 cups (4 to 5 servings)	½ cup equivalent is: • ½ cup fresh, frozen, or canned fruit • 1 med fruit • ¼ cup dried fruit • USDA: ½ cup fruit juice • DASH: ¾ cup fruit juice
Vegetable Group • Dark green vegetables • Orange vegetables • Legumes (dry beans) • Starchy vegetables • Other vegetables	2.5 cups (5 servings) 3 cups/week 2 cups/week 3 cups/week 3 cups/week 6.5 cups/week	2 to 2.5 cups (4 to 5 servings)	½ cup equivalent is: • ½ cup of cut-up raw or cooked vegetable • 1 cup raw leafy vegetable • USDA: ½ cup vegetable juice • DASH: ¾ cup vegetable juice
Grain Group • Whole grains • Other grains	6 ounce-equivalents 3 ounce-equivalents 3 ounce-equivalents	7 to 8 ounce-equivalents (7 to 8 servings)	1 ounce-equivalent is: • 1 slice bread • 1 cup dry cereal • ½ cup cooked rice, pasta, cereal • DASH: 1 oz dry cereal (½–1¼ cup depending on cereal type–check label)
Meat and Beans Group	5.5 ounce-equivalents	6 ounces or less meat, poultry, fish 4 to 5 servings per week nuts, seeds, and dry beans[‡]	1 ounce-equivalent is: • 1 of cooked lean meats, poultry, fish • 1 egg • USDA: ¼ cup cooked dry beans or tofu, 1 tbsp peanut butter, ½ oz nuts or seeds • DASH: 1½ oz nuts, ½ oz seeds, ½ cup cooked dry beans
Milk Group	3 cups	2 to 3 cups	1 cup equivalent is: • 1 cup low-fat/fat-free milk, yogurt • 1½ oz low-fat or fat-free natural cheese • 2 oz of low-fat or fat-free processed cheese
Oils	24 grams (6 tsp)	8 to 12 grams (2 to 3 tsp)	1 tsp equivalent is: • DASH: 1 tsp soft margarine • 1 tbsp low-fat mayo • 2 tbsp light salad dressing • 1 tsp vegetable oil
Discretionary Calorie Allowance • Example of distribution: Solid fat[§] Added sugars	267 calories 18 grams 8 tsp	~2 tsp (5 tbsp per week)	1 tbsp added sugar equivalent is: • DASH: 1 tbsp jelly or jam • ½ oz jelly beans • 8 oz lemonade

*All servings are per day unless otherwise noted. USDA vegetable subgroup amounts and amounts of DASH nuts, seeds, and dry beans are per week.
[†]The 2000-calorie USDA Food Guide is appropriate for many sedentary males 51 to 70 years of age, sedentary females 19 to 30 years of age, and for some other gender/age groups who are more physically active.
[‡]In the DASH Eating Plan, nuts, seeds, and dry beans are a separate food group from meat, poultry, and fish.
[§]The oils listed in this table are not considered to be part of discretionary calories because they are a major source of the vitamin E and polyunsaturated fatty acids, including the essential fatty acids, in the food pattern. In contrast, solid fats (i.e., saturated and trans fats) are listed separately as a source of discretionary calories.
From HHS/USDA Dietary Guidelines, 2005. Available at www.nhlbi.nih.gov/health/public/heart/obesity/wecan/downloads/intake.pdf

Table 7-2. Glycemic Index by Glycemic Load

Low GI	Medium GI	High GI
Low GL		
All-bran cereal (8, 42)	Beets (5, 64)	Popcorn (8, 72)
Apples (6, 38)	Cantaloupe (4, 65)	Watermelon (4, 72)
Carrots (3, 47)	Pineapple (7, 59)	Whole wheat flour bread (9, 71)
Chana dal (3, 8)	Sucrose (table sugar) (7, 68)	White wheat flour bread (10, 70)
Chick peas (8, 28)		
Grapes (8, 46)		
Green peas (3, 48)		
Kidney beans (7, 28)		
Nopal (0, 7)		
Oranges (5, 42)		
Peaches (5, 42)		
Peanuts (1, 14)		
Pears (4, 38)		
Pinto beans (10, 39)		
Red lentils (5, 26)		
Strawberries (1, 40)		
Sweet corn (9, 54)		
Medium GL		
Apple juice (11, 40)	Life cereal (16, 66)	Cheerios (15, 74)
Bananas (12, 52)	New potatoes (12, 57)	Shredded wheat (15, 75)
Buckwheat (16, 54)	Sweet potatoes (17, 61)	
Fettucine (18, 40)	Wild rice (18, 57)	
Navy beans (12, 38)		
Orange juice (12, 50)		
Parboiled rice (17, 47)		
Pearled barley (11, 25)		
Sourdough wheat bread (15, 54)		
High GL		
Linguine (23, 52)	Couscous (23, 65)	Baked Russet potatoes (26, 85)
Macaroni (23, 47)	White rice (23, 64)	Cornflakes (21, 81)
Spaghetti (20, 42)		

First number in parentheses is glycemic load, second is glycemic index.
GL: Low = 1–10, Med = 11–19, High = 20+
GI: Low = 1–55, Med = 56–69, High = 70–100
Available at: www.mendosa.com/common_foods.htm
From Revised International Table of Glycemic Index (GI) and Glycemic Load (GL). Am J Clin Nutrition July 2002.

or control group ($n = 1462$).[13] Women in the treatment group lowered their mean daily fat intake at 12 months to 33.3 g compared with 51.3 g in the control group. The intervention group also had a statistically significant mean 6-pound weight loss during the study period. After a median 5 years of follow-up, local, regional, distant, or ipsilateral breast cancer recurrence or new contralateral breast cancer had been reported in 9.8% of women in the dietary intervention group and in 12.4% of women in the control group, giving a statistically significant 0.76 relative risk (RR) of recurrence for the intervention group.[13]

Dairy Products

Eating low-fat dairy products may protect a woman from developing breast cancer, although the reasons this is so are not well elucidated. A prospective observational study, the Nurses' Health Study, followed up over 88,000 pre- and postmenopausal women and recorded dietary information at time of enrollment (1980) and every 4 years until the study's completion in 1994.[14] For *premenopausal* women, the study found an inverse association between breast cancer risk and intake of low-fat dairy products, calcium (owing mainly to dairy intake rather than supplement use), vitamin D (owing mainly to supplement use and not dairy intake), and lactose. The risk reduction comparing highest (>1 serving/day) and lowest ≤3 servings/month) intake categories were 0.68 (95% CI 0.55–0.86) for low-fat dairy foods and 0.72 (95% CI 0.56–0.91) for skim or low-fat milk. Risk reduction was also seen with dairy calcium (>800 mg/day versus ≤200 mg/day; RR 0.69, 95% CI 0.48–0.98), total vitamin D (>500 IU/day versus ≤150 IU/day; RR 0.72, 95% CI 0.55–0.94), and lactose (quintile 5 versus quintile 1; RR 0.68, 95% CI 0.54–0.86). No association was seen for any of these dietary factors with *postmenopausal* breast cancer risk, however.[14]

A nutrition cohort was begun in 1992 as a subset of a population followed up by the American Cancer Society, in which the Cancer Prevention Study II did find an inverse relationship between dietary calcium and breast cancer for postmenopausal women.[15] Over 68,500 postmenopausal women completed a dietary survey after enrollment (1992–1993) and were surveyed in 2001 for breast cancer status. Data were controlled for weight gain, hormone replacement therapy use, and other lifestyle factors. Analysis showed that women who consumed the most dietary calcium (>1250 mg/day) had a 20% lower risk of postmenopausal breast cancer compared with those in the lowest category of intake (<500 mg/day; RR 0.80, 95% CI 0.67–0.95; ptrend 0.02), but supplemental calcium did not change this risk. Neither dietary vitamin D intake nor supplementation with vitamin D was associated with decreased risk of breast cancer development overall, although the development of estrogen receptor-positive tumors was lower in the group with the most vitamin D intake (RR 0.74, 95% CI 0.59–0.93; ptrend 0.006).[15]

Soy Foods

Biologic Plausibility

Perhaps the most controversial area of nutrition is defining the relation of soy foods to risk of breast cancer development and growth. Soy foods are among the most potent food sources of isoflavones, compounds that are chemically very similar to estrogens. This fact, along with the epidemiologic data showing that Asian women, with a much higher per-capita consumption of soy foods, have a lower incidence of breast cancer than do women who do not eat an Asian diet, has intrigued scientists. A conference (sponsored by the soy industry) was convened in 2005 to review research on the subject of soy and breast cancer risk.[16] Researchers noted that soy isoflavones have been shown in some in vitro and animal studies to stimulate growth of breast cancer cell lines, yet isoflavones, by a nonhormonal mechanism, have also been shown to inhibit tumor growth.

Observational Studies

A case-control study of breast cancer among Chinese, Japanese, and Filipino women in Los Angeles County quantified intake of soy during adolescence and adult life. Controlling for other risks for breast cancer, researchers interviewed 501 breast cancer patients and 594 control subjects. The authors described a significant inverse association between soy intake during adolescence and adult life and the development of breast cancer, with consumption of soy during adolescence appearing to confer the greatest reduction in risk. They found that women who reported soy intake at least once per week during adolescence showed a statistically significant reduced risk of breast cancer. There was also a significant trend of decreasing risk with increasing soy intake during adult life. Subjects who were high soy consumers during both adolescence and adulthood showed the lowest risk (OR 0. 53, 95% CI 0.36–0.78) compared with those who were low consumers during both periods of their lives.[17]

A larger case-control study of non–Asian Americans, also in California and during the same time period, did not find an association between phytoestrogen consumption and breast cancer risk. Interviews were conducted with 1326 subjects and 1657 controls. Usual intake of specific phytoestrogenic compounds was assessed via a food frequency questionnaire and a nutrient database. In this study, phytoestrogen intake was not associated with breast cancer risk (OR 1.0, 95% CI 0.80, 1.3 for the highest versus lowest quartile). Subgroup analysis did not differ.[18]

A meta-analysis of 18 studies from 1978 to 2004 concluded that intake of soy may have a small protective effect against development of breast cancer, but the study urged caution in interpreting the results since the studies did not show a dose-response pattern and most had significant methodologic issues as well. Among all women, high soy intake was modestly associated with reduced breast cancer risk (OR 0.86, 95% CI 0.75–0.99).[19]

Fish Consumption

Omega-3 fatty acids have been noted in vitro and in animal studies to inhibit breast cancer cell growth, but case-control and cohort epidemiologic studies matching dietary fish intake—the biggest dietary source of omega-3 fatty acids—with breast cancer risk have yielded inconsistent results. As part of the EPIC study, 310,671 women between 25 and 70 years old completed a dietary survey at enrollment and then were followed up for an average of 6.4 years for the development of breast cancer. Though criticized for the short follow-up period, this study showed no association between fish intake and cancer development.[20]

Vitamins, Minerals, and Other Supplements

Vitamins are compounds essential for proper metabolism that the human body cannot synthesize; thus, they must be ingested in food or supplement form. Vitamin deficiency has been implicated in a number of chronic diseases and has been investigated for a role in breast cancer development.

Vitamin C (Ascorbic Acid)

Vitamin C is a strong antioxidant that provides reducing potential for biochemical reactions, especially those using iron or copper. Vitamin C is of interest in cancer prevention because it theoretically blocks or prevents some processes that may lead to carcinogenesis. Although epidemiologic reviews show increased cancer in vitamin C–deficient populations and animals, controlled trials of supplementation for cancer prevention have failed to show a definitive link. Vitamin C is a water-soluble vitamin; excess intake is excreted by the kidneys and may be associated with renal stones or diarrhea. A 1990 meta-analysis of 12 case-control studies investigated the link between dietary vitamin C intake and breast cancer risk and found a statistically significant inverse relationship.[21] However, further case-control studies as well as prospective studies, including some studies in which supplemental vitamin C was taken long term and at high doses, have failed to show a consistent association.[22]

Vitamin A and Carotenoids

Vitamin A—either from animal sources as preformed vitamin A (retinol and retinyl esters) or from plant sources as carotenoids converted into retinal—is involved with cell proliferation and differentiation, making it an attractive target of investigation in cancer research. Vitamin A has antioxidant properties as well. The Nurse's Health Studies and other case-control studies[23-25] have found inconsistent relationships between vitamin A intake and breast cancer risk. Though of short duration, the Women's Health Study randomized, in a double-blind fashion, almost 40,000 women to beta-carotene or placebo for 2 years, with 2 more years of follow-up, and did not find a decrease in risk of breast cancer. There is some suggestion that vitamin A may be protective among smokers and that vitamin A may reduce the chance that a breast cancer is estrogen receptor-negative; however, studies are not definitive.[22]

Vitamin E

Vitamin E has antioxidant and immunostimulant properties but has not been found by prospective or retrospective case-control study to decrease breast cancer risk.[22]

Calcium and Vitamin D

Vitamin D and its receptor have been shown in animal and tissue models to enhance differentiation and apoptosis in mammary gland tissue. Vitamin D deficiency is more common as people age, and estrogen deficiency is also associated with lower levels of vitamin D. Patients with breast cancer are more likely than patients without breast cancer to have low levels of vitamin D. In a meta-analysis of two retrospective case-control studies (1760 total subjects), Garland and associates[26] discovered a dose-response inverse relation between serum vitamin D levels and breast cancer risk. These researchers estimated that to reduce risk of breast cancer by 50%, an individual would have to consume 2700 IU of vitamin D daily, much higher than the U.S. median intake of 320 IU per day. Vitamin D is synthesized in the skin in response to sun exposure, and within the United States higher levels of breast cancer are seen in geographic areas with less sunshine compared with areas with more sunshine. All these factors make vitamin D, a supplement without risk of harm in patients with normal calcium metabolism, an attractive target for research in prevention of breast cancer. Indeed, the Women's Health Initiative is investigating this link in a prospective manner. Until these results are available, clinicians should encourage their patients to meet the RDA for vitamin D.[27]

DHEA

Dehydroepiandrosterone (DHEA) is an androgen produced by the adrenal glands; it is converted to estrogen and is one of the major sources of postmenopausal estrogen. As such, high levels of DHEA have been linked to an increased risk of postmenopausal (but not premenopausal) breast cancer and also to an increased risk of disease recurrence or progression in women treated with aromatase inhibitors or tamoxifen.[28] For obvious reasons, there have been no studies of DHEA in supplement form on risk of breast cancer. Unfortunately, DHEA is marketed in supplement form to promote good general health and to slow the effects of aging. Women seen by a primary care physician may be interested in taking this supplement and should be counseled to avoid it.

Recommendations

Overall recommendations for nutrition for people interested in prevention of primary or secondary breast cancer are to achieve and maintain a normal weight if they are overweight or obese and to follow a healthy diet as recommended by the American Cancer Society. Such a diet is high in plant-based foods, limiting fat to 20% to 35% of calories (less than 10% saturated fat, less than 3% trans-fatty acids), and incorporating lean protein sources, such as fish and low-fat dairy, nuts, seeds, and beans. Carbohydrates should be rich in essential nutrients and fiber, such as whole fruits and vegetables and unprocessed whole grains. It is recommended that individuals eat 2½ cups of fruits and vegetables daily, preferably of a variety of

---

Box 7-1. American Cancer Society Guidelines on Nutrition and Physical Activity for Cancer Prevention

Maintain a healthy weight throughout life.
- Balance caloric intake with physical activity.
- Avoid excessive weight gain throughout the life cycle.
- Achieve and maintain a healthy weight if currently overweight or obese.

Adopt a physically active lifestyle.
- Adults: engage in at last 30 minutes of moderate-to-vigorous physical activity, above usual activities, on 5 or more days of the week. Forty-five to 60 minutes of intentional physical activity are preferable.
- Children and adolescents: engage in at least 60 minutes per day of moderate-to-vigorous physical activity at least 5 days per week.

Consume a healthy diet, with an emphasis on plant sources.
- Choose foods and beverages in amounts that help achieve and maintain a healthy weight.
- Eat five or more servings of a variety of vegetables and fruits each day.
- Choose whole grains in preference to processed (refined) grains.
- Limit consumption of processed and red meats.

If you drink alcoholic beverages, limit consumption.
- Drink no more than one drink per day for women or two per day for men.

From Kushi LH, Byers T, Doyle C, et al: American Cancer Society Guidelines on nutrition and physical activity for cancer prevention: reducing the risk of cancer with healthy food choices and physical activity. CA Cancer J Clin 56:254–281, 2006, Table 1.

---

colors, since colorful vegetables and fruits have a variety of nutrients. Organic foods have not been shown to improve nutritional content or to prevent cancer development or recurrence[29] (Box 7-1).

LIFESTYLE

Many seemingly modifiable lifestyle factors that place a woman at higher risk for breast cancer are probably not risk factors in and of themselves but rather are markers of other known, less modifiable risk factors, such as age at menarche, parity, and age at first birth. Two examples are socioeconomic status and area of residence. Women of the highest socioeconomic status may have up to double the rate of breast cancer when compared with the incidence in women of the lowest socioeconomic classes, but it is felt that the risk is explained by lower parity and increased age at first birth. Similarly, although Hawaiians have the highest incidence of breast cancer (128 cases per 100,000 women) and women in Utah have a much lower incidence (98 cases per 100,000 women), this can probably be explained by the much higher parity rate and lower age at first birth in Utah.[30]

Adiposity

Biologic Plausibility

The higher the levels of circulating estrogens, the higher a woman's risk of developing breast cancer. Adipose (fat) tissue produces endogenous estrogens by aromatization of adrenal androgens. In addition, women with a higher BMI have lower levels of sex globulin-binding proteins, effectively further increasing the amount of bioavailable estrogens. Obesity is also associated with higher levels of insulin and insulin-like growth factor (IGF), which may contribute to the pathophysiology of cancer

growth. Many epidemiologic studies have linked being overweight with increased risk of breast cancer, particularly in postmenopausal women, in whom adipose conversion of adrenal androgens (DHEA) to estrogen provides the predominant circulating estrogen.[31]

Observational Studies

The Women's Health Initiative study estimated the magnitude of the effect of obesity on breast cancer risk by comparing over 87,000 postmenopausal women.[32] An association was found only for women who had never used hormone replacement therapy. In this group, women with a BMI at study enrollment of greater than 31.1 had an RR of postmenopausal breast cancer of 2.52 (95% CI 1.62–3.93) compared with women with a baseline BMI of less than 22.6 (Fig. 7-1).[32] Thus, it stands to reason that achieving or maintaining a normal body weight may help

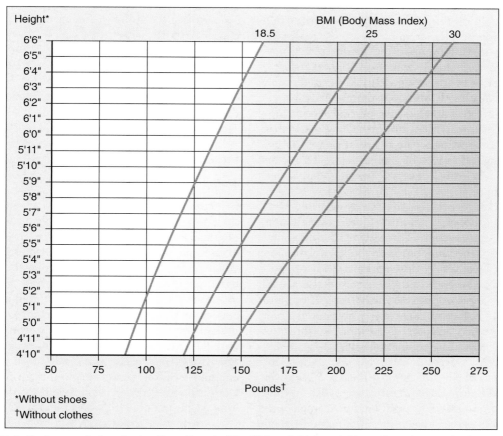

Figure 7-1. Body mass index chart. (From Report of the Dietary Guidelines Advisory Committee on the Dietary Guidelines for Americans, 2000, p 3.)

prevent breast cancer. Several large studies have investigated this premise.

Using data collected prospectively from the Nurses' Health Study,[33] researchers investigated the effects of weight change on breast cancer risk. Weight change since age 18 and weight change since menopause were assessed; nearly 50,000 women were followed up for an average of 24 years. Both weight gain since age 18 and weight gain after menopause were associated with higher risks of breast cancer development, with stronger associations seen in women who had *not* taken hormone replacement therapy. Taking exogenous hormones was thought to minimize differences due to excess weight as women would have had more equivalent circulating estrogen levels. In addition, women who had never used hormones and who lost at least 22 pounds (10 kg) after menopause had a lower risk of developing postmenopausal breast cancer than those who maintained their premenopausal weight (RR 0.43, 95% CI 0.21–0.86; P = .01 for weight loss trend).

Being overweight prepubescently and during young adulthood seems to have a *protective* effect for development of breast cancer, since obesity in this group often leads to irregular menstruation (and less estrogen exposure). Weight loss in the group that had been obese in young adulthood was not as dramatically associated with a decreased risk of cancer development. Overall, the authors concluded that 24.2% of postmenopausal breast cancer could be attributed to weight gain since age 18 and an additional 7.6% due to weight gain since menopause.[33]

If being overweight is associated with increased breast cancer risk, does severe underweight status confer protection? Adding evidence to the link between body weight and breast cancer was an observational study of 7303 Swedish women hospitalized before the age of 40 for anorexia nervosa between 1965 and 1998.[34] These women were compared in a case-matched fashion with women from the general Swedish population. The researchers found that women with hospitalization for anorexia before the age of 40 had a 53% lower incidence of invasive breast cancer, with an even more pronounced association for women who had a full-term pregnancy subsequent to their hospitalization (76% risk reduction, 95% CI 13–97).

An effect of weight on secondary prevention has also been observed. The Nurses' Health Study followed up over 5000 women who had been diagnosed with breast cancer and compared BMI at least 1 year after diagnosis with BMI before diagnosis.[35] For women who had never smoked, researchers found a significantly increased risk of recurrence and death linearly associated with weight gain after diagnosis (P = .03 for trend); a gain of 2 points in BMI (average weight gain of 17 pounds) was associated with RR of 1.64 (95% CI 1.0–2.51) compared with that for women who did not gain weight after diagnosis).[35] However, another recent study found no correlation between weight gain after diagnosis and secondary recurrence in over 3000 women studied.[36] Of note, many women gain weight during chemotherapy, with one third of women gaining more than 11 pounds (5 kg).[37]

Interventional Studies

Despite the links between adiposity and breast cancer risk, risk of breast cancer recurrence and poorer outcome with breast cancer, no randomized controlled trials of weight loss for any of these scenarios have been carried out. In a 2006 editorial, Byers and Sedjo[38] give an excellent overview of weight and breast cancer and issues that a good trial should address.

Exercise

Biologic Plausibility

Exercise is defined as planned, structured physical activity whose goal is to improve or maintain physical fitness. *Physical activity* is movement of the body and contraction of skeletal muscle, which increases energy expenditure above the basal energy expenditure level and includes exercise, household activity, job-related activity, and other activities. Physical activity can be measured in terms of metabolic equivalents (METs). METs provide an estimate of how much oxygen is used as a result of an activity and allow various physical activities to be compared with regard to their metabolic demand. One MET is defined as the metabolic rate at rest, which is approximately 3.5 mL O_2/kg/min for a seated adult. Table 7-3 shows METs for common physical activities.

Table 7-3. Metabolic Equivalents (METs) for Common Activities

Activities	METs
Leisure	
Mild	
Billiards	2.4
Canoeing (leisurely)	2.5
Dancing (ballroom)	2.9
Golf (with cart)	2.5
Horseback riding (walking)	2.3
Playing a musical instrument	
Accordion	1.8
Cello	2.3
Flute	2.0
Piano	2.3
Violin	2.5
Volleyball (noncompetitive)	2.9
Walking (2 mph)	2.5
Moderate	
Calisthenics (no weight)	4.0
Cycling (leisurely)	3.5
Golf (without cart)	4.4
Swimming (slow)	4.5
Walking (3 mph)	3.3
Walking (4 mph)	4.5
Vigorous	
Chopping wood	4.9
Climbing hills (no load)	6.9
Climbing hills (5 kg load)	7.4
Cycling (moderately)	5.7
Dancing	
Aerobic or ballet	6.0
Ballroom (fast) or square	5.5
Jogging (10 min mile)	10.2
Rope skipping	12.0
Skating	
Ice	5.5
Roller	6.5
Skiing (water or downhill)	6.8
Squash	12.1
Surfing	6.0
Swimming	7.0
Tennis (doubles)	5.0
Walking (5 mph)	8.0
Activities of daily living	
Gardening (no lifting)	4.4
Household tasks, moderate effort	3.5
Lifting items continuously	4.0
Loading/unloading car	3.0
Lying quietly	1.0
Mopping	3.5
Mowing lawn (power mower)	4.5

From Fletcher GF, Balady GJ, Amsterdam EA, et al: Exercise standards for testing and training: a statement for healthcare professionals from the American Heart Association. Circulation 104(14):1694–1740, 2001, Table 8.

Many factors suggest a biologic plausibility for an association between exercise and breast cancer risk[39] (Table 7-4). For example, strenuous exercise is associated with decreased production of estradiol and alteration of normal menses, occasionally inducing secondary amenorrhea. In addition, exercise is associated with decreased BMI and adiposity. Exercise increases insulin sensitivity and reduces insulin-like growth factor, which may play a role in tumor progression. Exercise may also enhance the body's ability to metabolize free radicals. Finally, moderate exercise improves markers of immune system function and has been shown to improve natural killer cell function and increase circulating T and B lymphocytes, monocytes, and macrophages.[40] Figure 7-2 shows many pathways through which exercise may directly and indirectly influence breast cancer risk.

Observational Studies

A large case-control study also found an inverse relation between breast cancer and exercise. The Women's Contraceptive and Reproductive Experiences Study was a multicenter (five large U.S. metropolitan areas) population-based, case-control study of black women and white women 35 to 64 years of age with newly diagnosed invasive breast cancer.[41] Over 4500 case patients were matched by age, race, and study site with over 4600 controls. Black women were oversampled to help provide more substantial data on race. Data were controlled for other known breast cancer risk factors, and estrogen receptor status was ascertained for cases. Study subjects were rigorously interviewed regarding lifetime physical activity. High levels of physical activity were defined as levels above the mean and were compared with those of inactive study subjects. Associations between exercise activity measures (metabolic equivalents of energy expenditure [MET]-hours per week per year) and breast cancer risk overall and among subgroups were examined. Among all women, increased levels of lifetime exercise were associated with approximately a 20% decrease in breast cancer risk: for 6.7 to 15.1 MET-hours/week/year, OR 0.82, 95% CI 0.71–0.93; for 15.2 MET-hours/week/year, OR 0.80, 95% CI 0.70–0.92. Results did not differ by race or for any breast cancer risk factor other than first-degree family history of breast cancer; for this

Table 7-4. Age-specific 15-year Incidence Rates of Breast Cancer of Former College Athletes and Non-athletes

Age at Time of Reporting Years	Athletes (*n* = 1935)*		Non-Athletes (*n* = 1973)*	
	Number	Rate/1000	Number	Rate/1000
<45	3	4.3	9	23.3
45–49	5	17.4	8	24.1
50–54	11	47.2	27	55.8
55–64	21	65.8	30	81.5
≥65	24	60.3	37	91.8
Total	64	32.9	111	56.3

*Excludes the 32 women (10 athletes and 22 non-athletes) who reported breast cancer in the earlier study.
From Wyshak G, Frisch RE: Breast cancer among former college athletes compared to non-athletes: a 15-year follow-up. Br J Cancer 82(3):726–730, 2000.

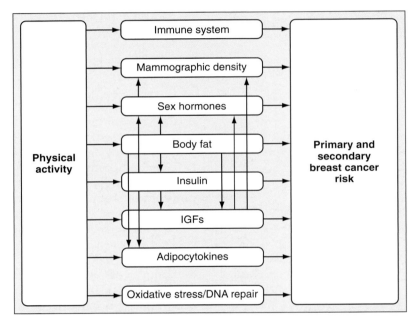

Figure 7-2. Hypothesized relation between physical activity and primary and secondary breast cancer risk. (From Irwin ML: Randomized controlled trials of physical activity and breast cancer prevention. Exerc Sport Sci Rev 34(4):182–193, 2006.)

group, no significant association between exercise and reduced risk was seen.[41]

Two large prospective observational studies have shown decreased risk for breast cancer for women who exercise. In the Women's Health Initiative study,[42] women who reported engaging in strenuous physical activity at least three times per week at age 35 had a 14% decreased risk of breast cancer compared with that for women who did not engage in regular strenuous activity (RR 0.86, 95% CI 0.78–0.95). Women who reported regular strenuous activity levels at ages 18 or 50 also had a slight reduction in breast cancer incidence, although the association did not reach statistical significance. This study, which prospectively followed up 74,147 postmenopausal women, also found that a higher level of current exercise (at time of study enrollment and over the almost 5-year follow-up) was also associated, in a dose-response relationship, with decreased breast cancer risk. Compared with women who were inactive, women who exercised the equivalent of 1.25 to 2.5 hours of brisk walking per week had an RR of 0.82 (95% CI 0.68–0.97). Protective effects of current exercise in this study were most pronounced in women who also had a BMI of less than 24.1.

In the Nurses' Health Study,[43] pre- and postmenopausal women were followed up for up to 16 years. Women who reported engaging in at least moderate physical activity for 7 or more hours per week had an RR of breast cancer of 0.82 (95% CI 0.70–0.97) compared with RR for those who engaged in moderate exercise for less than 1 hour per week.

The Iowa Women's Health Study sought to further define the relation between physical activity and breast cancer by looking at tumor hormone receptor status.[44] Over 41,800 postmenopausal women were followed up for 18 years for development of breast cancer. A baseline questionnaire ascertained physical activity level and differentiated activity into low, medium, and high activity levels. High levels of physical activity were associated with lower breast cancer risk, most pronounced for estrogen-positive/progesterone-negative tumors (RR controlled for BMI 0.66, 95% CI 0.46–0.94).

Based on these and other studies, the National Cancer Institute (NCI) states that "strenuous exercising more than 4 hours per week is associated with reduced breast cancer risk,"[45] with an average RR reduction of 30% to 40%. According to NCI, the effect may be greatest for premenopausal women of normal or low body weight.

Correlations have also been made between exercise and prevention of secondary breast cancer and breast cancer mortality. A prospective, observational trial published in 2005 showed a decreased risk of breast cancer death with an increase in exercise.[46] This study followed up 2987 women (most of whom were white) from the Nurses' Health Study who were diagnosed with stage I, II, or III breast cancer between 1984 and 1998 until death or June 2002, whichever came first. Women were stratified by physical activity into MET-hours per week. Three MET-hours are equivalent to walking at 2 to 2.9 mph for 1 hour. Less than 3 MET-hours per week constituted the lowest stratification; over 24 MET-hours, the highest. Compared with women who engaged in less than 3 MET-hours per week, any level of increased MET-hours per week higher than this reference was associated with a decreased risk of death from breast cancer.

Benefits of exercise were even more pronounced in women with hormone receptor-positive tumors. The RR of breast cancer death for women with hormone-responsive tumors who engaged in 9 or more MET-hours per week of activity compared with women with hormone-responsive tumors who engaged in less than 9 MET-hours per week was 0.50 (95% CI 0.34–0.74). Compared with women who engaged in less than 3 MET-hours per week of activity, the absolute unadjusted mortality risk reduction was 6% at 10 years for women who engaged in 9 or more MET-hours per week. The RR of adverse outcomes including death, breast cancer death, and breast cancer recurrence were 26% to 40% lower when women with the highest to the lowest category of activity were compared.

The American Cancer Society recommends 30 to 60 minutes of vigorous physical activity at least 5 days per week to reduce the risk for cancer. If a person is sedentary at baseline, however, this amount of exercise is not immediately attainable. As noted in the summary by Doyle and associates,[29] the message given to the patient should be that exercise is associated with reduced risk of cancer in a linear fashion; that is, doing even a little bit of exercise and increasing daily activity are better than doing nothing. (See Box 7-2 for suggestions for increasing physical activity.) Encouragement should be offered to all patients to help them to gradually achieve the recommended levels.

Interventional Studies

At this time, no prospective, randomized, controlled intervention trials of exercise and primary

---

Box 7-2. Suggested Ways to Increase Physical Activity

Use stairs rather than an elevator.
If you can, walk or bike to your destination.
Exercise with your family, friends, and coworkers.
Take an exercise break to stretch or take a short walk.
Walk to visit nearby friends or coworkers instead of sending an e-mail.
Plan active vacations rather than only driving trips.
Wear a pedometer every day and increase your daily steps.
Use a stationary bicycle or treadmill while watching TV.

From Doyle C, Kushi LH, Byers T, et al: Nutrition and physical activity during and after cancer treatment: an American Cancer Society guide for informed choices. CA Cancer J Clin 56:323–353, 2006, Table 4.

or secondary prevention of breast cancer have been published. A review of the NIH Research Portfolio Online Reporting Tool (RePORT) in February 2010 did not show any government-funded trials in progress (http://projectreporter. nih.gov/reporter.cfm).

Alcohol

Biologic Plausibility

Alcohol intake is associated with increases in circulating hormones (androgens and estrogens), increased susceptibility of mammary tissue to carcinogenesis, increased damage to mammary gland DNA, and greater potential for breast cancer cells, once formed, to become invasive.[47]

Observational Studies

An ambitious 2002 study combined data from approximately 80% of the world's case-control studies on alcohol and breast cancer and determined that as alcohol intake increases, the chance of developing breast cancer also rises, in a linear fashion.[48] The authors concluded that for each alcoholic drink (10 g) consumed by a woman on a daily basis, her risk of developing breast cancer rises by 7%. They further estimated that alcohol intake could account for 4% of breast cancers diagnosed in developed countries (Fig. 7-3).

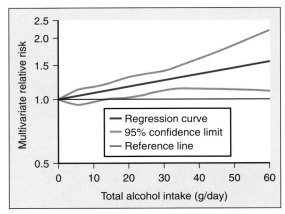

Figure 7-3. Alcohol intake and breast cancer. Nonparametric regression curve for the relation between total alcohol intake and breast cancer. (From Smith-Warner SA, Spiegelman D, Yaun SS, et al: Alcohol and breast cancer in women: a pooled analysis of cohort studies. JAMA 279:535–540, 1998.)

The NCI states that the RR of women consuming approximately four alcoholic drinks per day compared with that of nondrinkers is 1.32 (95% CI 1.19–1.45). The RR increases by 7% (95% CI 5.5–8.7) for each drink per day. People who drink large amounts of alcohol are more likely to have lower folate levels, but studies exploring the relation between folate consumption and breast cancer risk, adjusted for alcohol intake, have been inconclusive.

The risk of alcohol may be additive with the risk of hormone replacement therapy, as reported in the Nurses' Health Study.[49] In this group of 44,187 women followed up prospectively for 14 years, it was found that women who drank more than 20 g of alcohol per day and who had taken hormone replacement therapy for at least 5 years were two times more likely to develop breast cancer compared with women who neither drank alcohol nor used hormones (RR 1.99, 95% CI 1.42–2.79). As the authors put it, "A hypothetical postmenopausal woman whose lifetime risk for breast cancer is 4% could increase her risk to 8% with 5 or more years of current [hormone replacement therapy] use and consumption of more than one alcoholic drink daily."[49]

Two studies provide support for the proposed mechanism that alcohol may increase breast cancer risk through alterations in hormone levels. A 2003 study of postmenopausal older women in Washington state found that increased alcohol intake correlated with increased rates of breast cancer, with estrogen receptor-positive tumors being more likely than estrogen receptor-negative tumors.[50] Similarly, a Swedish study published in 2005 followed up 51,847 postmenopausal women and found an increased estrogen receptor-positive breast cancer risk associated with increasing alcohol intake.[51]

Stress

Biologic Plausibility

Patients often express concern that increased stress will lead to illness. In vivo and in vitro data do support the idea that stress can negatively affect the immune system; however, definitive links between stress and cancer have not been seen consistently, as illustrated by the following studies.

Observational Studies

A prospective cohort study of Finnish women surveyed self-perceived daily stress. Over 10,500 Finnish adult women were followed up for over 21 years, and no difference was seen between levels of perceived stress and risk of breast cancer.[52]

The same study group looked for a possible relation between stressful life events and the risk of breast cancer, using the same prospective Finnish twin cohort. They did find a statistically significant increased risk of breast cancer associated with three stressful life events that occurred in the 5 years before study enrollment: divorce, death of a husband, and death of a close relative. Hazard ratios for these events were 2.26 (CI 1.25–4.07), 2.00 (CI 1.03–3.88), and 1.36 (CI 1.00–1.86), respectively. The authors acknowledged that most studies of this subject had not found increased risk with stressful life events. Ratios did not change, however, when controls for possible confounders were added.[53]

Related to the issue of stress is the concept of a "cancer personality type." Some people believe that certain personality traits place a person at higher risk of developing cancer. However, such a link between personality type and cancer has not been found. In 1973, the Swedish Twin Cohort study administered the Eysenck Personality Inventory to 29,595 twins 15 to 48 years of age. They were followed up until 1999, and in twin pairs discordant for cancer, no relation between personality traits and cancer was seen.[54]

Exposures

Ionizing Radiation

A retrospective cohort study of 6068 women in the Childhood Cancer Survivor Study (CCSS), a multicenter study of persons who survived more than 5 years after childhood cancer diagnosed from 1970 to 1986, identified women in the cohort with breast cancer and compared their incidence of cancer with standardized incidence ratios for age-matched breast cancer in the general population. The evaluation showed that breast cancer risk was dramatically increased in survivors who had been treated with chest radiation therapy (standardized incidence ratio 24.7, 95% CI 19.3–31.0).

Perhaps it is also not surprising that exposure to pelvic radiation was protective for the development of breast cancer (RR 0.6, CI 0.4–0.9). The authors also noted that the risk may be underestimated, since the average age of the cohort had not yet reached an age at which the risk of breast cancer is greatest.[55] NCI summarizes: "Based on solid evidence, exposure of the breast to ionizing radiation is associated with an increased risk of developing breast cancer, starting 10 years after exposure and persisting lifelong. Risk depends on dose and age at exposure, with the highest risk occurring during puberty. [There is] approximately a 6-fold increase in incidence overall."[45]

This type of radiation, however, should not be considered a modifiable lifestyle factor because the women obviously needed this treatment for a current disease that presented an immediate risk to life, which would supersede consideration of a future potential risk. Screening recommendations for early diagnosis of breast cancer include childhood radiation as an indication for either earlier initiation of screening or more intensive screening, that is, magnetic resonance imaging (MRI).[56]

Women do have some control over exposure to other sources of ionizing radiation. For example, a woman may choose a career with radiation exposure, or she may choose to have (or not have) a procedure that uses ionizing radiation for diagnostic purposes (mammograms, computed tomography [CT] scans, plain radiographs). The association between exposure to ionizing radiation exposure in one's career and breast cancer seems to be negligible, and any increased risk with diagnostic radiation also appears to be zero or negligible.[57]

Sleep Cycle Issues

Some researchers believe that exposure to light at night may increase risk for breast cancer and that not sleeping at night may also increase risk. The biologic plausibility is thought to be related to decreased melatonin production in these situations; melatonin may protect against the development of breast cancer because it inhibits release of estrogen by the ovaries. Indeed, increased urinary melatonin levels have been associated with decreased breast cancer risk, but the strength of the associations has been variable.

Within the Nurses' Health Study II cohort, researchers paired breast cancer cases ($n = 147$) with controls ($n = 291$) and measured urinary melatonin metabolites in the first morning urine. Comparing women with the highest quartile of urinary metabolites with those with the lowest quartile showed a decreased RR of breast cancer of 0.59 (95% CI 0.36–0.97); the relationship held when controlled for common risk factors.[58] Another case-control study included 7035 Danish women with breast cancer and individually matched controls. Researchers found that the OR for breast cancer for women who had worked at night for at least half a year was 1.5 (95% CI 1.2–1.7), with a dose-response trend also seen.[59] Results were similar in another case-control study with over 1600 total patients.[60]

A more modest association between nighttime shift work and breast cancer risk was noted in a prospective cohort report from the Nurses' Health Study. This study followed up 78,562 women for 10 years in a prospective fashion and compared breast cancer cases with controls. Nurses were asked about the total number of years in which they had worked at least three night shifts per month. The risk of development of breast cancer was 1.08 for women who had worked 1 to 14 years or 15 to 29 years with night shifts, but in both cases the 95% CI included 1, making results nonstatistically significant. Statistically significant association was seen only after women had worked at least 30 years of night shifts (RR 1.36, 95% CI 1.04–1.78). There was a statistically significant relation for the trend, however.[61]

Chemicals and Pesticides

A number of environmental chemicals exist that seem with biochemical plausibility to increase the risk of breast cancer from a number of mechanisms; many of these have been shown to cause mammary cancer in rodents. Most of these chemicals would not be encountered by the average woman, however. Studies have looked at occupation and breast cancer risk, but these studies are by and large poorly designed. Organochlorides appear not to be associated with breast cancer risk, but organic solvents, such as those used in dry cleaning, may be associated with breast cancer; some studies have suggested an increased risk of breast cancer for dry cleaning workers. Some heavy metals, such as cadmium, copper, nickel, and lead, appear to activate the estrogen receptor and induce estrogenic effects, but studies on heavy metals and breast cancer risk have yet to be done.[62]

Given that industrialized nations have higher levels of breast cancer than nonindustrialized nations, researchers have looked for possible links between factors found in developed countries and breast cancer risk (Fig. 7-4). One possible risk factor is agricultural pesticides, since many of these compounds are known to be carcinogenic in lab animals and low levels can be detected in humans. One research group used the California Teacher's Cohort to investigate whether proximity to high levels of agricultural pesticide use would predict risk of breast cancer.[63] California was chosen because it has one of the highest rates of breast cancer in the nation and is a largely agricultural state. Over 130,000 women were followed prospectively between 1996 and 1999 for development of breast cancer; no links were found between proximity to pesticides and breast cancer.

Other Environmental Factors *Not* Associated with Increased Risk of Breast Cancer

Agents that have not been shown in well-designed trials not to be associated with increased breast cancer risk include deodorant, silicone breast implants, electromagnetic fields, electric blankets, hair dyes, underwire bras, and trauma to the breast. Other agents not associated with breast cancer risk exist, but these agents are the ones that have received the most media attention and are therefore a concern of many patients. The Susan G. Komen website[64] is an excellent resource for clinicians and patients who seek more information on this subject.

Tobacco

In the 2002 study by Hamajima and associates,[48] which investigated the relation between alcohol and breast cancer, the relation between tobacco and breast cancer was also analyzed. The authors noted that prior studies on tobacco and breast cancer had had mixed results, and they predicted that some of this discrepancy could likely be explained by confounding with alcohol intake. Indeed, when consumption of alcohol (higher in smokers versus nonsmokers) was controlled for, smoking status was not definitively associated

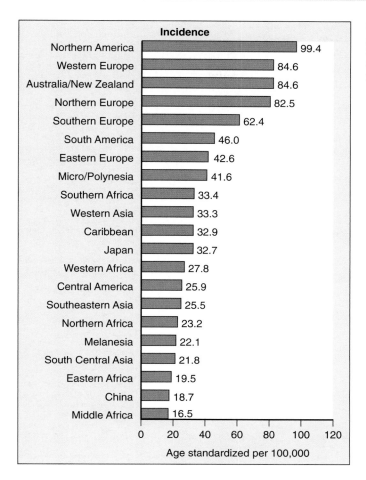

Figure 7-4. Breast cancer incidence by geographic area. (Adapted from Parkin DM, Bray F, Ferlay J, Pisani P: Global cancer statistics, 2002. CA Cancer J Clin 55:74–108, 2005.)

with breast cancer risk. However, the amount and duration of exposure to tobacco were not analyzed; just "never smoker" versus "ever smoker" were compared. Exposure to second-hand smoke was also not evaluated. Both of these conditions may have biased the results to a nonassociation.

Summary

The World Cancer Research Fund/American Institute for Cancer Research estimates that about one third of cancer cases worldwide can be prevented by good diet, physical activity, and avoidance of obesity. The preponderance of epidemiologic studies indicates that women who engage in 3 to 4 hours per week of moderate to vigorous levels of exercise have a 30% to 40% lower risk for developing breast cancer than do sedentary women as well as a lower risk of recurrence or death from breast cancer. Women who are overweight or obese have a 50% to 250% greater risk for postmenopausal breast cancer. Alcohol use, even at moderate levels (two drinks per day), increases the risk for both premenopausal and postmenopausal breast cancer. Certain dietary patterns, such as high fat consumption, low amounts of vegetables and fruits, low fiber, and high simple carbohydrates, may increase risk, but definitive data are lacking. Increasing the intake of low-fat dairy products and avoiding night shift work may be protective. These lifestyle factors are likely associated with breast cancer etiology through hormonal mechanisms. The worldwide trends of increasing obesity and decreasing physical activity may lead to an increasing incidence of breast cancer unless other means of risk reduction counteract these effects. Thus, adoption of lifestyle changes by individuals and populations may have a large impact on the future incidence of this disease.

References

1. Wold KS, Byers T, Crane LA, Ahnen D: What do cancer survivors believe causes cancer? (United States) Cancer Causes Control 16:115–123, 2005.
2. World Cancer Research Fund/American Institute for Cancer Research: Food, Nutrition, Physical Activity, and the Prevention of Cancer: a global perspective. Washington, DC: AICR, 2007. http://www.dietandcancerreport.org/downloads/chapters/prelims.pdf.
3. Lichtenstein P, Holm NV, Verkasalo PK, et al: Environmental and heritable factors in the causation of cancer. N Engl J Med 343:78–85, 2000.
4. Boyd NF, Stone J, Vogt KN, et al: Dietary fat and breast cancer risk revisited: a meta-analysis of the published literature. Br J Cancer 89:1672–1685, 2003.
5. Gonzalez CA: Nutrition and cancer: the current epidemiological evidence. Br J Nutr 96(Suppl 1):S42–S45, 2006.
6. Smith-Warner SA, Spiegelman D, Yaun SS, et al: Intake of fruits and vegetables and risk of breast cancer: a pooled analysis of cohort studies. JAMA 285:769–776, 2001.
7. Riboli E, Norat T: Epidemiologic evidence of the protective effect of fruit and vegetables on cancer risk. Am J Clin Nutr 78(Suppl 3):559S–569S, 2003.
8. van Gils CH, Peeters PH, Bueno-de-Mesquita BH, et al: Consumption of vegetables and fruits and risk of breast cancer. JAMA 293:183–193, 2005.
9. Lipscombe LL, Goodwin PJ, Zinman B, et al: Diabetes mellitus and breast cancer: a retrospective population-based cohort study. Breast Cancer Res Treat 98:349–356, 2006.
10. Tavani A, Giordano L, Gallus S, et al: Consumption of sweet foods and breast cancer risk in Italy. Ann Oncol 17:341–345, 2006.
11. Buzdar AU: Dietary modification and risk of breast cancer. JAMA 295:691–692, 2006.
12. Prentice RL, Caan B, Chlebowski RT: JAMA 295:629–642, 2006.
13. Chlebowski RT, Blackburn GL, Thomson CA: Dietary fat reduction and breast cancer outcome: interim efficacy results from the Women's Intervention Nutrition Study. J Natl Cancer Inst 98:1767–1776, 2006.
14. Shin MH, Holmes MD, Hankinson SE, et al: Intake of dairy products, calcium, and vitamin D and risk of breast cancer. J Natl Cancer Inst 94:1301–1311, 2002.
15. McCullough ML, Rodriguez C, Diver WR: Dairy, calcium, and vitamin D intake and postmenopausal breast cancer risk in the Cancer Prevention Study II nutrition cohort. Cancer Epidemiol Biomarkers Prev 14:2898–2904, 2005.
16. Messina M, McCaskill-Stevens W, Lampe JW: Addressing the soy and breast cancer relationship: review, commentary, and workshop proceedings. J Natl Cancer Inst 98:1275–1284, 2006.
17. Wu AH, Wan P, Hankin J, et al: Adolescent and adult soy intake and risk of breast cancer in Asian-Americans. Carcinogenesis 23:1491–1496, 2002.
18. Horn-Ross PL, John EM, Lee M, et al: Phytoestrogen consumption and breast cancer risk in a multiethnic population: the Bay Area Breast Cancer Study. Am J Epidemiol 154(5):434–441, 2001.
19. Trock BJ, Hilakivi-Clarke L, Clarke R: Meta-analysis of soy intake and breast cancer risk. J Natl Cancer Inst 98:459–471, 2006.
20. Engeset D, Alsaker E, Lund E, et al: Fish consumption and breast cancer risk. The European Prospective Investigation into Cancer and Nutrition (EPIC). Int J Cancer 119:175–182, 2006.
21. Howe GR, Hirohata T, Hislop TG, et al: Dietary factors and risk of breast cancer: combined analysis of 12 case-control studies. J Natl Cancer Inst 82:561–569, 1990.
22. Zhang SM: Role of vitamins in the risk, prevention, and treatment of breast cancer. Curr Opin Obstet Gynecol 16:19–25, 2004.
23. Dorjgochoo T, Gao YT, Chow WH, et al: Plasma carotenoids, tocopherols, retinol and breast cancer risk: results from the Shanghai Women Health Study (SWHS). Breast Cancer Res Treat 117:381–389, 2009.
24. Cho E, Spiegelman D, Hunter DJ, et al: Premenopausal intakes of vitamins A, C, and E, folate, and carotenoids, and risk of breast cancer. Cancer Epidemiol Biomarkers Prev 12:713–720, 2003.
25. Zhang S, Hunter DJ, Forman MR, et al: Dietary carotenoids and vitamins A, C, and E and risk of breast cancer. J Natl Cancer Inst 91:547–556, 1999.
26. Garland CF, Garland FC, Gorham ED, et al: The role of vitamin D in cancer prevention. Am J Public Health 96:252–261, 2003.
27. Welsh J, Wietzke JA, Zinser GM, et al: Vitamin D-3 receptor as a target for breast cancer prevention. J Nutr 133:2425S–2433S, 2003.
28. Calhoun KE, Pommier RF, Muller P, et al: Dehydroepiandrosterone sulfate causes proliferation of estrogen receptor-positive breast cancer cells despite treatment with fulvestrant. Arch Surg 138:879–883, 2003.
29. Doyle C, Kushi LH, Byers T, et al: Nutrition and physical activity during and after cancer treatment: an American Cancer Society guide for informed choices. CA Cancer J Clin 56:323–353, 2006.
30. Sturgeon SR, Schairer C, Gail M, et al: Geographic variation in mortality from breast cancer among white women in the United States. J Natl Cancer Inst 87:1846–1853, 1995.
31. Calle EE, Kaaks R: Overweight, obesity and cancer: epidemiological evidence and proposed mechanisms. Nat Rev Cancer 4:579–591, 2004.
32. Morimoto LM, White E, Chen Z, et al: Obesity, body size, and risk of postmenopausal breast cancer: the Women's Health Initiative (United States). Cancer Causes Control 13:741–751, 2002.
33. Eliassen AH, Colditz GA, Rosner B, et al: Adult weight change and risk of postmenopausal breast cancer. JAMA 296:193–201, 2006.
34. Michels KB, Ekbom A: Caloric restriction and incidence of breast cancer. JAMA 291:1226–1230, 2004.
35. Kroenke CH, Chen WY, Rosner B, et al: Weight, weight gain, and survival after breast cancer diagnosis. J Clin Oncol 23:1370–1378, 2005.
36. Caan BJ, Emond JA, Natarajan L, et al: Postdiagnosis weight gain and breast cancer recurrence in women with early stage breast cancer. Breast Cancer Res Treat 99:47–57, 2006.
37. Demark-Wahnefried W, Rock CL: Nutrition-related issues for the breast cancer survivor. Semin Oncol 30:789–798, 2003.
38. Byers T, Sedjo RL: A weight loss trial for breast cancer recurrence: pre-menopausal, post-menopausal, both, or neither? Cancer Causes Control 17:1–3, 2006.
39. Irwin ML: Randomized controlled trials of physical activity and breast cancer prevention. Exerc Sport Sci Rev 34:182–193, 2006.
40. Moldoveanu AI, Shephard RJ, Shek PN: The cytokine response to physical activity and training. Sports Med 31:115–144, 2001.
41. Bernstein L, Patel AV, Ursin G, et al: Lifetime recreational exercise activity and breast cancer risk among black women and white women. J Natl Cancer Inst 97:1671–1679, 2005.
42. McTiernan A, Kooperberg C, White E, et al: Recreational physical activity and the risk of breast cancer in postmenopausal women: the Women's Health Initiative Cohort Study. JAMA 290:1331–1336, 2003.
43. Rockhill B, Willett WC, Hunter DJ, et al: A prospective study of recreational physical activity and breast cancer risk. Arch Intern Med 159:2290–2296, 1999.
44. Bardia A, Hartmann LC, Vachon CM: Recreational physical activity and risk of postmenopausal breast cancer based on hormone receptor status. Arch Intern Med 166:2478–2483, 2006.
45. www.cancer.gov/cancertopics/pdq/prevention/breast/HealthProfessional#Section_178. This website gives information about breast cancer and interventions to prevent breast cancer.
46. Holmes MD, Chen WY, Feskanich D, et al: Physical activity and survival after breast cancer diagnosis. JAMA 293:2479–2486, 2005.
47. Singletary KW, Gapstur SM: Alcohol and breast cancer: review of epidemiologic and experimental evidence and potential mechanisms. JAMA 286:2143–2151, 2001.
48. Hamajima N, Hirose K, Tajima K, et al: Alcohol, tobacco and breast cancer—collaborative reanalysis of individual data from 53 epidemiological studies, including 58,515 women with breast cancer and 95,067 women without the disease. Br J Cancer 87:1234–1245, 2002.
49. Chen WY, Colditz GA, Rosner B, et al: Use of postmenopausal hormones, alcohol, and risk for invasive breast cancer. Ann Intern Med 137:798–804, 2002.

50. Li CI, Malone KE, Porter PL, et al: The relationship between alcohol use and risk of breast cancer by histology and hormone receptor status among women 65–79 years of age. Cancer Epidemiol Biomarkers Prev 12:1061–1066, 2003.

51. Suzuki R, Ye W, Rylander-Rudqvist T, et al: Alcohol and postmenopausal breast cancer risk defined by estrogen and progesterone receptor status: a prospective cohort study. J Natl Cancer Inst 97:1601–1608, 2005.

52. Lillberg K, Verkasalo P, Kaprio J, et al: Stress of daily activities and risk of breast cancer: a prospective cohort study in Finland. Int J Cancer 91:888–893, 2001.

53. Lillberg K, Verkasalo PK, Kaprio J, et al: Stressful life events and risk of breast cancer in 10,808 women: a cohort study. Am J Epidemiol 157:415–423, 2003.

54. Hansen PE, Floderus B, Frederiksen K, et al: Personality traits, health behavior, and risk for cancer: a prospective study of a Swedish twin cohort. Cancer 103:1082–1091, 2005.

55. Kenney LB, Yasui Y, Inskip PD, et al: Breast cancer after childhood cancer: a report from the Childhood Cancer Survivor Study. Ann Intern Med 141:590–597, 2004.

56. Saslow D, Boetes C, Burke W, et al: American Cancer Society guidelines for breast screening with MRI as an adjunct to mammography. CA Cancer J Clin 57:75–89, 2007.

57. Ronckers CM, Erdmann CA, Land CE: Radiation and breast cancer: a review of current evidence. Breast Cancer Res 7:21–32, 2005.

58. Schernhammer ES, Hankinson SE: Urinary melatonin levels and breast cancer risk. J Natl Cancer Inst 97:1084–1087, 2005.

59. Hansen J: Increased breast cancer risk among women who work predominantly at night. Epidemiology 12:74–77, 2001.

60. Davis S, Mirick DK, Stevens RG: Night shift work, light at night, and risk of breast cancer. J Natl Cancer Inst 93:1557–1562, 2001.

61. Schernhammer ES, Laden F, Speizer FE, et al: Rotating night shifts and risk of breast cancer in women participating in the nurses' health study. J Natl Cancer Inst 93:1563–1568, 2001.

62. Coyle YM: The effect of environment on breast cancer risk. Br Cancer Res Treat 84:273–288, 2004.

63. Reynolds P, Hurley S, Goldberg D, et al: Residential proximity to agricultural pesticide use and incidence of breast cancer in the California Teachers Study cohort. Environ Res 96:206–218, 2004.

64. Susan G. Komen website: http://www5.komen.org/BreastCancer/FactorsThatDoNotIncreaseRisk.html (accessed 2.7.10). This web page provides an extensive listing of other factors that do not increase the risk of breast cancer.

8

Radiologic Techniques for Early Detection and Diagnosis

John M. Lewin

KEY POINTS

- Mammography is still the best screening test for the early detection of breast cancer for most women.
- Women of average risk for breast cancer should begin annual mammographic screening at age 40.
- Digital mammography is equivalent to film screen mammography for most women and may be slightly better at detecting breast cancer in women under age 50 with dense breasts.
- Ultrasound is currently not used for screening but is an excellent diagnostic tool for further evaluation of an abnormal mammogram or clinical breast complaint.
- MRI is used for screening women at high risk for breast cancer and to evaluate the extent of disease in the ipsilateral and contralateral breast in a patient with a new diagnosis of breast cancer.
- Imaging techniques currently under investigation for screening or diagnosis include FDG-PET, sestamibi, tomosynthesis, contrast enhanced digital mammography, and dedicated breast CT.

Film Mammography

Despite no shortage of research on technologies meant to supplant it, mammography remains the mainstay of breast cancer screening. As such, any chapter on the early detection of breast cancer by imaging needs to include a discussion of this very important modality. A mammogram is an x-ray image of a compressed breast. For screening mammography, two mammograms are acquired in projections that are roughly 45 degrees apart. The signs of breast cancer on mammography include masses, architectural distortions, densities, and grouped calcifications (Fig. 8-1).

First proposed for use in widespread screening in the 1960s, mammography is the only screening test proven by randomized clinical trials to reduce breast cancer mortality. Eight large trials have been conducted to study the efficacy of screening mammography.[1-3] The results of these trials show an average 30% reduction in breast cancer mortality rate. Despite the success in the overall cohort, there remains a longstanding debate on the usefulness of screening average-risk women between 40 and 50 years old.[1,4,5] Although no trial had sufficient power to prove a significant difference in mortality for this age group, secondary analyses and meta-analyses have been put forward to support the use of screening mammography in this age group.[6-7] Currently, annual screening starting at age 40 is the recommendation of many professional organizations, including the American Cancer Society.[8]

Data supporting screening mammography can also be gleaned from population statistics on breast cancer mortality rates. In countries with screening programs, including the United States, Sweden, and the United Kingdom, decreases in breast cancer mortality are seen starting about 10 years after the initiation of widespread mammographic screening, in the mid-1970s in Sweden and in the mid-1980s in the United States and the United Kingdom.[9] In Denmark, however, which is just starting a screening program, breast cancer mortality rates continued to increase in that same period (Fig. 8-2), although there has been a decrease in Copenhagen, where a screening program was started in 1991.[10]

Digital Mammography

A much publicized development in mammography is the advent of digital mammography. This

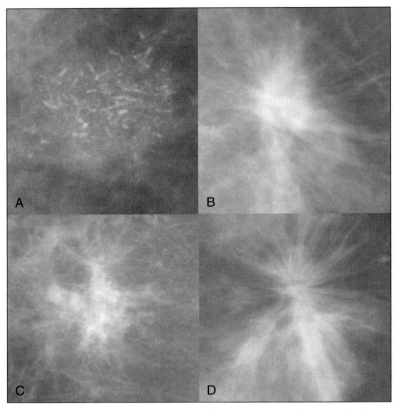

Figure 8-1. Signs of breast cancer on mammography. **A,** Grouped microcalcifications. **B,** Spiculated mass. **C,** Asymmetric density. **D,** Architectural distortion.

technology replaces the phosphorescent screen and film used in standard mammography with a digital detector. The advantages of the digital detector are greater contrast resolution and greater dynamic range, meaning that it is able to distinguish finer shades of gray in all parts of the image—light and dark. Digital mammography also enables digital image manipulation, as well as digital storage and retrieval. The disadvantage of digital mammography is a slightly lower spatial resolution. In addition, although digital mammography provides faster patient through-put per machine than film, it takes longer to interpret each study, primarily owing to the extra time spent manipulating the images.[11]

Because of both technical advantages and disadvantages of digital mammography compared with film mammography, clinical trials have been conducted to test the two modalities for cancer screening. Four prospective trials have been conducted to date. Three of these were paired trials, in which each subject received

both a film and a digital mammogram, allowing the subject to be used as her own control. The first two of these trials, the Colorado/Massachusetts trial and the Oslo I trial, showed no significant difference between film and digital mammography; in fact, both trials had trends favoring film for cancer detection (although both showed lower call-back rates for digital).[12,13] The most recent and largest paired trial, the Digital Mammographic Imaging Screening Trial (DMIST), conducted by the American College of Radiology Imaging Network (ACRIN), though not showing an overall difference, did show a significant advantage of digital mammography in certain subgroups of women, namely, premenopausal women with dense breasts under 50 years of age.[14,15] This is intuitively satisfying, since it is within dense breasts that one would expect the superior contrast resolution of digital mammography to have the greatest benefit. Table 8-1 summarizes the results of the DMIST trial. The one randomized trial, the Oslo II trial, in which

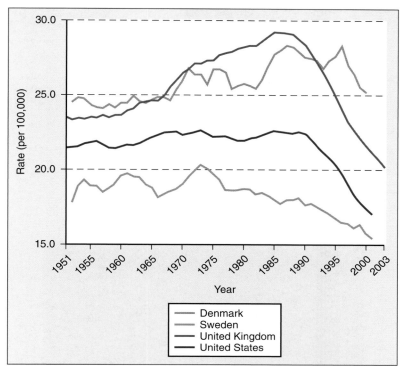

Figure 8-2. Graph showing age-adjusted breast cancer mortality in four countries. Note the dropoff in mortality occurring in the mid-1970s in Sweden and mid-1980s in the United States and the United Kingdom. In each case, the mortality decline begins about 10 years after the adoption of widespread mammographic screening. Denmark shows no decrease in that time period, although there may be a decline starting in 2000, possibly related to limited screening starting in 1991.

Cohort	Cancers Detected on Digital Only (n)	Cancers Detected on Film Only (n)	Cancers Detected on Both Modalities (n)	Cancers Detected on Neither Modality (n)	Area Under ROC Curve Digital	Area Under ROC Curve Film
All subjects	63	52	122	98	0.78 ± .02	0.74 ± .02
<50 years	22	6	26	18	0.84 ± .03	0.69 ± .05
Pre- or perimenopausal	33	11	32	24	0.82 ± .03	0.67 ± .05
Heterogeneously or extremely dense breasts	40	19	54	52	0.78 ± .03	0.68 ± .03

Table 8-1. Results of ACRIN DMIST[15]

ACRIN, American College of Radiology Imaging Network; DMIST, Digital Mammographic Imaging Screening Trial; ROC, receiver operating characteristic.
Reprinted with permission from Seminars in Breast Disease 9(3):105–110, 2006.

each subject was randomized to either film or digital mammography, originally showed no difference in cancer detection,[16] but the final analysis was revised to show a statistically significant improvement in cancer detection rate, but not sensitivity, by digital mammography.[17] This improved cancer detection rate was at the expense of an increased recall rate, however. Table 8-2 summarizes the results of the four clinical trials in digital mammography.

Despite no clear proven advantage in cancer detection for most women, digital mammogra-

Table 8-2. Comparison of Overall Results for Four Major Digital Mammography Screening Trials[12,13,15–17]

Trial	Cancer Detection/Sensitivity	Recall Rate/Specificity	Area under the ROC Curve
Colorado/Massachusetts	Trend for film	Digital superior	Trend for film
Oslo I	Trend for film	Film superior[b]	N/A[c]
Oslo II	Digital superior[d]	Film superior	N/A[c]
DMIST, Total cohort	Trend for digital	No difference	Trend for digital
DMIST, Subgroups[a]	Digital superior	No difference	Digital superior

[a]Subgroups are: <50 years old; pre-/ peri-menopausal; heterogeneously or extremely dense breasts.
[b]Large trend not tested for significance in published paper.
[c]ROC analysis not performed in the Oslo I and II studies.
[d]Final results revised to show digital superior in cancer detection rate but not sensitivity.
Modified with permission from Seminars in Breast Disease 9(3):105–110, 2006.

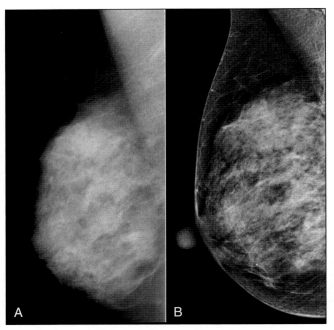

Figure 8-3. Dense breast imaged with film mammography (A) and digital mammography (B). Note the overall greater tissue detail and the improved depiction of tissue near the periphery of the breast on the digital mammogram.

phy is replacing film mammography. Most new systems sold are digital. The primary reason centers switch to digital is operational. Since the rest of radiology has long since done away with film, and therefore film processors and film storage, it makes operational sense to switch mammography to digital and take advantage of the digital infrastructure now present in most departments. The digital nature of the data also enables sophisticated postprocessing that allows the tissue to be optimally displayed in both the high-density and low-density portions of the image. Combined with the improved dynamic range and contrast resolution, this processing seems to make it possible to see through dense tissue in a way that was not possible with film mammography. At the same time, the periphery of the breast can be lightened digitally so that it is easily seen without any brightness adjustment by the user. Figure 8-3 shows a comparison of a dense breast imaged on both film and digital mammography. There is no question that digital mammography can create beautiful depictions of masses and microcalcifications; the question is whether these visually appealing images actually translate into a clinical benefit.

Ultrasound

Over the past 15 years, ultrasound has progressively increased in importance as a modality for diagnosing breast cancer. Ultrasound is used as a diagnostic tool to work up both mammographic findings and palpable abnormalities. Ultrasound has been used for over two decades to distinguish cysts from solid masses, but it is now commonly also used to characterize solid masses (Fig. 8-4) and to confirm questionable mammographic abnormalities. Ultrasound now serves as the primary modality for directing image-guided needle biopsies of masses. Stereotactic mammographic imaging is still the primary guidance for biopsies of microcalcifications.

One of the greatest diagnostic strengths of ultrasonography is in evaluating palpable abnor-

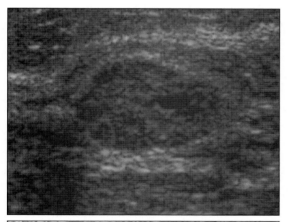

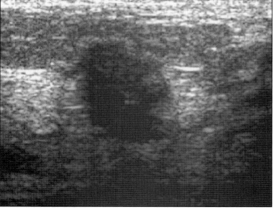

Figure 8-4. Benign versus malignant masses on ultrasound. Fibroadenoma (*top*) shows benign features including oval shape, circumscribed margins, and no posterior acoustic effect. Invasive ductal carcinoma (*bottom*) is irregularly shaped with indistinct margins and posterior acoustic shadowing.

malities. Most important is its high negative predictive value, which lies in the range of 99% to 100%.[18-20] In other words, the likelihood that a palpable abnormality is cancer falls to below 1% if no abnormality is detected on ultrasound examination of the palpable area. This contrasts with the relatively poor predictive value of a negative mammogram in the presence of a palpable abnormality. Cases of delayed diagnosis of palpable cancers because of a negative diagnostic mammogram are well known. For this reason, imaging evaluation of a palpable abnormality should always include ultrasound.

More recently, ultrasound has been studied for use in screening, especially of women with mammographically dense breasts. The impetus for this falls from the supposition that since there are mammographically occult palpable cancers that can be seen on ultrasound, there are almost certainly mammographically occult *non*-palpable cancers that could be picked up by ultrasound. Although ultrasound is being used increasingly as an ad hoc screening tool in many practices, it is not recommended for screening by any major organization and is not covered for screening by most insurance companies. For this reason, in clinical practice, a screening ultrasound is typically coded as a diagnostic ultrasound, with the indication being pain, lumps, or the ill-defined (but billable) fibrous mastopathy. Another, somewhat more forthright, strategy is to have patients who pay cash for their study with the extra screening.

Kolb and colleagues[21] performed 13,547 breast screening ultrasound examinations in women with dense breasts and normal mammograms and physical examinations. Thirty-seven cancers were found in 34 women for a yield of 0.27%, a percentage similar to the yield of screening mammography. A large ultrasound screening trial is underway under the auspices of ACRIN.

Magnetic Resonance Imaging

Contrast-enhanced magnetic resonance imaging (MRI) is a rapidly growing modality for evaluating the breast. The most common use at present is to evaluate the extent of disease in the ipsilateral and contralateral breast in a patient with a new diagnosis of cancer. MRI is superior to mammography and ultrasound in determining the size of the tumor, the presence of multifocal or multicentric disease (Fig. 8-5), and the presence of contralateral disease. In addition, MRI shows enlarged lymph nodes suggestive of metastatic spread (Fig. 8-6). This use of the technology is becoming more common throughout the world, but it is not supported by any studies showing improved outcomes. A knowledge of the extent of disease in the ipsilateral breast should improve the success of lumpectomy in obtaining negative surgical margins. It is not clear, however, whether additional foci of disease away from the index lesion are a common cause of ipsilateral recurrence after breast conserva-

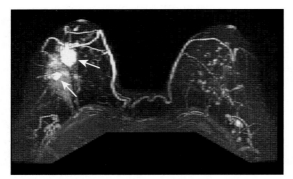

Figure 8-5. Maximum intensity projection rendering of a bilateral contrast-enhanced MRI shows two malignant masses in the right breast (*arrows*), consistent with multicentric breast cancer.

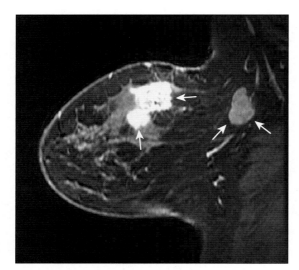

Figure 8-6. Contrast-enhanced sagittal breast MRI shows two adjacent malignant masses in the breast (*short arrows*) and a large abnormal axillary lymph node consistent with metastatic involvement (*long arrows*).

tion, since most such recurrence occurs at the lumpectomy site. A recent large multicenter trial looking at the contralateral breast found a 3% yield in detecting contralateral cancers.[22] This figure is actually lower than those reported in smaller single-institution series.[23,24] The difference is presumably due to the characteristics of the women studied. The earlier papers had a cohort skewed toward high-risk women, including those with *BRCA* mutations. Such patients are known to be more likely to have bilateral breast cancer. Of the 30 contralateral cancers in the multicenter trial, 12 were ductal carcinoma in situ (DCIS), and all but 1 of the 18 invasive cancers were smaller than 2 cm, with an average size of 9 mm. It is unknown how many of these cancers would have presented clinically.

Other common uses of MRI include monitoring neoadjuvant chemotherapy, searching for a breast primary in patients with adenocarcinoma of unknown origin in an axillary lymph node or a distant site, and evaluating a finding on mammography that cannot be sufficiently worked up with mammography and ultrasound alone. A typical example would be a one-view mammographic finding that cannot be localized stereotactically and has no ultrasound correlate. A major limitation of MRI is its relatively poor specificity. Benign areas of active normal breast tissue and fibrocystic change often enhance. To distinguish between enhancing cancers and benign enhancing tissue, both morphology and enhancement kinetics are used. The key indicators of malignancy are fast enhancement and washout. Unfortunately, most cancers do not show washout, and many benign lesions enhance rapidly. As an aid to distinguishing kinetics, parametric maps based on various features of the kinetic curve at each point can be created. Figure 8-7 shows an example of a cancer depicted with a parametric map.

MRI is also being used for screening high-risk women, a subject covered in detail in Chapter 9 of this book.

Nuclear Medicine Techniques

Two nuclear medicine imaging techniques are available for imaging breast cancers. Whole-body fluorodeoxyglucose-positron emission tomography (FDG-PET) is commonly used to image a variety of cancers, including breast, primarily to stage distant metastases. When

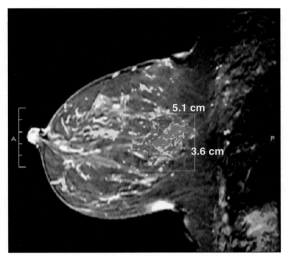

Figure 8-7. Parametric map of an invasive cancer shows different kinetics within the cancer. Color indicates a greater than 100% enhancement compared with surrounding background tissue at 90 seconds after contrast injection. Red and yellow areas show fast and medium washout, whereas blue areas show no washout.

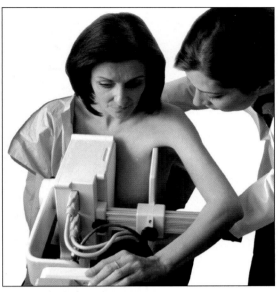

Figure 8-8. Breast-specific gamma camera for use with sestamibi breast imaging. (Courtesy of Dilon Technologies, LLC.)

used before definitive surgery, the primary breast tumor and any other focus of malignancy within the breasts may show up. Whole-body PET is not as accurate as MRI for evaluating extent of disease within the breasts, however, primarily because of limited sensitivity to tumors under 1 cm in diameter. To correct this, PET systems specific for the breast are being developed. Use of such devices has been shown to greatly increase the visibility of tumors under 1 cm.[25] Studies so far, however, have been small, and more clinical research is needed to fully understand how this technology could play a role in early detection and diagnosis.

Technetium-Tc 99m sestamibi (Cardiolite) has been used to evaluate myocardial ischemia and infarcts for decades, essentially replacing thallium for that indication. Sestamibi binds to mitochondria and thus, like FDG-PET, is an indication of metabolic activity. Imaged with a standard nuclear camera with both planar and single-photon emission computed tomography (SPECT) capabilities, the technique has been shown to be highly accurate for evaluating the heart. The breasts are naturally included in these views, and incidentally detected breast cancers, which are indicated by an area of high activity within a breast, are occasionally noted.

As with PET scanning, however, standard gamma cameras have limited sensitivity to tumors smaller than 1 cm. Just as with PET scanning, this limitation was overcome by the development of breast-specific gamma cameras, which allow the gamma detector to rest against the breast, increasing signal-to-noise ratio and spatial resolution (Fig. 8-8).

Results from these nuclear devices have been quite promising,[26,27] and at least one is available commercially for routine clinical use. Cancers appear as hot spots in the image (Fig. 8-9), which is acquired in the same planes as a mammogram and can thus be correlated to the mammographic images. Efforts are underway to develop a means to biopsy lesions visible only on the sestamibi scan. The primary indication for its use is currently to evaluate lesions with indeterminate mammographic appearance, but, as with all modalities, the indications are rapidly expanding.

Digital Breast Tomosynthesis

Although digital mammography has not been shown to be dramatically superior to film mammography, the advent of digital mammography opens the door to advanced applications not possible with film. The application likely to have the

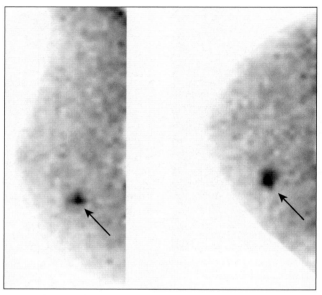

Figure 8-9. Sestamibi breast scan images show a malignant mass (*arrow*) in the inferomedial breast. The mediolateral oblique projection is on the right and the craniocaudal projection is on the left. (Courtesy of Dilon Technologies, LLC.)

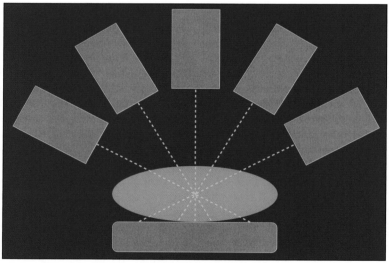

Figure 8-10. Schematic diagram showing one method of acquiring source images for tomosynthesis. In this method, the x-ray tube moves in an arc over a stationary detector/breast support. Typically, 7 to 11 projections are obtained.

earliest impact on breast cancer screening is digital breast tomosynthesis (DBT). DBT replaces the single projectional view used in standard mammography with a group of projections taken at slightly different angles over a small arc (Fig. 8-10). In practice, 7 to 11 images are acquired over about 30 degrees. From these images, a series of tomographic slices, similar in appearance to x-ray tomography, can be digitally produced. In this way, the problem of overlapping tissue obscuring masses and calcifications in mammography can be greatly reduced (Fig. 8-11). Also reduced is the creation of false-positive findings from the summation of unrelated overlapping areas of normal tissue (Fig. 8-12).

Clinical trials of tomosynthesis units from at least three manufacturers are underway, but no device has yet been approved for clinical use in

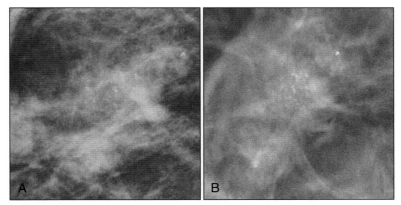

Figure 8-11. **Depiction of grouped microcalcifications on standard two-dimensional digital mammography (A) and digital breast tomosynthesis (B).** The calcifications are better seen on the tomosynthesis slice image than on the standard digital mammogram because of the removal of overlying tissue in the tomosynthesis image. (Courtesy of Loren Niklason, PhD, Hologic Inc. Reprinted with permission from *Seminars in Roentgenology* 42[4]:243–252, 2007.)

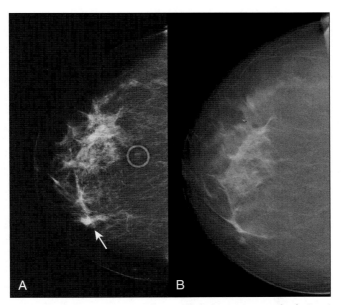

Figure 8-12. **Overlapping tissue causing an abnormality on digital mammography but not on tomosynthesis.** **A,** Standard two-dimensional digital mammogram shows a possible mass (*arrow*). **B,** Slice from digital tomosynthesis examination shows only normal tissue. By separating tissue in different planes of the breast, false-positive examinations due to overlapping tissue are reduced. (Courtesy of Loren Niklason, PhD, Hologic Inc. Reprinted with permission from *Seminars in Roentgenology* 42[4]:243–252, 2007.)

the United States. Introduction of this technology requires either hardware modifications to existing digital mammographic units or brand new designs. New software for image acquisition, processing, and viewing must also be introduced. Most important, unlike the transition from film to digital mammography, which produces similar images, the transition from mammography to tomosynthesis requires significant differences in image interpretation by the reader. The issue of how to train readers for this new modality is just one of many under debate. Other issues include the optimal way to process, reconstruct, and display the slices and whether both mammographic views will be needed or a single view will suffice.

At present, no results evaluating the use of DBT for cancer detection have been published in peer-reviewed literature. A series using DBT as an adjunct to mammography to decrease the recall rate did show that it could be used that way, but the primary result was a subjective comparison of image quality between mammography and DBT. DBT was judged to give a superior image compared with mammography in 37 of 99 cases, but in 51 cases there was no difference, and in 11 cases mammography was actually judged to be superior.[28] Although peer-reviewed data are few, a number of abstracts have been presented at meetings. The small series in these presentations have shown breast tomosynthesis to allow both improved lesion detection and decreased false-positive recalls. The results of what is expected to be the largest series—from the Massachusetts General Hospital—remain unpublished. Cases shown at meetings are extremely impressive and have generated much optimism about DBT.

Figure 8-13 demonstrates a spiculated mass much better depicted on tomosynthesis than on conventional mammography. Whether tomosynthesis will live up to its high expectations remains to be seen.

Contrast-Enhanced Digital Mammography

Another exciting application made possible by digital mammography is contrast-enhanced digital mammography (CEDM). In this technique, mammographic views are taken after the administration of an intravenous contrast agent. As with breast MRI and breast CT (see text that follows), the contrast agent preferentially collects in the interstitium of cancers rather than normal tissue. An iodine-based contrast agent, such as that used for routine clinical applications in body and brain CT scanning, is used for CEDM, although gadolinium[29] and even zirconium-based[30] agents have also been proposed.

The trick to CEDM is to make the contrast agent conspicuous enough to allow a diagnosis to be made. Although digital mammography is superior to film mammography in terms of contrast resolution, it is still a projection modality, just like other radiographic techniques. Liver lesions cannot be diagnosed on an excretory urogram, even with the latest digital radiography technology, despite their being easy to see on contrast-enhanced CT scans. Similarly, digital mammography does not compare with cross-

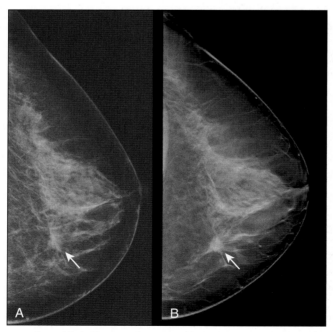

Figure 8-13. Spiculated cancer (*arrow*) is better seen in tomosynthesis image (**B**) than on standard digital mammogram (**A**) because of the removal of overlying tissue in the tomosynthesis image. (Courtesy of Loren Niklason, PhD, Hologic Inc. Reprinted with permission from *Seminars in Roentgenology* 42[4]:243–252, 2007.)

sectional modalities in its ability to show contrast enhancement. Fortunately, there are ways to optimize the visibility of the contrast agent by choosing an optimal energy for the x-ray beam and by using image subtraction.

Two methods of subtraction are being studied. In temporal subtraction, a precontrast image is subtracted from a postcontrast image. This method maximizes the effect of the subtraction on contrast visibility, but limits the study to a single projection of a single breast. Dual-energy subtraction makes use of the relative differences in the x-ray absorption spectra (i.e., the change in absorption with changing x-ray energy) of breast tissue and iodine. In this technique, two images are acquired at different energies after the contrast administration is complete. These two images are then combined to give a final image in which the breast tissue is subtracted out and only the contrast agent remains.

At least three small studies have been conducted to evaluate CEDM. All of the studies enrolled women with suspicious lesions who were scheduled for biopsy on the basis of clinical, mammographic, or ultrasound findings. Lewin and colleagues[31] studied 26 subjects with dual-energy subtraction CEDM. Of the 13 subjects later shown to have an invasive cancer at biopsy, CEDM identified all of the lesions. Eleven of them strongly enhanced; two weakly enhanced. The two studies resulting in weak enhancement of cancers both had technical limitations. On one the injection rate was decreased from the 4 mL/s used on the other studies down to 2 mL/s to accommodate a hand intravenous tubing. On the other, the intravenous tubing became decoupled, and only a fraction of the contrast was administered. The one case of DCIS in the study weakly enhanced. Of the 12 benign lesions, 2 weakly enhanced. One was a prior lumpectomy site, and the other was an area of atypical ductal hyperplasia. The other benign lesions showed no enhancement. Figure 8-14 shows an example from that paper.

By being able to obtain multiple projections, lesions can be localized within the breast using

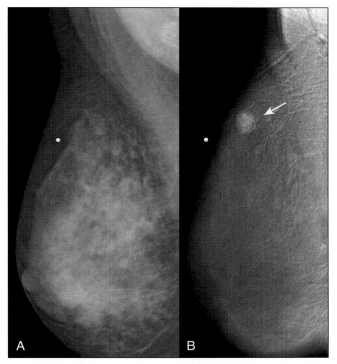

Figure 8-14. Invasive 12-mm lobular carcinoma is demonstrated with dual-energy contrast-enhanced digital mammography (CEDM). **A,** Digital mammogram is normal. A metal bead marks a palpable abnormality. **B,** Dual-energy CEDM image shows the cancer as a round enhancing mass in the superior breast (*arrow*). (© RSNA. Reprinted by permission. Originally published in Lewin JM, Isaacs PK, Vance V, Larke FJ: Dual-energy contrast-enhanced digital subtraction mammography: feasibility. Radiology 229:261–268, 2003.).

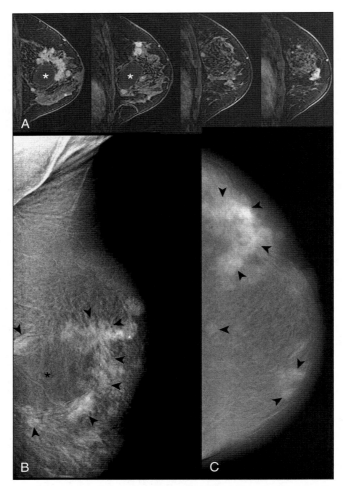

Figure 8-15. Sixty-one-year-old woman with multicentric invasive lobular carcinoma. Comparison of MR imaging and dual-energy contrast-enhanced digital mammography (CEDM) in two projections. **A,** Selected sagittal MR slices from lateral to medial. High-signal masses and foci on MRI are areas of cancer throughout the breast. A large cyst (*) is noted in the lateral breast. **B,** CEDM, mediolateral oblique (MLO) view. **C,** CEDM, craniocaudal (CC) view. Foci of high density are areas of malignancy. Cancer (*arrowheads*) surrounds the cyst (*) in the lateral breast, as shown on the MLO view, but is also present in the posterocentral and medial breast, as shown on the CC view. (Reprinted with permission from *Seminars in Breast Disease* 9[3]:105–110, 2006.)

dual-energy CEDM. Lesions depicted can therefore be correlated to those seen on an MRI. Figure 8-15 shows such a correlation in a case of multicentric cancer.

At the University of Toronto, Jong and colleagues[32] studied 22 subjects using temporal subtraction CEDM. Ten of these were shown at biopsy to have cancer. Eight of these cancers enhanced. Of the 12 benign lesions, 5 enhanced at CEDM. From these numbers, the calculated sensitivity and specificity using enhancement as the only criterion were 80% and 58%, respectively. The specificity is improved, however, by taking into account lesion shape and enhance-

ment kinetics. The protocol included imaging at multiple time points to allow analysis of a time-enhancement curve for each lesion.

At Charité Hospital in Berlin, Diekmann and colleagues[33] studied 21 subjects with 25 lesions including 14 cancers, using temporal subtraction CEDM. Three time points were studied for each lesion. All 11 invasive cancers enhanced as did 2 of the 3 cases of DCIS. One case of low-grade DCIS did not enhance.

Temporal subtraction was also performed in a recently published trial conducted in France.[34] Sixteen of the 20 cancers in the trial enhanced. The goal of the study was to compare the enhancement patterns with microvessel counts using CD34 immunostaining. The authors found that the correlation between enhancement pattern and microvessel count was poor. Although the authors did not compare their results with similar studies using MRI, these studies also show a poor correlation of enhancement kinetics to overall microvessel density,[35,36] although there is some correlation with the pattern of microvessel distribution within the tumor.

Intravenous contrast enhancement is also being studied with digital breast tomosynthesis with promising results.[37]

Dedicated Breast CT

Whereas MRI is the most common cross-sectional modality for imaging the breast in the United States and Europe, CT scanning has been used extensively for similar indications for years in Japan with great success. As with MRI, an intravenous contrast agent is used to obtain optimal results. The advantage of MRI over CT is the absence of ionizing radiation. The advantage of CT is lower cost, shorter exam times, and less claustrophobia.

CT scanners specifically designed for breast imaging have been developed and are in early clinical trials.[38] Unlike standard CT scanners, in which the tube and detectors rotate around a supine or prone patient in the axial plane, for these scanners the patient lies prone and only the breast lies within the gantry. Scanning is therefore in the coronal plain relative to the body and axial to the breast (Fig. 8-16). Because the entire torso does not need to be penetrated by the x-ray beam, the radiation dose to the breast from breast-specific scanners is much lower than that from conventional scanners. In the prototype systems currently being tested, the dose to the breast is equal to that of a conventional mammogram. Dedicated breast CT is being investigated for use both with and without intravenous contrast. With contrast, the technique can be expected to have properties similar to those of breast MRI. Such results have already been observed using conventional scanners similar to image the breasts. The dedicated scanners, in addition to a lower radiation dose, have higher spatial resolution, which should further improve on the results using contrast. A potential limitation of dedicated breast CT is decreased inclusion of posterior breast and chest wall tissues compared with both conventional CT and MRI. This limitation is the result of the scanner geometry.

The improved spatial resolution of dedicated breast CT compared with conventional CT and MRI may allow it to be useful for depicting cancers even without intravenous contrast. In this mode, it may compete with the other x-ray-based techniques, mammography and tomosynthesis, as a screening modality. As with those techniques, masses are identified by shape and margin, and groups of microcalcifications are used as an indication of DCIS. The advantage of CT over the other techniques is its true three-dimensional depiction of these lesions. As expected, breast CT is excellent at depicting the enhancement of cancers with iodinated contrast, further increasing its diagnostic usefulness (Fig. 8-17). Breast CT is being studied as a diagnostic modality, both in university and commercial settings. It has not yet been tested for screening in any systematic way.

Conclusion

Breast imaging remains a dynamic field, and several new technologies are in various stages of clinical trials or early clinical use. Despite all this activity, mammography remains the only test shown in randomized trials to lead to decreased breast cancer mortality and is still the cornerstone of breast imaging, as it has been for four decades. Given the excitement surrounding other modalities, however, it seems unlikely that two-dimensional mammography will be able to retain its place as the dominant imaging modality over the decade ahead.

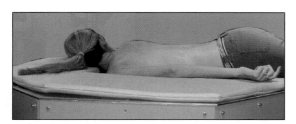

Figure 8-16. Patient positioned on dedicated breast CT scanner. The breast is imaged while in a dependent position so that it is extended by gravity and tissue is spread out. The scanner moves circularly around the breast. (Courtesy of J.M. Boone, University of California, Davis Medical Center.)

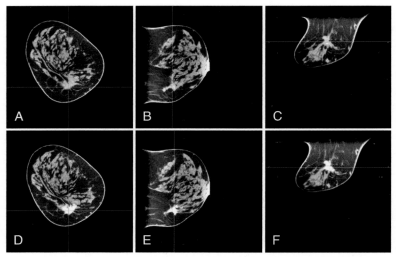

Figure 8-17. A–C, Invasive ductal carcinoma visible as a spiculated mass on unenhanced dedicated breast CT scan in axial, sagittal, and coronal planes (relative to the breast). The cancer lies at the intersection of the registration lines. **D–F,** Same slices after administration of intravenous iodinated contrast show enhancement of the cancer. (Courtesy of J.M. Boone, University of California, Davis Medical Center.)

References

1. Fletcher SW, Black W, Harris R, et al: Report of the International Workshop on Screening for Breast Cancer. J Natl Cancer Inst 85:1644–1656, 1993.
2. Nystrom L, Rutqvist LE, Wall S, et al: Breast cancer screening with mammography: overview of Swedish randomised trials. Lancet 341:973–978, 1993.
3. Tabar L, Fagerberg G, Duffy SW: Update of the Swedish two-county program of mammographic screening for breast cancer. Radiol Clin North Am 30:187–210, 1992.
4. Kerlikowske K: Efficacy of screening mammography among women aged 40 to 49 years and 50 to 69 years: comparison of relative and absolute benefit. J Natl Cancer Inst Monogr (22): 79–86, 1997.
5. Ringash J: Canadian Task Force on Preventive Health Care. Preventive health care, 2001 update: screening mammography among women aged 40–49 years at average risk of breast cancer. CMAJ 20;164(4):69–76, 2001. [Erratum in CMAJ 20;164(6):53, 2001.]
6. Tabar L, Yen MF, Vitak B, et al: Mammography service screening and mortality in breast cancer patients: 20-year follow-up before and after introduction of screening. Lancet 361(9367): 1405–1410, 2003.
7. Hendrick RE, Smith RA, Rutledge JH III, Smart CR: Benefit of screening mammography in women aged 40–49: a new meta-analysis of randomized controlled trials. J Natl Cancer Inst Monogr (22)87–92, 1997.
8. American Cancer Society Guidelines for the Early Detection of Cancer. www.cancer.org/docroot/PED/content/PED_2_3X_ACS_Cancer_Detection_Guidelines_36.asp
9. World Health Organisation databank, accessed through CANCERMondial. International Agency for Research on Cancer. www-dep.iarc.fr/
10. Olsen AH, Njor SH, Vejborg I, et al: Breast cancer mortality in Copenhagen after introduction of mammography screening: cohort study. BMJ 330:220, 2005. Epub 2005, Jan 13.
11. Berns EA, Hendrick RE, Solari M, et al: Digital and screen-film mammography: comparison of image acquisition and interpretation times. AJR Am J Roentgenol 187:38–41, 2006.
12. Lewin JM, D'Orsi CJ, Hendrick RE, Moss LJ, et al: Clinical comparison of full-field digital mammography to screen-film mammography for breast cancer detection. AJR Am J Roentgenol 179:671–677, 2002.

13. Skaane P, Young K, Skjennald A: Population-based mammography screening: comparison of screen-film and full-field digital mammography with soft-copy reading—Oslo I Study. Radiology 229:877–884, 2003.
14. Pisano ED, Gatsonis CA, Yaffe MJ, et al: American College of Radiology Imaging Network digital mammographic imaging screening trial: objectives and methodology. Radiology 236: 404–412, 2005.
15. Pisano ED, Gatsonis C, Hendrick E, et al: Digital Mammographic Imaging Screening Trial (DMIST) Investigators Group. Diagnostic performance of digital versus film mammography for breast-cancer screening. N Engl J Med 353:1773–1783, 2005.
16. Skaane P, Skjennald A: Screen-film mammography versus full-field digital mammography with soft-copy reading: randomized trial in a population-based screening program—the Oslo II Study. Radiology 232:197–204, 2004.
17. Skaane P, Hofvind S, Skjennald A: Randomized trial of screen-film versus full-field digital mammography with soft-copy reading in population-based screening program: follow-up and final results of Oslo II Study. Radiology 244:708–717, 2007.
18. Soo MS, Rosen EL, Baker JA, et al: Negative predictive value of sonography with mammography in patients with palpable breast lesions. AJR Am J Roentgenol 177(5):167–170, 2001.
19. Moy L, Slanetz PJ, Moore R, et al: Specificity of mammography and US in the evaluation of a palpable abnormality: retrospective review. Radiology 225(1):176–181, 2002.
20. Dennis MA, Parker SH, Klaus AJ, et al: Breast biopsy avoidance: the value of normal mammograms and normal sonograms in the setting of a palpable lump. Radiology 219(1):186–191, 2001.
21. Kolb TM, Lichy J, Newhouse JH: Comparison of the performance of screening mammography, physical examination, and breast US and evaluation of factors that influence them: an analysis of 27,825 patient evaluations. Radiology 2002;225: 165–175, 2002.
22. Lehman CD, Gatsonis C, Kuhl CK, et al; ACRIN Trial 6667 Investigators Group: MRI evaluation of the contralateral breast in women with recently diagnosed breast cancer. N Engl J Med 356(13):1295–1303, 2007.
23. Slanetz PJ, Edmister WB, Yeh ED, et al: Occult contralateral breast carcinoma incidentally detected by breast magnetic resonance imaging. Breast J 8(3):145–148, 2002.
24. Liberman L, Morris EA, Kim CM, et al: MR imaging findings in the contralateral breast of women with recently diagnosed breast cancer. AJR Am J Roentgenol 180(2):333–341, 2003.
25. Rosen EL, Turkington TG, Soo MS, et al: Detection of primary breast carcinoma with a dedicated, large-field-of-view FDG PET

mammography device: initial experience. Radiology 234(2): 527–534, 2005.

26. O'Connor MK, Phillips SW, Hruska CB, et al: Molecular breast imaging: advantages and limitations of a scintimammographic technique in patients with small breast tumors. Breast J 13(1): 3–11, 2007.

27. Brem RF, Fishman M, Rapelyea JA: Detection of ductal carcinoma in situ with mammography, breast specific gamma imaging, and magnetic resonance imaging: a comparative study. Acad Radiol 14(8):945–950, 2007.

28. Poplack SP, Tosteson TD, Kogel CA, Nagy HM: Digital breast tomosynthesis: initial experience in 98 women with abnormal digital screening mammography. AJR Am J Roentgenol 189(3): 616–623, 2007.

29. Sarnelli A, Elleaume H, Taibi A, et al: K-edge digital subtraction imaging with dichromatic x-ray sources: SNR and dose studies. Phys Med Biol 51:4311–4328, 2006.

30. Lawaczeck R, Diekmann F, Diekmann S, et al: New contrast media designed for x-ray energy subtraction imaging in digital mammography. Invest Radiol 38:602–608, 2003.

31. Lewin JM, Isaacs PK, Vance V, Larke FJ: Dual-energy contrast-enhanced digital subtraction mammography: feasibility. Radiology 229:261–268, 2003.

32. Jong RA, Yaffe MJ, Skarpathiotakis M, et al: Contrast-enhanced digital mammography: initial clinical experience. Radiology 228:842–850, 2003.

33. Diekmann F, Diekmann S, Jeunehomme F, et al: Digital mammography using iodine-based contrast media: initial clinical experience with dynamic contrast medium enhancement. Invest Radiol 40:397–404, 2005.

34. Dromain C, Balleyguier C, Muller S, et al: Evaluation of tumor angiogenesis of breast carcinoma using contrast-enhanced digital mammography. AJR Am J Roentgenol 187:528–537, 2006.

35. Su MY, Cheung YC, Fruehauf JP, et al: Correlation of dynamic contrast enhancement MRI parameters with microvessel density and VEGF for assessment of angiogenesis in breast cancer. J Magn Reson Imaging 18:467–477, 2003.

36. Teifke A, Behr O, Schmidt M, et al: Dynamic MR imaging of breast lesions: correlation with microvessel distribution pattern and histologic characteristics of prognosis. Radiology 239: 351–360, 2006.

37. Chen SC, Carton AK, Albert M, et al: Initial clinical experience with contrast-enhanced digital breast tomosynthesis. Acad Radiol 14(2):229–238, 2007.

38. Lindfoors KK, Boone JM, Nelson TR, et al: Dedicated breast CT: initial clinical experience. Radiology 246:725–733, 2008.

Screening of High-Risk Patients

9

James P. Borgstede and Brian M. Bagrosky

KEY POINTS

- Although most women who develop breast cancer have no elevated risk factors, a small group of women can be identified by personal and historical information as having a significantly elevated risk for developing breast cancer.
- More aggressive breast cancer screening of these high-risk women can lead to earlier breast cancer detection and improved survival.
- Mammography continues to be the mainstay for breast cancer screening in both average-risk and high-risk patients.
- The addition of annual magnetic resonance imaging (MRI) screening increases early detection for high-risk women.
- Several imaging technologies show promise in early detection of breast cancer in high-risk women, and research continues in this area.

Introduction

Screening for early detection of breast cancer aims to detect tumors at a stage when tumor size is smaller and there is less nodal involvement. Women with these earlier-stage tumors have a better prognosis than those diagnosed with tumors at a more advanced stage, thus decreasing mortality and improving survival. Although most women who develop breast cancer do not have identifiable factors that suggest they are high risk, a group of women can be identified through historical and family history information that suggests that they have a higher risk of developing breast cancer than the average woman. This group of high-risk patients may benefit from adjustments in their screening recommendations that would increase early detection and decrease breast cancer mortality.

Definition of High Risk

Identification of risk factors and stratification of patients for breast cancer risk are important for providing the best screening recommendations. Many factors that increase or decrease risk have been identified, and several statistical models, such as the Gail model and the Claus model, calculate risk based on these factors. The Gail model is the most commonly used methodology for calculating risk factors; however, some experts believe that the BRACAPRO or Tyrer-Cuzick models provide more accurate assessments of risk.[1] "High risk" has been arbitrarily defined as a 5-year Gail model risk of greater than 1.7% and a lifetime risk based primarily on family history of greater than 20%. Other situations or conditions that place a woman at high risk for breast cancer development are presented in Table 9-1. The National Cancer Institute and the National Surgical Adjuvant Breast and Bowel Project (NSABP) worked together to provide a free calculator based on the Gail model, which assesses some of these risk factors and provides an estimated 5-year and lifetime risk rate for a woman's developing breast cancer compared with the "average woman" (www.cancer.gov/bcrisktool/). The patient and her breast care provider should discuss the best screening plan based on the individual woman's estimated risk.

Mammography

Mammography, or breast x-ray, is the primary imaging modality used to screen women for occult breast cancer (Fig. 9-1). A standard screening mammogram involves two images of each breast (Figs. 9-2A and B and 9-3A and B).

Table 9-1. Recommendations for Breast MRI Screening as an Adjunct to Mammography

Recommend Annual MRI Screening (Based on Evidence*)

BRCA mutation
First-degree relative of *BRCA* carrier, but untested
Lifetime risk ~20–25% or greater, as defined by BRCAPRO or other models that are largely dependent on family history

Recommend Annual MRI Screening (Based on Expert Consensus Opinion†)

Radiation to chest between age 10 and 30 years
Li-Fraumeni syndrome and first-degree relatives
Cowden and Bannayan-Riley-Ruvalcaba syndromes and first-degree relatives

Insufficient Evidence to Recommend for or Against MRI Screening‡

Lifetime risk 15–20%, as defined by BRCAPRO or other models that are largely dependent on family history
Lobular carcinoma in situ (LCIS) or atypical lobular hyperplasia (ALH)
Atypical ductal hyperplasia (ADH)
Heterogeneously or extremely dense breast on mammography
Women with a personal history of breast cancer, including ductal carcinoma in situ (DCIS)

Recommend Against MRI Screening (Based on Expert Consensus Opinion)

Women with <15% lifetime risk

**Evidence from nonrandomized screening trials and observational studies.*
†*Based on evidence of lifetime risk for breast cancer.*
‡*Payment should not be a barrier. Screening decisions should be made on a case-by-case basis, since there may be particular factors to support MRI. More data on these groups are expected to be published soon.*
From Warner E, Yaffe M, Andrews KS, et al: American Cancer Society Guidelines for Breast Screening with MRI as an Adjunct to Mammography. CA Cancer J Clin 57:75–89, 2007, Table 1.

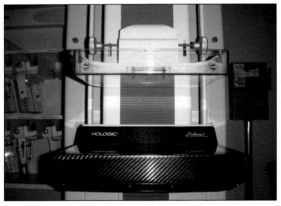

Figure 9-1. Digital mammography system. (Courtesy of Brian M. Bagrosky MD, Dianne O'Connor Thompson Breast Center, University of Colorado Hospital, Aurora, CO.)

Studies have shown that two views increase the rate of detection of small cancers (more favorable prognosis) and decrease the number of patients being called back for additional images.[2–4] The benefits just mentioned outweigh the minimal risks of additional radiation exposure received with only one view. The two images are named on the basis of the orientation of the view: MLO for mediolateral oblique (see Fig. 9-2) and CC for craniocaudal (Fig. 9-3). It is interesting that the effective whole body radiation dose from a screening mammogram is 40 mrem, which is equal to 10% of the annual background radiation and is within the range of normal background variation.

Many technologic advances to mammography units have dramatically improved the image quality and given radiologists a better ability to identify very small distortions in normal breast architecture, small masses, and microcalcifications.[5] Two of the most important advances have been compression paddles and the replacement of tungsten filament with molybdenum and rhodium. Although compression paddles (Fig. 9-4) can cause discomfort in some patients, they serve to spread the breast tissue out, creating less tissue thickness for the x-ray beam to penetrate and therefore decreasing scatter. Compression paddles also decrease motion during the imaging, which markedly improves the final images. Replacing tungsten filaments and aluminum filters (found in conventional x-ray units) with molybdenum and/or rhodium filaments and filters creates "softer" x-rays, which provide better imaging of very small differences in breast soft tissue attenuation. In addition to technologic advances in mammography units, the Mammography Quality Standards Act (MQSA) written by the Food & Drug Administration (FDA) and passed by Congress in October 1992 has created strict guidelines that all breast imaging centers must adhere to for accreditation. These guidelines include daily

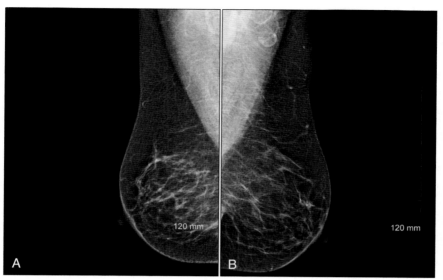

Figure 9-2. Bilateral digital screening mammogram: mediolateral oblique views of the left (**A**) and right (**B**) breasts. (Courtesy of Brian M. Bagrosky MD, Dianne O'Connor Thompson Breast Center, University of Colorado Hospital, Aurora, CO.)

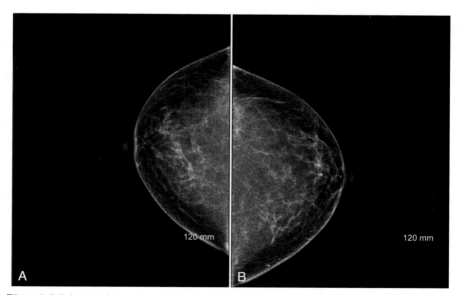

Figure 9-3. Bilateral digital screening mammogram: craniocaudal views of the left (**A**) and right (**B**) breasts of the same patient as in Figure 9-2. (Courtesy of Brian M. Bagrosky MD, Dianne O'Connor Thompson Breast Center, University of Colorado Hospital, Aurora, CO.)

film processor testing, weekly radiation dose testing, monthly image quality testing, and annual physics testing. The MQSA also sets a guideline on the minimum number of studies a radiologist must read every 2 years to be accredited. The MQSA guidelines have improved the specificity and sensitivity of all mammograms by an estimated 2% to 10%.[6]

Despite the technologic advances and the rigorous quality standards, mammography has skeptics. The National Breast Cancer Coalition

(NBCC) is a grassroots lobbying group with a stated mission of eradicating breast cancer. This coalition takes a guarded stance on mammography, stating: "The National Breast Cancer Coalition Fund (NBCCF) believes, on the basis of recently published reviews, that the benefits of screening mammography in reducing mortality are modest and there are harms associated with screening."[7] The NBCC cites the Cochrane review database, a respected meta-analysis, which has analyzed seven published studies on

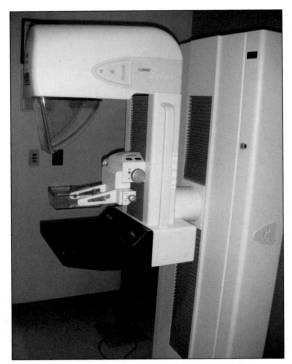

Figure 9-4. Compression paddle in mammography unit. (Courtesy of Brian M. Bagrosky MD, Dianne O'Connor Thompson Breast Center, University of Colorado Hospital, Aurora, CO.)

mammography screening for breast cancer. The conclusion of the Cochrane review in 2001 was that mass screening for breast cancer by mammography did not show a survival benefit. However, the later Cochrane review in 2006 concluded that mammography likely decreases breast cancer mortality, but that some women who partake in screening will undergo unnecessary further imaging and treatment because of false-positive results. This is a true and unfortunate part of any screening program for any disease.[8] Currently, it is estimated that mammography and early treatment of breast cancer are responsible for lowering breast cancer death rates by as much as 50% in the last 2 decades.[9]

Screening Recommendations

Women with Average Risk

Controversy over the age at which women should begin mammography screening existed until relatively recently. A multitude of research has settled this controversy, culminating in the 2003 American Cancer Society (ACS) breast cancer screening guidelines, which recommended annual mammogram screening for all women starting at

age 40.[10] The previous recommendation (1997) was a "baseline" mammogram at age 35, followed by screening every 1 to 2 years for women 40 to 50 years and then annual mammograms at age 50.[11] The change in these recommendations resulted from improved studies that looked specifically at breast cancer rates and mortality in women aged 40 to 50, which found that "screening mammograms are as important for women aged 40 to 49 as for women 50 years old and above. It was the improper use of retrospective, unplanned, subgroup analysis to advise women and their physicians that caused the controversy over mammograms for women under 50."

There was relative peace regarding breast cancer screening guidelines from 2003 until November 2009, when the U.S. Preventive Services Task Force released updated recommendations for breast cancer screening. Their recommendations were:

1. Biennial screening for women ages 50 to 74.
2. The decision to start regular, biennial screening mammography before the age of 50 years should be an individual one and take patient context into account, including the patient's values regarding specific benefits and harms.
3. Current evidence is insufficient to assess the additional benefits and harms of screening mammography in women 75 years or older.[12]

The release of these recommendations created an uproar in the breast cancer community. Most major organizations that provide breast cancer screening recommendations, such as the American Cancer Society, the American College of Radiology, and the American Society of Breast Surgeons, have made formal statements that this report has not changed their recommendation that women of average risk should begin annual mammography at age 40. We agree that most women will realize a significant early detection benefit when they begin their mammographic screening at age 40.

How long a woman should continue to undergo annual mammograms is also controversial, and less research is available to answer this question. Again, cost-effectiveness and anxiety from false-positives, with competing risks for death from other causes in the older populations, are issues that must be considered when deciding to cease annual screening. The percentage of

American women 65 years and older will continue to increase over the coming years, so this issue will continue to garner interest. The elderly population is very heterogeneous with regard to health and associated comorbidities, thus creating a large range of estimated life expectancies, further complicating this issue. Therefore, the ACS recommends that primary care physicians take into account competing risks of death and states that "as long as a woman is in reasonable good health and is a candidate for treatment she should continued to be screened with mammograms."[13] For routine screening to be warranted, a woman not only must be able to tolerate the mammographic screening itself but also must have baseline health sufficient to allow biopsy and/or surgery if the need arises. The ACS also advises that stopping screening is reasonable if a woman has severe functional limitations and/or comorbidities that would limit her life expectancy to 3 to 5 years.

Women with High Risk

Women with a high risk for developing breast cancer deserve special breast cancer screening consideration. Women with the highest risk of developing breast cancer are those with a known *BRCA1* and *BRCA2* gene mutation. Estimated lifetime risk for breast cancer development in this group of women may be as high as 85%. Effective screening for these patients is difficult because they develop breast cancer at an earlier age than other women, with 50% being diagnosed before the age of 50 and often before the usual age of recommended screening. Moreover, breast tissue in younger patients is more dense, which makes it more difficult to detect cancerous lesions by mammography alone. It has been suggested that the earlier age at onset combined with breasts that are more difficult to image is why cancers are often more advanced in these patients at presentation. It is also recognized that breast density is an independent risk factor for development of breast cancer.

Although annual mammography beginning at age 40 is the primary screening tool for women with an average risk of breast cancer, women at high risk because of a known gene defect or a family history that suggests an unidentified gene defect will need to begin screening at a much earlier age. Current recommendations are for screening to begin annually by age 30 (but not before age 25) if a gene defect has been identified

or, for those families without an identifiable gene defect, 10 years before the age of the youngest age at diagnosis, but not before 25, of a first-degree relative who has had breast cancer.[14]

There is some concern regarding early mammogram screening in high-risk patients and the consequences of radiation, even at very low doses. Because the *BRCA1* and *BRCA2* genes are DNA repair genes, there is a theoretical concern that radiation damage may be more significant in this group of women than in women with average risk. Such risks must be considered when recommending screening for these women. Because of the limitations of mammographic screening in this group, there is significant interest in using other imaging modalities for screening in this subset of patients.

Magnetic Resonance Imaging

MRI has the strongest data as an additional screening tool for screening high-risk patients (Table 9-2). MRI creates images by analyzing the different inherent magnetic field-induced spin properties of protons in various tissues (Fig. 9-5). MRI does not use ionizing radiation to create images as x-ray (mammography), computed tomography (CT), nuclear medicine, or positron emission tomography (PET) do. MRI offers increased sensitivity with its ability to use a variety of imaging pulse sequences and the use of intravenous gadolinium contrast.

Breast MRI is an expensive and time-consuming study that requires the administration of an intravenous contrast agent, gadolinium, special equipment, and specific imaging sequences. However, if these resources and knowledge are available, MRI images can show cancerous lesions that mammography does not detect. This increased sensitivity is particularly evident in dense breast tissue,[15] commonly present in younger women. The ACS recommends MRI screening for high-risk women beginning at age 30 for *BRCA1* or *BRCA2* mutation carriers, untested first-degree relatives of *BRCA* mutation carriers, women with a lifetime risk of greater than 20%, women who received thoracic radiation between the ages of 10 and 30, and women or first-degree relatives carrying a genetic mutation in the *TP53* or *PTEM* genes[16,17] (see Table 9-1). The increased breast tissue density found in younger patients is not problematic for MRI compared with mammography because MRI depends on tissue signal character-

Table 9-2. Published Breast MRI Screening Study Results

	The Netherlands	Canada	United Kingdom	Germany	United States	Italy
No. of centers	6	1	22	1	13	9
No. of women	1909	236	649	529	390	105
Age range	25–70	25–65	35–49	≥30	≥25	≥25
No. of cancers	50	22	35	43	4	8
Sensitivity (%)						
MRI	80	77	77	91	100	100
Mammogram	33	36	40	33	25	16
Ultrasound	n/a	33	n/a	40	n/a	16
Specificity (%)						
MRI	90	95	81	97	95	99
Mammogram	95	>99	93	97	98	0
Ultrasound	n/a	96	n/a	91	n/a	0

n/a, not applicable.
From Warner E, Yaffe M, Andrews KS, et al: American Cancer Society Guidelines for Breast Screening with MRI as an Adjunct to Mammography. CA Cancer J Clin 57:75–89, 2007, Table 2.

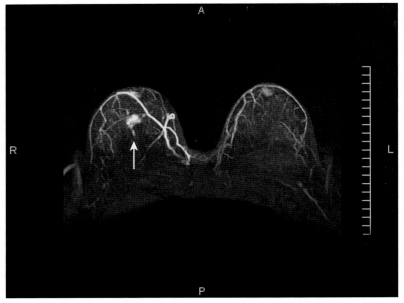

Figure 9-5. MRI of the breast with gadolinium contrast offers increased sensitivity for detecting breast cancer (*arrow*). (Courtesy of Brian M. Bagrosky MD, Dianne O'Connor Thompson Breast Center, University of Colorado Hospital, Aurora, CO.)

istics and not solely on density. Data are still lacking regarding the age at which high-risk women should start undergoing annual breast MRI. Because breast cancer develops earlier in these women, an age range of 25 to 35 years is usually recommended for initiation of MRI screening. Although MRI has an increased sensitivity for breast cancer detection, there is a significant incidence of false-positives, potentially increasing anxiety with further testing and biopsy of ultimately noncancerous lesions. Women

advised to undergo MRI screening should be aware of these possibilities (Table 9-3).

Whole Breast Ultrasound

Ultrasound creates images by recording the reflections of multiple sound waves arising from different surfaces. Ionizing radiation is not used to create these images. Ultrasound is best known for its use as a screening tool in pregnant women and in populations at risk for abdominal aortic

Table 9-3. Rates of Detection and Follow-up Tests for Screening MRI Compared with Mammography

	MRI		Mammography	
	The Netherlands	**United Kingdom**	**The Netherlands**	**United Kingdom**
Positives	13.7%	19.7%	6.0%	7.2%
Recalls	10.84%	10.7%	5.4%	3.9%
Biopsies	2.93%	3.08%	1.3%	1.33%
Cancers	1.04%	1.44%	0.46%	0.69%
False-negatives	0.23%	0.43%	0.81%	1.52%

From Warner E, Yaffe M, Andrews KS, et al: American Cancer Society Guidelines for Breast Screening with MRI as an Adjunct to Mammography. CA Cancer J Clin 57:75–89, 2007, Table 3.

aneurysms and carotid occlusive disease. Whole breast ultrasound was proposed in the early 1980s as a screening tool for breast carcinoma because of its relative ease of use, noninvasiveness, low cost, and the absence of ionizing radiation. Unfortunately, whole breast ultrasound has not been shown to be of value for the population at large. Whole breast ultrasound has been shown to be too insensitive compared with mammography for routine screening of cancer.[18] For women at high risk, whole breast ultrasound has shown promise. However, there is insufficient evidence to recommend for or against its use, and there are currently no published guidelines that include whole breast ultrasound as a recommended screening tool.

Nuclear Medicine

Positron emission tomography (PET) alone or combined with computed tomography (PET-CT) is being used to evaluate a variety of malignancies. PET detects the beta emissions of fluorodeoxyglucose (FDG) after it has been administered intravenously. FDG is actively taken up, but incompletely metabolized, by metabolically active cells. Cancer cells have increased metabolic activity compared with that of most cells in the body and thus have increased FDG uptake. Thus, these cells show up as an area of increased signal on PET scans.

Breast FDG-PET imaging has been shown to be insensitive, particularly for low-grade tumors and those less than 1 cm at the greatest diameter. Obviously, these lesions are the most important for a screening exam to identify, and therefore PET is not recommended for primary screening of breast cancer.[19] Note that FDG-PET should not be used in place of biopsy for lesions detected by mammography and/or ultrasound that are suspicious for neoplasm.[20] Currently, the only indications for FDG-PET and PET-CT are evaluation of the response of metastatic breast cancer to chemotherapy and staging recurrent or metastatic breast cancer. Continued research with alternative radiotracers that target estrogen receptors could add to these clinical indications in the future.

Tomosynthesis

As previously discussed, one of the biggest problems with mammography screening for breast cancer is the number of false-positive results. This problem is inherent in most disease-screening tests because the goal of these tests is not to miss any patients with the disease. Screening exams with high sensitivity result in some anxiety and more imaging—or even biopsy—for some women without breast cancer who have suspicious findings on mammograms. Breast tomosynthesis, a technique currently under trial, has as one potential goal the reduction in the number of false-positive results. Tomosynthesis allows three-dimensional acquisition of thin sections of tissue using a digital detector that receives x-rays emitted from a moving source. These data are reconstructed using algorithms such as CT (Fig. 9-6A and B). The main advantage of tomosynthesis is its ability to separate overlapping breast tissues. An important feature is that this technique allows for better differentiation of breast nodules on dense breasts than does standard mammography. Some researchers also think that tomosynthesis is better at depicting mass borders, microcalcifications, multiple masses, and distortion of adjacent ducts or vessels.[21] Finally, tomosynthesis provides better localization of skin findings. The challenges facing tomosynthesis are the expense of equip-

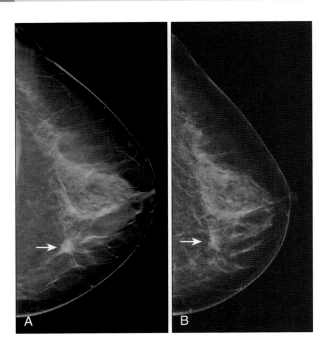

Figure 9-6. Spiculated cancer (*arrow*) better appreciated on tomosynthesis (**A**) than on digital mammography (**B**). Margins are much better seen with tomosynthesis. (From Lewin JM, Niklason L: Advanced applications of digital mammography: tomosynthesis and contrast-enhanced digital mammography. Semin Roentgenol 42:243–252, 2007, Fig. 3.)

ping breast imaging centers with these machines, the understanding of optimal imaging protocols, the determination of radiation dose to the patient, and the decision regarding whether this technology should be used for screening all patients or whether it should be focused only on high-risk and diagnostic patients.

Breast 1H MRI Spectroscopy

Proton MRI spectroscopy imaging gives a profile of the biochemical makeup of a selected portion of tissue. MRI spectroscopy has already been approved by the FDA and has been used for more than 20 years for evaluating brain masses. The most common metabolites evaluated with proton MRI spectroscopy are *N*-acetylcysteine (NAA), a neuronal marker; creatine (Cr), a measure of intracellular energy stores; lactate, a marker of anaerobic glycolysis; and choline (Cho), which is increased with high rates of cellular turnover or destruction. Therefore, with proton MRI spectroscopy, a radiologist can obtain information about the biochemical makeup of a suspicious-looking region of the breast. For example, if an area in the breast has a relatively elevated choline level (increased cell turnover), theoretically neoplasm would be more likely and the patient would proceed to surgical therapy. The principle behind MRI spectroscopy is essentially to obtain molecular information about a region of interest without an invasive biopsy. However, many technical problems must be addressed before this imaging method will benefit women being evaluated for breast cancer. The cost of spectroscopy is very high, and the time and number of scans necessary for lesion localization are burdensome, as is the difficulty in suppressing water and lipid signals to obtain an accurate biochemical profile. Finally, using the most current protocols, the breast lesion has to be $1\,cm^3$ for an accurate profile.[22] Stronger magnets and continued improvements in technical protocols will increase resolution and ultimately the usability of this powerful diagnostic tool for future use.

Conclusion

Mammography is still the primary screening tool for breast cancer. Women should be advised to have annual mammograms beginning at age 40. Women should be evaluated for breast cancer risk, and high-risk women should be more aggressively screened. Such screening should begin at an earlier age, and ACS recommendations for MRI screening should be considered.

Other imaging techniques including tomosynthesis, whole breast ultrasound, nuclear medicine, and MRI spectroscopy are being evaluated for their role in breast cancer detection. These advances in imaging are improving the survival rates of women who develop this disease.

References

1. Smith RA: Presentation to the Society of Breast Imaging 9th Post Graduate Course, April 27, 2009.
2. Bassett LW, Bunell DH, Jahanshahi R, et al: Breast cancer detection: one versus two views. Radiology 165(1):95–97, 1987.
3. Osborn GD, Beer H, Wade R, et al: Two-view mammography at the incident round has improved the rate of screen-detected breast cancer in Wales. Clin Radiol 61(6):478–482, 2006.
4. Blanks RG, Moss SM, Wallis MG, et al: Use of two view mammography compared with one view in the detection of small invasive cancers: further results from the National Health Service breast screening programme. J Med Screen 4(2):98–101, 1997.
5. Sickles EA: Breast imaging: from 1965 to the present. Radiology 215:1–16, 2000.
6. Burlington DB: Testimony on the Mammography Quality Standards Act of 1992 Before the House Committee on Commerce, Subcommittee on Health and the Environment. 5/8/1998. http://www.hhs.gov/asl/testify/t980508a.html
7. Mammography for Breast Cancer Screening: Harm/Benefit Analysis, Updated May 2007, National Breast Cancer Consortium, http://www.stopbreastcancer.org//index.php?option=com_content&task=view&id=133&Itemid=180. Accessed March 5, 2010.
8. Gøtzsche PC, Nielsen M: Screening for breast cancer with mammography. Cochrane Database of Systematic Reviews 2006, Issue 4. Art. No.: CD001877. DOI: 10.1002/14651858. CD001877.pub2.
9. Tabar T, Tot T, Dean P: Early detection of breast cancer: large-section and subgross thick-section histologic correlation with mammographic appearances. RadioGraphics 27:S5–S35, 2007.
10. Smith RA, Saslow D, Sawyer KA, et al: American Cancer Society Guidelines for Breast Cancer Screening: Update 2003 CA Cancer J Clin 53:141–169, 2003.
11. Kopans DB: An overview of the breast cancer screening controversy. J Natl Cancer Inst Monogr (22):1–3, 1997.
12. U.S. Preventive Services Task Force: Screening for Breast Cancer, released November 2009. http://www.ahrg.gov/clinic/uspstf/uspsbrca.htm. Accessed March 5, 2010.
13. American Cancer Society: Breast Cancer: Early Detection, Sept. 22, 2009. http://www.cancer.org/docroot/CRI/content/CRI_2_6x_Breast_Cancer_Early_Detection.asp?sitearea=. Accessed March 5, 2010.
14. Lee CH, Dershaw D, Kopans D, et al: Breast cancer screening with imaging: recommendations from the Society of Breast Imaging and the ACR on the use of mammography, breast MRI, breast ultrasound, and other technologies for the detection of clinically occult breast cancer. J Am Coll Radiol 7:18–27, 2010.
15. Warner E, Plewes DB, Hill KA, et al: Surveillance of BRCA1 and BRCA2 mutation carriers with magnetic resonance imaging, ultrasound, mammography, and clinical breast examination. JAMA 292(11):1317–1325, 2004.
16. Roubidoux MA: MR Screening of High Risk Patients, Society of Breast Imaging 9th Postgraduate Course, April 27, 2009.
17. Plevritis SK: Cost-effectiveness of screening BRCA1/2 mutation carriers with breast magnetic resonance imaging. JAMA 295(20):2374–2384, 2006.
18. Kopans DB, Meyer JE, Lindfors KK: Whole-breast US imaging: four-year follow-up. Radiology 157:505–507, 1985.
19. Kumar R, Chauhan J, Zhuang H, et al: Clinicopathologic factors associated with false negative FDG-PET in primary breast cancer. Breast Cancer Res Treat 98 (3):267–274, 2006.
20. Samson DJ, Flamm CR, Pisano ED, Aronson N: Should FDG PET be used to decide whether a patient with an abnormal mammogram or breast finding at physical examination should undergo biopsy? Acad Radiol 9(7):773–783, 2002.
21. Park JM, Franken EA Jr, Garg M, et al: Breast tomosynthesis: present considerations and future applications. RadioGraphics 27:S231–S240, 2007.
22. Bartella L, Huang W: Proton (1H) MR spectroscopy of the breast. RadioGraphics 27:S241–S252, 2007.

10 Minimally Invasive Breast Biopsy

Steve H. Parker, Terese I. Kaske, and Judy L. Chavez

KEY POINTS

- Significant improvements have been made in imaging and image-guided biopsy techniques in the past two decades.
- Most image-detected abnormalities can be diagnosed with an image-guided biopsy.
- Biopsy devices are larger and now include vacuum assistance, which aids in diagnostic accuracy.
- Atypical hyperplasia and lobular neoplasm identified by image-guided biopsy both have a high incidence of associated occult malignancy.
- MRI can increase the identification of occult disease.

Introduction

Significant improvements in both imaging modalities and biopsy devices have occurred in the past two decades, which have changed the standard care pathways in breast diagnosis. Vastly improved near-field ultrasound equipment, digital mammography, and breast MRI now allow for much better visualization of the breast tissue and any abnormality within. Surgical biopsy for diagnosis has been supplanted by minimally invasive tissue acquisition techniques. Image-guided fine-needle aspiration (FNA) has been replaced by histologic methods beginning in the 1980s with automated large-core biopsies. Subsequent improvements in tissue acquisition have been realized with vacuum-assisted biopsies (VABs) with their inherent ability to remove most, if not all, of the visualized lesion. These improvements have in turn raised the possibility of percutaneous or minimally invasive therapy.

Manufacturers of ultrasound equipment have realized the importance of breast-specific hardware and software. High-frequency, broadband width transducers (up to 17 MHz) have allowed for exquisite resolution of very small structures within the breast and the detection of subcentimeter cancer as well as ductal carcinoma in situ (DCIS) (Fig. 10-1). Coded harmonics and spatial compound imaging techniques reduce artifacts and allow for more confident lesion visualization. Color Doppler flow can be used in the setting of complex cysts and intraductal lesions to detect blood flow (Fig. 10-2). All these improvements have brought breast ultrasound to a level which makes it an indispensable tool in breast diagnosis.

Stereotactic mammographic units have digital imaging, which provides superior contrast resolution and near instantaneous image display compared with film screen imaging (Fig. 10-3). This has improved both efficiency and accuracy of the biopsy procedures. In addition, many manufacturers now offer digital mammographic spot-imaging capabilities. There are also units designed exclusively for specimen radiography (Fig. 10-4). These devices allow for immediate evaluation of breast tissue for the presence of calcifications and post-biopsy metallic markers, thus speeding the performance of both stereotactic biopsies as well as surgical lumpectomies. Finally, several manufacturers now have full-field digital mammography, which provides superior contrast resolution, increased throughput, and reduced radiation exposure compared with standard film screening mammography (Fig. 10-5). Full-field digital has also been shown to be superior to film screen for women with dense breasts, premenopausal women, and women under 50 years old.[1]

Breast MRI, though expensive, is an exceptionally helpful tool in treatment planning.

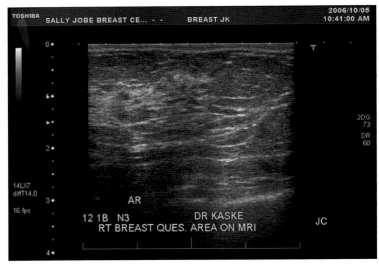

Figure 10-1. Biopsy-proven ductal carcinoma in situ (DCIS) as found at targeted second-look ultrasound after diagnostic breast MRI in patient with recent diagnosis of breast cancer.

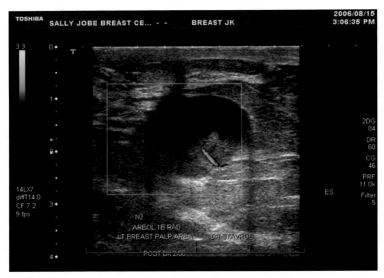

Figure 10-2. Complex cystic and solid mass with color Doppler flow proof of intracystic mass. Biopsy-proven papilloma with atypia.

There are in general two types of breast MRI, both of which use gadolinium contrast injection: dynamic breast MRI and high-resolution breast MRI (Fig. 10-6A through C). Dynamic breast MRI images the breast multiple times in the first few minutes after contrast injection. This allows for analysis of contrast uptake and washout with an improved specificity compared with the high-resolution breast MRI. High-resolution breast MRI results in very high sensitivity with impressive spatial resolution. The specificity is not as high as with dynamic imaging, however.[2,3] Most modern breast MRI equipment and software can do both dynamic and high-resolution imaging while imaging both breasts simultaneously.

Our experience has been that the increased specificity associated with dynamic imaging is not sufficient to eliminate the need for biopsy in enhancing lesions (Fig. 10-7A and B). However, in the patient with multiple enhancing nodules with benign morphology or diffuse fibroglandular enhancement, the dynamic information may assist in identifying the more suspicious lesion(s) to target. We rely heavily on the morphologic characteristics gleaned from the high-resolution images (Fig. 10-8A through D). We have found that MRI is most useful in the preoperative assessment of a patient with a biopsy-proven breast carcinoma.[4-7] In these instances, the true extent of disease is much better appreciated than with standard mammographic images, and the surgery can be appropri-

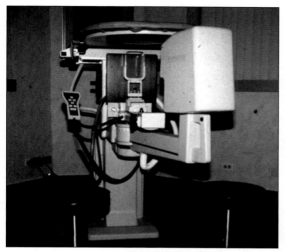

Figure 10-3. Mammo Test Stereotactic Biopsy Table. (Courtesy of Fischer Imaging, Inc. Denver, Colorado.)

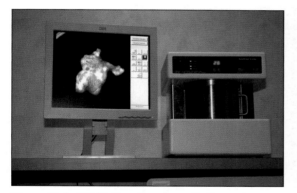

Figure 10-4. DX 50 Core Specimen Radiography System. (Courtesy of Faxitron X-Ray, Lincolnshire, Illinois.)

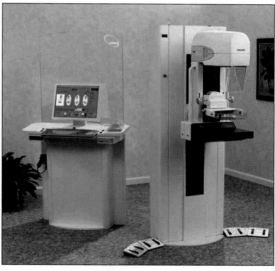

Figure 10-5. Selenia Digital Mammography. (Courtesy of Lorad, a Hologic Company, Bedford, Massachusetts.)

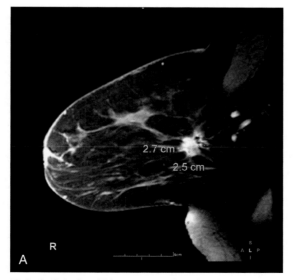

2.7 cm

2.5 cm

R

A

Figure 10-6. A, Spiculated biopsy-proven invasive ductal carcinoma (IDC).
(Continued)

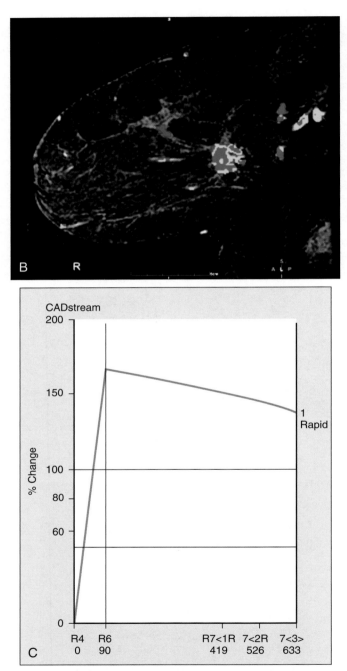

Figure 10-6, cont'd. B, Color map overlay of washout pattern of enhancement in IDC. **C,** Slope image-dynamic representation of suspicious pattern of enhancement—washout pattern.

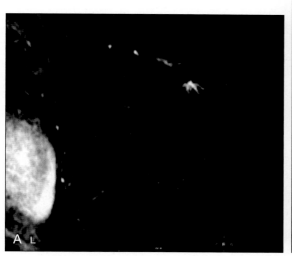
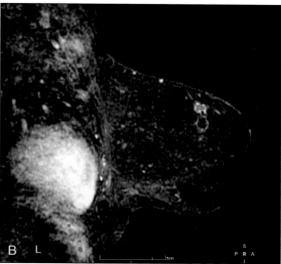

Figure 10-7. A, Sagittal breast MRI of known invasive ductal carcinoma at minimally invasive ultrasound-guided biopsy. **B,** Known cancer demonstrates blue/continuous pattern of dynamic enhancement.

ately tailored. In addition, in approximately 5% to 7% of patients, otherwise unsuspected carcinoma is detected in a different quadrant of the same breast (multicentric disease) (Fig. 10-9A and B). Also, in approximately 5% to 7% of patients, otherwise unsuspected carcinoma is found in the opposite breast[8-10] (Fig. 10-10A and B). More frequently, we are performing breast MRI on high-risk patients. These include patients with *BRAC 1* and *BRAC 2* genetic risk and patients with previous high-risk biopsy results or previous breast cancer[11-16] (Fig 10-11A through C). Occasionally, MRI is used for monitoring regression of disease during neoadjuvant chemotherapy. Other uses include postlumpectomy margin assessment[17,18] and evaluating patients with adenocarcinoma of an axillary node and an unknown primary.[19]

Two main issues must be decided in any minimally invasive breast biopsy: which guidance modality is to be used, and what needle is best suited for the lesion undergoing the biopsy. Of the three breast imaging modalities (ultrasound, stereotactic mammography, and MRI), we prefer ultrasound guidance in the majority of cases. Stereotactic guidance is reserved almost exclusively for targeting microcalcifications, and MRI is used for guidance only in those rare cases in which the MRI-detected abnormality cannot be seen on second-look ultrasound. Ultrasound guidance confers many advantages. It is performed in a more comfort-

able position than the other two guidance modalities, it uses no ionizing radiation, and it provides real-time visualization of the needle. It is our belief that a physician performing minimally invasive procedures should be facile with ultrasound and ultrasound-guided interventions to provide the patient with the advantages of this guidance modality enumerated above.

In concert with the improvements in imaging, there have been marked improvements in tissue acquisition. Percutaneous histologic tissue acquisition techniques currently in use, also referred to as minimally invasive breast biopsy, include large-core biopsy (typically 12–14 gauge) (Fig. 10-12A through C), including the Monopty and Maxcore by Bard and the Achieve needle by Cardinal Health; the vacuum-assisted biopsy (VAB) (typically 7–11 gauge), such as the Mammotome from Ethicon Endo-Surgery, the EnCor from SenoRx, and ATEC from Hologic (Fig. 10-13A through C), and larger tissue acquisition systems, such as the Halo from Rubicor and the en-bloc from Neothermia Corporation (Fig. 10-14A and B). Using smaller needles may risk the occurrence of higher false-negative rates. Fine-needle aspiration (FNA) techniques may be used for biopsy of axillary or internal mammary lymph nodes but are otherwise felt to be less desirable than histologic tissue acquisition techniques. The larger tissue acquisition systems (Rubicor and en-bloc) appear to offer little advantage over

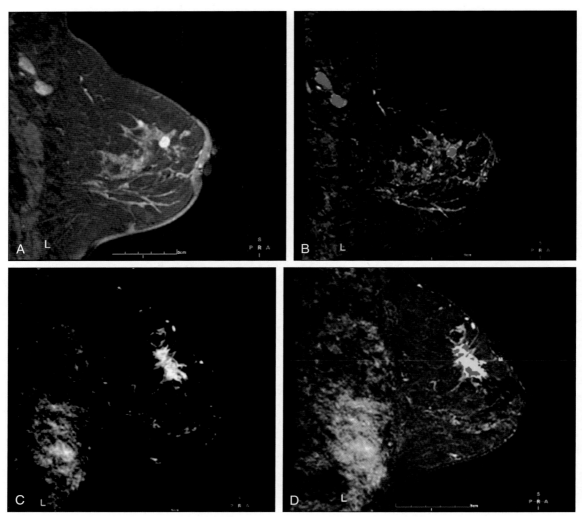

Figure 10-8. Atypical papilloma in the 6 SA location. Separate enhancing masslike lesion in the upper outer quadrant has slightly irregular margins and is an invasive ductal carcinoma (IDC) at targeted ultrasound-guided biopsy. **A,** IDC at 2:00 location. **B,** Color map applied to IDC at 2:00 location. **C,** Different patient with MRI image of classic IDC. **D,** MRI image with color map applied to IDC.

VAB for diagnostic procedures. Investigation of their therapeutic potential is ongoing.

Automated large-core breast biopsy (core needle biopsy) was used extensively by us and others performing minimally invasive breast biopsy in the infancy of the technique. Compared with FNA, core needle biopsy provided more reliable and consistent diagnostic results. However, core needle biopsy carries a substantial false-negative rate in the setting of stereotactic biopsy of microcalcifications[20–24] and a small false-negative rate in the setting of masses

less than 1.5 cm. In addition, core needle biopsy requires many, time-consuming needle insertions and sometimes yields only scant tissue.

The VAB was introduced as a result of the drawbacks of the standard automated core biopsy technique[25–29] (Fig. 10-15). We now use these needles for the majority of our biopsies. These devices allow a greater amount of breast tissue to be harvested in a much shorter amount of time. In addition, the tissue is obtained contiguously, leaving no region of the biopsied area unsampled. The "underestimation" of disease

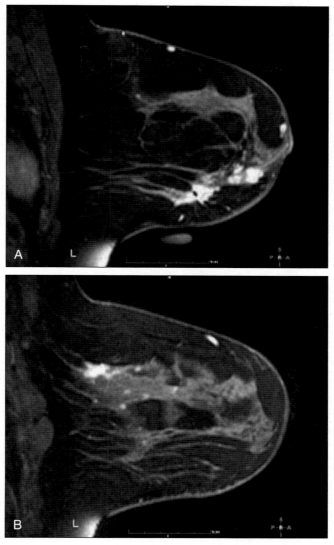

Figure 10-9. Unsuspected multifocal and multicentric breast cancer. A, Biopsied invasive ductal carcinoma (IDC) at 6:00 with targeted ultrasound biopsy-proven high nuclear grade ductal carcinoma in situ (DCIS) extending toward the nipple. **B,** Unsuspected small IDC with DCIS in upper outer quadrant identified with MRI and proven with targeted ultrasound-guided biopsy.

and occasional false-negative results that occurred with the standard automated core biopsy approach have been sharply reduced or eliminated with the VAB. We have found the VAB devices to be especially useful in cases of microcalcifications (Fig. 10-16A and B), ductal lesions, masses less than 1.5 cm, complex cysts (see Fig. 10-26), and any subtle or ill-defined region requiring biopsy (Fig. 10-17A through C). In these cases, most or the entire visualized lesion on the mammogram or ultrasound is removed. Because we have found that all of the

false-negatives that occurred after 14-gauge core biopsy of masses were in lesions less than 1.5 cm, we switched to VAB excisional biopsy of these small masses. For Breast Imaging and Reporting Data System (BIRADS) 5 masses greater than 1.5 cm, the standard 14-core biopsy is still performed, since we have found no false-negative diagnoses in this setting. Given the wide range of malignancy in ACR 4 lesions (3% to 89%), we use VAB to avoid the possibility of a false-negative result. VAB 7- and 8-gauge needles are now also available, which can easily remove

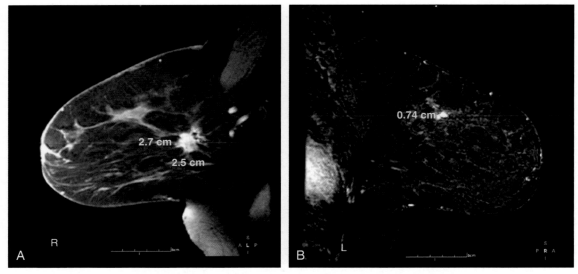

Figure 10-10. A, Known right breast invasive ductal carcinoma (IDC), sagittal MRI image. **B,** Unsuspected left intermediate nuclear grade ductal carcinoma in situ, identified and biopsied with targeted breast ultrasound, sagittal MRI subtraction image.

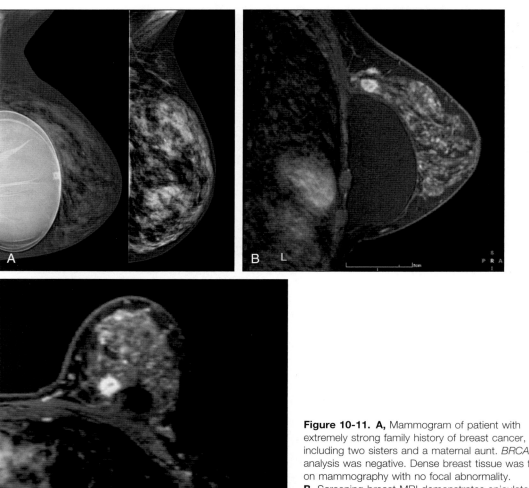

Figure 10-11. A, Mammogram of patient with extremely strong family history of breast cancer, including two sisters and a maternal aunt. *BRCA* analysis was negative. Dense breast tissue was found on mammography with no focal abnormality.
B, Screening breast MRI demonstrates spiculated enhancing mass in the upper inner quadrant of the left breast, sagittal view. **C,** MRI axial view. Targeted breast ultrasound and ultrasound-guided biopsy demonstrating an invasive ductal carcinoma.

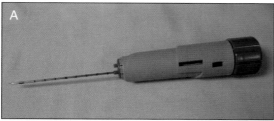

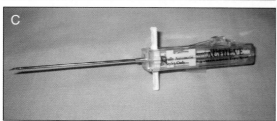

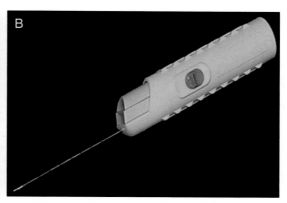

Figure 10-12. A, Monopty Disposable Biopsy System. (Courtesy of C.R. Bard, Covington, Georgia.) **B,** Maxcore Disposable Biopsy Instrument. (Courtesy of Bard Peripheral Vascular, Inc., Tempe, Arizona.) **C,** Achieve Automatic Biopsy System. (Courtesy of Cardinal Health, Dublin, Ohio.)

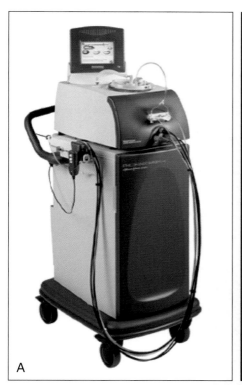

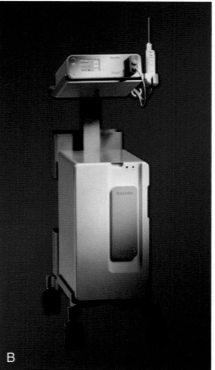

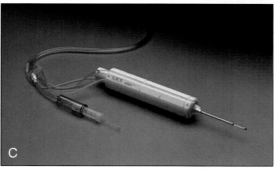

Figure 10-13. A, Mammotome Breast Biopsy System. (Courtesy of Ethicon Endo-Surgery, Cincinnati, Ohio.) **B,** EnCor Vacuum Biopsy Device. (Courtesy of SenoRx, Inc., Irvine, California.) **C,** ATEC Breast Biopsy and Excision System from Hologic. (Courtesy of Hologic, Bedford, Massachuestts.)

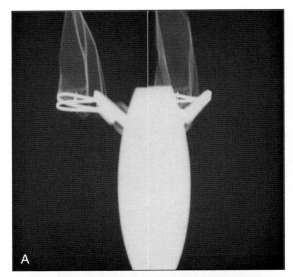

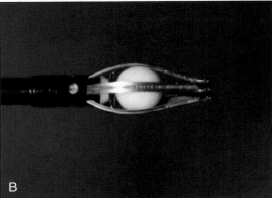

Figure 10-14. A, Halo Breast Biopsy Device. (Courtesy of Rubicor Medical, Inc., Redwood City, California.) **B,** en-bloc Breast Biopsy System. (Courtesy of Neothermia Corporation, Natick, Massachusetts.)

lesions up to 5 cm. For BIRADS, 3 masses (almost always fibroadenomas) greater than 1.5 cm (Fig. 10-18A through C), we use the 7- or 8-gauge VAB needles. Because most or the entire visualized lesion is removed in VAB biopsies, a metallic marker is placed (Fig. 10-19A and B). A post-biopsy mammogram should always be obtained to ensure that the metallic marker is adequately placed (Fig. 10-20A and B).

When multiple biopsies are performed and multifocal or multicentric cancer is diagnosed, the surgeon can identify the extent of disease mammographically. This allows for a lesion seen only on ultrasound to be identified mammographically as well. Modern post-biopsy metallic markers also have a component that can be visualized with ultrasound for a finite period of time (Fig. 10-21). The markers should also be able to be visualized on MRI as a signal void (Fig. 10-22A through C). This identifies the site of a cancer(s) on preop MRI so that additional disease can be confidently diagnosed distant from the index lesion. Unfortunately, manufacturers have used titanium in some of their post-biopsy markers, making them extremely difficult to visualize on subsequent breast MRI. We now believe that post-biopsy markers should be placed after all biopsies (including core needle biopsy) so that the biopsy site is easily identified on all future mammography and/or MRI if the biopsy result is a cancer.

After a minimally invasive breast biopsy, it is of paramount importance to correlate the

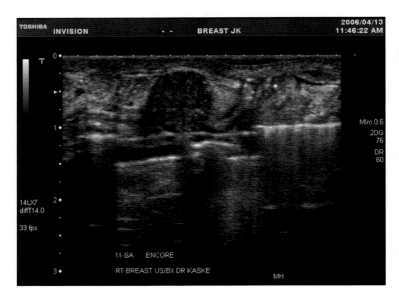

Figure 10-15. Ultrasound image of vacuum-assisted biopsy device in position posterior to lesion at the 11 SA location.

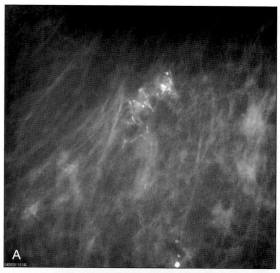

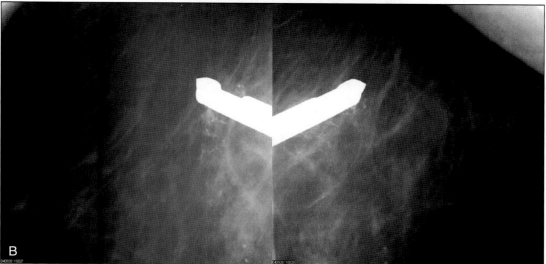

Figure 10-16. A, Scout view of stereotactic biopsy of microcalcifications. **B,** Stereo pair targeting prior to vacuum-assisted biopsy of microcalcifications.

pathologic/histologic diagnosis obtained from an image-guided breast biopsy with that from the imaging workup (Fig. 10-23). Before VAB, when there was discordance between the two, a re-biopsy (usually surgical) was necessary. In the age of VAB, however, this is no longer necessary. To avoid the necessity of re-biopsy in the setting of radiologic-pathologic discordance, it is essential to perform the VAB appropriately. That is, when a VAB is performed, it should not be viewed as a "sampling" procedure but rather as a biopsy that removes most, if not all, imaging evidence of the lesion. In this way, one can be certain that there was not a geographic miss or

an undersampling of a heterogeneous lesion. Even with VAB, it is still important to correlate the imaging and histology. When there is a discordance (e.g., a diagnosis of fibrocystic change in the setting of a BIRADS 5 lesion), then the radiologist needs to ensure that the pathologist reviews the histologic material again and, if necessary, cuts additional levels through the paraffin block to eliminate the possibility that the pathologist missed the lesion. If, after obtaining additional levels and extensive reevaluation of the histology from the VAB, there is still imaging-histologic discordance, the only possibility that remains is that the radiologist was

Text continued on p. 167

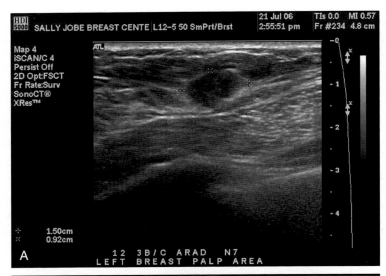

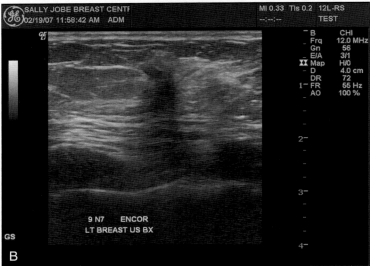

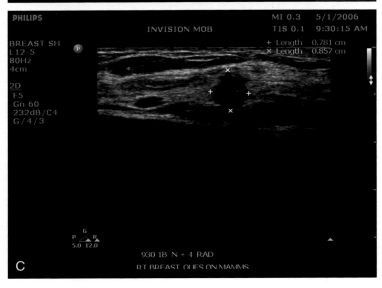

Figure 10-17. Three examples of ACR 4b or 4c lesions typical for vacuum-assisted biopsy. **A,** Small suspicious mass; largest dimension is 1.5 cm. **B,** Small subtle mass with shadowing. **C,** Small microlobulated mass, less than 1.0 cm.

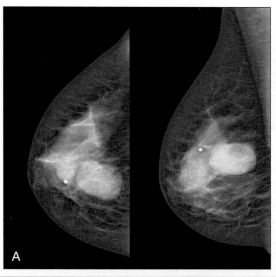

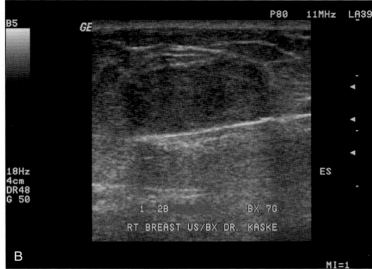

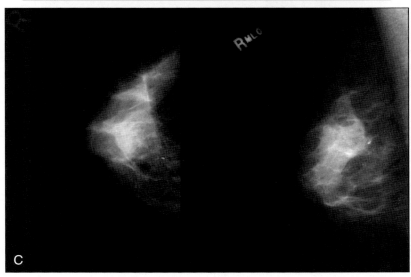

Figure 10-18. Thirty-two-year-old woman with large protruding palpable mass in upper inner quadrant of right breast. **A,** Diagnostic mammogram shows large mass with probable benign characteristics. **B,** Ultrasound image of vacuum-assisted biopsy device posterior to ACR 3 mass. **C,** Post-biopsy mammogram shows metallic marker in location of mass. The mass was excised and proved to be a fibroadenoma.

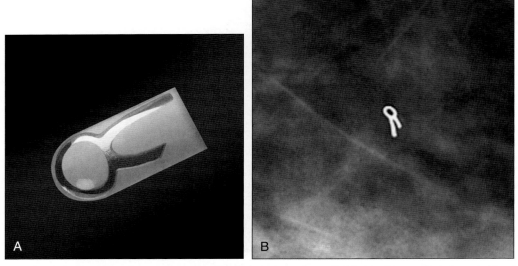

Figure 10-19. **A,** GelMark Ultra Breast Biopsy Marking System in package. **B,** Marking biopsy site in breast. (Courtesy of SenoRx, Inc., Irvine, California.)

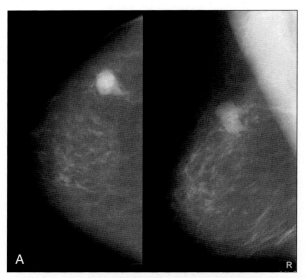

Figure 10-20. A, Pre-biopsy mammogram of mass in upper outer quadrant. **B,** Post-biopsy mammogram of biopsy cavity with metallic ribbon marker in place.

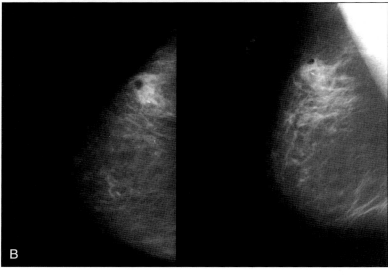

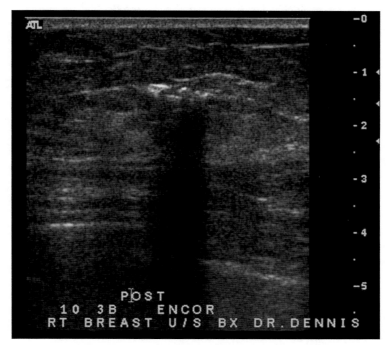

Figure 10-21. Post-biopsy ultrasound image of marker.

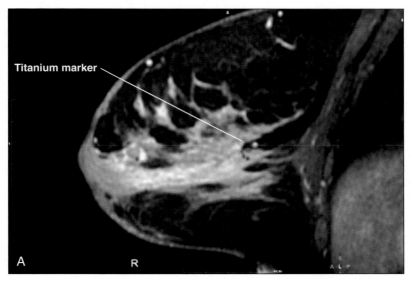

Figure 10-22. A, Sagittal MRI image of titanium marker signal void in deep central right breast.

(*Continued*)

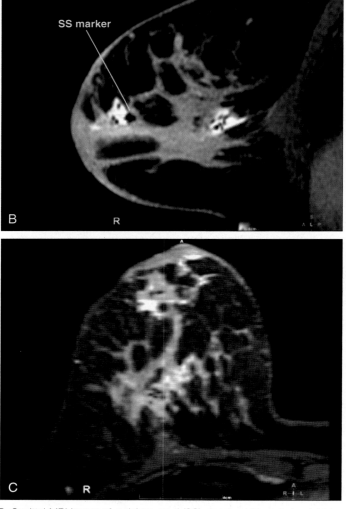

Figure 10-22, cont'd. B, Sagittal MRI image of stainless-steel (SS) signal void in anterior right breast. **C,** Axial MRI image shows both the deep titanium and more anterior stainless-steel marker signal voids.

Breast Procedures - Schedule

Add a Patient | Search | Reports

CX in Site column - procedure has been canceled; SU in Mod column - procedure is surgical; Call column is Results Called

Last Friday 11/13/2009	**Monday 11/16/2009**	Tuesday 11/17/2009	Wednesday 11/18/2009	Thursday 11/19/2009	Friday 11/20/2009

Pret	Time	Name	Site	Mod	Clip	DDX	Birads	Final Biop Path	Rad	Tech	Dict	Call
Y	7:30 am	Abbott, Thelma	L 4:30 N4	US	SenoRx Encor O / VAB	FC vs. DCIS	4a	FC / BCL	KA	JC	Y	JS
Y	8:00 am	Taylor, Louise	L 3:00 N3	US	SenoRx EnCor Ribbon / VAB	FC vs. DCIS	4a	FC / SA	KA	JC	Y	AE
Y	8:15 am	Brady, Marcia	L 11:30 N6	US	SenoRx EnCor Ribbon / NCB	FC vs. IDC	4a	FC	OB	GS	Y	AE
Y	8:30 am	Carlson, Jan	R 2:00 N4	US	SenoRx EnCor Ribbon / VAB	IDC vs. IP vs. FC	4b	IDC	KA	JW	Y	KA
			R Axilla	US	HydroMARK Titanium	ANM	5	ANM				
Y	9:00 am	Scottsdale, Cindy	R 1:00 N10	US	HydroMARK Titanium / NCB	IP vs. FC	4a	IP / FC	KA	GS	Y	JS
Y	9:30 am	Thomas, Alice	R 3:00 N5	ST	SenoRx Core X / VAB	FA	3	FA	OB	GS	Y	AE
N	10:00 am	Rochester, Betty	L 8:00 N8	US	SenoRx CorMark Ribbon / VAB	FN vs. FC vs. IDC	4a	FN / IF	KA	JW	Y	AE
Y	10:15 am	Beddingfield, Wilma	R 10:30 N7	US	SenoRx CorMark Ribbon / VAB	FC vs. DCIS	4a	FC / DHU / BCL	KA	JC	N	AE
Y	10:30 am	Pebbles, Dina	R 9:30 N9	US	SenoRx Core S / VAB	IDC	5	IDC / ILC	OB	JW	Y	OB
			R Axilla	US	JJ Core Mark / VAB	LN vs. ANM	4c	LN				
Y	11:30 am	Wilder, Laura	R 9:30 N7	US	SenoRx EnCor Ribbon / NCB	FC vs. FA vs. IDC	4b	FA	KA	GS	Y	JS
Y	1:00 pm	Engle, Mary	R 6:00 N6	ST	SenoRx EnCor Ribbon / NCB	FC vs. DCIS	4b	FC	KA	JC	Y	JS
Y	1:30 pm	James, Carrie	L 12:30 N9	US	SenoRx EnCor Ribbon / VAB	IDC vs. PSH	5	IDC	OB	GS	Y	OB
Y	2:00 pm	Frank, Janet	L 7:00 N7	US		FA vs. FC vs. DCIS	4a	FC / BCL	KA	JW	Y	JS
			L 7:00 N8	ST	SenoRx Encor M / VAB	FC vs. DCIS	4b	FC / BCL				
Y	3:00 pm	Snow, Chrissy	R Axilla	US	SenoRx Core S / NCB	FC vs. EBT vs. DCIS	4a	FC	KA	JC	Y	AE
Y	4:00 pm	Nichols, Jackie	L 9:00 N1	US	SenoRx StarchMark Ribbon / VAB	FC vs. IDC	4b	FC / IP / DHU	KA	GS	Y	JS

Figure 10-23. We utilize a web-based electronic "Big Board" (EWB) that all the breast imagers can access for follow-up and updates. The items included are biopsy date and time, patient's name, biopsy site, biopsy guidance method (ultrasound [US] or stereotactic [ST]), clip placed and biopsy needle type (vacuum-assisted biopsy [VAB] or needle core [NCB]), expected tissue results/differential diagnosis (DDX), the BIRADS code, final biopsy pathology, the initials of the radiologist who performed the biopsy and the assisting technologist, notation of dictation completed, and results called by the radiologist or the nurse. Follow-up information, notes, and referral to our high-risk program can be entered. The names on this example are fictitious.

wrong in his or her imaging diagnosis (after all, even in BIRADS 5 lesions, there is a 10% chance that the lesion is benign and therefore the radiologist's diagnosis was wrong). Regardless of what instrument is used, however, it should always be the radiologist's responsibility to determine the adequacy of the targeting and tissue acquisition from every biopsy. If a histologic discordance persists, a surgical biopsy should be performed.

To prevent imaging-histologic discordance due to undersampling, it is imperative that VAB be used in all stereotactic biopsies (in which the microcalcifications are almost always associated with a heterogeneous histology). As noted earlier, VAB should also be used for ultrasound-guided biopsy of small (less than 1.5 cm) masses or ill-defined/subtle lesions that cannot be confidently diagnosed with core biopsy sampling (Fig. 10-24A through F). Intraductal and other papillary lesions should undergo VAB rather than core biopsy (Fig. 10-25A through C). Surgical excision with localization may be necessary for extensive involvement but only after minimally invasive needle biopsy to make a diagnosis. Complex cysts requiring biopsy should be approached with VAB (Fig. 10-26A and B). In the setting of a complex cyst, one must be sure that any solid component of the lesion will be

harvested with the biopsy, unlike with a 14-gauge core biopsy in which, after the first pass and the decompression of the cystic part, any solid component may no longer be visualized for further sampling. In cases in which an automated core biopsy is performed and there is radiology-pathology discordance, then the re-biopsy should be performed with VAB, which probably should have been used in the first place.

One of the dilemmas encountered with percutaneous histologic breast biopsy is the diagnosis of atypical ductal hyperplasia (ADH), atypical lobular hyperplasia (ALH), or lobular carcinoma-in-situ (LCIS). Traditionally, ADH diagnosed at core needle biopsy has automatically undergone wide surgical excision because of the relatively high likelihood of finding DCIS associated with the ADH (50% of the time). On the other hand, it was felt that the diagnosis of ALH or LCIS following core needle biopsy did not require surgical excision. These lesions were believed to merely represent a fortuitous finding associated with a higher risk of developing breast cancer in either breast in the future, unrelated to the site of ALH or LCIS.

It has been shown that when the VAB is used for breast biopsy rather than core needle biopsy, the "underestimation of disease" (i.e., finding DCIS at surgery after the diagnosis of ADH at

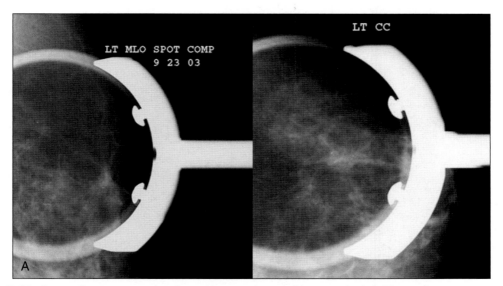

Figure 10-24. Case to illustrate proper imaging guidance and proper biopsy method. **A,** Diagnostic spot compression views demonstrate a spiculated mass in the upper outer quadrant of left breast.

(Continued)

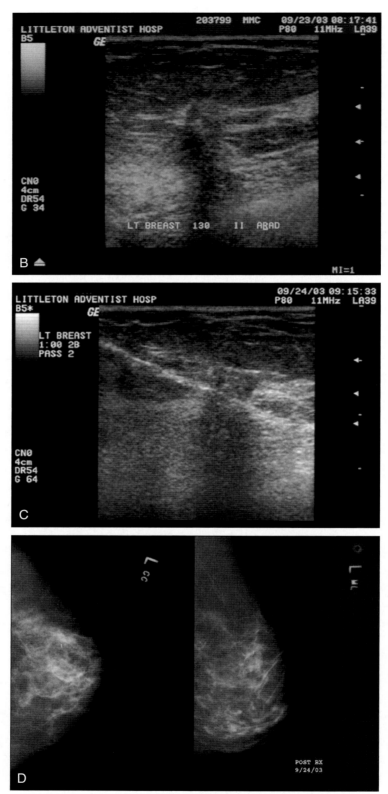

Figure 10-24, cont'd. B, Ultrasound image shows small spiculated mass with shadowing. **C,** Ultrasound-guided core biopsy image (proper image guidance with wrong biopsy device). **D,** Post-biopsy mammogram shows accurate location of metallic marker, but tissue diagnosis is fibrocystic change; therefore, there is image-histology discordance.

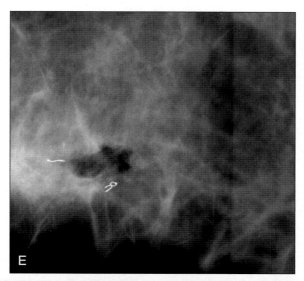

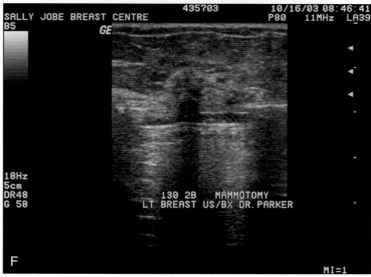

Figure 10-24, cont'd. E, Second biopsy attempt is stereotactic-guided vacuum-assisted biopsy (VAB; proper biopsy device with wrong imaging guidance). **F,** Proper biopsy method with VAB device performed with proper image guidance, ultrasound, obtains correct diagnosis, invasive ductal carcinoma grade I.

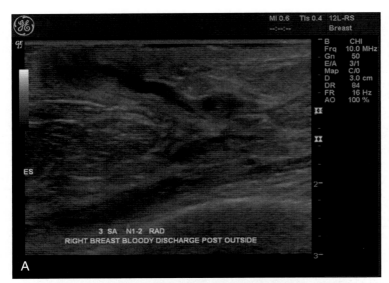

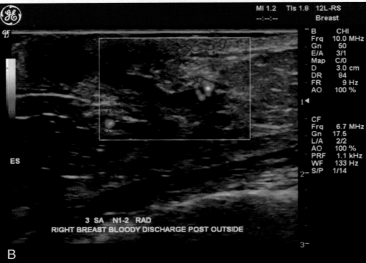

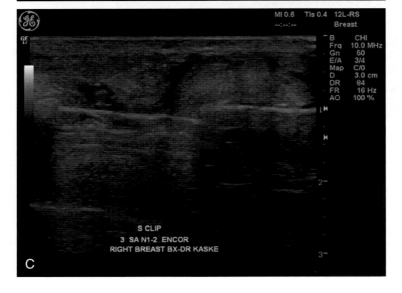

Figure 10-25. Intraductal mass in patient with bloody nipple discharge and abnormal ductogram showing filling defect in the medial right breast. **A,** Ultrasound image of dilated duct with intraductal mass. **B,** Ultrasound image of intraductal mass with internal Doppler flow. **C,** Ultrasound image of vacuum-assisted biopsy device posterior to intraductal mass.

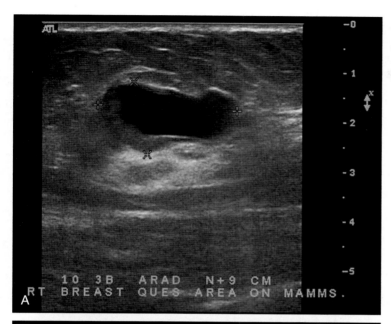

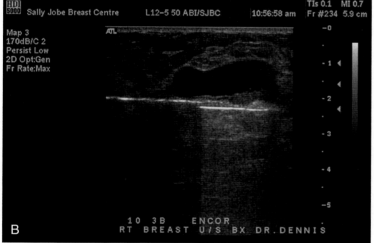

Figure 10-26. Complex cystic and solid mass is a vacuum-assisted biopsy (VAB)-proven intracystic papillary carcinoma. **A,** Ultrasound image of complex cystic and solid mass. **B,** VAB device posterior to complex cystic mass.

percutaneous biopsy) is reduced from 50% to 20% or less—a significant decrease but still a substantial incidence of occult disease. This calls into question the convention of always performing surgical excision following the percutaneous diagnosis with ADH. With regard to the high-risk lesions of ALH and LCIS, it has been recently suggested that the association of DCIS or invasive cancer is as high as 21% after the diagnosis of ALH and as high as 34% after the diagnosis of LCIS. This suggests that it might not be wise to simply follow these patients with mammography and clinical surveillance.[30–34] What seems to make the most sense is to apply

some logic to these situations rather than dogmatically sending all patients with ADH to wide surgical excision and dogmatically denying surgical excision to those patients with ALH and LCIS. At Sally Jobe Breast Centre, we perform MRI after the diagnosis of these borderline lesions. If the breast MRI is normal and there is no significant enhancement at the biopsy site or elsewhere in the remainder of the breast, then one can virtually exclude the possibility of a significant neoplasm in that breast. Conversely, if the breast MRI shows a significant degree of enhancement in the region of the biopsy, which yielded ADH, LCIS, or ALH, then we believe the patient would be well served with a wide surgical excision. Naturally, if there is suspicious enhancement anywhere else in either breast, a second look ultrasound with biopsy should be performed. In our experience, it is just as likely, if not more so, that a significant cancer is found elsewhere in the same breast or in the opposite breast as it is that a significant cancer is found at the exact site of the ADH, ALH, or LCIS (Fig. 10-27A through D).

In centers without breast MRI, one other consideration for determining the appropriate course of action following the diagnosis of ADH, LCIS, or ALH is to evaluate the context of the diagnosis before deciding the next step. If the ADH, LCIS, or ALH is a small focus within a generous vacuum-assisted biopsy and all or nearly all of the imaged abnormality (e.g., region of microcalcifications) has been removed, surgical excision is probably unnecessary. On the other hand, if an imaged abnormality has been subtotally sampled and the ADH, LCIS, or ALH is extensive, then that patient should go on to wide surgical excision. Liberman and colleagues have published their experience with LCIS and suggest that those lesions without any DCIS-like features and without any imaging discordance can be followed rather than excised.[34]

Thus, the standard dogma concerning the proper follow-up for the diagnosis of ADH, LCIS, or ALH may no longer be appropriate. Newer biopsy tools (e.g., VAB), newer data

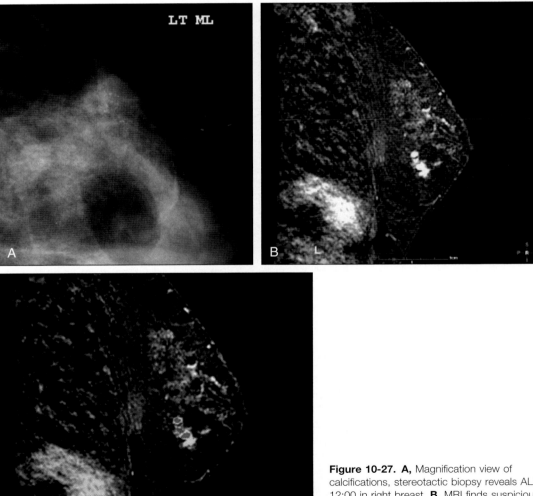

Figure 10-27. A, Magnification view of calcifications, stereotactic biopsy reveals ALH at 12:00 in right breast. **B,** MRI finds suspicious masslike enhancement at the 6:00 location in the left breast. **C,** Color map of suspicious masslike enhancement at 6:00.

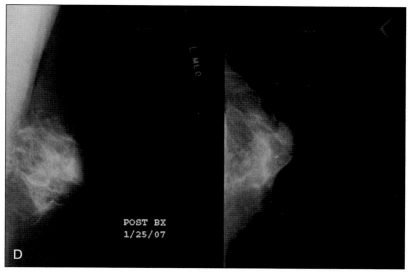

Figure 10-27, cont'd. D, Post-biopsy mammogram, ultrasound-guided biopsy identifies invasive ductal carcinoma at the 6:00 location.

regarding ALH and LCIS, and newer imaging capabilities (breast MRI) all combine to allow for a different, more logical approach to these lesions. As more information becomes available and newer diagnostic devices are developed, more changes may be forthcoming in the management of these interesting lesions.

With the introduction of the newer instruments for breast biopsy, there has come a realization that in some instances the image-guided diagnostic biopsy is successful in removing entire malignancies. Therefore, some clinicians have proposed using these devices for therapy rather than a standard surgical lumpectomy. Thus far, however, it has been difficult to predict the margin status and measure the pathologic tumor size with any of these instruments. Moreover, none is FDA-approved for therapy. The larger-specimen devices may be able to reliably evaluate margins. Other investigators are pursuing the possibility of in situ ablation with stereotactic or MRI-guided laser therapy and ultrasound-guided cryotherapy. It is likely that some form of percutaneous lesion removal, perhaps combined with in situ ablation, will be forthcoming. Physicians and other health care professionals involved with the diagnosis and treatment of breast cancer can look forward to many more exciting changes and improvements in their field.

Conclusion

Screening mammography has significantly advanced the time of diagnosis of breast cancer. As a result, the frequency of the diagnosis of DCIS and small invasive cancers has risen substantially over the past two decades. This ability to diagnose otherwise undetected additional DCIS and small invasive cancers has recently been supplemented by the expanded applications of ultrasound and MRI. The capability of interpreting all three imaging modalities and appropriately integrating these modalities with minimally invasive breast biopsy techniques such as FNA, core biopsy, or VAB is crucial to the locoregional staging of breast cancer. By using these techniques and applying the knowledge now available to diagnose otherwise unsuspected borderline lesions (ADH, ALH, LCIS, DCIS) and multifocal or multicentric infiltrating carcinoma, the women of the world can expect a reduction in breast cancer recurrence and a continued decline in breast cancer mortality rates.

References

1. Pisano ED, Gatsonis C, Hendrick E, et al: Diagnostic performance of digital versus film mammography for breast-cancer screening. N Engl J Med 353:1773–1783, 2005.

2. Viehweg P, Lampe D, Buchmann J, Heywang-Koebrunner SH: In situ and minimally invasive breast cancer: morphologic and kinetic features on contrast-enhanced MR imaging. MAGMA 11:129–137, 2000.

3. Kuhl CK, Mielcareck P, Kleschule S, et al: Dynamic breast MR imaging: are signal intensity time course data useful for differential diagnosis of enhancing lesions? Radiology 211:101–110, 1999.

4. Liberman L, Morris EA, Dershaw DD, et al: MR imaging of the ipsilateral breast in women with percutaneously-proven breast cancer. AJR Am J Roentgenol 180:901–910, 2003.

5. Berg WA, Nguyen TK, Gutierrez L, Segers A: Local extent of disease: preoperative evaluation of the breast cancer patient with mammography, ultrasound, and MRI. Radiology 221(P):230, 2001.

6. Tillman GF, Orel SG, Schnall MD, et al: Effect of breast magnetic resonance imaging on the clinical management of women with early-stage breast carcinoma. J Clin Oncol 20(16): 3413–3423, 2002.

7. Esserman L, Hylton N, Yassa L, et al: Utility of magnetic resonance imaging in the management of breast cancer: evidence for improved preoperative staging. J Clin Oncol 17(1):110–119, 1999.

8. Liberman L, Morris EA, Kim CM, et al: MR imaging findings in the contralateral breast of women with recently diagnosed breast cancer. AJR Am J Roentgenol 180:333–341, 2003.

9. Woo IJ, Orel SG, Schnall MD, et al: Breast MR imaging of the contralateral breast in patients with newly diagnosed breast cancer. Radiology 217(P):526, 2000.

10. Lee SG, Orel SG, Woo IJ, et al: MR imaging screening of the contralateral breast in patients with newly diagnosed breast cancer: preliminary results. Radiology 226(3):773–778, 779, 2003.

11. Kuhl CK, Schmutler RK, Leutner CC, et al: Breast MR imaging screening in 192 women proved or suspected to be carriers of a breast cancer susceptibility gene: preliminary results. Radiology 215:267–270, 2000,

12. Morris EA, Liberman L, Ballon DJ: MRI of occult breast carcinoma in a high-risk population. AJR Am J Roentgenol 181: 619–626, 2003.

13. Kriege M, Brekelsmans CTM, Boetes C, et al: Efficacy of MRI and mammography for breast cancer screening in women with a familial or genetic predisposition. N Engl J Med 351:427–437, 2004.

14. Warner E, Plewes DB, Shumak RS, et al: Comparison of breast MRI, mammography, and ultrasound for surveillance of women at high risk for hereditary breast cancer. J Clin Oncol 19: 3524–3531, 2001.

15. Stoutjesdijk MJ, Boets C, Barentsz JO, et al: MRI and mammography in women with a hereditary risk of breast cancer. J Natl Cancer Inst 93:1095–1102, 2001.

16. Blue Cross Blue Shield: MRI of the breast in high risk women. Dec 2003 bluecares.com/tec/vol18/18_15.html.

17. Lee JM, Orel SG, Czerniecki BJ, et al: MRI before re-excision in patients with breast cancer. AJR Am J Roentgenol 182: 473–480, 2004.

18. Soderstrom CE, Harms SE, Farrell RS, et al: Detection with MR imaging of residual tumor in the breast soon after surgery. AJR Am J Roentgenol 168:485–488, 1997.

19. Orel SG, Weinstein SP, Schnall MD, et al: Breast MR imaging in patients with axillary node metastases and unknown primary malignancy. Radiology 212:543–594, 1999.

20. Parker SH: Needle selection. In Parker SH, Jobe WE (eds): Percutaneous Breast Biopsy. New York: Raven Press, 1993, p 8.

21. Parker SH, Burbank F: A practical approach to minimally invasive breast biopsy. Radiology 200:11–20, 1996.

22. Parker SH, Burbank F, Jackman RJ, et al: Percutaneous large-core breast biopsy: a multi-institutional study. Radiology 193: 359–364, 1994.

23. Jackman RF, Nowels KW, Shepard MJ, et al: Stereotaxic large-core needle biopsy of 450 nonpalpable breast lesions with surgical correlation in lesions with cancer or atypical hyperplasia. Radiology 193:91–95, 1994.

24. Dowlatshahi K, Yaremko ML, Kluskens LF, Jokich PM: Nonpalpable breast lesions: findings of stereotaxic needle-core biopsy and fine-needle aspiration cytology. Radiology 181:745–750, 1991.

25. Parker SH, Klaus AJ, McVey PJ, et al: Sonographically guided directional vacuum-assisted breast biopsy using a handheld device. AJR Am J Roentgenol 177:405–408, 2001.

26. Perez-Fuentes JA, Longobardi IR, Acosta VF, et al: Sonographically guided directional vacuum-assisted breast biopsy. AJR Am J Roentgenol 177:1459–1463, 2001.

27. Parker SH, Jobe WE: Percutaneous Breast Biopsy. New York: Raven Press, 1993.

28. Parker SH, Stavros AT, Dennis MA: Needle biopsy techniques. Radiol Clin North Am 33:1171–1186, 1995.

29. Parker SH, Burbank F: State of the art: a practical approach to minimally invasive breast biopsy. Radiology 200:11–20, 1996.

30. Foster MD, Helvie MA, Gregory NE, et al: Lobular carcinoma in-situ or atypical lobular hyperplasia at core-needle biopsy: is excisional biopsy necessary? Radiology 231:813–819, 2004.

31. Lakhani SR: In-situ lobular neoplasia: time for an awakening. Lancet 361:96, 2003.

32. Page DL, Schuyler PA, Dupont WD, et al: Atypical lobular hyperplasia as a unilateral predictor of breast cancer risk: a retrospective cohort study. Lancet 361:125–129, 2003.

33. Cohen AM: Cancer upgrades at excisional biopsy after diagnosis of atypical lobular hyperplasia or lobular carcinoma in-situ at core-needle biopsy: some reasons why. Radiology 231:617–621, 2004.

34. Liberman L, Sama M, Susnik B, et al: Lobular carcinoma in situ at percutaneous breast biopsy: surgical biopsy findings. AJR Am J Roentgenol 173:291–299, 1999.

Surgical Biopsy

Elizabeth Prier

Introduction

Screening for breast cancer involves self-examination, physical examination by a clinician, and imaging. Palpable breast masses are identified by the patient or the patient's clinician or retrospectively after a positive imaging study. The proportion of patients identified in each category depends on the availability of health care services and the utilization of screening recommendations. Most patients presenting with a palpable breast mass have a benign finding, but malignancy is always in the differential diagnosis. Evaluation of a palpable breast mass requires a careful history and physical examination, imaging, and often a tissue biopsy. Other findings on physical examination that may require a surgical biopsy include a new nipple discharge, rashes or irregular lesions on the nipple, or changes to the color or texture of the breast skin.

Nonpalpable masses are identified by imaging, primarily screening mammography. The use of screening mammography has significantly increased over the last 20 years. The National Health Interview Survey showed that the percentage of eligible women undergoing mammography has increased from 29% in 1987 to 76% in 2000.[1] This significant escalation has led to an increase in the way in which breast biopsies are performed and has provided the impetus for changes in technology. Biopsies are performed for both palpable and nonpalpable lesions, and current techniques incur less morbidity with more accurate tissue sampling.

The use of breast biopsy as part of the algorithm in diagnosing breast cancer is a relatively new component in the workup of breast cancer. Only a few decades ago a woman with a breast mass would go to the operating room not knowing whether she would wake up with a mastectomy or an intact breast. The ability to biopsy both palpable and nonpalpable lesions as early as possible has led to a decrease in breast cancer mortality and morbidity. Current practice guidelines recommend core biopsy, if possible, before surgical intervention for both palpable and nonpalpable lesions.[2]

Evaluation of a Palpable Breast Lesion

Most palpable breast masses are benign (Box 11-1). Nevertheless, a breast mass that is palpable on physical examination requires careful evaluation. A thorough history, physical examination, and imaging are necessary before obtaining a sample of tissue for pathologic diagnosis (Boxes 11-2 and 11-3). Depending on the age of the patient and other risk factors, imaging might include mammography, ultrasound, or both. Mammography is performed to gather

Box 11-1. Most Common Breast Masses

Fibroglandular change
Cyst
Fibroadenoma
Lipoma
Abscess
Granuloma
Fat necrosis
Epidermal inclusion cyst
Lactational adenoma
Diabetic mastopathy
Malignancy—carcinoma, lymphoma, sarcoma

Box 11-2. Pertinent Information From Patient History

Patient's age
Length of time mass has been present
Pain
Menstrual history
Skin changes over breast
Nipple discharge
Personal history of previous masses or biopsies
Family history of breast cancer

Box 11-3. Pertinent Physical Examination Findings

Location
Size
Moveable within the breast
Tenderness
Fluctuance
Skin changes
Nipple discharge
Lymphadenopathy in the axillary, supraclavicular, or infraclavicular basins

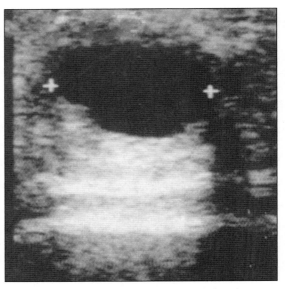

Figure 11-1. A simple cyst has smooth borders, no internal echoes, and good through transmission on ultrasound.

further information about the known lesion as well as screen the breast for other occult lesions. Although mammography is our best tool for screening, it has a high false-negative rate and cannot be relied on exclusively for diagnosis. Ultrasound is an important tool for evaluating a palpable abnormality and is very reliable in discriminating a solid mass from a cyst. It is also helpful in differentiating discrete masses from fibroglandular change, which can also have a lumpy texture. If a patient with a complaint of a palpable mass that has benign characteristics on clinician physical examination has a negative targeted ultrasound, the negative predictive value for cancer is 99.8%.[3] Nevertheless, a dis-

crete, persistent breast mass—whether or not it is visible on ultrasound—should have a tissue diagnosis.

A simple cyst identified by ultrasound does not require any further diagnostic evaluation or therapeutic intervention (Fig. 11-1). If the cyst is symptomatic, however, a cyst aspiration can be performed to relieve pain or to deflate the palpable abnormality. The technique for aspiration of a cyst involves infiltration of local anesthetic into the skin overlying the lesion. Using a 21- or 22-gauge needle attached to a 20-mL or larger syringe, the needle is advanced into the lesion and fluid is aspirated. Cyst aspirations can also be performed under ultrasound guidance.

Cyst fluid may be clear or cloudy yellow, green, gray, or brown. This fluid can be discarded, because many studies have shown that cytologic evaluation of benign cystic fluid has no value.[4] A purely blood aspirate or an aspirate of what appears to be old blood should be sent for cytology, and excision of the lesion should be performed. After aspiration of the cyst, the mass should disappear. A mass that persists, recurrent masses, or a bloody aspirate constitutes an indication for surgical excision.

Several techniques are available for biopsy of a palpable complex cyst or a solid mass. These include fine-needle aspiration (FNA),

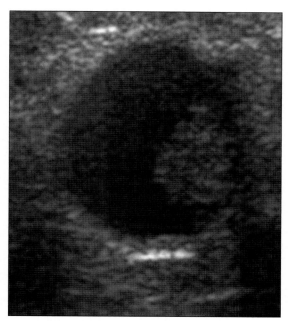

Figure 11-2. This complex cyst has a smooth wall with good through transmission, but there is an intraluminal mass that appears solid within the cyst.

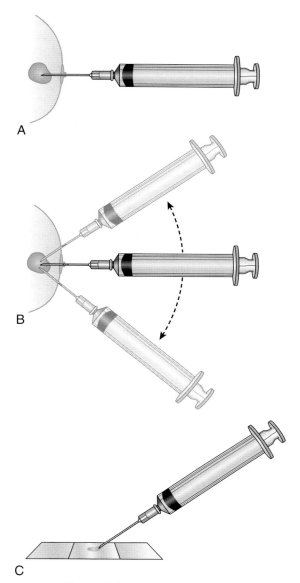

Figure 11-3. Fine-needle aspiration.

core biopsy, and surgical biopsy. The most appropriate technique is determined by the characteristics of the target lesion.

Complex Cyst

A complex cyst is a cystic lesion that contains a solid component, either extending from the wall of the cyst or contained within the cystic portion (Fig. 11-2). Careful consideration needs to be given to the biopsy technique selected for sampling a complex cyst. If the cystic component is ruptured and the fluid evacuates without obtaining an adequate sample of the solid component, the lesion may not be identifiable on subsequent ultrasound. Therefore, FNA would not be appropriate. If the solid component is significant so that evacuation of the cystic contents is not a concern, then an ultrasound-guided core biopsy is an option. If there is concern about loss of the landmarks, however, then a surgical excisional biopsy should be performed.

Biopsy Techniques

Several techniques are available for obtaining a tissue diagnosis of a palpable lesion. They vary in degree of invasiveness as well as risk of false-negative or false-positive results. The techniques that are described in the following text include FNA, core needle biopsy, and surgical biopsy.

Fine-Needle Aspiration

FNA is a simple procedure that can be performed in the office without anesthesia (Fig. 11-3). It can be helpful to identify fibroadenomas, other benign lesions, and cancers. Several advantages exist for using FNA as a first-line diagnostic test. It is simple and quick to perform, carries a low risk of morbidity, involves very little patient discomfort, and has a low cost. With a skilled cytopathologist, the false-positive rate can be as low as 0.5%. The disadvantages of FNA include an inability to discriminate between an in situ and an invasive lesion, a high false-negative rate in the hands of pathologists without significant experience, and the requirement of further biopsy to obtain histologic confirmation if the cells appear malignant.[5] The use of FNA versus core biopsy for initial diagnosis depends on the local resources of the practice. It is best applied in a practice that has quick access to an experienced cytopathologist who can provide a diagnosis with a very short turn-around time, that is, in less than 24 hours, or who can obtain a tissue diagnosis in a probable benign lesion such as a fibroadenoma, in which the patient wants to avoid a larger biopsy procedure. Non-diagnostic results, discordant results, papillary lesions, and hypercellular lesions need to proceed to a larger biopsy for definitive diagnosis. Malignant lesions, of course, need to proceed to further treatment planning.

Core Needle Biopsy

Core needle biopsy of a palpable lesion can be performed to obtain tissue suitable for histologic diagnosis (Fig. 11-4). False-negative results are rare and are usually related to small tumor size. The advantages of core needle biopsy over FNA include obtaining a more definitive histologic diagnosis, providing the distinction between invasive and in situ cancer, and usually providing adequate sampling for immunohisto-

chemistry evaluation. Core needle biopsy is performed most frequently with an automated 14-gauge core biopsy needle. It can also be done with a Tru-Cut biopsy needle. Automated core biopsy needles have the advantage of ease of use, better quality specimens, and higher sampling rate. A core biopsy can be performed by palpating the mass; however, improved results have been obtained with the addition of ultrasound, since the position of the needle in relation to the lesion before firing and within the lesion after firing can be visualized with the ultrasound.

Surgical Biopsy

If a preliminary diagnosis cannot be made by FNA or core needle biopsy, a surgical biopsy can be performed to obtain tissue for diagnosis as well as to provide treatment for most benign lesions. A surgical biopsy can be either incisional, which takes a subtotal piece of the lesion, or excisional, which completely removes the lesion. Incisional biopsies have been almost completely replaced with core biopsy techniques and are rarely used in a modern breast surgery practice.

Excisional biopsy involves the complete removal of a breast mass. These biopsies can be performed in a minor procedure room if the lesion is small and superficial, or in the operating room with local anesthetic and conscious sedation if a larger procedure is anticipated. The incision is usually placed along Langer lines for the best cosmetic result. If possible, a periareo-

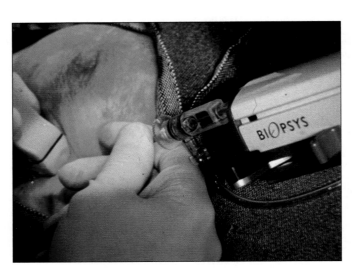

Figure 11-4. Ultrasound-guided core biopsy is performed freehand. The biopsy instrument map may be an automated gun or a vacuum assisted biopsy instrument. (Courtesy of Ethicon EndoSurgery, Inc. of Johnson and Johnson.)

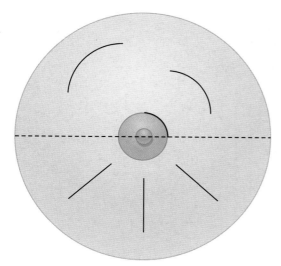

Figure 11-5. Incision placement.

lar incision should be used if the lesion is centrally located because the scar then blends in with the pigment change. In the lower half of the breast, radial incisions for malignant lesions are usually used. Even though the breast may be slightly narrowed by a radial incision in the lower half of the breast, incisions along Langer lines in the inferior pole can cause more cosmetic deformity by shortening the distance between the areolar complex and the inframammary fold (Fig. 11-5).

A breast biopsy is performed sharply using either a knife or scissors. Electrocautery is discouraged because it can leave char artifact, which makes margin interpretation difficult for the pathologist. A biopsy, as opposed to a lumpectomy, has the surgical goal of obtaining a diagnosis by removing the lesion while minimizing excessive tissue loss. Therefore, wide margins are not appropriate for a biopsy procedure. Lumpectomy, which is used to treat malignant disease, is discussed in Chapter 12.

Evaluation of a Nonpalpable Breast Lesion

The technique for biopsy of a nonpalpable breast lesion is a rapidly changing area of breast cancer treatment. Improvements in mammographic diagnostic capabilities, an increase in the number of women undergoing screening, and the addition of other screening modalities such as whole-breast ultrasound and MRI have significantly increased the number of nonpalpable breast abnormalities detected. This has, in turn, fueled the search for more accurate and cosmetically pleasing biopsy techniques. Mammographic abnormalities that are concerning for malignancy include lesions that contain microcalcifications, density lesions that include asymmetries, masses, and architectural distortions, or lesions containing a combination of both. Once identified by mammogram, these abnormalities require biopsy to determine their significance. Many modalities exist to biopsy these lesions, including stereotactic biopsy, ultrasound-guided biopsy, MRI-guided biopsy, and surgical excisional biopsy with image localization. Techniques for imaging guided biopsy are discussed in Chapter 10. Surgical excisional biopsy with image localization is an important tool in the surgeon's toolbox.

Image Localization Biopsy

Localization of nonpalpable lesions by imaging guidance is required to remove the target lesion while minimizing the loss of normal breast tissue. Before the advent of image-directed biopsies in the early 1990s, needle localization biopsy (NLBx) was the standard approach for obtaining a tissue diagnosis of lesions detected only by mammogram or ultrasound. In this era, it still has a role in the primary diagnosis of certain imaging abnormalities, primarily intraluminal ductal lesions and mammographic radial scars as well as indeterminate findings on image-guided core biopsy such as atypical hyperplasia, atypical columnar cell change, lobular neoplasia, and incompletely excised papillary lesions[6] (Box 11-4). Currently, the more common application of an image localized biopsy is after an image guided biopsy, either for further diagnosis or for treatment.

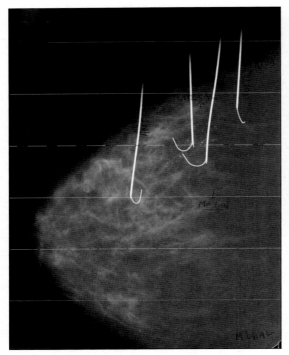

Figure 11-6. Multiple wires are used to localize and bracket a larger area of microcalcifications.

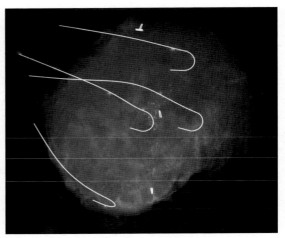

Figure 11-7. Imaging of the specimen confirms that the target lesion has been removed as well as documenting removal of the localizing wires.

Needle or wire localization of an image abnormality is the most common method for directing the surgeon to the target lesion. Other techniques that have been developed are direct ultrasound guidance, hematoma-directed excision,[7] and radioguided occult lesion localization.[8] Because these techniques are all performed as a variant of the needle localization biopsy, we focus here on this more common technique.

Needle localization biopsy requires close coordination among the radiologist, the surgeon, and the pathologist. The goal with this technique is to accurately pinpoint the lesion to completely remove the area of abnormality while minimizing the volume of tissue that is removed from the breast. For this to occur, the wire should be placed within 5 mm of the lesion. For larger lesions, many wires can be placed to "bracket" the lesion (Fig. 11-6).

The first stage of the needle localization biopsy is placement of the needle by the radiologist, although some surgeons are trained to place the wire themselves. The lesion is localized by mammogram or ultrasound. Several types of needles can be used for the localization, according to the preference of the physician perform-

ing the procedure. Needle types are hypodermic, hookwire, and anchored.

The hookwire needle is the most frequently used for localization. The wire is passed through a needle and the hook reforms after it has passed through the needle, allowing it to catch in the breast tissue. After needle placement, a mammogram is performed in the medial-lateral view as well as the cranial-caudal view to provide the operating surgeon with a three-dimensional location of the lesion.

There will be some change in the position of the breast between the mammogram table and the operating room table, but the position of the hook usually remains in the same place. The surgical incision should be placed as close to the lesion as possible, while still trying to create an incision that can be incorporated into a mastectomy incision if that proves necessary in the future. The dissection is then performed down to the wire and along its course to the site of the lesion. Once the lesion is removed, radiographic confirmation is required to prove the lesion is included within the specimen (Fig. 11-7).

Evaluation of Nipple Discharge

Mother Nature puts a great deal of emphasis on our ability to feed our young. The breast is designed to produce and secrete fluid that will provide the necessary nutrition for a new baby. This milk production occurs in response to hor-

Table 11-1. Characteristics of Nipple Discharge

Worrisome		Not Worrisome
Spontaneous	vs	Elicited
Unilateral	vs	Bilateral
Single duct	vs	Multiple ducts
Bloody	vs	Nonbloody

monal as well as physical (suckling) stimulation. Similar stimulation outside the lactational phase can result in an expressible nipple discharge. In addition, women who have completed breast-feeding can have a persistent discharge for years after weaning.

The challenge in the evaluation of nipple discharge is to determine whether the discharge is physiologic and benign or whether it represents a more worrisome situation—the most extreme of which is a breast malignancy. Several features are identifiable on the history and physical examination that can help direct further evaluation (Table 11-1). Four important history and physical examination features must be identified and sorted into worrisome or not-so-worrisome findings. The first is whether the discharge is spontaneous or elicited. An elicited discharge can be expressed only under manipulation. A spontaneous discharge may be seen on the bra or night clothes and is more worrisome than a discharge that is only elicited. Another finding is whether the discharge comes from one breast or both breasts. A discharge from both breasts suggests a physiologic condition. Similarly, if the discharge comes from one duct, it is more worrisome than if it arises from multiple ducts. Lastly, the characteristics of the discharge itself can lend a clue to its cause. A physiologic discharge has the same color and texture as fibrocystic fluid—gray, green, yellow, clear, white. More worrisome is a bloody discharge or a watery discharge.

The findings described in the history may or may not be reproduced on physical examination. If the discharge can be expressed, the fluid should not be sent for cytology. A benign discharge contains cellular debris that can be interpreted as atypical, and a malignant discharge can be acellular. Therefore, the information from cytology findings can only confuse the clinical picture and does not provide a definitive answer to the questions.

Further evaluation with imaging, however, should be pursued. Mammogram, if the patient is age-appropriate, and ultrasound are required. Ultrasound can concentrate on the retroareolar ducts to identify duct ectasia (physiologic dilation of the duct) or intraductal mass lesions. MRI is not appropriate for evaluation of nipple discharge. Ductography (galactography), which involves injection of the discharging duct with a contrast agent followed by mammography, can be performed if the discharge is reproducible in the clinical setting. A ductogram can demonstrate the caliber of the duct, can note the presence of filling defects that could represent papillomas or malignancy, and provide the distance of these filling defects from the nipple. Although most lesions that cause a nipple discharge are located within 2 cm of the nipple, about 20% are found more than 2 cm away, and this is important information for surgical treatment planning.

Appropriate treatment for each type of nipple discharge is described in Table 11-2. For a discharge that requires a surgical biopsy for diagnosis, a central duct excisional biopsy is performed. During this procedure, the discharging duct is cannulated and dilated using a lacrimal duct probe; then a small amount (0.1 mL) of methylene blue is instilled into the offending duct to allow easy visual identification of the duct and its branches. A circumareolar incision is made, limiting it to less than 50% of the circumference of the areola. Sharp dissection up to the underside of the nipple can identify the blue duct. If the discharge cannot be expressed in the operating room and a single duct identified, then all of the ducts need to be transected and excised. The patient needs to be counseled about the risks of central duct excision, including changes in sensation to the nipple, skin injury to the nipple, and interfer-

Table 11-2. Treatment of Nipple Discharge

Discharge	Treatment
Milky, unilateral	No treatment
Milky, bilateral	Check prolactin
Unilateral, spontaneous	Duct excision
Bloody	Duct excision
Bilateral, multiduct, or non–bloody-elicited	Reassurance, avoid trauma

ence with the ability to breastfeed in the future. Once the duct or ducts have been identified, they are dissected down to a depth of 2 to 2.5 cm, or to the depth of the lesion seen on ductogram, and excised. Typical pathologic findings are papillomas, duct ectasia, and less commonly ductal carcinoma in situ.

Skin Biopsy

Occasionally the first presenting symptom of breast cancer involves changes to the nipple or changes to the color or texture of the breast skin. Nipple changes that include an itchy, scaly, or erythematous rash must be evaluated for Paget disease, ductal carcinoma in situ of the nipple (Fig. 11-8). A biopsy of the nipple can be performed with local anesthesia using a sharp knife or punch biopsy tool. Because of the sensitive area for infiltration of the local anesthetic, conscious sedation may be required for the patient's comfort.

Inflammatory breast cancer is a clinical diagnosis made when a patient presents with an erythematous change to the skin of the breast that involves more than one third of the surface of the breast (Fig. 11-9). The skin may also be edematous from lymphatic obstruction creating the classic *peau d'orange* appearance (Fig. 11-10). Often, a discrete mass is not identified on physical examination or imaging. This clinical picture is often mistaken for mastitis, and prolonged antibiotic therapy can result in a delay in diagnosis. It is appropriate to initiate treatment with antibiotics, but if rapid resolution is not seen in 10 to 4 days, a biopsy of the skin that includes a small portion of underlying breast tissue must be performed. The skin changes in inflammatory breast cancer are caused by obstruction of the subdermal lymphatics with tumor cells, which is the diagnostic finding seen on pathologic evaluation (Fig. 11-11).

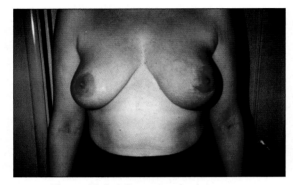

Figure 11-9. Inflammatory breast cancer.

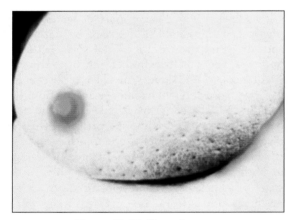

Figure 11-10. Peau d'orange.

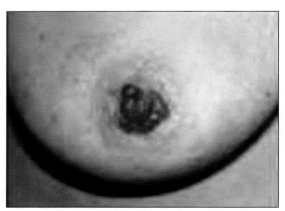

Figure 11-8. Paget disease of the nipple.

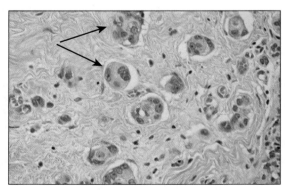

Figure 11-11. Inflammatory breast cancer. Tumor cells (*arrows*) are filling the subdermal lymphatic spaces.

Conclusion

The surgeon plays a vital role in the management of breast disease. From diagnosis to surgical therapy, there are several important tools in the surgical tool box. Knowing how to correctly choose the appropriate tool for the situation at hand is the hallmark of a thoughtful physician. Because breast diagnosis is one of the most rapidly changing areas of medicine, the techniques used 10 to 15 years ago are being altered or retired in place of current, more accurate, and cosmetically acceptable biopsy techniques. With the amount of research invested in breast cancer, these approaches will continue to change. The end goal ultimately is a timely and accurate diagnosis to decrease morbidity and mortality from breast cancer.

References

1. Humphrey LL, Helfand M, et al: Breast cancer screening: a summary of the evidence for the U.S. Preventive Services Task Force. Ann Intern Med 137:347–360, 2002.
2. NCCN guidelines for breast cancer screening, 2007. www.nccn.org/professionals/physician_gls/PDF/breast-screening.pdf, p 4.
3. Graf O, Helbich TH, Hopf G, et al: Probably benign breast masses at US: is follow-up an acceptable alternative to biopsy? Radiology 244(1):87–93, 2007.
4. Cowen PN, Benson EA: Cytological study of fluid from breast cysts. Br J Surg 66:209–211, 1979.
5. Kline TS, Joshi LP, Neal HS: Fine-needle aspiration of the breast: diagnosis and pitfalls: a review of 3545 cases. Cancer 44(4):1458–1464, 1979.
6. Tseng HS, Chen YL, Chen ST, et al: The management of papillary lesion of the breast by core needle biopsy. Eur J Surg Oncol 2008 Jul 17. [Epub ahead of print.]
7. Layeequr-Rahman R, Iuanow E, Crawford S, Quinlan R: Sonographic hematoma-guided vs wire-localized lumpectomy for breast cancer: a comparison of margins and volume of resection. Arch Surg 142(4):343–346, 2007.
8. Lavoue V, Nos C, Clough KB, et al: Simplified technique of radioguided occult lesion localization (ROLL) plus sentinel lymph node biopsy (SNOLL) in breast carcinoma. Ann Surg Oncol 15(9):2556–2561, 2008.

12

Surgical Therapy of Early Breast Cancer

Michael Ford and Christina A. Finlayson

KEY POINTS

- Surgical therapy of early breast cancer is a required component of multidisciplinary care.
- The primary surgical options for the breast are mastectomy or breast conservation.
- Carefully conducted clinical trials have identified which patients require mastectomy and which patients can achieve equivalent outcomes with breast conservation.
- Although many more women can be successfully treated with breast conservation, there are still several situations in which breast conservation is not appropriate and mastectomy is required.

Introduction

The breast begins development as a ridge of tissue that is visible 7 to 8 weeks after conception and has identifiable structures by 16 weeks. Beginning at puberty, estrogen and progesterone cause the breast to enlarge and mature over a period lasting 3 to 4 years.

The breast is composed of skin, the nipple-areola complex, fat, connective tissue, milk ducts, and lobules. Each breast has approximately 15 lobules arranged in a radial pattern from the nipple, with a higher concentration in the superior and lateral quadrant extending out to the tail of Spence. The breast is supported by Cooper's ligaments, which originate from the pectoralis fascia and extend to the dermis overlying the breast in the inferior aspect. Over time, these ligaments relax, causing ptosis of the breast.

Breast tissue is broadly distributed along the milk line from the axilla to the groin, and breast cancer can arise at any of these ectopic locations (Fig. 12-1). Ectopic breast cancer, however, is rare, and surgical treatment is local excision. Most breast cancers occur in the breast proper, and surgical treatment of these tumors is the focus of this chapter.

Breast cancer can arise from any of the breast structures. The most common cell type, adenocarcinoma, arises from the terminal ductal-lobular unit. Other epithelial tumors include squamous cell carcinoma and metaplastic carcinoma. The stromal components of the breast can give rise to benign and malignant phylloides tumors and various types of sarcomas.

Breast cancer treatment requires both locoregional control in the breast and axilla as well as prevention and control of distant metastatic disease. Distant control of metastatic disease is obtained through chemotherapy, hormone therapy, or biologic therapy. Locoregional control is attained through surgery and radiation therapy to the breast, chest wall, and axilla. Surgical procedures for early breast cancer therapy are mastectomy or lumpectomy. Sentinel lymph node biopsy and axillary lymph node dissection are used to provide staging information as well as local control of metastatic disease in the axilla; these are discussed further in Chapter 15.

History

In this century, surgery remains the central aspect of breast cancer treatment, as it has for millennia. In the mid-1860s, Edwin Smith acquired an ancient manuscript thought to have originated in Egypt around 1600 BC and believed to be a copy of a text 1000 years older.[1] It includes the first recorded description of breast cancer and, although the author concluded that breast cancer was not treatable, this didn't stop others from trying. Around 2000 BC, physicians on the Indian subcontinent were treating breast cancer with surgery, cautery, and arsenic compounds.[2] By

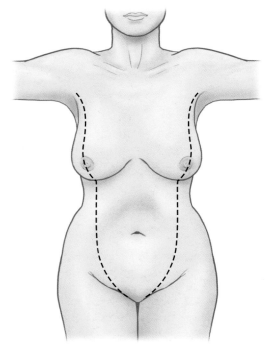

Figure 12-1. Distribution of breast tissue along milk lines. (From Marshall MB, Moynihan JJ, Frost A, Evans SRT: Ectopic breast cancer: case report and literature review. Surg Oncol 3:295–304, 1994, Figure 1.)

460 BC, Hippocrates was describing breast tumors as a buildup of "black bile" (melanchole). Around 200 BC, Galen, the surgeon to Roman Emperor Marcus Aurelius, noted that the only way to cure breast cancer is complete surgical excision in early-stage disease. Another Roman surgeon, Aulus Cornelius Celsus, knew the problem of local recurrence in 100 BC "after excision, even when a scar has formed, none the less the disease has returned."[3] Whether "complete excision" could be done sufficiently with lumpectomy or required mastectomy was debated in the surgical literature until the mid-1900s.

In 1894, Halsted[4] published his experience with a procedure subsequently labeled the Halsted radical mastectomy for the local control of breast cancer (Fig. 12-2). He developed this procedure based on the work of other contemporary surgeons of his day. He used anesthesia, antisepsis, and strict hemostasis to remove the skin, breast, pectoralis major and minor muscles, and the axillary contents, including infraclavicular and supraclavicular nodes en bloc. One of the most important but often overlooked aspects of this achievement was that none of Halsted's patients died from sepsis. Before this report, up to 50% of the women undergoing mastectomy died from infection within the first 2 weeks after surgery. Information about aseptic technique had just recently been incorporated in surgical procedures, and this, combined with Halsted's early practice of leaving the chest wound open to heal by secondary intention,

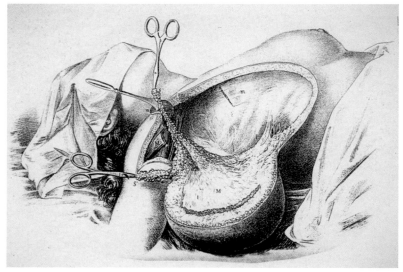

Figure 12-2. Halsted mastectomy. (From Halsted W: The Results of Operations for the Cure of Cancer of the Breast Performed at The Johns Hopkins Hospital from June 1889 to January 1894. The Johns Hopkins Hospital Reports. The Johns Hopkins Press, 1894, p 33)

increased short-term survival to 100%. He subsequently used skin grafts to cover the large open wound.

Dr. Halsted's patients were left with disfiguring and large wounds with minimal impact on long-term, cancer-specific survival: breast cancer left untreated has a 2.7-year average survival, whereas Halsted's patients had a 3-year average survival. In addition, his patients experienced significant morbidity. Differences in sociologic norms of the day are best expressed in Halsted's own words:

> After all, disability, ever so great, is a matter of very little importance as compared with the life of the patient. Furthermore, these patients are old. Their average age is nearly 55 years. They are no longer very active members of society. We should, perhaps, sacrifice many lives if we were to consider the disability which might result from removing a little more tissue from here and there.[4]

Currently, we still have a limited arsenal of surgical procedures for treating breast cancer. Simply, there are two fundamental choices to make: (1) mastectomy or lumpectomy for local control in the breast and (2) axillary node dissection or sentinal node biopsy for axillary staging and local control. All other treatment decisions stem from these two key choices.

Mastectomy

In modern practice, the Halsted radical mastectomy is mostly a historical footnote. Nevertheless, Halsted set an important precedent in carefully documenting his technique and outcomes, which laid the foundation for the next step forward, the prospective, randomized, controlled clinical trial. By the mid-1900s, many surgeons and institutions were analyzing their retrospective outcomes and wondering if "more" really was "better."[5] In the United States, the National Surgical Adjuvant Breast and Bowel Project (NSABP) pioneered the concept of collecting and comparing outcomes data from large, multi-institutional studies to guide appropriate surgical therapy. In 1971, they began a study that randomized women to radical mastectomy or total mastectomy with or without radiation therapy. The initial publication announcing no difference in survival at 10 years of follow-up was presented in 1985.[6] This was in keeping with Halsted's observation that local control is important for disease management but does not impact ultimate survival. The treatment changing information from the B-04 study was that, in most instances, radical mastectomy did not improve local control over total mastectomy and the best local control was achieved in women with clinically negative lymph nodes who received total mastectomy and radiation therapy (Fig. 12-3).

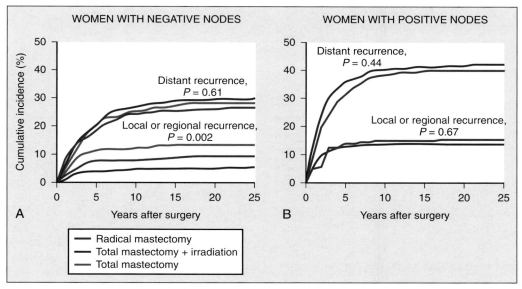

Figure 12-3. Recurrence rates for women with negative nodes (A) versus positive nodes (B). (From Fisher B, Jeong JH, Anderson S, et al: Twenty-five-year follow-up of a randomized trial comparing radical mastectomy, total mastectomy, and total mastectomy followed by irradiation. N Engl J Med 347(8):567–575, 2002, Figure 2.)

During this time the radical mastectomy gave way to the modified radical mastectomy (MRM). More recently, MRM has been replaced by total mastectomy combined with sentinel lymph node biopsy. The modified radical mastectomy involves removal of the breast, the nipple-areolar complex, enough skin to allow the remaining skin flaps to close without tension, the pectoralis fascia, and the axillary lymph nodes. Total mastectomy includes all the components of this procedure except axillary lymph node dissection. The borders of the breast dissection are the clavicle superiorly, lateral border of the sternum medially, the latissimus dorsi laterally, and the inframammary fold inferiorly. The fascia overlying the pectoralis major is removed, but the muscle is left intact. Because breast tissue extends beyond these borders as well as interdigitating with the subcutaneous fat of the skin, even the most radical of mastectomies leaves residual breast tissue in situ (Fig. 12-4).

A modification of this procedure when immediate reconstruction is planned is the skin-sparing mastectomy (SSM). This procedure involves performing an oncologically sound operation while leaving as much skin as possible. In the appropriate patient, the SSM is an excellent treatment option. In one study, 286 patients were randomized to SSM or MRM and followed up for a mean 59 months. Of the 112 patients with SSM, six (5.4%) had a recurrence, whereas the MRM group had 11 recurrences (8.2%).[7] The originally described SSM included removal of the nipple-areola complex, but some surgeons are pushing that boundary by using methods to preserve even the nipple and still reporting low local recurrence rates. See Chapter 13, Breast Reconstruction After Mastectomy.

Mastectomy has historically been indicated for tumors larger than 5 cm. A more patient-specific criterion is applying mastectomy when the tumor is large for the size of the remaining breast and when an oncologically acceptable lumpectomy would not leave a cosmetically acceptable outcome. Increasingly, patient desire, particularly for bilateral mastectomy, has influenced a recent increase in mastectomy for early breast cancer.[8]

Partial Mastectomy (Lumpectomy)

After successfully completing accrual to the B-04 study evaluating the extent of mastectomy

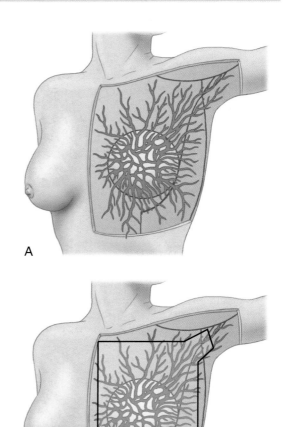

A

B

Figure 12-4. Extent of breast tissue (**A**) versus extent of mastectomy (**B**).

for invasive breast cancer, the NSABP turned their attention to defining the role of partial mastectomy with the B-06 study initiated in 1976. The study compared, in a prospective, randomized fashion, total mastectomy with lumpectomy with and without whole breast radiation therapy (Fig. 12-5). This landmark study in breast cancer surgery demonstrated equivalent overall and disease-free survival for appropriately selected tumors (smaller than 4 cm). The results demonstrated similar survival for all groups; however, lumpectomy without radiation had significantly higher ipsilateral breast cancer recurrence rates than the other two groups. The conclusion, after 20 years of follow-up, is that mastectomy versus lumpectomy with radiation offers similar

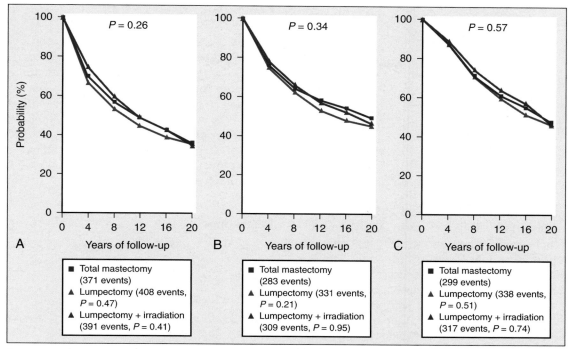

Figure 12-5. Disease-free survival (**A**), distant-disease-free survival (**B**) and overall survival (**C**) among 589 women treated with total mastectomy, 634 treated with lumpectomy alone, and 628 treated with lumpectomy plus irradiation. In each panel, the P value above the curves is for the three-way comparison among the treatment groups. The P values below the curves are for the two-way comparisons between lumpectomy alone or with irradiation and total mastectomy. (From Fisher B, Anderson S, Bryant J, et al: Twenty-year follow-up of a randomized trial comparing total mastectomy, lumpectomy, and lumpectomy plus irradiation for the treatment of invasive breast cancer. N Engl J Med 347:1233–1241, 2002, Figure 2.)

long-term outcomes.[9] Simultaneous with the work of the NSABP in the United States and Canada, similar studies were performed in Europe, which also supported breast conservation as an appropriate therapy in the appropriately selected patient.

Since the mid-1980s when these data first became available, the number of women whose breast cancer has been able to be successfully treated while preserving their breast has increased. Initial barriers of patient and physician education and preference, as well as access to radiation therapy, have crumbled over the years. The indications for breast conservation have expanded now to many women who would have historically required mastectomy at the time of original presentation. Many of these women who would previously have been relegated to the loss of a breast can now be treated by breast conservation by the use of neoadjuvant chemotherapy.[10]

Current practice now considers breast conservation rates a quality indicator for breast surgeons. When breast tumors are small in relation to the size of the breast, only the offending lesion with a rim of surrounding normal tissue needs to be excised. It must be emphasized, however, that when breast conservation is performed, radiation is required postoperatively to achieve local recurrence rates similar to those with mastectomy.

Although lumpectomy allows breast conservation for most patients, there are several populations for whom it is not indicated (Box 12-1). The surgical principle is that all identified malignant tissue is removed with a margin of normal breast tissue but leaving a breast that is cosmetically pleasing. Because cosmetic outcomes are subjective, one patient's excellent result may be another patient's deformity. Therefore, no absolute guidelines on size can be stated, although the previous studies evaluated

---

Box 12-1. Contraindications to Breast Conservation

Relative

Tumor >5 cm
Multiple tumors
Pregnancy

Absolute

Persistent positive margins
Collagen vascular disease
Previous history of breast radiation
Inability to access or refusal of radiation therapy

---

tumors smaller than 5 cm. Mastectomy is usually required for women with multiple tumors in the same breast, diffuse malignant-appearing calcifications, or positive margins with attempts at breast conservation. Repeat local excision can be attempted, but if margins remain positive when as much breast tissue as possible has been removed, then mastectomy is required. Limitations to radiation therapy access are diminishing with the advent of shorter courses of radiation therapy, including partial breast radiation techniques.

Radiation is usually contraindicated during pregnancy; however, judicious timing of other adjuvant therapies can often postpone the need for radiation treatments until after delivery. Remaining contraindications to radiation therapy include a history of breast radiation given in situations such as previous breast cancer treatment or mantle radiation for the treatment of lymphoma, or collagen vascular disease such as systemic lupus erythematosus, which can result in an unpredictable tissue response to radiation therapy.

Conclusion

Surgical therapy remains a mainstay for the local control of breast cancer. Carefully conducted clinical trials performed in the last century have delineated the criteria for determining whether a patient requires a mastectomy for optimal therapy or whether breast conservation can provide an equivalent outcome. This has provided greater options for the management of breast cancer and has decreased the morbidity that women experience after treatment for this disease.

References

1. Bishop W: The Early History of Surgery. New York: Barnes & Noble Publishing, 1995, pp 31–35.
2. Rayter Z, Mansi J: Medical Therapy of Breast Cancer. Cambridge: Cambridge University Press, 2003, p 2.
3. Celsus AC: De Medicina. (Transl. by Spencer W). 1938. Loeb Classical Library, vol II, p 133.
4. Halsted W: The Results of Operations for the Cure of Cancer of the Breast Performed at The Johns Hopkins Hospital from June 1889 to January 1894. The Johns Hopkins Hospital Reports. The Johns Hopkins Press, 1894, p 33.
5. Payne WS, Taylor WF, Khonsari S, et al: Surgical treatment of breast cancer: trends and factors affecting survival. Arch Surg 101(2):105–113, 1970.
6. Fisher B, Redmond C, Fisher ER, et al: Ten-year results of a randomized clinical trial comparing radical mastectomy and total mastectomy with or without resection. N Engl J Med 312:674–681, 1985.
7. Gerber B, Krause A, Reimer T, et al: Skin-sparing mastectomy with conservation of the nipple-areola complex and autologous reconstruction is an oncologically safe procedure. Ann Surg 238(1):120–127, 2003.
8. Tuttle T, Habermann E, Grund EH, et al: Increasing use of contralateral prophylactic mastectomy for breast cancer patients: a trend toward more aggressive surgical treatment. J Clin Oncol 25(33):5203–5209, 2007.
9. Fisher B, Anderson S, Bryant J, et al: Twenty-year follow-up of a randomized trial comparing total mastectomy, lumpectomy, and lumpectomy plus irradiation for the treatment of invasive breast cancer. N Engl J Med 347:1233–1241, 2002.
10. Bonadonna G, Veronesi U: Primary chemotherapy to avoid mastectomy in tumors with diameters of three centimeters or more. J Natl Cancer Inst 82(19):1539–1545, 1990.

13 Breast Reconstruction after Mastectomy

Alex Colque, Hanjoon Song, and Erica D. Anderson

KEY POINTS

- Breast reconstruction should be offered to all patients undergoing mastectomy.
- Immediate breast reconstruction offers many advantages over delayed reconstruction.
- Reconstruction options include prosthetic implants, pedicled flaps, and free and perforator flaps.
- The choice of reconstruction method should be made with a plastic surgeon.
- Partial breast reconstruction should be offered to patients undergoing lumpectomy resulting in a deformity.
- Physical examination is the most important modality in detecting cancer recurrence in the reconstructed breast.

Introduction

Breast reconstruction after mastectomy remains an essential part of the treatment for breast cancer. The improvements in the outcomes of breast cancer treatment lead more women to be concerned about the appearance of their breasts when treatment is complete. Also, with the increase in screening for genetic mutations of the *BRCA1* and *BRCA2* genes, reconstruction after prophylactic mastectomy has become more common. Studies have demonstrated that most women desire surgical breast reconstruction after mastectomy. Furthermore, since 1998, federal law has mandated that insurance companies cover breast reconstruction.[1,2] Therefore, all health care providers who treat patients with breast cancer need to have a basic knowledge of the different types of breast reconstruction and inform their patients that such options are available. This will aid in the understanding and treatment of the "whole patient," coordina-tion of treatment with the ablative and reconstructive surgeons, and surveillance of local recurrence.

Excellent aesthetic results have been obtained with many types of breast reconstruction (Fig. 13-1). Breast reconstruction has also been shown to provide psychological and emotional benefit to reconstructed patients.[3,4] Despite these facts, breast reconstruction rates after mastectomies are surprisingly low. Only 8.1% of patients in the United States undergo breast reconstruction, and these rates are lower in patients older than 50 years.[5] This may be due in part to the lack of knowledge about breast reconstruction by oncologists and general surgeons who may incorrectly believe that it interferes with adjuvant treatment and detection of local recurrences.[6] Proper knowledge of the benefits and risks of breast reconstruction should improve the rates of referral of mastectomy patients to plastic surgeons and the rate of reconstruction.

Reconstruction of the breast after mastectomy is an option that should be given to all breast cancer patients. Breast reconstruction should be discussed with any patient who is considering the treatment options of lumpectomy versus mastectomy. It should also be part of every discussion about prophylactic mastectomy. The knowledge of reconstruction options gives patients the information they need to make an educated decision about their choices in breast cancer therapy. The federal law mandating that insurance companies cover mastectomy be required to also cover reconstruction should alleviate patient concerns over the cost of reconstruction.[1]

The choices for breast reconstruction are numerous and involve many factors. Breast

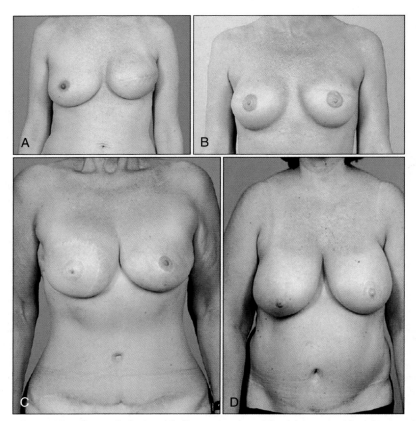

Figure 13-1. Breast reconstruction techniques.   A, Reconstruction of the left breast with an implant. **B,** Bilateral breast reconstruction with implants and subsequent nipple-areola reconstruction. **C,** Right breast reconstruction with a TRAM flap. The patient also underwent reduction mammoplasty of the left breast. **D,** Left breast reconstruction with a unilateral, free TRAM flap following skin-sparing mastectomy. Subsequent reconstruction of the nipple-areola complex was also completed. (From Cordeiro PG: Breast reconstruction after surgery for breast cancer. N Engl J Med 359(15):1590–1601, 2008, Fig. 5.)

reconstruction involves either volume replacement (e.g., implant or autologous breast reconstruction) or volume-displacing procedures (e.g., local tissue rearrangement for partial mastectomy defects). In addition, breast reconstruction can be further categorized into (1) *immediate* versus *delayed* reconstruction and (2) *prosthetic* versus *autologous* reconstruction. It is important for health care providers to know that there is no single best choice for breast reconstruction. Each patient has a best option based on her needs, wishes, and the size and shape of her breast. Ultimately, the decision regarding the optimal type of breast reconstruction for an individual should be made between the patient and the reconstructive surgeon. The need for adjuvant therapy and the desire to augment the contralateral breast in unilateral mastectomy are also important factors in determining the best

option for patients. All of these issues, the risks and benefits of each, and the expectations of the patient should be fully discussed with a plastic surgeon before a decision is made about the type of breast reconstruction.

The options for patients who choose breast reconstruction have increased over the last four decades. Implant reconstruction has been available since the 1960s, and the cosmetic results have improved with new plastic surgery techniques and improvements in newer generation of breast implants. In the 1970s and 1980s, pedicled flaps were developed and used in breast reconstruction. Over the last two decades, advancements in microsurgical techniques have led to free tissue flaps and perforator tissue flaps in which a portion of the body and its blood supply are detached, transferred to the chest, and reconnected to blood vessels

Table 13-1. Recurrence Rate after Skin-Sparing Mastectomy

Study	No. of SSM	Local Recurrence (%)	Follow-up (Months)
Newman et al.[9]	372	6.2	26
Simmons et al.[10]	77	3.9	60
Kroll et al.[11]	114	7.0	72
Medina-Franco et al.[12]	176	4.5	73
Spiegel and Butler[13]	177	5.6	118

SSM, skin-sparing mastectomy.
From Chung AP, Sacchini V: Nipple-sparing mastectomy: where are we now? Surg Oncol 17(4):261–266, 2008, Table 1.

at the recipient site. These advancements have helped to reduce donor site morbidity and to increase the options for patients pursuing breast reconstruction.

The total course of breast reconstruction almost always involves more than one procedure. In either the implant or autologous tissue pathway, the first procedure involves transferring tissue or placing an implant or expander to give the reconstructed breast volume and shape for symmetry. After this is complete, secondary procedures are carried out 3 to 6 months later to modify the shape, size, and scars of the breast. A nipple-areola complex can also be reconstructed at this time. Finally, tattooing of the nipple-areola complex is performed, usually under local anesthetic, resulting in the final reconstructed breast. It is important for all patients considering breast reconstruction to know that more than one procedure is necessary to achieve the final appearance and that this can take up to 1 year to complete.

Breast-conserving therapy is now a common way to treat early-stage breast cancer. Patients who undergo breast-conserving therapy with lumpectomy may suffer from postoperative breast deformities. Several techniques are also available for partial breast reconstruction to treat these patients.

The decision about reconstructive options is best made for each individual patient by the patient and her reconstructive surgeon. Reconstruction after mastectomy increases the operative time, blood loss, and prolongs recovery. The method of breast reconstruction depends on patient preference, the shape and size of the native breast, the condition of the recipient site, the availability of donor sites, the patient's comorbidities, and the expertise of the plastic surgeon.

Regardless of the reconstruction method, the technique used during mastectomy is important in achieving adequate symmetry. Maintaining the skin envelope and the inframammary fold guides size and preserves landmarks for breast positioning. Three types of mastectomy techniques allow this. Skin-sparing mastectomy is resection of the breast tissue and the nipple-areola complex that still preserves the breast skin envelope and inframammary fold. Areola-sparing mastectomy is similar, but also preserves the areola with resection of the nipple. Subcutaneous mastectomy, which is offered in prophylactic mastectomy, preserves the entire nipple-areola complex. Note that skin-sparing mastectomy does not increase the incidence of local recurrence rates when compared with simple mastectomy[7,8] (Table 13-1).

Immediate versus Delayed Reconstruction

The decision to have immediate reconstruction after mastectomy involves the preference of the patient, the availability of the plastic surgeon, and the anticipated postoperative chemotherapy and radiation therapy that are part of the oncologic treatment. Immediate breast reconstruction has been shown to be cost-effective, to have psychological and cosmetic benefits, and not to increase operative or oncologic risk.[3] Patients who receive immediate reconstruction feel that it aids in the emotional healing of mastectomy. It leads to improved self-esteem, sexuality and femininity, and less depression.[4,14] It also improves postoperative breast symmetry and sensation.[15] It is important that immediate reconstruction does not increase the risk of local recurrence or difficulty with surveillance[16,17]

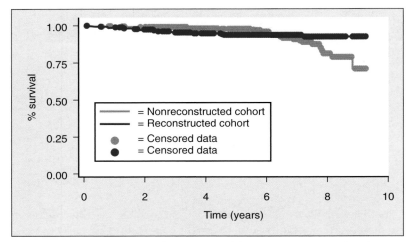

Figure 13-2. Local recurrence-free survival curves for patients with immediate reconstruction after mastectomy (the reconstructed cohort) and those with no postmastectomy reconstruction (the nonreconstructed cohort). (From McCarthy CM, Pusic AL, Sciafani L, et al: Breast cancer recurrence following prosthetic, postmastectomy reconstruction: incidence, detection, and treatment. Plast Reconstr Surg 121:381–388, 2008.)

Table 13-2. Summary of Postradiation Cosmetic Outcomes

Institution	Type of Reconstruction	Median Age (Years)	Median Follow-up (Months)	Cosmetic Outcome Good/Excellent
Memorial Sloan-Kettering[24]	TEI	45	64	80%
Kaohsiung Medical University Hospital[25]	TRAM	43	40	70%
Massachusetts General Hospital/Boston University[26]	TRAM & TEI	47	32	70%
Fox Chase Cancer Center[27]	TRAM & TEI	45	28	85%

TEI, tissue expander/implant; TRAM, transverse rectus abdominis myocutaneous flap.

(Fig. 13-2). It has also been shown not to delay further treatment of breast cancer.[18]

Immediate reconstruction also has surgical benefits. When combined with skin-sparing mastectomy, immediate reconstruction allows the reconstructed breast to have the most natural look and feel. By maintaining the breast envelope and the inframammary fold, the final breast appearance is more likely to match the patient's other breast. The natural envelope and tissue landmarks are lost in delayed reconstruction. This is due to scarring of the chest and wound contracture that pose challenges in breast symmetry. Another advantage of skin-sparing mastectomy is less need for tissue expansion. These benefits are lost in delayed reconstruction.

Patients with a relative contraindication to immediate breast reconstruction are patients who will receive postoperative radiation as part of their oncologic treatment. Radiation therapy

after implant reconstruction has been shown to cause increased rates of severe capsular contracture and overall increased perioperative complications, including infections and exposure of the implant.[19,20] In addition, studies have also demonstrated that autologous breast reconstruction leads to poorer aesthetic outcomes and higher complications in patients receiving postmastectomy radiation after immediate reconstruction compared with those with delayed reconstruction[21–23] (Table 13-2). In one study comparing immediate and delayed free TRAM (transverse rectus abdominis myocutaneous) reconstruction in patients receiving postmastectomy radiation, the authors found that the incidence of late complications was significantly higher in the immediate reconstruction group compared with the delayed reconstruction group.[23] Overall, close to one third of patients in the immediate reconstruction group required an additional flap to correct the radiation-induced distortion from flap shrinkage and contraction.[23]

Although uncommon, partial or total flap loss of autologous tissues used for breast reconstruction has significant consequences. Partial flap loss may lead to areas of fat necrosis and skin loss, which may result in scarring and significant deformities that may require surgical revision and/or additional flap reconstruction. Total flap loss is more common with free flaps. When the whole flap is lost, it is no longer an option for the patient and another flap from a different donor site is needed. If the patient is a candidate, she may also opt to switch to implant reconstruction. One option for patients undergoing postoperative radiation is to have immediate tissue expanders placed at the time of mastectomy to preserve the breast envelope and skin. After the course of radiation is complete, the patient can then undergo a second-stage implant or autologous tissue reconstruction.

Oftentimes, if it is unclear whether the patient will require postmastectomy radiation, immediate tissue expanders can be placed at the time of the mastectomy. After review of permanent sections, a determination is made about whether postmastectomy radiation is needed. If radiation therapy is needed, standard delayed reconstruction is carried out. However, if no radiation therapy is necessary, then the reconstructive surgeon will proceed with definitive breast reconstruction. Using this delayed-immediate approach allows patients who do not need postmastectomy radiation to achieve aesthetic results comparable to immediate breast reconstruction without significant sequelae.[28]

Prosthetic Reconstruction

Prosthetic implant reconstruction is the most common form of breast reconstruction in the United States (Fig. 13-3). Implant reconstruction is appealing to patients who do not want autologous tissue removed from other portions of their body. It is also the recommended method for thin women who do not have adequate tissue volume in potential donor sites. Implant reconstruction requires a shorter operation and gives a good cosmetic result with symmetry, but usually requires a two-stage operation. The first operation is the placement of a tissue expander. This is a submuscular implant that can be placed immediately after

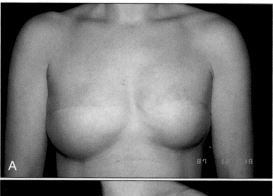
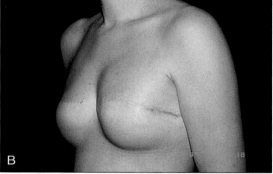

Figure 13-3. Frontal and side views of a patient after bilateral implants. (From Eberlein TJ, Tsangaris TN: Breast cancer surgery. In Hayes DF (ed): Atlas of Breast Cancer, 2nd ed. London: Mosby, 2000, Figure. 6.23.)

mastectomy. It has a port that can be serially inflated during postoperative office visits (Fig. 13-4). The expander is inflated to a size symmetric to the contralateral breast—or in the case of bilateral mastectomy with reconstruction—to the patient's desired size. When the desired size is reached, the expander is exchanged for the implant in a second operation.

Implant reconstruction is generally recommended for patients with smaller breasts with little ptosis to their shape and for patients who undergo skin-sparing mastectomy. This allows for patients to achieve optimal symmetry after reconstruction. However, tissue expansion provides larger breast envelopes that allow for larger implants. When compared with autologous tissue, implant reconstruction gives the breast a more youthful appearance and a fuller upper pole. Patients who wish to have implant reconstruction but have large breasts or more ptosis may also consider implant augmentation or a breast lift with or without reduction in the contralateral breast to further facilitate breast symmetry.

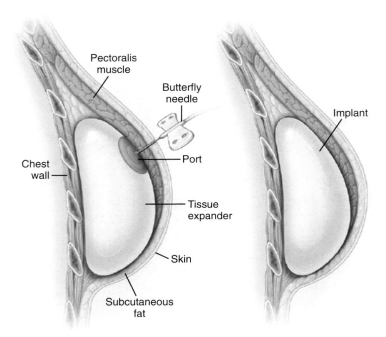

Figure 13-4. Breast reconstruction involving a tissue expander and implant. A tissue expander is placed in a submuscular position and filled with saline injected into a self-sealing port. When expansion is complete, the permanent implant is placed under the expanded muscle and skin. (From Cordeiro PG: Breast reconstruction after surgery for breast cancer. N Engl J Med 359(15):1590–1601, 2008, Fig. 1.)

The disadvantages of implant reconstruction are mostly due to foreign body implant. Early after implant placement, patients may develop exposure, extrusion, or infection of the implant. Implant contracture, rupture, rippling, migration, or pain may also develop over time with breast implants. The overall complication rate for implant reconstruction in a nonirradiated breast is less than 10%.[29] In patients who undergo postoperative radiation, this rate increases to 18% to 50%.[29,30] A recent study identified smoking, obesity, hypertension, and age over 65 as independent risk factors for perioperative complications after expander/implant breast reconstruction.[31] Significantly, active smokers were twice as likely to develop perioperative complications and five times more likely to fail reconstruction compared to non-smokers[31] (Table 13-3).

The two options for implants that patients can choose from are saline and silicone gel. The Food and Drug Administration (FDA) put a moratorium on silicone gel implants in 1992 and allowed their use only in breast reconstruction patients who entered a clinical trial. This was due to concerns that silicone gel implants cause other medical problems. Studies now have proved that these implants do not increase the risk for patients to develop cancer or connective tissue diseases.[32–38] As a result of these findings, the FDA lifted this restriction in November 2006. Silicone gel implants are now being evaluated in post-approval studies to confirm their safety.

Autologous Reconstruction

Pedicled Flaps

Pedicled flaps transfer tissue from one part of the body to another by rotating around an intact vascular pedicle. Transverse rectus abdominis myocutaneous (TRAM) and latissimus dorsi flaps are the most common pedicle flaps used to reconstruct the breast. The main advantage of autologous flaps in general is a longer-lasting, more natural look and feel. This also prevents an implant and the associated risk of complications.

The TRAM flap is the more commonly used of these two methods. The rectus muscle has two main blood supplies arising from the superior epigastric and deep inferior epigastric vessels. In the pedicled TRAM flap, the deep inferior epigastric vessels are ligated. Thus, the TRAM flap relies solely on the superior epigastric vessels for its blood supply. The fat, skin, rectus muscle, and a portion of the abdominal fascia between the umbilicus and pubis are used,

rotated based on the superior epigastric pedicle, and transferred to the chest to replace the breast volume (Fig. 13-5). The pedicled TRAM flap has better results in patients without diabetes, hypertension, obesity, or a smoking history. If the blood flow is questionable, the flap may be "supercharged" (i.e., augmentation of blood flow to the flap) by performing a microvascular anastomosis between the ligated ends of the deep inferior epigastric artery to the thoracodorsal or internal mammary systems. This method of supercharging the pedicled TRAM has been successfully used in high-risk patients such as the obese population.[39]

The TRAM flap uses the abdominal skin, fat, and rectus muscle to give a reconstructed breast with excellent shape, ptosis, and contour. It offers a more natural look and feel than implant reconstruction (Fig. 13-6). The limit in size depends on the amount of fat tissue that a patient has; however, the TRAM flap can be combined with an implant if more volume is necessary. It can be used in patients who have an adequate amount of abdominal tissue to

Table 13-3. Factors Associated with Poor Outcome with Tissue Expander/Implant Reconstruction

Risk Factor	Relative Greater Risk of Complications	Relative Greater Risk of Implant Failure
Smoking	2.2	4.9
Age over 65 years	2.5	NS
Obesity	1.8	6.9
Hypertension	1.8	4.3

From McCarthy CM, Mehrara BJ, Riedel E, et al: Predicting complications following expander/implant breast reconstruction: an outcomes analysis based on preoperative clinical risk. Plast Reconstr Surg 121(6):1886–1892, 2008.

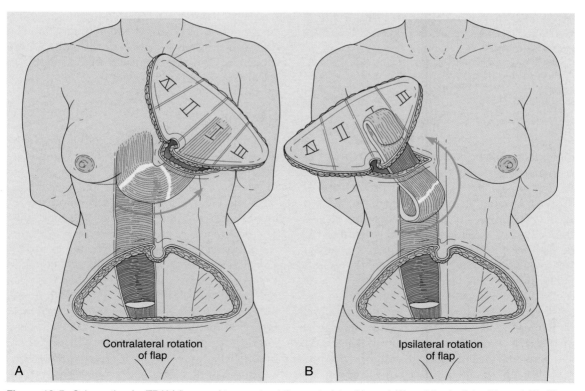

Figure 13-5. Schematic of a TRAM flap used to construct the contralateral breast (**A**) and the ipsilateral breast (**B**). (From Vasconez LO, LeJour H, Gamboa-Bobadilla M: Atlas of Breast Reconstruction. New York: Gower Medical Publishing, 1991.)

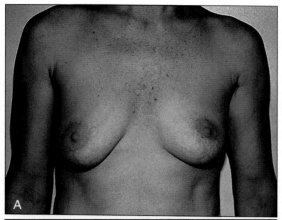

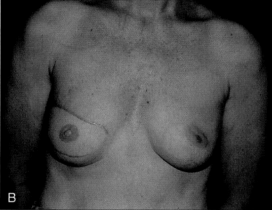

Figure 13-6. Patient before mastectomy (**A**) and after mastectomy and a TRAM flap reconstruction (**B**). (From Eberlein TJ, Tsangaris TN: Breast cancer surgery. In Hayes DF (ed): Atlas of Breast Cancer, 2nd ed. London: Mosby, 2000, Figure 6.30.)

reconstruct one or both breasts. The TRAM flap is a long-lasting and reliable choice for patients. It also can be performed in an immediate or delayed fashion. Although patients do have a second operative site, the patients also receive the benefit of an abdominoplasty as part of the procedure. TRAM flaps do not delay adjuvant treatment for breast cancer or increase the difficulty in detecting local recurrence.[40–42]

The disadvantages of the TRAM flap are increased operative time, potential flap failure, fat necrosis, donor site incision, and the removal of the rectus muscle. Flap failure, fat necrosis, and impaired healing are increased in patients who are obese or use tobacco. Patients are instructed to abstain from tobacco products for at least 1 month before the operation. Thin patients may not have adequate donor tissue to

be used for reconstruction. Abdominal muscle strength is decreased after TRAM flap procedures to about 60% for unilateral and 30% for bilateral flaps. TRAM flaps are also contraindicated in patients who have had previous abdominal surgery that would disrupt the blood supply to the abdominal tissues such as a previous TRAM or abdominoplasty. The flap also has the increased complications of skin necrosis and fibrosis if it is radiated postoperatively.[43]

Latissimus dorsi flaps use the latissimus muscle and overlying tissue supplied by the thoracodorsal artery and vein. This option can also be used for immediate or delayed reconstruction. This flap is reliable and can make a nicely contoured breast. The amount of tissue is less than the TRAM flap, so the latissimus dorsi flap is better used in reconstruction of smaller breasts. However, the amount of autologous tissue obtained from the back may not be adequate and may require an underlying implant as well to help achieve better symmetry in patients with large breasts. Minimally invasive harvesting of the flap has been described.[44] This allows for decreased morbidity at the donor site. The latissimus dorsi flap should not be used in patients who have had this muscle divided in a previous surgery, such as a lateral thoracotomy, or who have had previous radiation to the axilla. These procedures can compromise the blood supply to the flap and lead to flap failure.

Free Flaps

Free flap reconstructions refer to the transfer of tissue to another site of the body by completely excising it and reconnecting the artery and vein to vessels at the recipient site. The main advantages of free flaps are increased blood supply, less fat necrosis, and less donor site morbidity. The disadvantages are increased operative time, the need for a surgeon with greater expertise, and increased incidence of complete flap failure versus pedicled autologous flaps. Free flaps can also be done in an immediate or delayed procedure. The common types of free flaps used in breast reconstruction are free TRAM flaps, deep inferior epigastric perforator (DIEP) flaps, superficial inferior epigastric artery (SIEA) flaps, and superior and inferior gluteal artery perforator (SGAP, IGAP) flaps.

The free TRAM flap uses skin, fat, and a decreased amount of rectus abdominis muscle compared with the pedicled TRAM flap. Contrary to the pedicled TRAM, the free TRAM relies on the deep epigastric artery and vein rather than on the superior epigastric vessels. The deep inferior epigastric vessels are completely ligated and reconnected to the thoracodorsal or internal mammary artery and vein by microsurgical techniques. The increased blood supply to this flap makes it more reliable in high-risk patients such as active smokers and the obese.[45] It also uses less muscle which leads to less reduction in abdominal strength. Each rectus muscle can be used in bilateral breast reconstruction. The major risk is total flap loss, which occurs in less than 3% of cases. The technical expertise required for free TRAM reconstruction is greater than with pedicled TRAM, but less than is needed for the DIEP flap.

Perforator Flaps

Perforator flaps were first introduced in 1992 and were developed out of a desire to further mimimize donor site morbidity and possibly recovery time without compromising safety or aesthetic outcomes.[46] The DIEP (deep inferior epigastric perforator) flap relies on the perforating blood vessels arising from the deep inferior epigastric vessels to supply the abdominal skin and fat used to reconstruct the breast. Thus, the DIEP flap perfuses the same abdominal tissue as a TRAM flap without sacrificing the rectus muscle or fascia leading to less donor site morbidity and potentially less recovery time.[47] Like the free TRAM flap, the recipient vessels are either the internal mammary or thoracodorsal vessels. Perforator flaps yield a reliable result with good cosmetic symmetry (Fig. 13-7). This flap should not be performed in patients who have had previous abdominal liposuction or those who are active smokers (less than 1 month before surgery). Perforator flap breast reconstruction is an advanced procedure and is generally offered by plastic surgeons with advanced training or experience in microsurgery.

The SIEA (superficial inferior epigastric artery) flap, like the TRAM and DIEP flaps, uses the skin and fat of the abdomen. In terms of donor site morbidity, the SIEA flap is superior to either the free TRAM or DIEP flaps, since no incision is made in the abdominal fascia and the rectus muscle remains undisturbed. Unfortunately, the SIEA flap is not as reliable as flaps

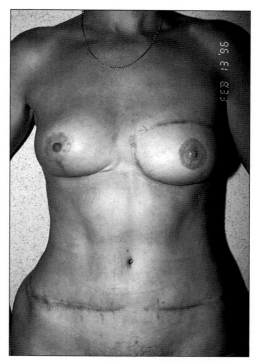

Figure 13-7. A patient 15 months after a DIEP flap reconstruction on the left side. (Photo courtesy of Dr. Philip N. Blondeel.)

that are based on the deep inferior epigastric system (i.e., free TRAM, DIEP flaps) The SIEA is present in approximately 60% to 70% of patients, of whom only 50% have adequate vessels needed to make use of this technique. The presence of SIEA with both a palpable pulse and a diameter greater than 1.5 mm has been reported to correlate with the successful use of this flap for breast reconstruction.[48] This decision is determined intraoperatively. In addition, since the vascular territory covered by the superior epigastric system is variable, the amount of abdominal tissue that can be supported by the SIEA is consequently variable as well. Finally, surgeons have reported that insetting the flap with microvascular anastomosis to the recipient vessels is more difficult than with either the free TRAM or DIEP flaps owing to the position of the superior inferior epigastric vessels.

Although the abdomen is the most commonly used soft tissue donor site for autologous free flap breast reconstruction, for those patients whose abdomen is not an option as a donor site, the buttock area (i.e., inferior gluteal artery perforator [IGAP] flap or superior gluteal artery

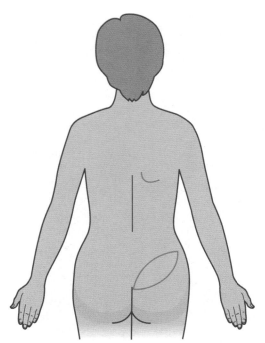

Figure 13-8. Location of the tissue source for an SGAP flap reconstruction. (From Stephan P: SGAP breast reconstruction: plastic surgery to restore breast symmetry. About.com; http://breastcancer.about.com/od/reconstructivesurgery/tp/sgap_flap.htm; accessed 10/2/08.)

perforator [SGAP] flap) provides another potential source of donor tissue for autologous breast reconstruction (Fig. 13-8). The IGAP and SGAP flaps are based on perforators from either the superior or inferior gluteal artery. The skin and fat of either the upper or lower buttock is used to reconstruct the breast. Some surgeons favor the IGAP over the SGAP flap due to an improved donor site contour and scar.[49] Patients usually have enough tissue in this area to use this flap even if they do not have adequate abdominal tissue for a TRAM, DIEP, or SIEA flap. This flap also spares underlying muscle. Similar to the DIEP flap, SGAP flaps are contraindicated in patients with previous liposuction to the buttocks or a history of active smoking (within 1 month). As with DIEP flaps, donor site morbidity for SGAP and IGAP flaps is minimal.

Although microvascular perforator breast reconstructions are technically demanding, surgeons who have expertise in microvascular techniques and who perform a high volume of perforator flaps have excellent results, with flap failures generally reported to be less than 2%.[50]

Nipple Areola Reconstruction

Nipple areola reconstruction is a critical component of breast reconstruction and contributes to the impression of realism that any reconstruction achieves. Morbidity surrounding nipple areola reconstruction is minimal. It can be performed using local nonspecialized tissues under local anesthesia in virtually any setting.

Nipple reconstruction is typically performed as a component of the second stage of breast reconstruction that involves adjustment of the reconstructed and/or contralateral breast in pursuit of optimal symmetry. Some surgeons advocate primary reconstruction of the nipple at the time of the mound reconstruction, although there is no obvious advantage. Proper position of the nipple areola complex is critical, since even small degrees of asymmetry are noticed by the least observant viewer. Optimal nipple areola position, therefore, is best pursued after optimal symmetry between the breast mounds has been accomplished. An asymmetric nipple areola reconstruction is difficult to correct secondarily.

A spectrum of techniques is available for reconstruction of the nipple, including local flaps with or without skin grafts. When trying to create a particularly projecting or substantial nipple, a composite graft from the contralateral breast may have some appeal. Augmenting the reconstructed nipple by inserting filler materials, such as dermal fat grafts, AlloDerm, or cartilage grafts, at the time of the initial procedure can also aid with long-term projection.

Areolar reconstruction is accomplished by intradermal tattoo alone, as is colorization of the final nipple (Fig. 13-9). Pigmented grafts from the contralateral areola, genitalia, or paragenital regions are outdated and undesirable. These full-thickness grafts are more rigid than the natural areola or a tattooed patch of skin. Although exact color match with the opposite side remains an artistic challenge, the results achieved by even the beginner surgeon/tattooist exceed those available by other means. The tattoo procedure is performed some time after the nipple reconstruction—typically 3 or 4 months later. This simple stage of reconstruction, performed in the office under local anesthesia, offers one final opportunity to adjust nipple areola position in pursuit of optimal symmetry.

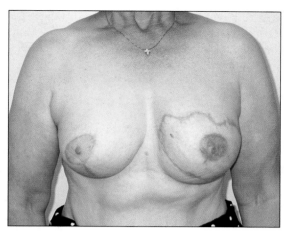

Figure 13-9. Reconstruction of the nipple and subsequent tattooing for the areola. (From Bland KI, Copeland EM: The Breast: Comprehensive Management of Benign and Malignant Diseases, 4th ed. Philadelphia: Saunders, 2009, Figure 48-55B.)

Partial Breast Reconstruction

As more breast cancers that were once thought to be poor candidates for lumpectomies are now being considered for breast conservation therapy (BCT), the potential for unfavorable breast deformities has increased. Furthermore, the addition of radiation in breast conservation therapy increases the risk of disfigurement and may adversely affect subsequent reconstructive procedures.[51] To address the potential for unfavorable aesthetic outcomes, simultaneous reconstruction after partial mastectomy has become more popular.

Delayed partial breast reconstruction is performed after lumpectomy or quadrantectomy leaves the breast with a significant defect. Lumpectomy results in a deformity of the breast in 5% to 40% of patients.[52] This percentage is increased in patients with larger tumors, lower quadrant tumors, and larger breasts. The deformity may be due to volume loss, skin retraction, or nipple deviation. Volume loss of more than 20% of the breast usually requires partial reconstruction to fill this defect. This is more important in patients with smaller breasts. The degree of deformity is subjective to the patient, and there are options for partial reconstruction based on her desires. There are various methods for breast reconstruction after partial mastectomy, including local tissue rearrangement, breast reductions, and latissimus and thoracoepigastric

flaps. Local tissue rearrangement can be sufficient for small defects. Latissimus flaps previously described are also an option to help fill in larger defects.[53] Fat from other areas of the body can also be grafted into the defect to fill the deformity. Breast reductions of the lumpectomy breast or the contralateral breast are also options to match size and symmetry.[54]

The timing of partial breast reconstruction is controversial. Partial breast reconstruction performed 1 to 2 weeks after lumpectomy allows assurance of negative margins around the tumor. However, immediate partial breast reconstruction may allow for a wider resection of the tumor and safe margins. As a general rule, reconstruction with local tissue transfers or breast reduction should be done before radiation treatment to avoid manipulation of radiated tissue.[43] Aesthetic outcomes have been shown to be better and the risk for complications lower with immediate breast reconstruction of partial mastectomy defects, since the local tissue that is being used to fill the defect is nonirradiated.[55,56] Theoretically, there are oncologic advantages to this procedure because this method has been shown to result in larger resective specimens than with partial mastectomy alone.[57] Also, sampling of the contralateral breast tissue is made possible if a simultaneous contralateral breast reduction is performed for maintaining symmetry and balance. Indeed, the incidence of occult breast carcinoma in breast reduction specimens approximates between 0.2% and 0.8%, and is theoretically higher in patients with known breast cancer.[58]

Surveillance after Breast Reconstruction

After completion of primary treatment of breast cancer, patients are routinely placed under surveillance to identify and treat any recurrence of cancer or to discover any new breast cancer in the opposite breast at the earliest stage. Women who develop breast cancer have an increased risk of cancer in the opposite breast. For women over 50, this risk is about 4% for their remaining years; for those under 50, it is about 14%. Therefore, careful evaluation with a targeted history and physical at routine intervals is mandatory.

Detecting a new breast tumor in the opposite breast is accomplished by a familiar triad: monthly breast self-examination, clinical evaluation by a physician or nurse practitioner every 6 to 12 months, and annual mammography. This combination provides the greatest assurance of early diagnosis.

There is no evidence that reconstruction causes any significant delay in detecting recurrent cancer in a reconstructed breast.[59–62] Surveillance of a reconstructed breast is also a collaborative effort on the part of the patient and her surgeon, the medical or radiation oncologist, and the primary physician. The goal of self-examination of the reconstructed breast, like examination of the normal breast, is to detect an area that feels different to the examining fingers or looks different in the mirror. However, the reconstructed breast may present unique problems. In patients with implants, there may be capsule formation that could interfere with the examination. With autologous tissue reconstruction, there also may be areas of scarring and/or fat necrosis. These palpable abnormalities in the reconstructed breast occasionally may be suspicious enough to require biopsy, but this has not proved to be a common clinical problem.

Routine mammography of the reconstructed breast is not needed if a complete mastectomy has been done. Monthly self-examination of the reconstructed breast has proved to be the best method for detecting a recurrence. In a patient who has undergone breast reconstruction with a silicone gel-filled implant, a magnetic resonance imaging (MRI) study is the most useful imaging study to monitor the integrity of the device.

Conclusion

All patients who choose to undergo mastectomy for the treatment of breast cancer should be offered reconstruction. Many reconstruction options are available for patients, including oncoplastic surgical techniques, implants, pedicled flaps, free flaps, and perforator flaps. The decision regarding which option is best for each patient depends on the comorbidities, the size and shape of the breasts, the patient's desires, and available donor sites. This decision should be made with a plastic surgeon who can offer his or her expertise. Partial breast reconstruction should also be offered to patients undergoing lumpectomy resulting in a deformity. Physical examination is the most important modality in detecting recurrence in recon-

structed patients. All providers who care for patients with breast cancer should have basic knowledge of the reconstructive techniques used in breast cancer therapy.

References

1. National Cancer Institute. Stat bite: states requiring inpatient insurance coverage after mastectomy. J Natl Cancer Inst 90:1035, 1998.
2. Granzow JW, Levine JL, Chiu ES, Allen RJ: Breast reconstruction using perforator flaps. J Surg Oncol 94:441–454, 2006.
3. Brandberg Y, Malm M, Blomqvist L: A prospective and randomized study, "SVEA," comparing effects of three methods for delayed breast reconstruction on quality of life, patient-defined problem areas of life, and cosmetic result. Plast Reconstr Surg 105:66, 2000.
4. Stevens LA, McGrath MH, Druss RG, et al: The psychological impact of immediate breast reconstruction for women with early breast cancer. Plast Reconstr Surg 73:619, 1984.
5. Polednak AP: Geographic variation in post mastectomy breast reconstruction rates. Plast Reconstr Surg 106:298, 2000.
6. Wanzel KR, Brown MH, Anastakis DJ, et al: Reconstructive breast surgery: referring physician knowledge and learning needs. Plast Reconstr Surg 110:1441, 2002.
7. Toth BA, Forley BG, Calabria R, et al: Retrospective study of skin-sparing mastectomy in breast reconstruction. Plast Reconstr Surg 104:77, 1999.
8. Carlson GW, Bostwick J III, Styblo TM, et al: Skin-sparing mastectomy: oncologic and reconstructive considerations. Ann Surg 225:570, 1997.
9. Newman LA, Keurer, HM, Hunt KK, et al: Presentation, treatment, and outcome of local recurrence after skin-sparing mastectomy and immediate reconstruction. Ann Surg Oncol 5:620–626, 1998.
10. Simmons RM, Fish SK, Gayle L, et al: Local and distant recurrence rates in skin-sparing mastectomies compared with non-skin-sparing mastectomies. Ann Surg Oncol 6:676–681, 1999.
11. Kroll SS, Khoo A, Singletary SE, et al: Local recurrence risk after skin-sparing and conventional mastectomy: a 6-year follow-up. Plast Reconstr Surg 104:421–425, 1999.
12. Medina-Franco H, Vasconez LO, Fix RJ, et al: Factors associated with local recurrence after skin-sparing mastectomy and immediate breast reconstruction for invasive breast cancer. Ann Surg 235:814–819, 2002.
13. Spiegel AJ, Butler CE: Recurrence following treatment of ductal carcinoma in situ with skin-sparing mastectomy and immediate breast reconstruction. Plast Reconstr Surg 111:706–711, 2004.
14. Wellisch DK, Schain WS, Noone RB, et al: Psychosocial correlates of immediate versus delayed reconstruction of the breast. Plast Reconstr Surg 76:713, 1985.
15. Losken A, Carlson GW, Bostwick J III, et al: Trends in unilateral breast reconstruction and management of the contralateral breast: the Emory experience. Plast Reconstr Surg 110:89, 2002.
16. Trabulsy PP, Anthony JP, Mathes SJ: Changing trends in postmastectomy breast reconstruction: a 13-year experience. Plast Reconstr Surg 93:1418, 1994.
17. Slavin SA, Love SM, Goldwyn RM: Recurrent breast cancer following immediate reconstruction with myocutaneous flaps. Plast Reconstr Surg 93:1191, 1994.
18. Allweis TM, Boisvert ME, Otero SE, et al: Immediate reconstruction after mastectomy for breast cancer does not prolong the time to starting adjuvant chemotherapy. Am J Surg 183:218, 2002.
19. Forman DL, Chiu J, Restifo RJ, et al: Breast reconstruction in previously irradiated patients using tissue expanders and implants: a potentially unfavorable result. Ann Plast Surg 40:360, 1998.
20. Vandeweyer E, Deraemaecker R: Radiation therapy after immediate breast reconstruction with implants. Plast Reconstr Surg 106:56, 2000.
21. Javaid M, Song F, Leinster S, et al: Radiation effects on the cosmetic outcomes of immediate and delayed autologous breast reconstruction: an argument about timing. J Plast Reconstr Aesthet Surg 59(1):16–26, 2006.

22. Rogers NE, Allen RJ: Radiation effects on breast reconstruction with the deep inferior epigastric perforator flap. Plast Reconstr Surg 109:1919–1924, 2002.

23. Tran NV Chang DW, Gupta A, et al: Comparison of immediate and delayed free TRAM flap breast reconstruction in patients receiving postmastectomy radiation therapy. Plast Reconstr Surg 108(1):78–82, 2001.

24. McCormick B, Wright J, Cordiero P: Breast reconstruction combined with radiation therapy: long-term risks and factors related to decision making. Cancer J 14(4):264–268, 2008.

25. Huang CJ, Ming-Feng H, Sin-Daw L, et al: Comparison of local recurrence and distant metastases between breast cancer patients after postmastectomy radiotherapy with and without immediate TRAM flap reconstruction. Plast Reconstr Surg 118:1079–1086, 2006.

26. Chawla AK, Kachnic LA, Taghian AG, et al: Radiotherapy and breast reconstruction: complications and cosmesis with TRAM versus tissue expander/implant. Int J Radiat Oncol Biol Phys 54(2):520–526, 2002.

27. Anderson PR, Hanlon AL, McNeeley SW, et al: Low complication rates are achievable after postmastectomy breast reconstruction and radiation therapy. Int J Radiat Oncol Biol Phys 59(4):1080–1087, 2004.

28. Kronowitz SJ, Hunt KK, Keurer HM, et al: Delayed-immediate breast reconstruction. Plast Reconstr Surg 113(6):1617–1628, 2004.

29. Spear SL, Majidian A: Immediate breast reconstruction in two stages using textured, integrated-valve tissue expanders and breast implants: a retrospective review of 171 consecutive breast reconstructions from 1989 to 1996. Plast Reconstr Surg 101:53, 1998.

30. Evans GR, et al: Reconstruction and the radiated breast: is there a role for implants? Plast Reconstr Surg 96:1111, 1995.

31. McCarthy CM, Mehrara BJ, Riedel E, et al: Predicting complications following expander/implant breast reconstruction: an outcomes analysis based on preoperative clinical risk. Plast Reconstr Surg 121(6): 1886–1892, 2008.

32. Brinton LA, Brown SL: Review: breast implants and cancer. J Natl Cancer Inst 89:1341, 1997.

33. Deapen DM, Bernstein L, Brody GS: Are breast implants anti-carcinogenic? A 14-year follow up of the Los Angeles study. Plast Reconstr Surg 99:1346, 1997.

34. Berkel H, Birdsell DC, Jenkins H, et al: Breast augmentation: a risk factor for breast cancer? N Engl J Med 326:1649, 1992.

35. Petit JY, Lê MG, Mouriesse H, et al: Can breast reconstruction with gel-filled silicone implants increase the risk of death and second primary cancer in patients treated by mastectomy for breast cancer? Plast Reconstr Surg 94:115, 1994.

36. Gabriel SE, O'Fallon WM, Kurland LT, et al: Risk of connective tissue disease and other disorders after breast implantation. N Engl J Med 330:1697, 1994.

37. Sanchez-Guerrero J, Colditz GA, Karlso EW, et al: Silicone implants and the risk of connective-tissue diseases and symptoms. N Engl J Med 332:1666, 1995.

38. Hennekens CH, Lee IM, Cook NR, et al: Self-reported breast implants in connective tissue diseases in female health professionals. A retrospective cohort study. JAMA 275:616, 1996.

39. Wu LC, Iteld L, Song DH: Supercharging the transverse rectus abdominis musculocutaneous flap: breast reconstruction for the overweight and obese population. Ann Plast Surg 60(6):609–613, 2008.

40. Godfrey PM, Godfrey NV, Romita MC: Immediate autogenous breast reconstruction in clinically advanced disease. Plast Reconstr Surg 95:1039, 1995.

41. Styblo TM, Lewis MM, Carlson GW, et al: Immediate breast reconstruction for stage III breast cancer using transverse rectus abdominis musculocutaneous (TRAM) flap. Ann Surg Oncol 3:375, 1996.

42. Sultan MR, Smith ML, Estabrook A, et al: Immediate breast reconstruction in patients with locally advanced disease. Ann Plast Surg 38:345, 1997.

43. Hidalgo DA: Aesthetic refinement in breast reconstruction: complete skin-sparing mastectomy with autogenous tissue transfer. Plast Reconstr Surg 102:63, 1998.

44. Fine NA, Orgill DP, Pribaz JJ: Early clinical experience in endoscopic-assisted muscle flap harvest. Ann Plast Surg 33:456, 1994.

45. Kroll SS, et al: Fat necrosis in free and pedicle TRAM flaps. Plast Reconstr Surg 102:1502, 1998.

46. Allen RJ, Treece P: Deep inferior epigastric perforator flap for breast reconstruction. Ann Plast Surg 32:32, 1994.

47. Blondeel N, Vanderstraeten GG, Manstrey SJ, et al: The donor site morbidity of free DIEP flaps and free TRAM flaps for breast reconstruction. Br J Plast Surg 50:322, 1997.

48. Spiegel AJ, Khan FN: An intraoperative algorithm for use of the SIEA flap for breast reconstruction. Plast Reconstr Surg 120(6):1450–1459, 2007.

49. Allen RJ, Levine JL, Granzow JW: The in-the-crease inferior gluteal artery perforator flap for breast reconstruction. Plast Reconstr Surg 118(2):333–339, 2006.

50. Tran NV, Buchel EW, Convery PA: Microvascular complications of DIEP flaps. Plast Reconstr Surg 119(5):1397–1405, 2007.

51. Clough KB, Lewis JS, Couturaud B, et al: Oncoplastic techniques allow extensive resections for breast-conserving therapy for breast carcinomas. Ann Surg 237:26, 2003.

52. Nahabedian M: Determining the optimal approach to breast reconstruction after partial mastectomy. Plast Reconstr Surg 117:12, 2006.

53. Losken A, Schaefer TG, Carlson GW, et al: Immediate endoscopic latissimus dorsi flap: risk or benefit in reconstructing partial mastectomy defects. Ann Plast Surg 53:1, 2004.

54. Losken A, Elwood ET, Styblo TM, et al: The role of reduction mammaplasty in reconstructing partial mastectomy defects. Plast Reconstr Surg 109:968, 2002.

55. Mandi M, Wolfli J, Van Landuyt K: Partial mastectomy reconstruction. Clin Plast Surg 34:51, 2007.

56. Clough KB, Kroll SS, Audretsch W: An approach to the repair of partial mastectomy defects. Plast Reconstr Surg 104(2): 409–420, 1999.

57. Giacalone PL, Roger R, Dubon O, et al: Comparative study of the accuracy of breast resection in oncoplastic surgery and quadrantectomy in breast cancer. Ann Surg Oncol 14(2):605–614, 2007.

58. Colwell AS, Kukreia J, Breuing KH, et al: Occult breast carcinoma in reduction mammaplasty specimens: 14-year experience. Plast Reconstr Surg 113(7):1984–1988, 2004.

59. Howard MA, Polo K, Pusic AL, et al: Breast cancer local recurrence after mastectomy and TRAM flap reconstruction: incidence and treatment options. Plast Reconstr Surg 117:1381, 2006.

60. Shaikh N, LaTrenta G, Swistel A, et al: Detection of recurrent breast cancer after TRAM flap reconstruction. Ann Plast Surg 47:602, 2001.

61. Taylor CW, Horgan K, Dodwell D: Oncological aspects of breast reconstruction. The Breast 14:118, 2005.

62. Tuli R, Flynn RA, Brill KL, et al: Diagnosis, treatment, and management of breast cancer in previously augmented women. Breast J 12:343, 2006.

14 Oncoplastic Surgical Techniques for the Partial Mastectomy

Chin-Yau Chen, Kristine E. Calhoun, and Benjamin O. Anderson

KEY POINTS

- Oncoplastic surgery is a technique that achieves wide surgical margins while at the same time preserving the shape of the breast.
- Ductal carcinoma in situ (DCIS) is often segmentally distributed in the breast. Within the ductal system, DCIS is commonly multifocal but is not usually multicentric.
- Because breast segments vary in size and extent, some segmentally oriented cancers are amenable to partial mastectomy, whereas other cancers inevitably require mastectomy for complete excision.
- Invasive cancer commonly arises peripherally rather than centrally within a segmentally distributed field of in situ disease. Understanding the cancer distribution is mandatory.
- A combination of imaging modalities (including sonogram, mammogram, and in some circumstances MRI) can best evaluate the extent of the cancer.
- Bracketing wires can be helpful in directing surgical excision.
- Parallelogram mastopexy lumpectomy using local breast tissue for repair of the defect after partial mastectomy is the basic oncoplastic surgery technique.

Introduction to Oncoplastic Surgery

For breast conservation to be efficacious, the surgeon needs (1) to obtain complete excision of the cancer with adequate surgical margin width and (2) to achieve a surgical result that maintains the breast's shape and appearance over time.[1] For larger cancers, it can be technically challenging to simultaneously address both of these goals in the same operation. Simple flap advancement "mastopexy" techniques developed by plastic surgeons for breast reduction can reshape the breast immediately after larger breast cancer resections, while minimizing deformities that can develop during radiation therapy.[2] This novel approach was first referred to as "oncoplastic surgery" by W. Audretsch[3] in 1994.

Until recently, the term "oncoplastic surgery" had various meanings depending on the expertise and specialty training of the surgeon. In the plastic surgery literature, oncoplastic surgery typically refers to large partial mastectomy combined with myocutaneous flap reconstruction, such as the latissimus dorsi flap or the transverse rectus abdominis myocutaneous (TRAM) flap. Major reconstructive procedures using myocutaneous flaps are technically demanding and time consuming and require special training to learn and apply properly. Scheduling conflicts between oncologic and plastic surgeons can also be problematic, making true immediate reconstructions difficult to coordinate.

By contrast, small- or intermediate-sized cancers can generally be managed nicely using simple oncoplastic techniques that facilitate wide excision of the cancer and preserve the shape and appearance of the breast. In oncoplastic surgery, by advancing locally available fibroglandular tissue along the chest wall, the defect created by partial mastectomy is closed with a breast "fibroglandular flap," called mastopexy closure. Multiple technically simple techniques have been described, all following these same surgical principles. These basic oncoplastic operations are easily taught to and used by surgeons with experience in breast surgery. In a review of 84 women who underwent partial mastectomy and radiation therapy, Kronowitz and colleagues[4] showed that immediate repair of partial-mastectomy defects with local tissues results in a lower risk of complications (23% to 67%) and better aesthetic outcomes (57% to 33%) than that with a latissimus dorsi flap. The latissimus dorsi flap is preferred for delayed reconstruction, and the TRAM flap is best reserved for total mastectomy defects in case of local recurrence.[5] In this chapter, we describe a collection of oncoplastic procedures that apply local breast tissue flap advancement.

Anatomic Distribution of Cancer in the Breast

The design of the traditional lumpectomy commonly used in the United States originated mainly from the NSABP (National Surgical Adjuvant Breast and Bowel Project) B-06 study initiated in 1976 under the direction of Dr. Bernard Fisher. This large trial helped establish the equivalency of breast-conserving surgery and mastectomy in terms of survival.[6] In the traditional lumpectomy, a curvilinear incision is placed directly over the cancer, no skin island is removed, the cancer is excised in a minimalist fashion with the intention of obtaining negative but not necessarily wide margins, and the skin is closed without any formal attempt to obliterate the lumpectomy pocket. In the B-06 trial, there was no predefined amount of normal tissue to be removed around the tumor; a tumor-free margin of 1 mm—or even less—was considered adequate. Fisher[6] hypothesized that breast cancer is fundamentally a systemic disease, and in the course of doing so, he minimized the issues surrounding local control of disease.

With the use of more limited resections, a higher risk of local recurrence would be expected. Multiple studies have confirmed this hypothesis. In the Milan trial, for example, 705 patients were randomized to receive lumpectomy (excision with narrow margin) or quadrantectomy (excision of surrounding normal tissue of 2 to 3 cm). Even though the rates of distant metastases and survival were no different between the two groups, the rate of local recurrence at 5 years was much higher in the lumpectomy group (7% compared with 2.2%).[7] However, since lumpectomy was developed for breast conservation, little thought was given to understanding the anatomic orientation of cancers in the breast. For good oncoplastic surgical technique, understanding of common patterns of cancer distribution is mandatory.[8]

Segmental Anatomy of the Breast

In 1840, English surgeon and anatomist Sir Astley Paston Cooper (1768–1841) published his book, *On the Anatomy of the Breast*.[9] Cooper, who became the namesake for the breast's suspensory ligaments, provided technically precise descriptions of breast anatomy that remain surprisingly accurate even by modern standards (Fig. 14-1A).

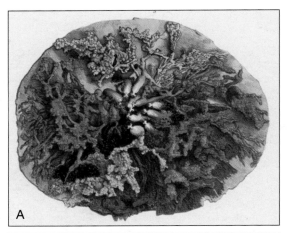

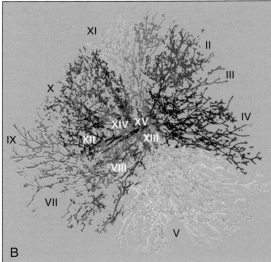

Figure 14-1. A, Breast ducts injected with colored wax, published by Cooper in 1840. (Reproduced courtesy of Jefferson Digital Commons, Scott Memorial Library, Thomas Jefferson University.) **B,** Three-dimensional computer modeling images of all ducts and branches in an autopsy breast, viewed en face, based on 2-mm serial subgross sections in an autopsied breast. (Published by Going and Moffat in 2004. Copyright Pathological Society of Great Britain and Ireland. Reproduced with permission of John Wiley & Sons on behalf of the Pathological Society.)

The number of ductal orifices and ductal segments in the breast has been a subject of controversy. The number of central ducts terminating as ductal orifices at the nipple has variably been quoted as 15 to 20 and 15 to 25 or more, although these figures have not been based on documented anatomic studies.[10] To the contrary, Cooper reported, "The greatest number of lactiferous tubes I have been able to inject has been twelve, and more frequently from seven to ten." Cooper suggested that the radiation of one of the mammary tubes commonly occupied one-sixth to one-fifth of the circumference of the breast, findings that have been verified by modern investigators. Dr. Susan Love used a combination of in vivo and ex vivo analyses to show that more than 90% of all nipples examined contained only five to nine ductal orifices, generally arranged as a central group and a peripheral group.[11]

Another set of investigators, Going and Moffat from the University of Glasgow, used 2-mm serial subgross sections to generate three-dimensional computer modeling images of the ductal tree in an autopsied breast.[10] They described three populations of ducts: (1) seven major ducts that maintained a wide lumen up to the skin surface; (2) 20 ducts that tapered to a minute lumen at their origin in the vicinity of skin appendages of the nipple; and (3) a minor duct population arising at the base of the papilla. Going and Moffat found one dominant branching duct that drained as much as 23% of the total breast's volume and observed that the largest six systems drain 75% of the total breast's volume in most cases (Fig. 14-1B). These observations all suggest that the number of major ductal systems is fewer than 10 and that the anatomy is variable, with ductal segments of differing sizes and distributions throughout the breast. Accordingly, a major ductal system can represent either a very small percentage of the breast's glandular tree or up to one fourth of the total breast volume.

In some regions of the breast, the ductal branches extend full thickness from skin to chest wall, but in other regions, the ductal branches are layered from anterior to posterior. Cooper noticed, "On the sternal (medial) and clavicular (superior) aspect of the breast, a single duct radiates to the margin; but upon the axillary (lateral) and abdominal (inferior) aspects, two or three ducts ramify to the circumference of the gland, so that two or three ducts are placed upon each other."[9] Moffat and Going[12] also found that some of the ducts pass back from the nipple for a much longer distance before ramifying in the deep part of the breast. Similarly, Ohtake[13] also found several ductal systems overlapping one another in the same region of the breast.

Not all ducts pass radially from the nipple to the periphery of the breast. Cooper noted one group of central ducts which branched directly toward the chest wall without extensive arborization into the periphery of the breast. In another retrospective study of 1312 archival ductograms collected by Sartorius, the ducts did not all extend in a radial fashion from the nipple; rather, some traveled directly back from the nipple toward the chest wall, with the peripheral ducts draped over the central ducts in a radial fashion.[11] For a cancer found centrally, therefore, it is possible that only a central duct is involved.

Cooper[9] stated that, with rare exception, the ducts ramify but do not communicate with each other. Cooper had observed a single instance of two intercommunicating ductal branches among 200 cases, which he described as a rare deviation from a general law. Ductal anastomoses were found in 4 of 16 ductal systems in Ohtake's computer model. However, similar anastomoses could not be identified in other studies.[10–12,14] The communication between different ductal systems, previously suspected to be the cause of multicentricity in DCIS, is a rare event, if it exists at all.

Cooper was the first to observe that the breast's arterial supply comes from multiple sources, with plentiful anastomotic interconnections. He noted, "The most common supply of arterial blood in the human subject is derived from the axillary and internal mammary arteries. . . . The posterior or axillary branch may be seen to form a circle around the nipple, and a network with frequent communications upon the surface of the breast."[9] The well-collateralized vasculature of the breast has made it possible to move and remodel its glandular tissue safely without resultant tissue ischemia or loss.

Common Patterns of Cancer Distribution

DCIS and lobular carcinoma in situ (LCIS) generally arise in terminal ductal-lobular units or in the lobules themselves.[15] In a study of 119 mastectomy specimens, Holland[16] found that the distribution of DCIS is typically segmental within one ductal system. DCIS was often multifocal and on histologic examination was found to contain many small tumor foci within a single ductal branch. In poorly differentiated DCIS, 90% showed predominantly continuous growth. In contrast, only 30% of well-differentiated DCIS demonstrated a continuous distribution. Eight percent (5 of 60) showed a discontinuous (multifocal) growth with a gap wider then 10 mm.

In cases of poorly differentiated DCIS, preoperative margin assessment may be more reliable than with well-differentiated DCIS, because the microcalcifications associated with higher-grade lesions often appear mammographically as linear, branching, or coarse granular calcifications. This finding generally corresponds well to the amorphous calcifications seen at histology. In contrast, the microcalcifications associated with well-differentiated DCIS are typically seen on imaging studies as multiple clusters of fine granular microcalcifications, which correspond to the clusters of laminated, crystalline calcifications found at histology. The fine granular microcalcifications seen with lower-grade disease, which at times are subtle, may result in an underestimation of the extent of disease on mammogram.[17]

Finally, in terms of invasive breast cancers, most lesions have been shown to have an associated component of in situ carcinoma.[18] Holland[14] found that 12% of the patients had prominent DCIS (defined as six or more microscopic low-power fields of intraductal carcinoma) beyond 2 cm of the edge of the invasive tumor. This common finding should be taken into consideration when planning one's operative conduct.

By correlating three-dimensional MRI with precise histopathologic maps, Amano and colleagues[19] classified the distribution of breast cancer into three patterns: (1) localized (n = 30), (2) segmentally extended (n = 19), and (3) irregularly extended (n = 5). The segmentally extended pattern showed diffuse enhancement along duct-lobular segments, forming a cone shape. Histologically, DCIS was distributed segmentally. Mai and colleagues[20] studied the pattern of distribution of intraductal and infiltrating ductal carcinoma in 30 mastectomy specimens with infiltrating carcinoma less than 3 cm in diameter. Intraductal carcinomas showed a "fanned out" pattern of distribution and frequently extended toward the nipple (with involvement of the nipple or subareolar tissue in 7 of 30 cases). In their study of 62 lumpectomy specimens for DCIS, the margins were identified as proximal (closest to the nipple), distal (farthest from the nipple), or peripheral (neither proximal nor distal). They found that positive or close margins were associated with proximal lesions in 6 cases and peripheral lesions in 13 cases, whereas none was found with distal cancer.[21] These findings demonstrate that invasive ductal carcinoma more commonly arises at the periphery rather than in the center of the originating DCIS bed. Thus, cancer resection intending only to remove palpable invasive carcinoma often produces inadequate surgical margins for noninvasive cancer and leaves residual tumor cells in the remaining breast.

Preoperative Assessment of Disease Distribution

MRI of the Breast

When based only on the extent of microcalcifications, mammography underestimates the size of DCIS by an average of 1 to 2 cm, especially when the fine-granular microcalcifications seen with low-grade lesions are present.[14] Boetes and colleagues[22] reported on the histologic results and preoperative imaging findings (mammography, ultrasound, MRI) of 61 tumors in 60 women undergoing mastectomy for carcinoma. In 10% of cases, the index tumors were not seen at mammography, and ultrasound missed 15% of the tumors. In contrast, breast MRI missed only 2% of the index tumors. On mammographic and ultrasound images, tumor size was significantly underestimated in 14% and 18% of cases, respectively, whereas MRI showed no significant difference in size compared with that found in a pathologic evaluation.

Although MRI has the lowest false-negative rate in detecting invasive lobular carcinoma and the highest accuracy in measuring its size,[22] the high overall false-positive rate has inhibited some surgeons from incorporating MRI into routine breast surgical practice.[23] In 2004, the International Breast MRI Consortium published that among 821 patients referred for breast biopsy, breast MRI examinations had a sensitivity of 88.1% but a specificity of only 67.7%.[24]

This study also showed that, though sensitive, 12% of cancers identified by mammography or clinical breast exam were negative on MRI. Although a negative or benign MRI should not be used to replace a recommendation for biopsy based on other traditional imaging modalities, MRI is proving to be valuable in the assessment of extent of disease in patients with a recent diagnosis of breast cancer.[25]

A consensus report from the American Society of Breast Surgeons in 2005 supports the use of MRI for determining ipsilateral tumor extent or the presence of contralateral disease in patients with breast cancer (especially those with invasive lobular carcinoma) when dense breast tissue precludes an accurate mammographic assessment.[26] A combination of imaging methods (mammography with magnification views, ultrasonography, MRI, or all) may yield the best estimates of overall tumor size.[27]

Multiple Bracketing Wires

Because more than 90% of DCIS currently diagnosed is nonpalpable, the surgeon often requires preoperative localization to accurately identify the area warranting resection. Silverstein and colleagues[28] suggested that preoperative placement of bracketing wires, defined as multiple wires to delineate the boundaries of a single lesion, may be useful in this regard (Fig. 14-2). In a study by Liberman and colleagues,[29] of 42 calcific lesions that were bracketed, complete removal of suspicious calcifications was accomplished in 34 (81.0%). Bracketing wires may assist the surgeon in achieving complete excision of calcifications.

Oncoplastic Partial Mastectomy

In breast conservative surgery, margin width has been shown to be the single most important predictor of local recurrence.[30-32] Oncoplastic surgery offers a better chance of wide anatomic resection while preserving overall cosmesis.

Parallelogram Mastopexy Lumpectomy: A Basic Technique

The parallelogram mastopexy lumpectomy offers a technically simple method for designing full-thickness segmental resection (Figs. 14-3 and 14-4). Localized and/or small segmental

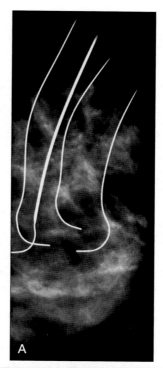

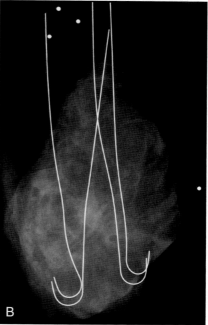

Figure 14-2. A, Bracketed multiwire localization of segmentally distributed ductal carcinoma. **B,** Specimen radiograph of resected ductal carcinoma.

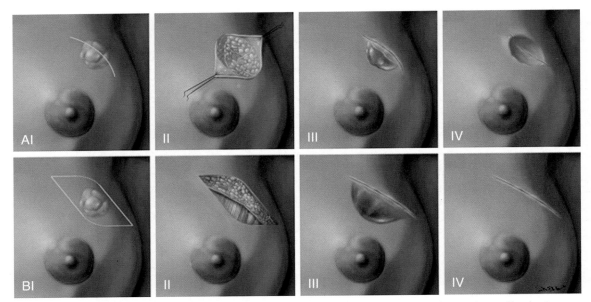

Figure 14-3. Comparison of the standard lumpectomy and parallelogram mastopexy lumpectomy: (I) prior to incision, (II) after excision of the lesion, (III) after wound closure with seroma, and (IV) after seroma reabsorption. **A,** With a standard lumpectomy incision, the removal of underlying fibroglandular tissue creates a defect that ultimately can cause a visible tissue deficit ("saucerization") at the site of the incision. **B,** By contrast, with a parallelogram mastopexy lumpectomy, wider resection margins are achieved while the shape of the breast is preserved without an underlying divot of breast tissue. Care needs to be taken not to remove so much skin that it causes excessive deviation of the nipple relative to the contralateral breast. (Courtesy of University of Washington.)

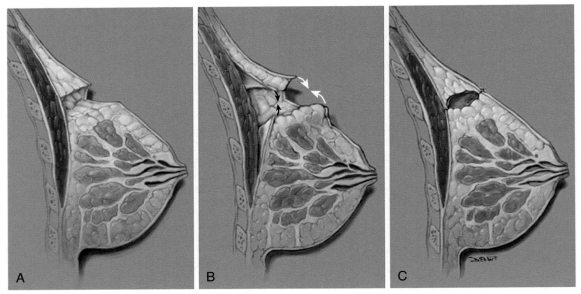

Figure 14-4. Breast flap mastopexy advancement closure in an oncoplastic partial mastectomy resection.
A, The fibroglandular tissue is resected full thickness from pectoralis fascia to skin, including an overlying skin island to allow proportional reduction in skin and fibroglandular tissue. **B,** The remaining fibroglandular tissue is elevated off the pectoralis muscle to permit its advancement over the chest wall. The undermining of fibroglandular tissue at the pectoralis fascia is adequate to permit breast tissue advancement over the muscle without being so extensive as to threaten the blood supply to the residual breast tissue. **C,** The fibroglandular tissue is closed at its deepest level and at the skin to effectively close the significant defect created by the wide surgical excision. (Courtesy of University of Washington.)

cancers can be excised using this procedural design. Skin incisions in the upper breast should follow transverse Kraissl's lines; those in the lower half (including the 3-o'clock and 9-o'clock positions) of the breast should be radial.[33–35]

With the help of wire localization or preoperative sonogram, the location and distribution of the tumor are marked. The parallelogram incision design is a rounded parallelogram whereby the two margins are of equal length[2] (see Fig. 14-3). An island of skin is excised, which prevents leaving behind redundant skin over the defect, because this can induce infolding of the skin, adherence to the chest wall, and nipple deviation.[2] To prevent substantial shifting of the nipple-areolar complex, the surgeon needs to ensure that the ellipse of the skin is not too wide compared with the length of the incision. After excision of the skin island, short skin flaps are raised along both sides of the wound. Then, based on the extent of cancer, dissection is carried down to the chest wall, and the breast is lifted up and off the pectoralis muscle with preservation of the fascia. A notable advantage of this posterior dissection of tissue is that it permits bimanual palpation of the target lesion, thus allowing the surgeon to find where the breast tissue should best be divided.

After lesion excision, the breast tissue is undermined at the level of the pectoralis muscle to permit the mobilization of the surrounding fibroglandular flaps. The mobilized fibroglandular tissue, now advanced over the chest wall to close the defect, is sutured at its deepest level, taking care to avoid deformity or undesired traction of the peripheral breast skin.[2] Since most breast surgeons have been taught to avoid suturing of the breast parenchyma in an effort to obliterate dead space after excising a tumor, this technique at first seems contrary to habit. In oncoplastic breast surgery, however, the fibroglandular tissues are appropriately mobilized and reapproximated to facilitate maximally round and natural-appearing results (see Fig. 14-4).

Batwing Mastopexy Lumpectomy

The batwing mastopexy lumpectomy (Fig. 14-5) is an ideal approach for resection of cancers that are located deep or adjacent to, but that do not directly involve, the nipple.[31] Two similar half-circle incisions are made with angled

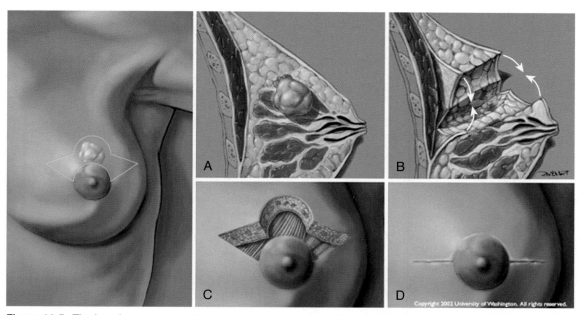

Figure 14-5. The batwing mastopexy lumpectomy.   For cancers adjacent or deep to the nipple-areolar complex, this approach creates equidistant upper and lower skin margins to facilitate cosmetic closure. **A,** Preoperative view. **B,** Two similar half-circle incisions are made with angled wings on each side of the areola and full-thickness excision is performed. **C,** The remaining fibroglandular tissue is advanced to close the subsequent defect. **D,** Final result at closure. This approach causes some uplifting of the nipple, which can cause asymmetry relative to the contralateral breast. (Courtesy of University of Washington.)

wings on each side of the areola. Full-thickness excision is then performed, and the fibroglandular tissue is advanced to close the subsequent defect. Because this approach causes some upward deviation of the nipple, excessive asymmetry may require a contralateral lift at a later time to restore symmetry. Since the batwing mastopexy lumpectomy involves an incision that centers around the nipple-areolar complex, it can be revised to a central lumpectomy with resection of the nipple-areolar complex itself when necessary due to margin issues.[36] Of note, since the blood supply of the external nipple arises from the underlying fibroglandular tissue

investing the major lactiferous sinuses rather than as collateral circulation from the surrounding areolar skin, when dissection extends high up inside the backside of the nipple, nipple necrosis can occur.

Donut Mastopexy Lumpectomy

The donut mastopexy lumpectomy is a unique breast resection technique in which a segmental area of tissue is removed through a periareolar incision (Fig. 14-6).[1,37,38] For segmentally distributed cancers of the upper or lateral breast, donut mastopexy lumpectomy can offer

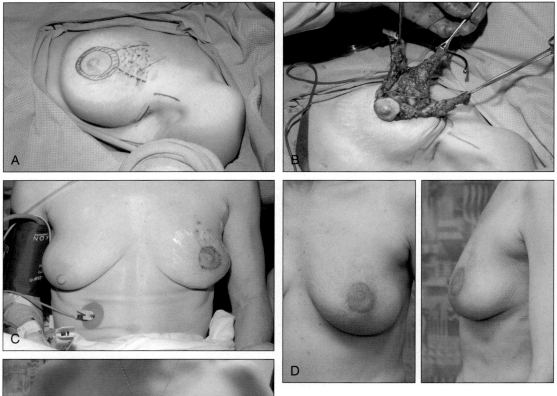

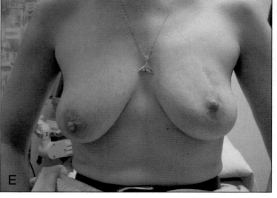

Figure 14-6. Donut mastopexy lumpectomy.   A, The periareolar incision is planned. Multiple bracketing wires are placed around the segmentally distributed cancer. The sentinel node biopsy is completed before performing the lumpectomy. **B,** Full-thickness segmental excision of the lesion is performed. **C,** After the operation is completed, only a periareolar incisional wound is noted. **D,** The shape and appearance of the breast are well preserved 6 months after operation. (*Left*) Anteroposterior view. (*Right*) Lateral view. **E,** Two years after operation, the shape and appearance of the breast are well preserved. Slight upward deviation of left nipple-areolar complex is noted.

complete cancer excision without sacrifice of too much skin or nipple-areolar deviation. The donut mastopexy lumpectomy uses a modification of the skin-sparing mastectomy in which only a segment of the breast is removed. Because it is a more complex operation involving wide skin-sparing dissection, the donut mastopexy lumpectomy should not be undertaken until the more basic oncoplastic techniques are fully understood and mastered.

Initially, a donut of skin is excised around the nipple-areolar complex using a Benelli-type "round block" incision, a technique commonly used in breast reduction surgery.[39] Care is taken not to excessively separate the areola from the underlying tissues to avoid devascularization of the periareolar skin. Up to half of the breast volume is delivered full thickness through the incision, and a wedge of tissue, which includes the entire segment of breast tissue with associated disease, is removed. The remaining fibroglandular tissue is returned to the cavity and sutured together to close the resulting defect. A purse string around the nipple completes the closure, leaving only a periareolar incision at the conclusion of the operation.

Because it requires a more complex dissection, the donut mastopexy lumpectomy is gen-erally reserved for more extensive, segmentally distributed cancers in the upper half of the breast. As a result, most patients require mastectomy if donut mastopexy lumpectomy surgical margins are found to be inadequate. Since the incision is exclusively periareolar, a skin-sparing total mastectomy with immediate flap reconstruction remains an excellent option for salvage in these situations.

Reduction Mastopexy Lumpectomy

Standard lumpectomy in the lower breast frequently results in significant defect and down-pointing of the nipple. For radially oriented lesions in the lower hemisphere of the breast (4-o'clock to 8-o'clock position, going clockwise), reduction mastopexy lumpectomy is a useful technique for excision that prevents deviation of nipple (Fig. 14-7). Large amounts of breast tissue can be removed while simultaneously obtaining excellent cosmetic results and widely clear margins.[40]

Like the donut mastopexy lumpectomy, the reduction mastopexy lumpectomy is an advanced oncoplastic technique based on the more basic skills of full-thickness excision and breast flap advancement. As such, surgeons without

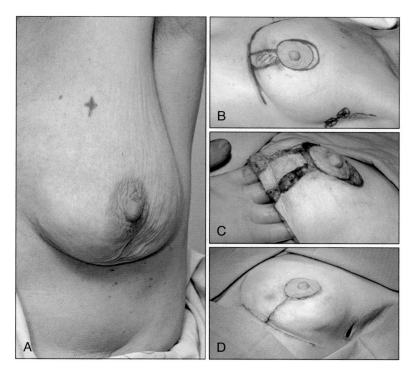

Figure 14-7. The reduction mastopexy lumpectomy.
A, Preoperative image of lower pole cancer at 6 o'clock showing tenting of breast skin overlying an invasive cancer. **B,** Skin marking showing location of cancer and design of operative incision. **C,** Intraoperative development of incision prior to fibroglandular excision. **D,** Final result at closure.

specific oncoplastic training should be cautious when attempting this approach. A significant limitation of this approach is that if the patient is found to have positive surgical margins, the surgeon may find it technically challenging to include both the initial incisions and the nipple-areolar complex in a subsequent total mastectomy.

Conclusions

Oncoplastic surgical techniques, a fairly new concept in breast conservation therapy, are designed with the cancer's contour in mind. Breast surgeons planning breast-conserving surgery should consider how the disease is distributed within the breast before making an incision. Knowledge of normal ductal anatomy and common patterns of cancer distribution, as well as the use of different imaging modalities (including sonogram, mammogram, and MRI), can help delineate the extent of cancer before operation. In addition, bracketing wires can be exceptionally helpful intraoperatively to design resection areas. Basic oncoplastic techniques, such as the parallelogram, batwing, donut, and reduction mastopexy lumpectomies, can be easily learned and used by experienced breast surgeons.

References

1. Masetti R, Pirulli PG, Magno S, et al: Oncoplastic techniques in the conservative surgical treatment of breast cancer. Breast Cancer 7:276–280, 2000.
2. Anderson BO, Masetti R, Silverstein MJ: Oncoplastic approaches to partial mastectomy: an overview of volume-displacement techniques. Lancet Oncol 6:145–157, 2005.
3. Audretsch W, Rezai M, Kolotas C: Onco-plastic surgery: "target" volume reduction (BCT-mastopexy), lumpectomy reconstruction (BCT-reconstruction), and flap-supported operability in breast cancer. Proceedings 2nd European Congress on Senology. Vienna, Austria, October 2–6, 1994, Bologna, Italy, Monduzzi, 1994, pp 139–157.
4. Kronowitz SJ, Feledy JA, Hunt KK, et al: Determining the optimal approach to breast reconstruction after partial mastectomy. Plast Reconstr Surg 117:1–11, 2006.
5. Nahabedian MY: Determining the optimal approach to breast reconstruction after partial mastectomy: discussion. Plast Reconstr Surg 117:12–14, 2006.
6. Fisher B: Lumpectomy (segmental mastectomy) and axillary dissection. In Bland KI, Copeland EM (eds): The Breast: Comprehensive Management of Benign and Malignant Diseases, 2nd ed. Philadelphia: WB Saunders, 1998, pp 917–939.
7. Veronesi U, Volterrani F, Luini A, et al: Quadrantectomy versus lumpectomy for small size breast cancer. Eur J Cancer 26:671–673, 1990.
8. Chen CY, Calhoun KE, Masetti R, et al: Oncoplastic breast conserving surgery: a renaissance of anatomically-based surgical technique. Minerva Chir 61:421–434, 2006.
9. Cooper AP: On the anatomy of the breast. London, Longman, Orme, Green, Brown, and Longmans. (Special Collections, Scott Memorial Library, Thomas Jefferson University. Available at http://jdc.jefferson.edu/cooper/) 1840.
10. Going JJ, Moffat DF: Escaping from Flatland: clinical and biological aspects of human mammary duct anatomy in three dimensions. J Pathol 203:538–544, 2004.
11. Love SM, Barsky SH: Anatomy of the nipple and breast ducts revisited. Cancer 101:1947–1957, 2004.
12. Moffat DF, Going JJ: Three dimensional anatomy of complete duct systems in human breast: pathological and developmental implications. J Clin Pathol 49:48–52, 1996.
13. Ohtake T, Kimijima I, Fukushima T, et al: Computer-assisted complete three-dimensional reconstruction of the mammary ductal/lobular systems: implications of ductal anastomoses for breast-conserving surgery. Cancer 91:2263–2272, 2001.
14. Holland R, Faverly DRG: Whole-organ studies. In Silverstein MJ (ed): Ductal Carcinoma in Situ of the Breast. Baltimore: Williams & Wilkins, 1997, pp 233–240.
15. Wellings SR, Jensen HM, Marcum RG: An atlas of subgross pathology of the human breast with special reference to possible precancerous lesions. J Natl Cancer Inst 55:231–273, 1975.
16. Holland R, Hendriks JH: Microcalcifications associated with ductal carcinoma in situ: mammographic-pathologic correlation. Semin Diagn Pathol 11:181–192, 1994.
17. Holland R, Hendriks JH, Verbeek AL, et al: Extent, distribution, and mammographic/histological correlations of breast ductal carcinoma in situ. Lancet 335:519–522, 1990.
18. Schnitt SJ, Guidi AJ: Pathology of invasive breast cancer. In Harris JR, Lippman ME, Morrow M, et al (eds): Diseases of the Breast, 3rd ed. Philadelphia: Lippincott Williams & Wilkins, 2004, pp 541–584.
19. Amano G, Ohuchi N, Ishibashi T, et al: Correlation of three-dimensional magnetic resonance imaging with precise histopathological map concerning carcinoma extension in the breast. Breast Cancer Res Treat 60:43–55, 2000.
20. Mai KT, Yazdi HM, Burns BF, et al: Pattern of distribution of intraductal and infiltrating ductal carcinoma: a three-dimensional study using serial coronal giant sections of the breast. Hum Pathol 31:464–474, 2000.
21. Mai KT, Perkins DG, Mirsky D: Location and extent of positive resection margins and ductal carcinoma in situ in lumpectomy specimens of ductal breast carcinoma examined with a microscopic three-dimensional view. Breast J 9:33–38, 2003.
22. Boetes C, Veltman J, van Die L, et al: The role of MRI in invasive lobular carcinoma. Breast Cancer Res Treat 86:31–37, 2004.
23. Morrow M: Magnetic resonance imaging in breast cancer: is seeing always believing? Eur J Cancer 41:1368–1369, 2005.
24. Bluemke DA, Gatsonis CA, Chen MH, et al: Magnetic resonance imaging of the breast prior to biopsy. JAMA 292:2735–2742, 2004.
25. Lehman CD, Schnall MD: Imaging in breast cancer: magnetic resonance imaging. Breast Cancer Res 7:215–219, 2005.
26. Dardik A: Use of magnetic resonance imaging in breast oncology. J Am Coll Surg 200:742, 2005.
27. Silverstein MJ, Lagios MD, Recht A, et al: Image-detected breast cancer: state of the art diagnosis and treatment. J Am Coll Surg 201:586–597, 2005.
28. Silverstein MJ, Gamagami P, Rosser RJ, et al: Hooked-wire-directed breast biopsy and over penetrated mammography. Cancer 59:715–722, 1987.
29. Liberman L, Kaplan J, Van Zee KJ, et al: Bracketing wires for preoperative breast needle localization. AJR Am J Roentgenol 177:565–572, 2001.
30. MacDonald HR, Silverstein MJ, Mabry H, et al: Local control in ductal carcinoma in situ treated by excision alone: incremental benefit of larger margins. Am J Surg 190:521–525, 2005.
31. Silverstein MJ: An argument against routine use of radiotherapy for ductal carcinoma in situ. Oncology (Williston Park) 17:1511–1533; discussion 1533–1534, 1539, 1542 passim, 2003.
32. Smitt MC, Nowels K, Carlson RW, et al: Predictors of reexcision findings and recurrence after breast conservation. Int J Radiat Oncol Biol Phys 57:979–985, 2003.
33. Wilhelmi BJ, Blackwell SJ, Phillips LG: Langer's lines: to use or not to use. Plast Reconstr Surg 104:208–214, 1999.
34. Borges AF: Relaxed skin tension lines (RSTL) versus other skin lines. Plast Reconstr Surg 73:144–150, 1984.
35. Kraissl CJ: The selection of appropriate lines for elective surgical incisions. Plast Reconstr Surg 8:1–28, 1951.

36. Pezzi CM, Kukora JS, Audet IM, et al: Breast conservation surgery using nipple-areolar resection for central breast cancers. Arch Surg 139:32–37; discussion 38, 2004.
37. Amanti C, Moscaroli A, Lo Russo M, et al: [Periareolar subcutaneous quadrantectomy: a new approach in breast cancer surgery]. G Chir 23:445–449, 2002.
38. Amanti C, Regolo L, Moscaroli A, et al: [Total periareolar approach in breast-conserving surgery]. Tumori 89:169–172, 2003.
39. Benelli LC: Periareolar Benelli mastopexy and reduction: the "round block." In Spear SL (ed): Surgery of the Breast: Principles and Art, 2nd ed. Philadelphia: Lippincott Williams & Wilkins, 2006, pp 977–990.
40. Clough KB, Lewis JS, Couturaud B, et al: Oncoplastic techniques allow extensive resections for breast-conserving therapy of breast carcinomas. Ann Surg 237:26–34, 2003.

15

Axillary Management

M. Catherine Lee and Michael S. Sabel

KEY POINTS

- Axillary assessment by clinical examination alone is extremely inaccurate. Ultrasound evaluation of axillary lymph nodes is a growing practice with higher sensitivity and specificity, especially when combined with fine-needle aspiration of abnormal-appearing nodes.
- Sentinel lymph node (SLN) biopsy is the initial axillary staging procedure of choice for women with clinically node-negative invasive breast cancer; however, surgeons and patients should be prepared to do an axillary lymph node (ALN) dissection at the time of surgery if the mapping procedure fails.
- SLN biopsy should be strongly considered in women undergoing mastectomy for ductal carcinoma in situ (DCIS).
- Patients with micrometastases less than 0.2 mm on sentinel node biopsy are considered node-negative (N0mic) and should not be considered for completion dissection or adjuvant chemotherapy based on their nodal status. Patients with metastases larger than 0.2 mm should continue to be treated as node-positive.
- SLN biopsy is feasible in the assessment of recurrent breast cancers; however, surgeons and patients should be prepared for aberrant sentinel node drainage and operate accordingly.
- Although it is associated with a higher rate of complications than SLN biopsy alone, axillary nodal clearance is indicated in patients with clinically positive nodes or a positive SLN biopsy.

Introduction

The importance of the regional lymph nodes in the origin, prognosis, and management of breast cancer has been an area of controversy for hundreds of years. Shortly after the discovery of the lymphatic system in the 17th century, René Descartes proposed a lymph theory for the origin of breast cancer. This was in contrast to Galen's theory that cancer arises from an excess of black bile in the body. In the 18th century, John Hunter, often referred to as the father of scientific surgery, was a proponent of the lymph theory of breast cancer, suggesting that a coagulative defect in the lymph ultimately leads to the appearance of breast cancer. Although his reasoning may have been incorrect, he was one of the first surgeons to focus attention on the regional lymph nodes in the management of breast cancer, calling for the need for removal of the cancer along with the potential areas of lymphatic spread, preceding Halsted's theory by over a century.

Axillary dissection was introduced clinically by Lorenz Heister in the 19th century, although it was not soon adopted. The strongest argument for the surgical excision of the axillary lymph nodes (ALNs) came in 1867, when Charles Hewitt Moore described, in a treatise entitled "On the Influence of Inadequate Operations on the Theory of Cancer,"[1] the importance of removing involved ALNs en bloc with the cancer. He later went on to prescribe full axillary dissection for all patients with breast cancer, noting that involved nodes may not be detected clinically. Ernst G.F. Kuster and Richard von Volkmann also described a virtual elimination of axillary recurrences when axillary clearance was routinely performed. The work of these surgeons, as well as Joseph Lister and Samuel D. Gross, who were also strong proponents of detailed axillary dissection, had a significant influence on William Stewart Halsted.

Halsted[2] most radically changed the surgical management of breast cancer after he first described the radical mastectomy in 1882, arguing for not only the removal of the breast and both pectoral muscles, but also an extensive axillary dissection incorporating levels I through III. Although the radical mastectomy was associated with significant postoperative deformity and diminished upper extremity function and the operative procedure itself resulted in significant intraoperative blood loss, it had a dramatic impact on locoregional control and was quickly adopted. In the 1930s, D.H. Patey of London popularized the modified radical mastectomy, which spared the pectoral muscle while removing the breast, axillary contents (levels I and II), and a large ellipse of skin. The safety of the modified radical mastectomy was demonstrated when long-term follow-up failed to demonstrate any breast cancer recurrences in the preserved pectoral muscles, rarely in the level III or interpectoral nodes, and no difference in survival compared with radical mastectomy.

The end of Halsted's radical mastectomy arrived when it became apparent that although dramatically affecting local recurrence rates, the procedure had no significant impact on overall survival.[3] This called into question the relative impact that local or regional control had on overall survival. These questions would be addressed when, in a tremendous step forward for the treatment of breast cancer, the National Surgical and Adjuvant Breast Project (NSABP) was established by Dr. Rudolph Noer under the supervision of the National Cancer Institute (NCI). Under the leadership of Dr. Bernard Fisher, the NSABP has performed numerous multicenter, randomized clinical trials examining the effects of surgery, chemotherapy, and radiation on breast cancer outcomes. These

large randomized trials represent the most solid evidence-based information available, and the results of these studies continue to have a marked influence on clinical decision making worldwide. In one of the first trials that the NSABP conducted, NSABP B-04, the project sought to specifically address the controversy surrounding the ideal management of the ALNs.

The NSABP B-04 trial, conducted between July 1971 and September 1974, took patients with operable invasive breast cancers and clinically negative nodes ($N = 1079$) and randomized them to one of three arms: (1) total mastectomy with ALN dissection; (2) total mastectomy with postoperative radiation; and (3) total mastectomy with a delayed axillary dissection only if clinically positive axillary nodes developed. An additional 586 women with clinically positive nodes were randomized to either radical mastectomy or total mastectomy without axillary surgery, but with postoperative radiation. Twenty-five-year follow-up of the B-04 trial has demonstrated no survival difference among either the node-negative treatment groups and the node-positive treatment groups.[4] Table 15-1 summarizes the results of the trial to date.

The NSABP B-04 trial did demonstrate the necessity of surgical lymph node dissection in identifying regional disease (clinical axillary staging was incorrect in 25% to 40% of cases) and also the superiority of surgical lymph node dissection compared with axillary radiation for local disease control among clinically node-positive patients.[4,5] However, the trial also revealed that the ALN dissection as part of the

Table 15-1. Results of NSABP B-04: Survival Equivalence of All Three Node-Negative Groups and of Both Node-Positive Groups

	Node-Negative			Node-Positive	
	RM	TM	TM + XRT	RM	TM + XRT
No. of patients	362	365	352	292	294
OS at 25 years	25%	26%	19%	14%	14%
OS at 10 years	58%	54%	59%	38%	39%
OS at 5 years	75%	74%	75%	62%	58%

19% of clinically node-negative patients underwent delayed ALN dissection for axillary relapse (median time to development of positive axillary nodes 14.8 months).

11.9% of clinically node-positive patients randomized to TM + XRT developed axillary relapse compared with 1.0% in RM arm.

OS, overall survival; RM, radical mastectomy; TM, total mastectomy; TM + XRT, total mastectomy and external-beam radiation.

surgical management of breast cancer was not associated with any survival benefit. Despite this finding, surgical management did not change, and axillary dissection remained the standard of care. There were several reasons for this. Although the therapeutic benefit may have been called into question, the prognostic information provided by ALN dissection was still crucial for adjuvant therapy decisions. In addition, the study was not powered to detect a small survival benefit for those who had ALN dissection, and critics of the study point out that in the mastectomy-alone arm, many surgeons still included a large number of axillary nodes with the specimen.

Surgical management of the ALNs did not change, even while local management transformed dramatically, and ALN dissection remained the standard of care for the woman with invasive breast cancer whether she underwent lumpectomy or mastectomy. The approach to the regional nodes, however, took a striking turn in 1994 when Giuliano and associates[6] first described the use of sentinel lymph node (SLN) biopsy in breast cancer. At that point in time, axillary sampling was being investigated as a means of staging the axilla without subjecting patients to the complications of axillary clearance. Sentinel node biopsy using blue dye was being widely investigated in melanoma staging when Giuliano described it as an accurate method for interrogating the axilla in clinically node-negative breast cancer patients.

Noninvasive Axillary Assessment

Clinical Examination

The initial evaluation of any woman with known or suspected breast cancer centers on a detailed history and physical examination and a thorough examination of the regional lymph nodes, including the axillary, supraclavicular, and cervical basins. With the patient sitting up, the examination should begin with the cervical lymph nodes along the anterior border of the sternocleidomastoid muscle. As the examiner moves downward, adenopathy should be sought in the supraclavicular fossa and possibly some infraclavicular nodes within the deltopectoral groove. To examine the axillary nodes, the examiner should face the patient or stand slightly to her side. The examiner uses the nonpalpating hand either to steady the patient's shoulder, or to support her arm, asking her to let it go loose. This relaxes the pectoralis major and axillary fascia, allowing for a better examination of the axilla. Physical examination of the axilla involves palpation of the anterior, deep, and posterior axillary surfaces. Enlarged or firm nodes may sometimes be detected on firm compression of the axillary tissues against the smoother surface of the pectoral muscles, the lateral chest wall, or the subscapular musculature. The examination should start high in the axilla. In this way, the axillary nodes are trapped lower rather than initially being pushed upward. Gently palpate back and forth to feel whether any nodes are apparent. Several passes should be made from top to bottom, both anteriorly and posteriorly in the axilla. If any lymph nodes are detected, their size, consistency, and fixation should be noted.

Physical examination alone is highly inaccurate for clinical staging, lacking in both sensitivity and specificity. Approximately one third of clinically node-negative axillae are falsely negative. False-positives are also a significant problem. A recent study from Memorial Sloan-Kettering Cancer Center examined 106 patients believed to have clinically positive axillary nodes.[7] Of 62 patients believed to have moderately suspicious findings on exam, 53% were falsely positive. Even among 44 patients whose nodes were deemed highly suspicious, 23% were node-negative. Overall, 41% of all the clinical exams were inaccurate, further reinforcing the position that clinical examination, even in very experienced hands, is only moderately useful in assessing both the absence and the presence of nodal involvement. Given that today women who are node-negative can be spared the morbidity of ALN dissection, the impact of a false-positive physical exam can be significant. Therefore, fine-needle aspiration biopsy should be used to confirm the presence of metastatic disease in any breast cancer patient with palpable ALNs. This can be done freehand or with ultrasound guidance.

Axillary Ultrasound

Imaging of the axilla with ultrasound is rapidly becoming standard practice for preoperative axillary assessment in patients with biopsy-proven invasive cancers. The technique of

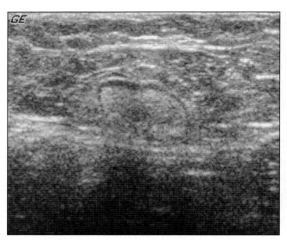

Figure 15-1. A normal axillary lymph node in a patient with ipsilateral breast cancer. It is a true negative. (Courtesy of Dr. Alexis Nees, Department of Radiology, University of Michigan, Ann Arbor, Michigan.)

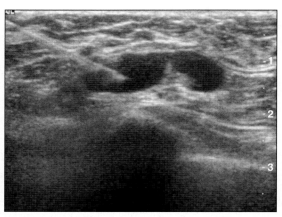

Figure 15-2. An ultrasound-guided fine-needle aspiration of a suspicious lymph node. (Courtesy of Dr. Alexis Nees, Department of Radiology, University of Michigan, Ann Arbor, Michigan.)

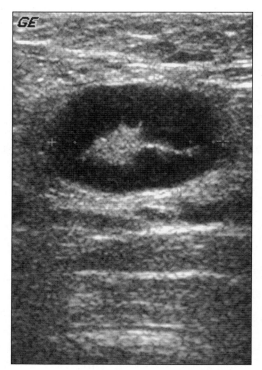

Figure 15-3. Ultrasound of a suspicious axillary lymph node. This node demonstrates cortical thickening with flattening and compression of the fatty hilum. (Courtesy of Dr. Alexis Nees, Department of Radiology, University of Michigan, Ann Arbor, Michigan.)

axillary ultrasound for breast cancer evaluation was first described in the European literature and was rapidly adopted as a diagnostic modality in conjunction with fine-needle aspiration biopsy of abnormal-appearing lymph nodes. Specificity of axillary ultrasound in identifying involved lymph nodes is between 87% and 95%, with a sensitivity of 50% to 70%. The specificity is significantly improved with the addition of fine-needle aspiration biopsy of any abnormal lymph nodes, increasing to nearly 100% in some studies.[8-12] Preoperative diagnosis of axillary metastasis is an excellent tool for staging and operative planning, especially with regard to patient selection for neoadjuvant chemotherapy.

Abnormal lymph nodes are identified either by their size or by a change in their general appearance on ultrasound (Figs. 15-1 through 15-4). Size is felt to be the weakest predictor of abnormality; normal nodes generally measure between 4 and 6 mm in length, and although nodes greater than 10 mm are generally considered abnormal, changes in morphology are significantly more useful in diagnosing metastasis. Rounding of the normal elliptical shape is considered an indication of neoplastic infiltration. Obliteration of the normally hypoechoic nodal cortex, irregularities of the cortical or medullary contours, and eccentric compression of the hyperechoic nodal medulla are also suggestive of metastatic disease. Loss of the nodal capsule is also an indicator of tumor invasion. The addition of color-flow Doppler may also enhance the diagnostic sensitivity of axillary ultrasound; hypervascularity and visualization of multiple feeding vessels for a single lymph node are strong indicators of neoplastic activity. Table 15-2 summarizes the sonographic findings indicative of metastatic nodal disease. Any abnormal lymph nodes identified on axillary ultrasound should undergo ultrasound-guided fine-needle aspiration to confirm the presence of metastases. Patients with fine-needle aspiration–proven regional disease can be spared the time and expense of SLN biopsy and proceed directly to ALN dissection at the time of their lumpectomy or mastectomy.

Management of the Clinically Negative Axilla

Sentinel Lymph Node Biopsy

Considering the potential long-term morbidity of axillary node dissection, the SLN biopsy has become the standard of care in the staging of the clinically node-negative breast cancer patient. The SLN biopsy involves removing only the node(s) that first receive lymphatic drainage from the breast without removing all of the lymph node-bearing fibrofatty tissue of the axilla. The sentinel nodes are the most likely nodes to harbor micrometastatic disease and therefore accurately reflect whether the patient is node-negative or node-positive. Today, ALN dissection is reserved for the patient with demonstrated regional disease, or for those patients whose SLN cannot be accurately identified.

When the SLN biopsy was first proposed for invasive breast cancer—although it promised an improved quality of life for breast cancer

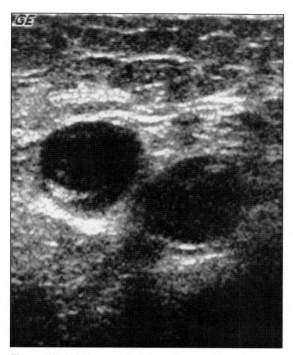

Figure 15-4. Ultrasound of two abnormal lymph nodes. The node on the left side of the image demonstrates cortical thickening with severe flattening and compression of the fatty hilum. The lymph node on the right demonstrates loss of the fatty hilum. (Courtesy of Dr. Alexis Nees, Department of Radiology, University of Michigan, Ann Arbor, Michigan.)

Table 15-2. Sonographic Findings of Abnormal Lymph Nodes

Criteria	Findings
Size	Enlarged diameter
Shape	Rounding (unlike normal ovoid)
Echogenicity	Markedly hypoechoic cortex
Relationship	Obviously abnormal node adjacent to normal node consistent with malignancy; inflammation tends to affect multiple adjacent nodes in a cluster
Symmetry	Right-to-left asymmetry or symmetry
Color Doppler	Flow patterns may indicate hypervascularity, consistent with malignancy
Pulsed Doppler	Systolic/diastolic waveforms may be indicative of inflammation vs. malignancy
Morphologic abnormalities	Cortical thickening: uniform vs. eccentric
	Hilar compression: uniform vs. eccentric
	Hilar indentation: convex "rat bite"
	Hilar displacement
	Hilar obliteration
	Loss of echogenic outer capsule and angular margins

Adapted from Stavros AT: Breast Ultrasound. Philadelphia: Lippincott, 2004, Table 19-1.

patients—there were a number of valid concerns regarding its use. The most obvious concern was the accuracy of the procedure. False-negatives, caused by inadequate uptake of dye or nuclear colloid by lymphatics blocked by tumor emboli, were a very legitimate concern. Failure to properly identify the sentinel node can lead to missed axillary disease and inaccurate staging. This could lead not only to an increased axillary recurrence rate, but also to an increased distant recurrence rate if adjuvant chemotherapy decisions were based on erroneous information. These concerns prompted multiple studies involving SLN biopsy followed by complete axillary node dissection, examining the sensitivity, specificity, and accuracy of sentinel node biopsy. A multicenter validation study of sentinel node biopsy in breast cancer demonstrated a 93% identification rate, with 97% accuracy for determining positive or negative axillary involvement and a 100% specificity.[13] Subsequent studies have demonstrated false-negative rates ranging from 0% to 29%, with an average of 7.3% overall and up to 100% accuracy in determining axillary nodal status.[6,14-17] Table 15-3 lists the results of several studies published between 1997 and 1999 that examined the accuracy of sentinel node biopsy with radionuclide and blue dye lymphoscintigraphy.

Based on these reports, the SLN biopsy began to be adopted as clinical practice despite the fact that these studies were all pathologic in nature: looking for micrometastatic disease among the nonsentinel lymph nodes when the SLN showed no evidence of disease. As data accumulated, retrospective studies also suggested the safety of the procedure. A series of 2458 breast cancer patients treated at the Moffitt Cancer Center suggested that there is no survival or disease-free survival difference ($P = .98$) among node-negative patients treated by axillary node dissection compared with those treated with sentinel node biopsy alone.[18] The median follow-up for patients in the sentinel node group was relatively brief at 2 years.

No clinical trial of sentinel node biopsy compared with ALN dissection had been performed establishing sentinel node biopsy as the standard of care. NSABP B-32 opened in May 1999 and closed to accrual in February 2004 after randomizing 5611 patients. This study randomized women with surgically resectable invasive breast cancers and clinically negative axillae to undergo either sentinel node biopsy immediately followed by complete axillary dissection (group 1) versus SLN biopsy followed by ALN dissection only if the SLN biopsy was positive (group 2). All of the operations in this study were performed by surgeons who had undergone a standardized training program for axillary sentinel node biopsy procedures prior to patient randomization.[19]

The B-32 study was designed to address a number of issues concerning axillary management for breast cancer, specifically the accuracy of sentinel node biopsy in axillary staging and

Table 15-3. Results of Sentinel Lymph Node Biopsy Feasibility Studies Using Both Isosulfan Blue and Radioactive Isotope Injection for Mapping, 1997–1999

Author (Year of Publication)	No. of Patients	Identification Rate (%)	Accuracy (%)	Comments
Albertini[109] (1997)	62	92	100	
O'Hea[108] (1998)	60	93	95	
Barnwell[110] (1998)	42	90	100	
DeCicco[111] (1998)	382	98.7	96.8	Used combination of blue + tracer in 54/382 cases
Schneebaum[112] (1998)	30	93	NR	Both failed mappings had prior axillary radiation therapy
Nwariaku[113] (1998)	119	81	98.6	
Czerniecki[114] (1999)	42	95	100	
van der Ent[115] (1999)	70	100	NR	93–100% sensitivity
Bass[116] (1999)	700	95	99.2	
Burak[117] (1999)	50	90	100	
Jaderborg[118] (1999)	91 (79 analyzed)	81	98	

NR, not reported.

the impact on disease-free and overall survival of SLN biopsy alone among node-negative patients. Another goal of the B-32 study was a standardized assessment of the side effects of sentinel node biopsy compared with axillary clearance. Quality of life and formal measurements of function are being assessed as part of the study, examining specifically arm edema, arm mobility, and sensory neuropathy.

Julian and colleagues[20] presented the preliminary results from the B-32 study in December 2004. Initial review of the data demonstrated that sentinel node identification was 97%. Twenty-six percent of patients were found to have positive sentinel nodes. Of the patients who had positive sentinel node biopsies and went on to have complete lymph node dissections, 61.5% had disease limited to the sentinel nodes only. Looking at group 1, the overall accuracy of SLN biopsy was 97.2% with a negative predictive value of 96.1%. The false-negative rate was 9.7%. These data suggest that sentinel node biopsy is both a reliable and accurate method of axillary staging in experienced surgical hands. The follow-up period at the time of this publication has not been sufficient to produce further results; a comprehensive analysis of the patients will be performed after 300 deaths have been recorded.[5]

Patient Selection

Patients with invasive cancer and no clinical evidence of axillary disease are candidates for SLN biopsy. Patients with palpable axillary nodes or suspicious lymph nodes on axillary ultrasound should be initially evaluated by fine-needle aspiration, with or without ultrasound guidance. A positive needle aspirate is helpful in confirming a diagnosis of regional metastases and precluding the need for sentinel node biopsy. Negative or inconclusive needle aspirates, however, call for more invasive biopsy techniques. In some cases, the patient may proceed with SLN biopsy, but it is important for the surgeon to carefully examine the axilla for abnormal lymph nodes and excise these, even if they do not take up the radioactive colloid or the blue dye. In other cases, image-guided core needle biopsy or surgical lymph node excisional biopsy can be performed if the presence or absence of lymph node metastasis is a key component of the therapeutic algorithm.

Although SLN biopsy is primarily indicated in patients with invasive breast cancer, in some situations it may be considered in patients with ductal carcinoma in situ (DCIS). Patients undergoing mastectomy for DCIS are candidates for SLN biopsy. This is primarily done as a method for staging the axilla if an unexpected invasive component is identified within the mastectomy specimen. If invasive cancer is incidentally identified in a patient with DCIS undergoing a simple mastectomy without SLN biopsy, the only option for staging the axilla is a complete ALN dissection. Patients undergoing lumpectomy for DCIS do not require SLN biopsy because if an invasive component is discovered, they may return to the operating room. It is not unreasonable, however, to consider SLN biopsy in DCIS patients undergoing breast conservation in whom there is a strong clinical suspicion for an invasive component, such as in patients with DCIS presenting as a palpable mass or in those with extensive high-grade DCIS with comedonecrosis.

When SLN biopsy was first introduced clinically, its use was limited to small unicentric, invasive cancers. However, the success rates and accuracy of the procedure have subsequently been described in patient populations in which SLN biopsy was considered contraindicated. These include patients with multicentric cancers, patients with large (over 5 cm) primary tumors, and even patients with previous axillary surgery or breast irradiation. Many of these changes were prompted by alterations in the method of injection of the tracer (see below). In any such case, however, it falls on the judgment of the surgeon to decide whether SLN biopsy will give an accurate representation of the nodal status. If there is reasonable concern, either before or during the procedure, then ALN dissection should be performed.

Sentinel Lymph Node Procedure

Sentinel node biopsy is a multistep procedure, involving perioperative localization followed by intraoperative nodal excision. The method of nodal localization has been a subject of much investigation, using different timing sequences, agents, and injection techniques to determine the optimum procedure for identifying the sentinel node.[21]

The initial description of the sentinel node procedure used blue dye only as a method of localizing the SLN. Today, the most common approach to SLN biopsy is the use of a combination of tracers, most commonly technetium-99m (^{99m}Tc) and isosulfan blue dye (Lymphazurin). The application of both a nuclear tracer and blue dye does increase the sensitivity, specificity, and accuracy of sentinel node identification.[15,22–24] However, blue dye alone has a sentinel node identification rate ranging from 77% to 92%, making sentinel node biopsy feasible in facilities that lack nuclear medicine capabilities.[15,23,25,26]

The timing and technique of the injection of these tracers for sentinel node localization have been extensively researched. The procedure typically begins with the injection of the ^{99m}Tc, a radiotracer bound to a colloid substance that travels through the lymphatic system. Sulfur colloid is the molecule commonly used in the United States; albumin is often the preferred compound overseas. In the United States, ^{99m}Tc sulfur colloid is available as unfiltered or filtered, having been passed through a 22 μm filter. Filtration eliminates much of the heterogeneity found in the sulfur colloid molecules, theoretically producing a more concentrated and easily localized radioactive signal when explored with a gamma probe.[27] A number of studies have been performed examining the clinical benefit of using filtered versus unfiltered ^{99m}Tc. However, the results have failed to demonstrate a clear advantage of one over the other.[27–29]

Often the injections are performed on the morning of surgery, with lymphoscintigraphy performed 2 hours after injection. This can complicate surgical scheduling because cases involving SLN biopsies cannot begin until late morning. Several studies have demonstrated no difference in node identification rates using ^{99m}Tc between 2 and 24 hours after injection, a fact that often simplifies the logistics of scheduling surgery by allowing the injection to take place the night before.[30–32]

The technique of injection for sentinel node localization has also been examined by several institutions for both the radioactive colloid and the blue dye. Originally, injections were always performed peritumorally based on the concept that this would be the most accurate anatomically. The peritumoral technique involves injection of the tracer in the breast parenchyma surrounding the tumor or the cavity of the excisional biopsy. However, this requires that the person injecting the tracer (often a nuclear medicine technician) knows where the tumor is, which for nonpalpable lesions can be an issue. In addition, accidental injection into the biopsy cavity results in a failure of localization. Subsequent studies have shown that other methods of injection are equally accurate, if not more so. Periareolar, subareolar, and intradermal injections all have been used in various studies with blue dye as well as radioactive colloid. Intradermal injections still require knowledge of the tumor location, and unless the skin overlying the tumor is resected, they leave residual radiation and blue dye. For tumors in the upper outer quadrant, false gamma counter signals—colloquially referred to as "shine-through"—from a peritumoral or intradermal ^{99m}Tc injection can make identification of the SLN difficult.[33,34] Many surgeons advocate periareolar or subareolar injections for the radioactive colloid. This simplifies the procedure since the person injecting the tracer does not need to know the location of the breast tumor. This also prevents the shine-through phenomenon for upper outer quadrant tumors.

Before coming to the operating room, the patient typically undergoes lymphoscintigraphy (Fig. 15-5). Imaging of the sentinel node with nuclear lymphangiography is a useful but not essential aspect of axillary staging. Several large multicenter studies demonstrated that lymphangiographic imaging does not add significantly to the identification rates of sentinel nodes. The sensitivity of the hand-held gamma probe and visualization of the blue dye are more important factors in sentinel node identification, since a number of patients without sentinel nodes on lymphoscintigram are likely to have focal nodal uptake on intraoperative examination. Nuclear lymphoscintigraphy plays a greater role in patients undergoing reoperative axillary surgery, who may have aberrant drainage pathways, and for assessing extra-axillary nodal drainage patterns (see text that follows).[35]

Once the patient is in the operating room, injection of the blue dye takes place. Although most surgeons use isosulfan blue dye for this, some centers report using methylene blue, citing fewer allergic reactions, with similar efficacy.[36,37] Allergic reaction to the blue dye is an important complication for the surgeon to keep in mind

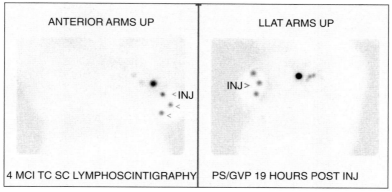

Figure 15-5. Nuclear lymphoscintigraphy demonstrating an ipsilateral sentinel node. Note the lymphatic drainage channels that demonstrate fainter uptake along the chest wall. LLAT, left lateral. (Courtesy of Dr. John Cahill, Department of Nuclear Medicine, University of Michigan, Ann Arbor, Michigan.)

during this portion of the procedure and to discuss preoperatively with the patient. Allergic reactions can occur in 1% to 2% of patients. Most involve urticaria, blue hives, or pruritus; however, about 0.5% may have bronchospasm and hypotension.[38] If the patient is undergoing general anesthesia, it is reasonable to delay the injection of the blue dye until the airway is secured. Allergic reaction should be considered in any patient experiencing hypotension in whom blue dye was used and is readily managed with fluid resuscitation and short-term pressor support.

The method of injection for the blue dye can be peritumoral, intradermal, or subareolar. Many studies suggest the superiority of intradermal injection compared with subdermal or deeper peritumoral breast injections. Injection of the dermal lymphatics is felt to drain the marker faster to the axilla than does injection into the breast parenchyma.[21,39-41] However, intradermal or subareolar injections of blue dye may cause tattooing of the nipple or skin, which may persist for months in patients undergoing breast conservation. In a patient undergoing a mastectomy, either an intradermal or subareolar injection of the blue dye seems ideal. For the patient undergoing lumpectomy, intradermal injection can be used if the overlying skin is to be resected with the tumor. Otherwise, a peritumoral injection of the blue dye provides adequate localization without leaving the breast tattooed for an extended period of time. Table 15-4 summarizes the advantages and disadvantages of the various injection substances and techniques.

Nodal excision is typically performed through a small axillary incision, posterior to the lateral border of the pectoral muscle. Preoperative scanning with the gamma probe is often helpful in planning the incision. The incision should be easily incorporated into an incision for a subsequent ALN dissection. Nodes stained blue or with attached blue lymphatic channels, or with evidence of radioactivity on the gamma probe, are excised intact and sent in formalin for pathologic review (Figs. 15-6 and 15-7). In addition, nodes that are palpably firm or enlarged should also be excised. The procedure is considered complete after scanning with the gamma probe fails to reveal further radioactive counts greater than 10% of the highest count detected.

Pathologic Examination of Sentinel Lymph Nodes

A key feature of sentinel node biopsy is the detailed pathologic review. By focusing on a few nodes rather than the entire axilla, which may contain up to 40 lymph nodes, a more thorough examination of each node in the sentinel node specimen is feasible. Sentinel nodes are routinely multiply sectioned and examined on routine hematoxylin and eosin (H&E) staining (Figs. 15-8 through 15-10). Compared with bivalving the SLN, several studies have demonstrated the importance of obtaining multiple sections in detecting axillary metastases. Many centers also examine nodal sections with immunohistochemistry (IHC), a more sensitive method of detecting metastatic cells. The usefulness of immunohistochemistry staining is discussed in further detail later in the text.

Table 15-4. Potential Advantages and Disadvantages of Various Lymphatic Mapping Techniques

Issue	Advantages	Disadvantages
Use of filter for radiocolloid Unfiltered (average particle size 50–1000 nm)	Fewer SLNs; less extensive nodal extraction Less uptake to higher echelon nodes	Fewer SLNs; ?increased risk of SLN nonidentification Slower transit
Filtered (average particle size <200 nm)	More SLNs; lower risk of SLN nonidentification More rapid transit	More SLNs; possible increased risk of morbidity related to larger volume of lymphatic tissue resected Increase uptake to higher echelon nodes
Mapping injection site Intraparenchymal (peritumoral)	Conceptually the "purest" mapping route in replicating intramammary lymphatic path from breast tumor to sentinel node(s)	Difficult for nonpalpable tumors Risk of injecting into Bx cavity ?Accuracy with multiple tumors Shine-through/background counts
Dermal	Rapid lymphatic uptake ↑ SLN identification rate Easier with nonpalpable tumors, but requires marking of skin overlying lesion Less shine-through	?Accuracy with multiple tumors ?Accurate reflection of lymphatic pathway for underlying breast parenchyma May require image-guided marking of skin site overlying nonpalpable tumor
Subareolar	Rapid lymphatic uptake Less shine-through Can be used for multiple breast tumors ?More physiologic, based on embryologic lymphatic system development	?Accurate reflection of lymphatic pathway for underlying breast parenchyma "Blue breast" syndrome
Preop lymphoscintigraphy Yes; routine use of preop scan	Documents primary drainage pattern and volume of SLNs Guides internal mammary SLN dissection, if deemed appropriate Guides timing of surgery when performed on same day	Time Cost Less sensitive than intraoperative probe; radioactive SLN frequently identified in cases of negative preop scan
No preop scan	Saves time Saves cost	Uncertainty regarding lymphatic drainage pattern
Timing of isotope injection Same day as surgery	Single visit for patient Single intervention/wire localization if patient has nonpalpable lesion and IP mapping is desired	May prolong and complicate day of surgery in cases of slow lymphatic transit Disruptive to surgery schedule
One day preop	Facilitates planning/timing of operating room schedule Extends mapping period for cases of slow lymphatic transit	Additional hospital visit required Additional intervention/wire localization necessary if patient has nonpalpable lesion and IP mapping is desired ?Increased drainage to higher-echelon nodes

IP, intraparenchymal; SLN, sentinel lymph node; XRT, radiation therapy.
From Newman LA: Lymphatic mapping and sentinel lymph node biopsy in breast cancer patients: a comprehensive review of variations in performance and technique. J Am Coll Surg 199(5):804–816, 2004.

Intraoperative evaluation of sentinel nodes has been investigated in a number of studies in hopes of sparing patients from multiple operations for axillary staging and clearance. Frozen-section analysis of SLNs has proved to be accurate for identifying macrometastatic lesions. However, this adds considerable time to the procedure, and there is some concern that frozen section significantly decreases the subsequent detection of micrometastases.[42–44] Touch-prep protocols provide a rapid approach to sentinel node diagnosis, with sensitivity ranging from 40% to 95.7%.[44–46] Combining immunohisto-chemistry with intraoperative touch-prep

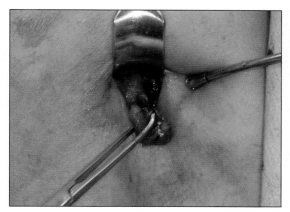

Figure 15-6. This photograph illustrates a blue lymphatic channel leading into a normal-colored lymph node. (Courtesy of Dr. M. Catherine Lee, Department of Surgery, University of Michigan, Ann Arbor, Michigan.)

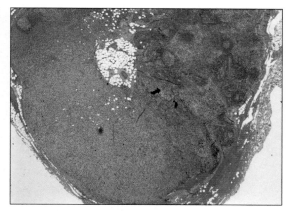

Figure 15-8. This lymph node shows reactive follicles on the right, but is replaced by metastatic lobular carcinoma on the lower left side. The loss of normal nodal architecture indicates malignancy. (Courtesy of Dr. Michael Hayes, Department of Pathology, University of Michigan, Ann Arbor, Michigan.)

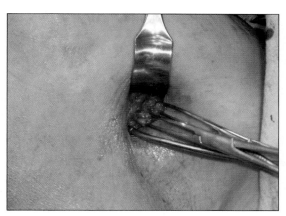

Figure 15-7. A blue-stained sentinel node (*left*) next to a normal-appearing unstained lymph node. (Courtesy of Dr. M. Catherine Lee, Department of Surgery, University of Michigan, Ann Arbor, Michigan.)

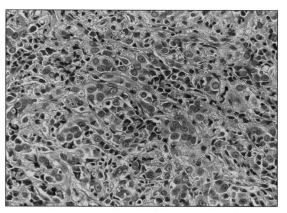

Figure 15-9. High-power view of metastatic lobular carcinoma cells seen in Figure 15-7. The malignant cells demonstrate enlarged monotonous nuclei with prominent nucleoli. (Courtesy of Dr. Michael Hayes, Department of Pathology, University of Michigan, Ann Arbor, Michigan.)

increases the sensitivity to around 80%. Although a negative SLN biopsy result intraoperatively does not completely preclude a return to the operating room for subsequently discovered metastases, it does spare many women the need for a second operation.

Controversies in Sentinel Lymph Node Biopsy

Immunohistochemistry-Detected Micrometastases

With increased scrutiny of the SLN, smaller and smaller metastases can be identified. Although it seems reasonable to presume that the discovery

of any disease in a lymph node would portend a worse prognosis, this is not necessarily the case. Several retrospective studies of patients with negative ALN dissection have involved reexamining the lymph nodes by serial sectioning and immunohistochemistry, and the outcomes of patients with occult metastases were compared with those without occult metastases. Although some studies found a worse outcome associated with micrometastases,[47–50] most found no negative impact on prognosis[51–58] (Table 15-5).

The significance of immunohistochemistry-detected micrometastases is further called into

Table 15-5. Studies of Micrometastases in Node-Negative Invasive Breast Cancer

Author (Year of Publication)	Total Patients	Patients with Micrometastatic-only Nodes	Conclusions
Langer et al[58] (2005)	234	27	All patients with micrometastatic-only SLN disease were disease-free at mean follow-up of 42 months
Carcoforo et al[65] (2002)	210	18	Tumor cells unlikely in non-SLN with small primary and only micrometastatic involvement in SLN; ALN dissection likely not necessary
Liang et al[126] (2001)	227	15	No evidence of local recurrence after mean follow-up of 13.5 months
Clare et al[50] (1997)	86	11	Occult metastases shorten the disease-free interval; recommend more thorough axillary staging
de Mascarel et al[56] (1992)	1680 89 129	120 (SMS) 37 (ILC by IH only) 13 (IDC by IH only)	Micrometastasis on SMS have prognostic significance. Micrometastasis of ILC has no clinical significance; IDCs are of uncertain prognostic significance
Chen et al[127] (1991)	80	23	3 of 17 patients developed distant metastases less than 3 years from surgery
Attiyeh et al[128] (1977)	105		Survival at 10 and 14 years = 85% and 77% with micrometastasis only

ALN, axillary lymph node; IDC, infiltrating ductal carcinoma; IH, immunohistochemistry; ILC, infiltrating lobular carcinoma; SLN, sentinel lymph node; SMS, serial macroscopic sectioning.

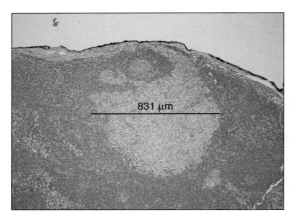

831 μm

Figure 15-10. Micrometastatic (0.831 mm) focus of ductal carcinoma in an axillary lymph node (greater than 0.2 mm but less than 2.0 mm). A small cluster of benign macrophages is seen at the lower left of the micrometastasis; note the similar cytoplasmic color but less crowded nuclei. (Courtesy of Dr. Michael Hayes, Department of Pathology, University of Michigan, Ann Arbor, Michigan.)

question by the DCIS literature. Micrometastatic disease can be detected in up to 10% of patients undergoing SLN biopsy for DCIS, which has a nearly 99% survival rate and for which axillary recurrences are extremely rare.[59,60] In addition, three studies have demonstrated that immunohistochemistry-detected micrometastases correlate more with the method of biopsy than with the biology of the cancer, sug-

gesting that they may be an artifact rather than a biologic phenomenon.[61-63] Thus, the available evidence does not support the routine use of immunohistochemistry in the evaluation of the SLN.[64] Immunohistochemistry may be used selectively, such as in the case of lobular carcinoma, which may be difficult to identify in the lymph node. If metastases are detected by immunohistochemistry, their presence should be confirmed on H&E.

Patients with micrometastases less than 0.2 mm are considered node-negative (current American Joint Committee on Cancer [AJCC] staging stages these patients as N0mic) and have not been considered for completion dissection or adjuvant chemotherapy based on their nodal status. Recent data, however, suggest that micrometastases may be associated with a reduced 5-year rate of disease-free survival and may benefit from adjuvant chemotherapy.[66] Pending data from recent prospective trials are hoped to help clarify these issues.

Drainage to Internal Mammary Lymph Nodes

The updated AJCC staging system expanded the nodal classifications based on the presence of the internal mammary node (IMN) involvement. Patients with gross disease in the internal mammary node chain on clinical exam or on nonlymphoscintigraphic imaging are considered N2b; patients with concurrent gross axillary and internal mammary node involvement have N3 disease. Microscopic evidence of tumor in a clinically normal-appearing internal mammary nodal basin alone is staged pN1b.

With the advent of lymphoscintigraphy, biopsy of clinically silent internal mammary nodes has become a point of much contention. Between 5% and 10% of patients undergoing lymphoscintigraphy have evidence of radioactivity at the ipsilateral internal mammary node chain. This is partly dependent on the method of injection. Internal mammary drainage is more commonly seen after peritumoral injection and much less so after subareolar or intradermal injection. Intraoperative identification and biopsy of internal mammary nodes are technically challenging, and a significant percentage of patients with positive lymphoscintigraphy do not have localizable nodes at the time of surgery.[65,67–69] Furthermore, the clinical significance of microscopic internal mammary node metastases is still unclear. In the few studies examining internal mammary node sampling, between 0% and 6% of patients with positive lymphoscintigraphy have tumor involvement of the internal mammary node, and its impact on adjuvant therapeutic decision making is variable since many patients with internal mammary node disease have axillary involvement as well.[65,67–69] However, the presence of metastases is critical for proper staging and adjuvant planning, and detection of internal mammary nodes may alter the decision-making process.[70] Some studies even suggest that internal mammary node evaluation may be more accurate than axillary nodal staging.[71] Unfortunately, little consensus exists regarding the ideal management when the lymphoscintogram demonstrates drainage to the internal mammary lymph nodes. In patients who drain only to the internal mammary node, or to both the internal mammary node and axillary nodes, the surgeon should consider each patient individually and consider the possible impact on subsequent therapy decisions if internal mammary node metastases are identified.

Axillary Management in Neoadjuvant Chemotherapy Patients

Before the introduction of SLN biopsy as a method of staging the axilla, there was little consequence surgically regarding whether or not patients received neoadjuvant chemotherapy, because either way they would be receiving an ALN dissection. The most significant impact of preoperative therapy was that some patients who may have been node-positive initially were node-negative after chemotherapy. Therefore, their true nodal status remained unknown. This did not alter their surgery, and at the time there was less use of nodal status in guiding radiation therapy. This changed dramatically as lymphatic mapping and SLN biopsy became standard in the surgical therapy of breast cancer. Now patients who opted for neoadjuvant chemotherapy to shrink their primary tumor were obligated to undergo ALN dissection as part of their surgery, whereas those who had surgery first could opt for a sentinel node biopsy and avoid ALN dissection if they were node-negative.

Another change that has taken place has been larger role of the nodal status in therapy decisions. Two examples include reserving the use of taxanes or dose-dense regimens for patients known to be node-positive and the use of postmastectomy radiation or the inclusion of the internal mammary nodes in the radiation fields of node-positive patients. These practices made it more important to know prior to therapy whether the patient was node-positive. Thus, the question arose of how to best integrate SLN biopsy with neoadjuvant chemotherapy for clinically node-negative breast cancer.

Sentinel node biopsy is necessary only in clinically node-negative patients. Patients with palpable disease in the lymph nodes can have this confirmed by fine-needle aspiration and proceed with neoadjuvant chemotherapy with a planned ALN dissection at the completion of systemic therapy. Clinically node-negative candidates for neoadjuvant chemotherapy should have an ultrasound of the axilla to check for abnormal lymph nodes. Ultrasound-guided fine-needle aspiration can then document these patients to be node-positive prior to neoadjuvant chemotherapy.[72,73] For patients who are clinically and ultrasonographically node-negative, there are two options for the use of SLN biopsy if they are candidates for neoadjuvant chemotherapy.

The first option is to perform the SLN biopsy before beginning chemotherapy[74–76] Among the several advantages of this approach is that the true nodal status is known before initiating chemotherapy, which may be important in deciding what regimen and schedule to use. This may also help the radiation oncologist decide whether to recommend postmastectomy radiation if the patient does not become a candidate for breast conservation. This is why these decisions are often best made in a multidisciplinary setting. Another advantage of sentinel node biopsy before chemotherapy is that it can give physicians increased confidence in the feasibility and accuracy of the procedure because of concern that chemotherapy may affect the lymphatic drainage and make identification of the SLN more difficult. Performing SLN biopsy after chemotherapy presumes that any disease in the lymph nodes will either completely disappear from all the nodes, or will remain in the sentinel node. However, if disease is eradicated from the sentinel node, but not the nonsentinel nodes, this can lead to a false-negative finding. There are, however, disadvantages to this approach, primarily that performing SLN biopsy before beginning chemotherapy means an extra procedure and a delay in the initiation of therapy.

The second option is to perform the SLN biopsy *after* completing chemotherapy.[77-80] Several studies of SLN biopsy performed after neoadjuvant chemotherapy have suggested an unacceptably high false-negative rate, but overall this approach seems to be reasonable.[81] Although a clear disadvantage of postchemotherapy sentinel node biopsy is not knowing the true pretreatment nodal status, if it does not impact the chemotherapy or radiation decisions, it is less of a factor. Regarding postmastectomy radiation, an argument could be made that the nodal status after chemotherapy might serve as a better indicator of whether to offer radiation to the chest wall. Delaying the SLN biopsy until after chemotherapy also allows the chemotherapy to start immediately and may preclude the need for additional surgery. The most important advantage of SLN biopsy after chemotherapy is that patients who may have been node-positive before chemotherapy and node-negative after chemotherapy can be spared from ALN dissection. Approximately 20% of patients may be converted from node-positive to node-negative,[82,83] and SLN biopsy *before* chemotherapy would obligate those patients to undergo ALN dissection.

Sentinel Node Biopsy and Breast Reconstruction

Sentinel node biopsy may be performed in the setting of breast conservation or in conjunction with a total mastectomy. In patients with a known plan for postoperative radiation therapy, breast reconstruction is often delayed until the completion of radiation. This is particularly true when reconstruction is to be performed with tissue expanders and implants, but reconstruction with autologous flaps is also commonly delayed when it is known that chest wall radiation is needed. Postreconstruction radiation therapy may have significant deleterious effects, including poor wound healing, infection, flap atrophy, and implant extrusion, in addition to suboptimal cosmetic outcomes.[84]

The use of SLN biopsy with mastectomy and immediate reconstruction opens up the possibility that if the SLN is positive, the patient may be a candidate for postmastectomy radiation (see Chapter 16, Radiation Oncology). Thus, the implementation of SLN biopsy in a woman undergoing mastectomy with immediate reconstruction is one of timing. Many institutions opt to perform the SLN biopsy as a separate procedure before the mastectomy. If the result is negative, the patient may proceed with mastectomy and reconstruction. If positive and the patient desires postmastectomy radiation, the reconstruction can be delayed. An alternate approach has been the immediate delayed reconstruction for highly selected patients.[84-86] Finally, there is the option for women with invasive disease to simply undergo mastectomy and SLN biopsy alone, delaying reconstruction until the results of the pathologic axillary review are known.[87] Patients undergoing total mastectomy and sentinel node biopsy for DCIS are often considered good candidates for immediate breast reconstruction, since the likelihood of postmastectomy radiation is extremely low.

Re-Staging of the Axilla after In-Breast Recurrence

Accompanying the improved overall survival of breast cancer patients and the increasing role of breast conservation therapy is the growing population of women with in-breast recurrences. For patients who have undergone previous breast conservation followed by locoregional radiation, salvage mastectomy is the operation of choice with regard to the breast itself. However, the appropriate axillary staging procedure for these patients is not as clear-cut. Patients previously treated for invasive cancer have all undergone some form of axillary staging with their prior operation. In the past, this was always an ALN dissection, but an increasing population of patients with in-breast recurrences have intact ALNs, having previously had a negative SLN biopsy.

The initial SLN studies were performed in patients with primary breast cancers; sentinel node techniques were discouraged in previously operated axillae because of concerns regarding altered drainage patterns and the resulting potential inaccuracy.[88] Therefore, a woman treated by lumpectomy and SLN biopsy who had an in-breast recurrence had two options: simple mastectomy alone, which may ignore metastases from the recurrence to the regional nodes, or a modified radical mastectomy, with the resultant risk of lymphedema. Recently, a number of small studies have demonstrated the feasibility and accuracy of sentinel node biopsy for in-breast recurrence.

The feasibility of sentinel node biopsy in patients with recurrent breast cancer has been addressed in several retrospective studies (Table 15-6), the first being a landmark study from Memorial Sloan-Kettering Cancer Center in 2002.[89] There is a markedly lower sentinel node identification rate in reoperative lymphatic mapping compared with initial lymphatic mapping procedures, with most studies having an identification rate in the 60% to 68% range, compared with 93% to 97% identification in primary sentinel node biopsies. Although the sentinel node identification rate for these patients is significantly lower than in primary breast cancers, this is still a reasonable success rate that can spare a large number of women from unnecessary ALN dissection.

For patients who have had a negative SLN biopsy, intraoperative lymphatic mapping and SLN biopsy is reasonable, with ALN dissection reserved for patients with demonstrated metastases. The surgeon plans ahead of time what will occur if the lymphatic mapping is unsuccessful. It must also be remembered that patients with previous axillary surgery may have aberrant axillary drainage, including drainage to the internal mammary or supraclavicular

or contralateral axilla. Again, when planning remapping of a patient with a local recurrence, the surgeon must be prepared to chase the SLN to more unusual locations. For patients with a previous lumpectomy and ALN dissection presenting with an in-breast recurrence, the success rate of SLN biopsy is much lower and the incidence of aberrant axillary drainage is much higher (Fig. 15-11). Although intraoperative lymphatic mapping and SLN biopsy may still be attempted, the decision to proceed must be based on how the information will affect further treatment. Again, presentation of these patients in a multidisciplinary setting facilitates these decisions.

Management of the Clinically Positive Axilla

Axillary Lymph Node Dissection

Whether the disease was identified by physical examination, axillary ultrasound, or SLN biopsy, ALN dissection remains the standard of care for patients with known involvement of the ALNs. The few patients in whom a sentinel node cannot be identified, even intraoperatively, are also candidates for primary complete axillary lymphadenectomy for staging purposes. The axillary dissection for breast cancer involves en bloc resection of the level I and level II lymph nodes. The axilla is anatomically defined posteriorly by the subscapularis and latissimus dorsi muscles, medially by the chest wall and the overlying serratus anterior muscle, laterally by the skin and subcutaneous tissue of the underarm area, and superiorly by the axillary vein. These anatomic boundaries do not imply that lymph nodes do not reside above the vein, but that they rarely possess metastases from breast cancer, and their routine dissection exposes the brachial plexus to injury. This area encompasses the intercostobrachial nerve(s), the thoracodorsal bundle, and the long thoracic nerve, which are often intimately involved with the soft tissue and lymphatics of the surgical specimen.

The thoracodorsal bundle, consisting of a nerve, artery, and vein, contains the major blood supply and innervation to the latissimus dorsi. Disruption of the thoracodorsal nerve results in weakness during abduction and medial rotation of the shoulder. The long thoracic nerve is the sole motor nerve to the serratus anterior, a thin,

Table 15-6. Reported Series of Sentinel Lymph Node Biopsy for Locally Recurrent Breast Cancer

Study	Institution	N	SLN ID Rate			Proportion of Local Recurrence Cases with Aberrant Lymphatic Drainage			Proportion of Local Recurrence Cases with Metastatic SLNs	
			Total	Cases with Prior ALN Dissection	Cases with Prior SLN	Total	Cases with Prior ALN Dissection	Cases with Prior SLN	Total	Metastases in Aberrant SLNs
Port[89] (2002)	Memorial Sloan-Kettering	22	15/22	8/14	7/8	NR	NR	NR	3/22	NR
Dinan[119] (2005)	Beaumont Hospital	16	11/16	9/14	2/2	7/11	5/9	2/2	0	0
Intra[120] (2005)	European Institute of Oncology	18	18/18	0/0	18/18	0/18	0/0	0/18	2/18	0/0
Agarwal[121] (2006)	University of Pittsburgh Cancer Institute	2	2/2	2/2	0/0	2/2	2/2	0/0	1/2	1/2
Taback[122] (2006)	John Wayne Cancer Institute	15	11/15	6/9	5/6	7/11	4/5	3/5	3/11	2/7
Newman[123] (2006)	University of Michigan	10	9/10	6/7	1/1	7/9	0/0	7/7	0/9	0/7
Boughey[124] (2006)	M.D. Anderson Cancer Center	21*	13/21	6/12	5/5	6/21	5/12	1/5	1/21	0/6
Port[125] (2006)	Memorial Sloan-Kettering	117	117/117	24/63	40/54	19/63†	NR‡	NR‡	10/64	2/19

Stratification of results by clinicopathologic features has been extrapolated from reports in studies in which these features were not directly reported.

ALN, axillary lymph node; SLN, sentinel lymph node.

*Four patients had no prior axillary surgery at time of local recurrence.

†Sixty-three patients from total study sample had successful lymphoscintigraphy.

‡Number of cases with prior ALN dissection versus prior SLN and reoperative aberrant SLN not specified, but report comments on higher risk for aberrant drainage among cases of prior ALN dissection.

From Newman LA: Lymphatic mapping and sentinel lymph node biopsy for locally-recurrent breast cancer: new clues to understanding the biology of chest wall relapse. *Ann Surg Oncol* 14:2182–2184, 2007.

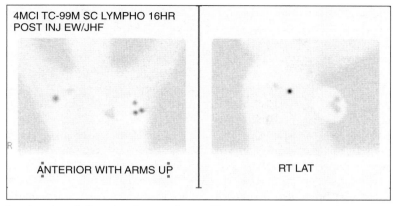

4MCI TC-99M SC LYMPHO 16HR
POST INJ EW/JHF

ANTERIOR WITH ARMS UP   RT LAT

Figure 15-11. Nuclear lymphoscintigraphy after previous axillary surgery demonstrating contralateral axillary and ipsilateral internal mammary sentinel node uptake. (Courtesy of Dr. John Cahill, Department of Nuclear Medicine, University of Michigan, Ann Arbor, Michigan.)

flat muscle primarily responsible for anchoring the scapula to the posterior chest wall. Injury to the long thoracic nerve results in "winging" of the scapula, in which the medial edge of scapula protrudes involuntarily and uncomfortably from the posterior thorax.

Axillary dissection is accomplished in concert with mastectomy (modified radical mastectomy) via an oblique elliptical mastectomy incision or through a separate incision through a curvilinear incision connecting the anterior and posterior axillary lines, just inferior to the axillary hairline (Fig. 15-12). Adequate exposure and careful dissection are vital for the preservation of the delicate structures passing through the axilla. The upper extremity is routinely prepped and draped into the field for intraoperative mobility of the shoulder and arm region, providing improved exposure of the apical axillary structures.

Superior and inferior flaps are raised, taking care not to make the flaps too thin because this does not increase the amount of lymph nodes removed and can lead to a more pronounced cosmetic defect in the axilla. Once the flaps are raised, the next step is to identify three landmarks: the pectoralis major and minor muscles, the axillary vein, and the latissimus dorsi muscle. There are several approaches to the ALN dissection, which involve identifying the relevant structures in varying order, each of which is acceptable. With the pectoralis major muscle retracted medially, the pectoralis minor muscle is exposed and the investing fascia opened. During the exposure of the muscles, it is impor-

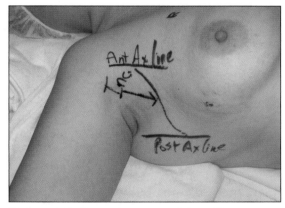

Figure 15-12. External anatomy of the axilla.
Exposure of the axilla for clearance is obtained via an incision (Inc), which spans the anterior to posterior axillary lines, just caudal to the inferior hairline. (Courtesy of Dr. Lisa A. Newman, Department of Surgery, University of Michigan, Ann Arbor, Michigan.)

tant to identify and preserve the medial pectoral neurovascular bundle. Cutting the nerve causes atrophy of a portion of the pectoralis muscle. The latissimus dorsi muscle is identified at the inferior aspect of the axilla and then exposed superiorly, staying on the anterior edge of the muscle to avoid injury to the thoracodorsal bundle. The latissimus dorsi muscle should be exposed to the point at which the axillary vein crosses it. During this dissection, the intercostobrachial nerves are encountered. Preserving these nerves, though adding time to the procedure, prevents numbness of the upper inner arm.

The axillary vein is often encountered during the exposure of the latissimus dorsi and can be cleared in a lateral to medial fashion. Dissection superior to the axillary vein can result in injury to the brachial plexus, which is one of the most debilitating complications of the procedure. Once the vein is identified, dissection should be along the inferior aspect, since skeletonizing the entire anterior surface of the vein may increase the potential for lymphedema. This dissection is greatly facilitated by retracting the axillary contents caudally. As the fat is dissected from the vein, the branches of the axillary vein are divided and ligated with 3–0 silk sutures.

The thoracodorsal vein is usually identified as the first deep branch off the axillary vein as one moves medially. The artery is often seen in close proximity. At this point, the nerve is not typically running with the vein, but located more medially. It eventually joins the vein and artery as they course toward the latissimus dorsi muscle. An alternate method involves identifying the bundle medial to the latissimus and tracking it toward the vein. The long thoracic nerve is identified along the serratus anterior muscle. With these structures identified, the fibrofatty tissue can be safely excised. With medial rotation of the arm and relaxation of the pectoralis major and minor muscles, the level II nodes are included in the dissection. Failure to satisfactorily mobilize the pectoralis minor muscle and include the underlying level II nodes results in an increased regional recurrence rate. The highest level of the axilla should be marked for the pathologist because involvement of these nodes by cancer may impact the radiation fields. A closed-suction drain is placed in the axillary fossa at the end of the operation to prevent seroma formation and is left in place until the drainage decreases sufficiently.

Complications of Axillary Surgery

Patients undergoing axillary surgery—either SLN biopsy or ALN dissection—may experience short-term or long-term complications. Most common are seroma formation in the immediate postoperative period and numbness and paresthesias of the upper arm, especially if the intercostobrachial nerve is divided during the course of the operation. However, the most common complication—and the most feared—is lymphedema. Although uncommon after SLN biopsy alone, the incidence of lymphedema in patients undergoing axillary clearance ranges from 2% to 30%.[90-92] Part of the difficulty in estimating the incidence of lymphedema lies in the variability of the assessment tools used to determine the degree of swelling. In some reports, lymphedema is defined as a subjective complaint by the patient or by an examiner documenting a noticeable difference in arm circumference. In other reports, all patients underwent routine circumferential measurements, typically performed at 10 cm above and 10 cm below the elbow. Lymphedema is defined as a difference in limb circumference of more than 2 cm in some studies and more than 4 cm in others. In still other cases, volumetric measurements are obtained by submerging the arms in water, with lymphedema defined as a greater than 20% difference between the two limbs. Obviously, the way one looks for and defines lymphedema impacts the reported incidence.[93]

Lymphedema may have an indolent course, developing years after the initial surgery. Limb trauma, cellulitis, and obesity may all further impair the lymphatic drainage of the arm, increasing the risk of lymphedema. The addition of radiation to an axillary dissection field also increases the risk of postoperative lymphedema.[94-96] A retrospective review performed at Roswell Park investigated the incidence of lymphedema in patients receiving postmastectomy radiation therapy (PMRT) for locally advanced breast cancer. In 105 of these patients, 27% developed lymphedema. Total dose and posterior axillary boost doses were significantly associated with upper extremity lymphedema.[96]

Lymphedema prevention and treatment are multifaceted. Although up to 20% to 30% of women may develop some lymphedema after ALN dissection, only a small percentage develop lymphedema severe enough to impair the range of motion in their upper extremity or otherwise decrease the function of their upper extremity. All patients undergoing axillary dissection should be instructed that postoperatively it is important to maintain an ideal body weight, avoid tight or constricting garments or jewelry, and avoid even minor injuries to the hand and arm. Box 15-1 is a summary of recommendations for preventing lymphedema. If swelling develops,

Box 15-1. Recommendations after Axillary Lymph Node Dissection to Avoid Lymphedema

- Use the opposite arm for intravenous cathethers, blood draws, injections, and blood pressure measurements. Always inform all doctors and nurses that you have had a lymph node dissection on that side.
- Avoid cuts, scratches, and burns to your hand and arm by wearing long sleeves and/or gloves when doing cooking, gardening, household projects, etc. If you cut yourself, wash immediately with soap and water and apply an antiseptic. Notify your physician about any redness or swelling.
- Do not wear tight or constricting jewelry or clothing. Bra straps should be wide and padded and should not cut into the skin.
- Avoid heavy lifting with the dissected arm. Try not to carry a purse or suitcase on that side when possible. Avoid repetitive heavy lifting in particular, and wear a compression sleeve if lifting is necessary.
- Avoid sunburn of the arm by wearing long sleeves and sunscreen.
- Do not pick at cuticles or hangnails.
- Use insect repellents.
- Avoid high temperatures (saunas or hot tubs, reaching into hot ovens or clothes driers).
- Shave under the arm with an electric razor rather than a blade.
- Wear a compression sleeve on the arm when traveling on an airplane.
- Maintain an ideal body weight.

limb elevation and compression garments are commonly prescribed for the affected hand, forearm, or upper arm. Special massage techniques may also be applied by trained therapists to try to improve lymphatic drainage from the arm.

Alternatives to Axillary Lymph Node Dissection for the Sentinel Lymph Node–Positive Patient

Just as lumpectomy greatly minimized the morbidity of breast surgery compared with mastectomy, SLN biopsy has done the same for axillary surgery compared with ALN dissection. As described in the previous text, ALN dissection may be safely avoided in the 80% of women with negative sentinel nodes. What about the 20% of patients with a positive sentinel node? Nearly 50% of patients with a positive SLN biopsy result have additional disease in the non-SLNs.[97–100] Documenting the number of involved nodes provides further staging information,

which may impact adjuvant chemotherapy and radiation decisions, since multiple involved lymph nodes are associated with increased recurrence rates and decreased survival. In many patients, however, simply knowing that the patient is node-positive or node-negative may be enough information to determine the remainder of the therapy. In such patients, is there a therapeutic benefit to gaining regional control, or can these patients be observed, with ALN dissection performed only if they recur?

Since almost all patients with node-positive SLN receive adjuvant systemic therapy, regional recurrence in this situation may be extremely low. However, even if recurrence does occur and the patient undergoes a delayed ALN dissection, would this have an impact on survival? As previously mentioned, the NSABP B-04 trial specifically addressed this issue, and after a 25-year follow-up, did not demonstrate any difference in overall survival among patients undergoing axillary dissection, axillary radiation, or delayed axillary clearance for recurrence.[101] This is the strongest argument against the need for ALN dissection. However, the study was not large enough to detect a small but meaningful difference in survival rates, and many surgeons, in the habit of routinely performing modified radical mastectomies, still removed a substantial number of ALNs when performing a simple mastectomy, thus clouding the results. Other studies suggest a survival benefit for the early removal of micrometastatic disease in the lymph nodes.

One of the largest of these studies was conducted at the Institut Curie from 1982 to 1987.[102] The Curie study randomized 658 patients to either lumpectomy and axillary dissection or lumpectomy with postoperative radiation. Enrollment was limited to clinically node-negative patients with tumors less than 3 cm. Five-year follow-up demonstrated a 4.0% survival benefit ($P = .014$) for patients undergoing axillary dissection compared with those with axillary radiation only. A meta-analysis of six randomized controlled trials examining axillary node dissection in early breast cancer demonstrated a 5.4% overall survival benefit for clinically node-negative patients undergoing axillary dissection.[102]

However, these studies have limitations. The meta-analysis included several sizable European studies (including the Curie study) conducted from the 1950s to the 1980s. Since that time, there have been significant advances in screening, surgical management, and adjuvant therapy. It is unclear whether these results translate to today. More important, in some of these studies patients who were found to be node-positive were treated with adjuvant chemotherapy, an option not available to women who did not undergo ALN dissection. Thus, a significant treatment bias exists between the two groups.

Although these data suggest a possible benefit to controlling regional disease, one cannot assume that the results obtained with the omission of ALN dissection among clinically node-negative patients from years ago would be the same as among SLN-positive patients today. Neither the risk of distant disease nor the amount of residual disease in the axillary nodes is directly comparable. The only way to determine whether ALN dissection may be safely omitted for patients with a positive SLN biopsy would be a randomized trial, which was initiated by the American College of Surgeons Oncology Group (ACOSOG), but unfortunately closed prematurely owing to poor accrual. Therefore, the therapeutic benefit of completion ALN dissection remains unknown.

Rather than declaring whether ALN dissection is or isn't necessary, if one could accurately predict which patients are so unlikely to harbor additional disease in the non-SLN, a selective approach to completion ALN dissection could be applied. Although some clinicopathologic features such as the size and grade of the primary tumor, the size of the lymph node metastases, and the ratio of positive SLN to the number of SLN removed may help stratify risk, no factor appears sufficient to select patients who may avoid dissection.[103] Even the lowest-risk groups have a 10% to 20% chance of harboring additional disease. The use of statistical models or nomograms may better select patients with a low likelihood of harboring disease in the non-SLN,[104,105] but it must be cautioned that these studies underestimate the risk of additional disease, since the non-SLN are not subjected to the histologic scrutiny to which the sentinel node is subjected.

Completion ALN dissection is not the only option available to patients with a positive SLN biopsy. Axillary radiation may be a reasonable alternative, as evidenced by data collected before the emergence of SLN biopsy. In a series of 418 women treated with axillary radiation therapy after either no or limited ALN dissection, only 1.4% developed a regional failure after 8 years of follow-up.[106] Of the subset of patients who had a limited ALN dissection with positive nodes, the regional failure rate was 7% (3 of 42 cases). A randomized trial in Italy of ALN dissection versus axillary radiation therapy accrued 435 patients; after a mean follow-up of 66 months, only one axillary recurrence was recorded in the radiation arm and two axillary recurrences in the surgery arm.[107] Although these data suggest that axillary radiation may be effective in obtaining regional control, it is difficult to transpose these numbers to the SLN-positive population. A randomized trial of axillary radiation versus ALN dissection for SLN-positive patients is presently accruing patients and will not only answer these questions, but it will also help to determine whether axillary radiation truly decreases the morbidity of treatment compared with surgery.

References

1. Moore CH: On the influence of inadequate operations on the theory of cancer. Med Chr Trans 50:245, 1867.
2. Halsted WS: The results of operations for the cure of cancer of the breast performed at the Johns Hopkins Hospital from June 1889 to January 1894. The Johns Hopkins Reports 4: 297–350, 1894.
3. Adair F, Berg J, Joubert L, Robbins GF: Long-term follow-up of breast cancer patients: the 30 year report. Cancer 33: 1145–1150, 1974.
4. Fisher B, Jeong J-H, Anderson S, et al: Twenty-five year follow-up of a randomized trial comparing radical mastectomy, total mastectomy, and total mastectomy followed by irradiation. N Eng J Med 347:567–575, 2002.
5. Wickerham DL, Constantino JP, Mamounas EP, Julian T: The landmark surgical trials of the National Surgical Adjuvant Breast and Bowel Project. World J Surg 30:1138–1146, 2006.
6. Giuliano AE, Kirgan DM, Guenther JM, Morton DL: Lymphatic mapping and sentinel lymphadenectomy for breast cancer. Ann Surg 220:391–398, 1994.
7. Specht MC, Fey JV, Borgen PI, Cody H: Is the clinically positive axilla in breast cancer really a contraindication to sentinel lymph node biopsy? J Am Coll Surg 200(1):10–14, 2005.
8. de Kanter AY, van Eijck CHJ, van Geel AN, et al: Multicentre study of ultrasonographically guided axillary node biopsy in patients with breast cancer. Br J Surg 86(11):1459–1462, 1999.
9. Lam WW, Yang WT, Chan YL, et al: Detection of axillary lymph node metastases in breast carcinoma by technetium-99m sestamibi breast scintigraphy, ultrasound, and conventional mammography. Eur J Nucl Med Mol Imaging 23(5):498–503, 1996.
10. Bonnema J, van Geel AN, van Ooijen B, et al: Ultrasound-guided aspiration biopsy for detection of nonpalpable axillary node metastases in breast cancer patients: new diagnostic method. World J Surg 21(3):270–274, 1997.
11. Walsh JS, Dixon JM, Chetty U, Paterson D: Colour Doppler studies of axillary node metastasis in breast carcinoma. Clin Radiol 49(3):189–191, 1994.
12. Ciatto S, Brancato B, Risso G, et al: Accuracy of fine needle aspiration cytology (FNAC) of axillary lymph nodes as a triage

test in breast cancer staging. Breast Ca Res Treat 103(1):85–91, 2007.

13. Krag DN, Weaver D, Ashikaga T, et al: The sentinel node in breast cancer: a multicenter validation study. N Engl J Med 339(14):941–946, 1998.

14. Veronesi U, Paganelli G, Viale G, et al: A randomized comparison of sentinel-node biopsy with routine axillary dissection in breast cancer. N Engl J Med 349(6):546–553, 2003.

15. Tafra L, Lannin DR, Swanson M, et al: Multicenter trial of sentinel node biopsy for breast cancer using both technetium sulfur colloid and isosulfan blue dye. Ann Surg 233(1):51–59, 2001.

16. Kim T, Giuliano AL, Lyman GH: Lymphatic mapping and sentinel lymph node biopsy in early stage breast carcinoma: a metaanalysis. Cancer 106(1):4–16, 2006.

17. Sabel MS, Zhang P, Barnwell JM, et al: Accuracy of sentinel node biopsy in predicting nodal status in patients with breast carcinoma. J Surg Oncol 77(4):243–246, 2001.

18. Cox C, White L, Allred N, et al: Survival outcomes in node-negative breast cancer patients evaluated with complete axillary node dissection versus sentinel lymph node biopsy. Ann Surg Oncol 13(5):708–711, 2006.

19. Krag DN, Julian TB, Harlow SP, et al: NSABP-32: Phase III, randomized trial comparing axillary resection with sentinel lymph node dissection: a description of the trial. Ann Surg Oncol 11(3):208S–210S, 2003.

20. Julian TB, Krag D, Brown A, et al: Preliminary technical results of NSABP B-32, a randomized phase III clinical trial to compare sentinel node resection to conventional axillary dissection in clinically node-negative breast cancer patients. San Antonio Breast Cancer Symposium. San Antonio, Texas, 2004.

21. Newman L: Lymphatic mapping and sentinel lymph node biopsy in breast cancer patients: a comprehensive review of variations in performance and technique. J Am Coll Surg 199(5):804–816, 2004.

22. Dupont EL, Kamath VJ, Ramnath EM, et al: The role of lymphoscintigraphy in the management of the patient with breast cancer. Ann Surg Oncol 8(4):354–360, 2001.

23. Kelley MC, Hansen N, McMasters KM: Lymphatic mapping and sentinel lymphadenectomy for breast cancer. Am J Surg 188(1):49–61, 2004.

24. Linehan DC, Hill AD, Akhurst T, et al: Intradermal radiocolloid and intraparenchymal blue dye injection optimize sentinel node identification in breast cancer patients. Ann Surg Oncol 6(5):450–454, 1999.

25. Degnim AC, Oh K, Cimmino VC, et al: Is blue dye indicated for sentinel lymph node biopsy in breast cancer patients with a positive lymphoscintigram? Ann Surg Oncol 12(9):712–717, 2005.

26. Varghese P, Mostafa A, Abdel-Rahman AT, et al: Methylene blue dye versus combined dye-radioactive tracer technique for sentinel lymph node localisation in early breast cancer. Eur J Surg Oncol 33(2):147–152, 2007.

27. Linehan DC, Hill ADK, Tran KN, et al: Sentinel lymph node biopsy in breast cancer: unfiltered radioisotope is superior to filtered. J Am Coll Surg 188(4):377–381, 1999.

28. Tafra L, Chua AN, Ng PC, et al: Filtered versus unfiltered technetium sulfur colloid in lymphatic mapping: a significant variable in a pig model. Ann Surg Oncol 6(1):83–87, 1999.

29. Lloyd L, Wesen C, McCallum S: An analysis of filtration and volume of radionucleotide in sentinel lymph node biopsy in breast cancer patients. Am J Surg 68(4):373–375, 2002.

30. White DC, Schuler FR, Pruitt SK, et al: Timing of sentinel lymph node mapping after lymphoscintigraphy. Surgery 126(2):156–61, 1999.

31. Schneebaum S, Stadler J, Cohen M, et al: Gamma probe-guided sentinel node biopsy—optimal timing for injection. Eur J Surg Oncol 24(6):515–519.

32. Yeung HWD, Cody III HS, Turlakow A, et al: Lymphoscintigraphy and sentinel node localization in breast cancer patients: a comparison between 1-day and 2-day protocols. J Nucl Med 42(3):420–423, 2001.

33. Klimberg VS, Rubio IT, Henry R, et al: Subareolar versus peritumoral injection for location of the sentinel lymph node. Ann Surg 229(6):860–865, 1999.

34. Layeeque R, Kepple J, Henry-Tillman RS, et al: Intraoperative subareolar radioisotope injection for immediate sentinel lymph node biopsy. Ann Surg 239(6):845–848, 2004.

35. Kawase K, Gayed IW, Hunt KK, et al: Use of lymphoscintigraphy defines lymphatic drainage patterns before sentinel lymph node biopsy for breast cancer. J Am Coll Surg 203(1):64–72, 2006.

36. Simmons R, Thevarajah S, Brennan M: Methylene blue dye as an alternative to isosulfan blue dye for sentinel lymph node localization. Ann Surg Oncol 10:242–247, 2003.

37. Simmons RM, Smith SM, Osborne M: Methylene blue dye as an alternative to isosulfan blue dye for sentinel lymph node localization. Breast J 7:181–183, 2001.

38. Montgomery LL, Thorne AC, Van Zee KJ, et al: Isosulfan blue dye reactions during sentinel lymph node mapping for breast cancer. Anesth Analg 95:385–388, 2002.

39. McMasters KM, Wong SL, Martin R, et al: Dermal injection of radioactive colloid is superior to peritumoral injection for breast cancer sentinel lymph node biopsy: results of a multiinstitutional study. Ann Surg 233(5):676–687, 2001.

40. Shimazu K, Tamaki Y, Taguchi T, et al: Comparison between periareolar and peritumoral injection of radiotracer for sentinel lymph node biopsy in patients with breast cancer. Surgery 131(3):277–286, 2002.

41. Motomura K, Komoike Y, Hasegawa Y, et al: Intradermal radioisotope injection is superior to subdermal injection for the identification of the sentinel node in breast cancer patients. J Surg Oncol 82(2):91–97, 2003.

42. Turner RR, Ollila DW, Krasne DL, Giuliano AE: Histopathologic validation of the sentinel lymph node hypothesis for breast carcinoma. Ann Surg 226:271–278, 1997.

43. Wada N, Imoto S, Hasebe T, et al: Evaluation of intraoperative frozen section diagnosis of sentinel lymph nodes in breast cancer. Jpn J Clin Oncol 34(3):113–117, 2004.

44. Menes TS, Tartter PI, Mizrachi H, et al: Touch preparation or frozen section for intraoperative detection of sentinel lymph node metastases from breast cancer. Ann Surg Oncol 109(10):1166–1170, 2003.

45. Dabbs D, Fung M, Johnson R: Intraoperative cytologic examination of breast sentinel lymph nodes: test utility and patient impact. Breast J 10(3):190–194, 2004.

46. Rubio IT, Korourian S, Cowan C, et al: Use of touch preps for intraoperative diagnosis of sentinel lymph node metastases in breast cancer. Ann Surg Oncol 5(8):689–694, 1998.

47. International (Ludwig) Breast Cancer Study Group: Prognostic importance of occult axillary lymph node micrometastases from breast cancers. Lancet 335:1565, 1990.

48. Hainsworth PJ, Tjandra JJ, Stillwell RG, et al: Detection and significance of occult metastases in node-negative breast cancer. Br J Surg 80:459–463, 1993.

49. McGuckin MA, Cummings MC, Walsh MD, et al: Occult axillary node metastases in breast cancer: their detection and prognostic significance. Br J Cancer 73:88–95, 1996.

50. Clare SE, Sener SF, Wilkens W, et al: Prognostic significance of occult lymph node metastases in node-negative breast cancer. Ann Surg Oncol 4:447–451, 1997.

51. Cote RJ, Peterson HF, Chaiwun B, et al: Role of immunohistochemical detection of lymph-node micrometastases in management of breast cancer. International Breast Cancer Study Group. Lancet 354:896–900, 1999.

52. Pickren JW: Significance of occult metastases: a study of breast cancer. Cancer 14:1266–1271, 1961.

53. Fisher ER, Swamidoss S, Lee CH, et al: Detection and significance of occult axillary node metastases in patients with invasive breast cancer. Cancer 42:2025–2031, 1978.

54. Rosen PP, Saigo PE, Braun DW, et al: Occult axillary lymph node metastases from breast cancers with intramammary lymphatic tumor emboli. Am J Surg Pathol 6:639–641, 1982.

55. Wilkinson EJ, Hause LL, Hoffman RG, et al: Occult axillary lymph node metastases in invasive breast carcinoma: characteristics of the primary tumor and significance of the metastases. Pathol Annu 17(Pt 2):67–91, 1982.

56. de Mascarel I, MacGrogan G, Picot V, Mathoulin-Pelissier S: Prognostic significance of immunohistochemically detected breast cancer node metastases in 218 patients. Br J Cancer 87:70–74, 2002.

57. Chagpar AB, Middleton LP, Sahin AA, et al: Clinical outcome of patients with lymph node-negative breast carcinoma who have sentinel lymph node micrometastases detected by immunohistochemistry. Cancer 103(8):1571–1580, 2005.

58. Langer I, Marti WR, Guller U, et al: Axillary recurrence rate in breast cancer patients with negative sentinel lymph node

(SLN) or SLN micrometastases: prospective analysis of 150 patients after SLN biopsy. Ann Surg 241:152–158, 2005.

59. Klauber-DeMore N, Tan LK, Liberman L, et al: Sentinel lymph node biopsy: is it indicated in patients with high-risk ductal carcinoma in situ and ductal carcinoma in situ with microinvasion? Ann Surg Oncol 7(9):636–642, 2000.

60. Edge SB, Sheldon DG: Sentinel lymph node biopsy is not indicated for ductal carcinoma in situ. J Natl Comprehens Ca Netw 1(2):207–212, 2003.

61. Hansen NM, Ye X, Grube BJ, Guiliano AE: Manipulation of the primary breast tumor and the incidence of sentinel node metastases from invasive breast cancer. Arch Surg 139: 634–640, 2004.

62. Newman EL, Kahn A, Diehl KM, et al: Does the method of biopsy affect the incidence of sentinel lymph node metastases? Breast J 12(1):53–57, 2006.

63. Moore KH, Thaler HT, Tan LK, et al: Immunohistochemically detected tumor cells in the sentinel lymph nodes of patients with breast carcinoma: biologic metastasis or procedural artifact? Cancer 100:929–934, 2004.

64. Lyman GH, Guiliano AE, Somerfield MR, et al: American Society of Clinical Oncology guideline recommendations for sentinel lymph node biopsy in early-stage breast cancer. J Clin Oncol 23:7703–7720, 2005.

65. Carcoforo P, Bergossi L, Basaglia E, et al: Prognostic and therapeutic impact of sentinel node micrometastasis in patients with invasive breast cancer. Tumori 88(3):S4–S5, 2002.

66. de Boer M, van Deurzen CHM, van Dijck JAAM, et al: Micrometastases or isolated tumor cells and the outcome of breast cancer. N Engl J Med 361:653–663, 2009.

67. Paredes P, Vidal-Sicart S, Zanon G, et al: Clinical relevance of sentinel lymph nodes in the internal mammary chain in breast cancer patients. Eur J Nucl Med Mol Imaging 32(11): 1283–1287, 2005.

68. Lawson LL, Sandler M, Martin W, et al: Preoperative lymphoscintigraphy and internal mammary sentinel lymph node biopsy do not enhance the accuracy of lymphatic mapping for breast cancer. Am Surg 70(12):1050–1055, 2004.

69. Mansel RE, Goyal A, Newcombe R, ALMANAC Trialists Group: Internal mammary node drainage and its role in sentinel lymph node biopsy: the initial ALMANAC experience. Clin Breast Cancer 4:279–284, 2004.

70. van Rijk MC, Tanis PJ, Nieweg OE, et al: Clinical implications of sentinel nodes outside the axilla and internal mammary chain in patients with breast cancer. J Surg Oncol 94(4):281–286, 2006.

71. Carcoforo P, Sortini D, Feggi L, et al: Clinical and therapeutic importance of sentinel node biopsy of the internal mammary chain in patients with breast cancer: a single-center study with long-term follow-up. Ann Surg Oncol 13(10):1338–1343, 2006.

72. van Rijk MC, Deurloo EE, Nieweg OE, et al: Ultrasonography and fine-needle aspiration cytology can spare breast cancer patients unnecessary sentinel lymph node biopsy. Ann Surg Oncol 13(1):31–35, 2006.

73. Khan A, Sabel MS, Nees A, et al: Comprehensive axillary evaluation in neoadjuvant chemotherapy patients with ultrasonography and sentinel lymph node biopsy. Ann Surg Oncol 12(9):697–704, 2005.

74. Sabel MS, Schott AF, Kleer CG, et al: Sentinel node biopsy prior to neoadjuvant chemotherapy. Am J Surg 186(2): 102–105, 2003.

75. Jones JL, Zabicki K, Christian RL, et al: A comparison of sentinel node biopsy before and after neoadjuvant chemotherapy: timing is important. Am J Surg 190(4):517–520, 2005.

76. Schrenk P, Hochreiner G, Fridrik M, Wayand W: Sentinel node biopsy performed before preoperative chemotherapy for axillary lymph node staging in breast cancer. Breast J 9(4): 282–287, 2003.

77. Breslin TM, Cohen LF, Sahin AA, et al: Sentinel lymph node biopsy is accurate after neoadjuvant chemotherapy for breast cancer. J Clin Oncol 18(20):3480–3486, 2000.

78. Brady EW: Sentinel lymph node mapping following neoadjuvant chemotherapy for breast cancer. Breast J 8(2):97–100, 2002.

79. Mamounas EP, Brown A, Smith R, et al: Accuracy of sentinel node biopsy after neoadjuvant chemotherapy in breast cancer: updated results from NSABP B-27. Proc Am Soc Clin Oncol 21:140, 2002.

80. Stearns V, Ewing CA, Slack R, et al: Sentinel lymphadenectomy after neoadjuvant chemotherapy for breast cancer may reliably represent the axilla except for inflammatory breast cancer. Ann Surg Oncol 9(3):235–242, 2002.

81. Xing Y, Foy M, Cox DD, et al: Meta-analysis of sentinel lymph node biopsy after preoperative chemotherapy in patients with breast cancer. Br J Surg 93:539–546, 2006.

82. Kuerer HM, Sahin AA, Hunt KK, et al: Incidence and impact of documented eradication of breast cancer axillary lymph node metastases prior to surgery in patients treated with neoadjuvant chemotherapy. Ann Surg 230:72–78, 1999.

83. Hennessy BT, Hortobagyi GN, Rouzier R, et al: Outcome after pathologic complete eradication of cytologically proven breast cancer axillary node metastases following primary chemotherapy. J Clin Oncol 23(36):9304–9311, 2005.

84. Pomahac B, Recht A, May J, et al: New trends in breast cancer management: is the era of immediate breast reconstruction changing? Ann Surg 244(2):282–288, 2006.

85. Kronowitz SJ, Kuerer HM: Advances and surgical decision-making for breast reconstruction. Cancer 107(5):893–907, 2006.

86. Mokbel R, Mokbel K: Skin-sparing mastectomy and radiotherapy: an update. Internatl Semin Surg Oncol 3(1):35, 2006.

87. Schrenk P, Woelfl S, Bogner S, et al: The use of sentinel node biopsy in breast cancer patients undergoing skin sparing mastectomy and immediate autologous reconstruction. Plast Reconstr Surg 115(5):1278–1286, 2005.

88. Agarwal A, Heron DE, Sumkin J, Falk J: Contralateral uptake and metastases in sentinel lymph node mapping for recurrent breast cancer. J Surg Oncol 92(1):4–8, 2005.

89. Port ER, Fey J, Gemignani ML, et al: Reoperative sentinel lymph node biopsy: a new option for patients with primary or locally recurrent breast carcinoma. J Am Coll Surg 195(2): 167–172.

90. Karakousis CP: Surgical procedures and lymphedema of the upper and lower extremity. J Surg Oncol 93(2):87–91, 2006.

91. Querci della Rovere G, Ahmad I, Singh P, et al: An audit of the incidence of arm lymphoedema after prophylactic level I/II axillary dissection without division of the pectoralis minor muscle. Ann R Coll Surg Engl 85(3):158–161, 2003.

92. Petrek JA, Heelan MC: Incidence of breast carcinoma-related lymphedema. Cancer 83(S12B):2776–2781, 1998.

93. Francis WP, Abghari P, Du W, et al: Improving surgical outcomes: standardizing the reporting of incidence and severity of acute lymphedema after sentinel lymph node biopsy and axillary lymph node dissection. Am J Surg 192(5):636–639, 2006.

94. Recht A, Edge SB, Solin LJ, et al: Postmastectomy radiotherapy: clinical practice guidelines of the American Society of Clinical Oncology. J Clin Oncol 19:1539–1569, 2001.

95. Pierce L: Use of radiotherapy after mastectomy: a review of the literature. J Clin Oncol 23:1706–1717, 2005.

96. Hinrichs CS, Watroba NL, Rezaishiraz H, et al: Lymphedema secondary to postmastectomy radiation: incidence and risk factors. Ann Surg Oncol 11:573–580, 2004.

97. Krag D, Weaver D, Ashikaga T, et al: The sentinel node in breast cancer: a multicenter validation study. N Engl J Med 339:941–946, 1998.

98. Guiliano AE, Kirgan DM, Guenther JM, et al: Lymphatic mapping and sentinel lymphadenectomy for breast cancer. Ann Surg 220:391–401, 1994.

99. Borgstein PJ, Pijpers R, Comans EF, et al: Sentinel lymph node biopsy in breast cancer: guidelines and pitfalls of lymphoscintigraphy and gamma probe detection. J Am Coll Surg 186: 275–283, 1998.

100. Albertini JJ, Lyman GH, Cox CE, et al: Lymphatic mapping and sentinel node biopsy in the patient with breast cancer. JAMA 276:1818–1822, 1996.

101. Fisher B, Jeong J-H, Anderson S, et al: Twenty-five year follow-up of a randomized trial comparing radical mastectomy, total mastectomy and total mastectomy followed by irradiation. N Engl J Med 347:567–575, 2002.

102. Orr R: The impact of prophylactic axillary node dissection on breast cancer survival—a bayesian meta-analysis. Ann Surg Oncol 6(1):109–116, 1999.

103. Degnim AC, Griffith KA, Sabel MS, et al: Clinicopathologic features of metastasis in nonsentinel lymph nodes of breast carcinoma patients. Cancer 98(11):2307–2315, 2003.

104. Van Zee KJ, Manasseh DM, Bevilacqua JL, et al: A nomogram for predicting the likelihood of additional nodal metastases in breast cancer patients with a positive sentinel node biopsy. Ann Surg Oncol 10:1140–1151, 2003.

105. Degnim AC, Reynolds C, Pantvaidya G, et al: Nonsentinel node metastasis in breast cancer patients: assessment of an existing and a new predictive nomogram. Am J Surg 190(4):543–550, 2005.

106. Galper S, Recht A, Silver B, et al: Is radiation alone adequate treatment to the axilla for patients with limited axillary surgery? Implications for treatment after a positive sentinel node biopsy. Int J Radiat Oncol Biol Phys 48(1):125–132, 2000.

107. Zurrida S, Orecchia R, Galimberti V, et al: Axillary radiotherapy instead of axillary dissection: a randomized trial. Italian Oncological Senology Group. Ann Surg Oncol 9:117–119, 2002.

108. O'Hea BJ, Hill ADK, El-Shirbiny AM, et al: Sentinel lymph node biopsy in breast cancer: initial experience at Memorial Sloan-Kettering Cancer Center. J Am Coll Surg 186(4):423–427, 1998.

109. Albertini JJ, Lyman GH, Cox C, et al: Lymphatic mapping and sentinel node biopsy in the patient with breast cancer. JAMA 276(22):1818–1822, 1996.

110. Barnwell JM, Arredondo MA, Kollmorgen D, et al: Sentinel node biopsy in breast cancer. Ann Surg Oncol 5(2):126–130, 1998.

111. De Cicco C, Chinol M, Paganelli G: Intraoperative localization of the sentinel node in breast cancer: technical aspects of lymphoscintigraphic methods. Semin Surg Oncol 15(4):268–271, 1998.

112. Schneebaum S, Stadler J, Cohen M, et al: Gamma probe-guided sentinel node biopsy–optimal timing for injection. Eur J Surg Oncol 24(6):515–519, 1998.

113. Nwariaku FE, Euhus DM, Beitsch PD, et al: Sentinel lymph node biopsy, an alternative to elective axillary dissection for breast cancer. Am J Surg 176(6):529–531, 1998.

114. Czerniecki BJ, Scheff AM, Callans LS, et al: Immunohistochemistry with pancytokeratins improves the sensitivity of sentinel lymph node biopsy in patients with breast carcinoma. Cancer 85(5):1098–1103, 1999.

115. van der Ent FW, Kengen RA, van der Pol HA, Hoofwijk AG: Sentinel node biopsy in 70 unselected patients with breast cancer: increased feasibility by using 10 mCi radiocolloid in combination with a blue dye tracer. Eur J Surg Oncol 25(1):24–29, 1999.

116. Bass SS, Cox CE, Ku NN, et al: The role of sentinel lymph node biopsy in breast cancer. J Am Coll Surg 189(2):183–194, 1999.

117. Burak WE, Jr, Walker MJ, Yee LD, et al: Routine preoperative lymphoscintigraphy is not necessary prior to sentinel node biopsy for breast cancer. Am J Surg 177(6):445–449, 1999.

118. Jaderborg JM, Harrison PB, Kiser JL, Maynard SL: The feasibility and accuracy of the sentinel lymph node biopsy for breast carcinoma. Am Surg 65(8):699–703, 1999.

119. Dinan DD, Nagle CE, Pettinga J: Lymphatic mapping and sentinel lymph node biopsy in women with an ipsilateral second breast carcinoma and a history of breast and axillary surgery. Am J Surg 190:614–617, 2005.

120. Intra M, Gatti G, Luini A, et al: Surgical technique of intraoperative radiotherapy in conservative treatment of limited-stage breast cancer. Arch Surg 137(6):737–740, 2002.

121. Agarwal A, Heron D, Sumkin JH, Falk J: Contralateral uptake and metastases in sentinel lymph node mapping for recurrent breast cancer. J Surg Oncol 92:4–8, 2006.

122. Taback B, Nguyen P, Hansen N, et al: Sentinel lymph node biopsy for local recurrence of breast cancer after breast-conserving therapy. Ann Surg Oncol 13(8):1099–1104, 2006.

123. Newman EA, Cimmino VM, Sabel MS, et al: Lymphatic mapping and sentinel lymph node biopsy for patients with local recurrence after breast-conservation therapy. Ann Surg Oncol 13(1):52–57, 2006.

124. Boughey JC, Ross MI, Babieri GV, et al: Sentinel lymph node surgery in locally recurrent breast cancer. Clin Breast Ca 7:248–253, 2006.

125. Port E, Park J, Fey J, et al: Reoperative sentinel lymph node biopsy: a new frontier in the management of ipsilateral breast tumor recurrence. Ann Surg Oncol 14:2209–2214, 2007.

126. Liang W, Sickle-Santanello B, Nims T: Is completion axillary dissection indicated for micrometastases in the sentinel lymph node? Am J Surg 182:365–368, 2001.

127. Chen ZL, Wen DR, Coulson WF, et al: Occult metastasis in the axillary lymph nodes of patients with breast cancer node negative by clinical and histologic examination and conventional histology. Dis Markers 9:239–248, 1991.

128. Attiyeh FF, Jensen M, Huvos AG, Fracchia A: Axillary micrometastasis and macrometastasis in carcinoma of the breast. Surg Gynecol Obstet 144(6):839–842, 1977.

Radiation Oncology

16

Richard Zellars, Timothy George, and Lee Myers

KEY POINTS

- Outcomes in overall survival with mastectomy and breast-conserving therapy (BCT) are similar.
- Results of the National Surgical Adjuvant Breast and Bowel Project (NSABP) trial B-06 on women receiving mastectomy alone, lumpectomy with adjuvant radiation, and lumpectomy without adjuvant radiation showed no difference in overall survival among the three treatment groups.
- There is clear evidence that radiation reduces local recurrence and improves overall survival when applied after BCT when compared with BCT alone.
- Partial breast irradiation (PBI) appears to be a promising alternative to whole breast irradiation, but more long-term follow-up studies are needed before this technique is widely used.
- Although studies clearly show that radiation reduces local recurrences after breast-conserving surgery, a population may exist for whom conservative surgery alone should be considered.
- Therapeutic radiation administered after mastectomy is considered somewhat controversial in women with 1–3 positive lymph nodes.
- The social and physical effects of radiation therapy must be considered when a plan of treatment is being outlined.

Introduction

In general, the treatment for breast cancer consists of surgery with or without radiation and with or without systemic therapy. Most women with breast cancer have two distinct local therapy options: mastectomy or breast-conserving therapy (BCT), which is defined as limited surgery and adjuvant whole breast irradiation. The choice of local therapy depends on several factors, not the least of which is patient preference. In a review of over 16,000 patients with stages I and II breast cancer treated in 1994, Morrow and associates reported that only 42%

were treated with BCT.[1] Using 11 SEER (Surveillance Epidemiology and End Results) registries of women diagnosed with breast cancer between 1988 and 1999, researchers found that 51% and 49% were treated with mastectomy and breast-conserving surgery (BCS), respectively.[2] Ninety-six percent of the patients undergoing BCS also received adjuvant radiation. In contrast, researchers in France reported that in 2002 78% of eligible breast cancer patients were treated with BCT.[3] The increase in BCT over the years is perhaps due to the comfort of patients and physicians with the results of several randomized trials comparing BCT with mastectomy. Although some studies failed to show an improvement in overall survival with BCT, it is clear that outcomes in overall survival are similar with mastectomy and BCS. In addition, there have been reports of improved quality of life in women treated with BCT when compared with those treated with mastectomy.[4] The indications and contraindications of radiation after BCS and mastectomy are discussed in the following sections.

Traditionally, radiation therapy follows surgery, but the sequencing with systemic therapy may have more variability. The sequencing of radiation and chemotherapy does not appear to affect disease-free or overall survival. The term *systemic therapy* refers to chemotherapy, hormonal therapy, and biologics (e.g., trastuzumab). These agents may be administered at different times during the management of breast cancer. They may be administered before definitive surgery (neoadjuvant), after surgery but before radiation, concurrent with radiation, or after radiation. The sequence chosen depends on the agent used and its associated toxicities. There is no clear evidence that sequencing affects overall survival.[5-7] Neoadjuvant chemotherapy has been most influential in predicting a patient's ultimate response to chemotherapy and increasing the rates of BCT. In the National Surgical Adjuvant Breast and Bowel Project (NSABP) trial B-18, 27% of the patients originally considered ineligible for BCT and for whom mastectomies were planned were able to have lumpectomies following tumor shrinkage as a response to chemotherapy.[6-9]

Breast-Conserving Therapy

The most common use of therapeutic radiation with respect to breast cancer is in BCT. There have been seven randomized prospective trials in women with invasive breast cancer comparing mastectomy with limited breast surgery (lumpectomy) with or without adjuvant whole breast irradiation.[10,11] These trials showed not only that there were similar survival rates between the mastectomy and lumpectomy patients but also that whole breast irradiation after lumpectomy significantly reduced the incidence of local failures when compared with that for patients treated with lumpectomy alone (Table 16-1). Based on the strength of these findings, the National Cancer Institute (NCI) put forth the following consensus statement: "Breast conservation treatment is an appropriate method of primary therapy for the *majority* of women with stage I–II breast cancer and is preferable because it provides survival rates equivalent to those of total mastectomy and axillary dissection while preserving the breast."[17]

Invasive Disease and Breast-Conserving Therapy

Several prospective randomized trials have shown that local failure (LF) after lumpectomy alone may be as high as 30% to 40%. However, if radiation is administered, local failure is reduced to approximately 6% to 15%[9,11-14] (see Table 16-1). Perhaps the most quoted American study is the NSABP B-06. In this trial, women with tumors smaller than 4 cm were randomized to mastectomy or lumpectomy with or without adjuvant radiation. With 20 years' median follow-up, there was no difference in overall survival among the three treatment groups. However, there was a significant difference in local failure between the conservative surgery groups. The incidence of ipsilateral breast recurrence was 14% in the women who underwent lumpectomy and radiation compared with 39% in the women who underwent lumpectomy alone.[21]

Approximately 75% of all local failures occur within the first 5 years after treatment. However, late local recurrences have been reported at 15 to 20 years after treatment. Factors predictive of local failure after conservative breast surgery and radiation include positive/close margins, young age (less than 35 to 40 years old), extensive intraductal component, and lymph vascular invasion.[22-24]

Until recently, most evidence supported equivalent overall survival rates in patients treated with either modified radical mastectomy (MRM) or lumpectomy with or without radiation. However, there is now evidence to the contrary. The Early Breast Cancer Trialists' Cooperative Group (EBCTCG) evaluated seven prospective randomized trials comparing BCS with and without adjuvant radiation. With 15 years' follow-up, the authors showed a statistically significant 5% absolute survival benefit in women who received radiation after BCS compared with survival in women who underwent BCS alone.[10] Another meta-analysis, by Vinh-Hung and Vershraegen, showed a similar statistically significant survival benefit of 8.5% in favor of adjuvant radiation therapy.[25] It is now clear

Table 16-1. Lumpectomy Alone versus Lumpectomy with Radiation Therapy (RT)

| Trial | No. of Patients | Local Failure | | | Survival | | | Follow-up |
		No RT (%)	RT (%)	P value	No RT (%)	RT (%)	P value	Years
NSABP B-06 (Fisher et al, 1986)[21]	1851	39.2	14.3	<.001	46	46	NS	20
Ontario COG (Clark et al, 1996)[13]	837	35	11	<.0001	76	79	NS	7.6
Milan (Veronesi et al, 1993)[14]	579	23.5	5.8	<.001	77	82	NS	10
Sweden BCG (Malmstrom et al, 2003)[15]	1187	14	4	<.001	93	94	NS	5
Danish CTG (Forrest et al, 1996)[16]	585	24.5	5.8	<.05	99	97	NS	5

that radiation not only reduces local recurrence after BCS but also provides a real survival benefit when compared with BCS alone.

Ductal Carcinoma in Situ and Breast-Conserving Therapy

Unlike invasive breast cancer, there are no randomized trials comparing BCT with mastectomy in patients with ductal carcinoma in situ (DCIS). The closest study to an ideal randomized trial was a trial essentially by error. When reviewing the pathology of patients treated in NSABP B-06, a trial in which patients were randomized to lumpectomy alone, lumpectomy and radiation, or mastectomy, it was discovered that some of the patients enrolled in this invasive breast cancer trial in reality had DCIS.[12] The DCIS patients were evenly distributed among the three treatment groups. With a median follow-up of 39 months, the local failure rates in the lumpectomy patients with and without adjuvant radiation were 7% and 23%, respectively. There was no difference in survival rates among the three groups. The lack of survival differences suggests that DCIS could be equally well managed with mastectomy or conservative surgery and radiation.

Additional support for BCT in patients with DCIS comes from two large randomized prospective trials comparing lumpectomy alone with lumpectomy and radiation—NSABP B-17 and European Organisation for Research and Treatment of Cancer (EORTC) 10853 (Bijker 2006).[26,27] Both trials revealed that the rate of local recurrence was significantly reduced by approximately 50% with adjuvant radiation. In B-17, with a median follow-up of 8 years, the rates of local recurrence in the lumpectomy alone and lumpectomy and radiation groups were 31% and 13%, respectively. In the EORTC trial, with a median follow-up of 10 years, the local failure rates were 15% and 26% in patients who did and did not receive adjuvant radiation, respectively. Factors associated with an increased rate of local failure in patients with DCIS receiving BCT include young age, solid and cribriform subtypes, positive margins, and symptomatic detection of DCIS.[28–32]

Alternative Breast-Conserving Therapies

Partial Breast Irradiation

Because of the physical and social costs of whole breast irradiation, there has been much interest in developing ways of facilitating BCT.[33–39] One such method is partial breast irradiation (PBI). Because most local recurrences after BCT have been in the vicinity of the original tumor, one may question the need to treat the whole breast. Several large ongoing randomized trials in both North America and Europe are attempting to answer this question. In general, there are three ways to deliver radiation to the lumpectomy bed plus the margin while minimizing the dose to the remainder of the breast (PBI). The methods can be divided into two general techniques: brachytherapy and teletherapy. *Brachytherapy* is the placement of radioactive source close to, next to, or through the target organ/tissue. *Teletherapy* refers to treatment in which the radioactive source is at some distance from the target organ/tissue. The benefit of brachytherapy is that the radiation dose decreases rapidly with increasing distance from the source. Thus, this technique is uniquely suitable for treating small areas with high doses while sparing surrounding tissue.

Brachytherapy may be delivered via interstitial or intracavitary techniques.[37,40,41] The interstitial technique consists of placing hollow needles through the breast and lumpectomy bed in multiple planes. At some later time, radioactive sources are placed in those needles to treat the lumpectomy bed. This can be achieved with low-dose-rate or high-dose-rate brachytherapy. In the intracavitary brachytherapy technique, a balloon is placed in the lumpectomy bed at the time of surgery. The balloon is inflated to approximate the walls of the cavity. A source is then placed in the balloon to deliver radiation to the walls of the lumpectomy bed. High-dose-rate brachytherapy is commonly used in the intracavitary technique.

The remaining PBI techniques are via an external source (teletherapy). Teletherapy PBI is delivered either intraoperatively or postoperatively. The intraoperative technique delivers one large dose of radiation to the exposed lumpectomy bed with either photons or electrons.[42–44] The postoperative technique uses three-dimensional conformal or intensity-modulated radiation therapy (IMRT) to deliver radiation to the lumpectomy bed with margin.[38] The duration of postoperative PBI may range from 5 days of twice-daily treatments to 15 once-daily fractions.[38,45,46] See Figure 16-1 for an example of postoperative external beam PBI.

All of the latter PBI techniques concentrate on decreasing the duration of the radiation portion

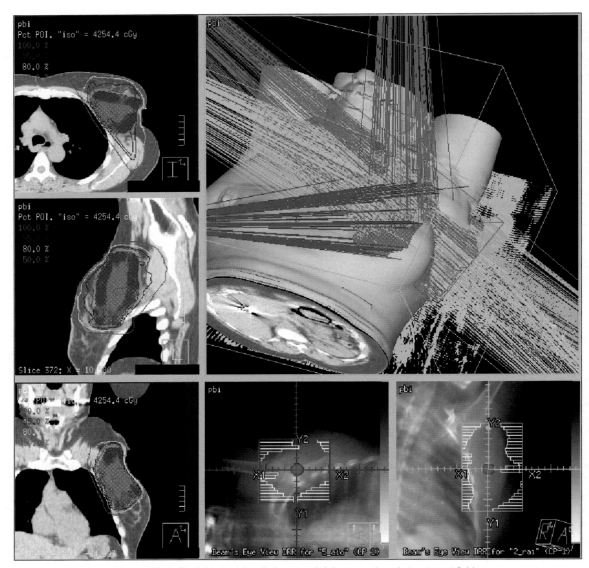

Figure 16-1. Partial breast irradiation on a left breast using six treatment fields.

of BCT. However, if one considers the entire adjuvant course of therapy for many women, then decreasing only the radiation is of little consequence to those facing several months of systemic therapy. In the hope of facilitating the entire course of adjuvant breast cancer therapy, researchers at Johns Hopkins are combining PBI with concurrent dose-dense chemotherapy (doxorubicin and cyclophosphamide) (PBICC).[45] A typical course of chemotherapy every 3 weeks followed by adjuvant radiation can range from 5 to 7 months or longer. With PBICC, the complete course of chemotherapy and radiation could be reduced to just 2 to 4 months. Although PBI

and PBICC appear attractive, one must remember that they are still experimental therapeutic techniques and regimens. Trials rigorously comparing PBI with standard whole breast irradiation are in progress. Until long-term follow-up is available, PBI and PBICC should not be offered off-study.

Lumpectomy Alone for Invasive Breast Cancer

Several studies attempted to identify a subset of breast cancer patients for which radiation is not necessary. Despite these many attempts, all studies showed that radiation reduced the rate of local failure when compared with limited surgery alone. However, recent studies suggest that certain elderly women may safely consider foregoing radiation. In a trial by Hughes and colleagues, women older than 70 years were randomized to receive adjuvant radiation or no radiation after lumpectomy for estrogen receptor-positive tumors less than 2 cm.[35] Nodal status was not evaluated in all patients. All patients received tamoxifen. With 5 years of follow-up, the authors reported a statistically significant difference in local failure of 1% in favor of radiation compared with 4% with no radiation. The authors argue that the absolute local failure difference between the two arms is small; thus, radiation could be safely avoided in this group.[35] Fyles and coworkers reported a similarly designed trial that evaluated the efficacy of adjuvant radiation in women older than 50 years. In this trial, with a median of 5.6 years, the rate of local failure was 0.6% and 7.7% in those who did and did not receive adjuvant radiation, respectively.[36] In both studies, there was a several-fold increase in local control with the addition of radiation. Although this is promising, longer follow-up is needed, and currently conservative surgery alone may be best considered for the elderly woman with multiple comorbidities whose life expectancy is relatively short.

Lumpectomy Alone for Ductal Carcinoma in Situ

Once factors are identified as predictive of local failure after BCT, it is only natural to attempt to identify patients who have a risk of local failure so small that they may avoid radiation. Probably the most well-known decision tool in this regard is the Van Nuys Prognostic Index (VNPI) first published by Silverstein and colleagues.[47] This prognostic index is used to divide patients into three risk groups, each with different needs for radiation or mastectomy. Unfortunately, though very attractive, the VNPI has not been reliably verified in other studies. Mascarel and associates were unable to reproduce the VNPI results, nor were Fisher and coworkers when this classification system was applied to patients treated in NSABP B-17.[29,48] Nonetheless, there is such great interest in defining a group that could be treated with conservative surgery alone that there are two large American

trials addressing this topic. Eastern Cooperative Oncology Group registry trial E5194 monitored patients with DCIS who refused radiation after lumpectomy.[49] The other trial sponsored by the Radiation Therapy Oncology Group (RTOG) 98-04, randomizes women with DCIS to radiation or no radiation, with or without adjuvant tamoxifen.

Although the results of RTOG 98-04 are not yet available, early results of E5194 have been published.[50] Eligible patients ($n = 711$) who were entered in this study had to have a low-/intermediate-grade DCIS of 2.5 cm or less or a high-grade DCIS of 1.0 cm or less. All patients had to have a 3.0 mm or greater margin. After a median 5.4 years of follow-up, rates of 6.1% and 14.8% of ipsilateral breast events were found in patients with low-/intermediate- and high-grade DCIS, respectively. The authors state that carefully selected patients with low-/intermediate-grade DCIS treated with surgery alone have an acceptably low rate of ipsilateral breast events. Patients with high-grade DCIS do not appear to be candidates for conservative surgery alone. However, they also recognize that these results are preliminary and that further follow-up is necessary.

Contraindications to Breast-Conserving Therapy (Invasive or DCIS)

Although the NCI consensus statement declares that the majority of women with early-stage breast cancer are eligible for BCT, one must ask who are the minority of women for which BCT is not an option? In other words, what are the contraindications to the use of BCT in this group? These contraindications may be divided into three general categories: unacceptable cosmetic result, unacceptable complication rate, and high probability of recurrence (Box 16-1). We briefly discuss here each of these categories.

The main motivation behind BCT, as the name implies, is preservation of the breast while maximizing survival. However, if the preserved breast is cosmetically unacceptable, the patient has not fully benefited from this therapy. Therefore, factors associated with poor cosmetic outcome are considered contraindications to BCT. An unacceptable cosmetic result may occur in women with small breasts who undergo complete resection of a large tumor. In these patients, there is very little remaining breast

---

Box 16-1. Relative Contraindications to Breast Conservation Therapy

High probability of poor cosmetic results

Surgical considerations:
  Small breast remnant after lumpectomy
  Large volume of resection
  Subareolar resection
  Poor scar placement
Radiotherapy consideration:
  Large breasts
  Radiation dose
  Radiation technique

High probability of complications

Previous radiation
Collagen vascular disease
Pregnancy

High probability of recurrence

Positive/close margins
Multicentric disease
Lymphovascular invasion
Invasive disease with extensive ductal carcinoma in situ

---

tissue, and they would be better served with a mastectomy and reconstruction. Women with very large breasts are also at risk of having a poor cosmetic outcome, since it is technically difficult to deliver a homogeneous dose of radiation. As a consequence of the large differential doses across the breast, these women may develop fibrosis and other soft tissue toxicities associated with radiation. Surgical treatment factors associated with poor cosmetic outcome include large volume of resection, subareola resection, and poor scar orientation. Radiation treatment factors that may affect cosmetic outcome include fraction size, total dose, type of radiation, and concurrent chemotherapy and radiation therapy.[51–57] For these reasons, one must use optimal surgical and radiation techniques.

Another category of contraindications to BCT addresses factors associated with a high rate of complications. These complications may also affect cosmetic outcome. Previous radiation to the breast is considered a contraindication because it has been associated with fibrosis and tissue necrosis.[58] However, evidence suggests that, in certain cases, additional limited radiation may be possible.[59,60] Another factor associated with an unacceptably high rate of complications is the presence of collagen vascular diseases (connective tissue diseases) such as systemic lupus erythematosus or scleroderma.[61–63] BCT,

in the setting of connective tissue disorders, may also result in breast fibrosis or tissue necrosis. Note that the literature supporting a link between collagen vascular disease and increased radiation toxicity is somewhat tenuous. The conclusions are not uniform, and the published reports contain relatively small numbers of patients.[61,62] Thus, some refer to collagen vascular diseases as a relative contraindication. Finally, because of the fear of complications, pregnancy is also included in this category. Although studies have shown that the theoretical exposure to the fetus during breast/chest wall irradiation would be minimal, many still consider pregnancy an absolute contraindication to radiation therapy.[64,65] A pregnant woman may have a lumpectomy or mastectomy and receive chemotherapy after the first trimester.[66] After delivery, she may then receive breast irradiation. With the advent of neoadjuvant chemotherapy, one could argue to treat the pregnant patient with chemotherapy until she delivers and then to perform either a lumpectomy or mastectomy.

The third and final category of contraindications specifically addresses in-breast recurrence risk. When the risk of a recurrence in the breast is greater than 30% to 40% at 5 years, perhaps the patient is not well served by BCT and may be better served by mastectomy. This is especially true when one considers the growing literature linking in-breast recurrence with increased mortality.[67] Factors associated with a high rate of in-breast recurrence after BCS and radiation include positive or close margins, multiple sites of disease involving more than one quadrant (multicentric disease), lymph-vascular invasion (LVI), and invasive disease with an extensive DCIS component.[11,31,68,69] Patients who have the *BRCA1* or *BRCA2* mutation do not have a higher rate of in-breast failures and thus are candidates for BCT.[70,71] Women younger than 35 to 40 years have an increased rate of local failure when compared with that of their older counterparts for reasons that are not exactly clear.[30–32] Nonetheless, when BCT is compared with mastectomy, in younger patients there is no difference in overall survival.[72] Therefore, young age alone is not a contraindication to BCT.

Breast-Conserving Technique

In most of the studies previously discussed, BCS was followed by whole breast irradiation, which did not routinely include regional nodes (supraclavicular, axillary, and internal mammary lymph nodes). Some of the lower axillary nodes are included in the breast tangents by default. However, there are occasions in which regional nodal irradiation is purposely added to whole breast radiation therapy. At our institution, the indications for nodal radiation are presently extrapolated from the postmastectomy radiation therapy trials and are discussed in the following section.

Typically, the entire breast is treated to a microscopic disease dose of 45–50 Gray in 25–28 fractions. The tumor bed then receives an additional 10–16 Gy (boost). Two prospective randomized trials have shown an improvement in local control when patients received a boost to the lumpectomy bed after whole breast radiation.[73,74]

See Figures 16-2 and 16-3 for examples of patient positioning and planning for standard breast-conserving therapy.

Postmastectomy Radiation

The second most common use of therapeutic radiation in the management of breast cancer occurs after mastectomy (postmastectomy radiation [PMXRT]). Some of the earliest randomized prospective trials in oncology addressed the role of radiation after mastectomy for breast cancer. These early trials clearly showed a local control benefit with postmastectomy radiation. Unfortunately, evidence of a survival benefit was lacking. In fact, a meta-analysis of these early trials showed a survival detriment.[75] Most of these deaths were believed to be associated with radiation damage to the heart. As a consequence, PMXRT was reserved only for the most advanced cases.

In 1997 and 1999, three randomized prospective trials of PMXRT were published. All three trials showed not only a local control benefit with PMXRT, as already seen in many of the earlier trials, but also a statistically significant survival benefit. These trials, in contrast to their predecessors, benefited from modern standardized radiation therapy techniques as well as from modern chemotherapy (Table 16-2).[18–20,76]

Many criticized these trials on both systemic and local therapeutic grounds. The criticisms concerning systemic therapy centered on the use of CMF (cyclophosphamide, methotrexate, 5-fluorouracil [5-FU]) in two of the trials and tamoxifen in the third. One may argue that the results of these PMXRT trials are not applicable to today's breast cancer patient because (1) CMF is no longer the most common first-line chemotherapy in breast cancer and (2) tamoxifen was prescribed for only 1 year as opposed to today's recommended 5-year regimen.

The high rate of local failure is at the core of the remaining criticisms. In all three trials, an unusually high rate of local regional failure was seen in the patients with one to three positive lymph nodes who did not receive radiation—30% to 33%. This rate stands in contrast to a local regional failure rate of 13%, as reported in a review of many prospective American trials.[77] Some have argued that inadequate surgery, specifically an inadequate axillary dissection, may be the cause of the high rate of local failure in these trials. As a consequence, radiation compensated for less than ideal surgery. An attempt to specifically address these concerns was made via a large phase III trial randomizing women with one to three positive lymph nodes to radiation or no radiation. Unfortunately, because of poor accrual, the trial was closed prematurely.

The controversy over whether to offer PMXRT to patients with one to three positive

Table 16-2. Mastectomy Alone versus Mastectomy with Radiation Therapy (RT)

| Trial | No. of Patients | Local Failure | | | Survival | | | Follow-up |
		RT (%)	No RT (%)	P value	RT (%)	No RT (%)	P value	Years
Overgaard et al (1997)[18]	1708	9	32	<.001	54	45	<.001	9.5
Ragaz et al (2005)[19]	318	10	26	.002	47	37	.03	20
Overgaard et al (1999)[20]	1375	8	35	<.001	45	36	.03	10

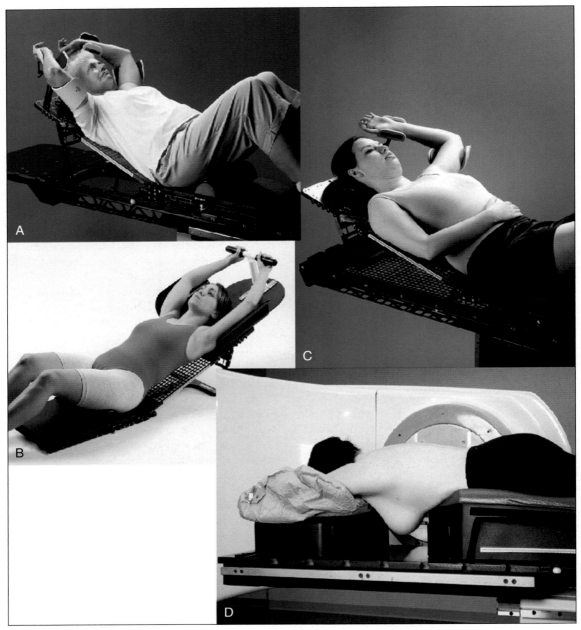

Figure 16-2. Immobilization devices for standard breast setups. **A,** Breast board with double indexed arm supports. **B,** Foam (alpha) cradle. **C,** Breast wing board with overhead handle. **D,** Breast board with single indexed arm support. (Reprinted with permission from Cardinal Health Systems.)

lymph nodes may soon be ending (Table 16-3).[18–20,78,79] In 2006, the Early Breast Cancer Trialists' Cooperative Group presented the results of a meta-analysis of more than 3000 women with pathologically proven one to three positive lymph nodes, treated with mastectomy and axillary clearance with or without adjuvant radiation. The majority of the patients received

systemic therapy. In this study, the authors reported a statistically significant overall survival benefit in favor of adjuvant radiation.[80] This survival benefit was also seen in women with four or more positive nodes. The report strongly suggests that when deciding whether to offer adjuvant radiation therapy, the distinction made among one and three and four or more positive

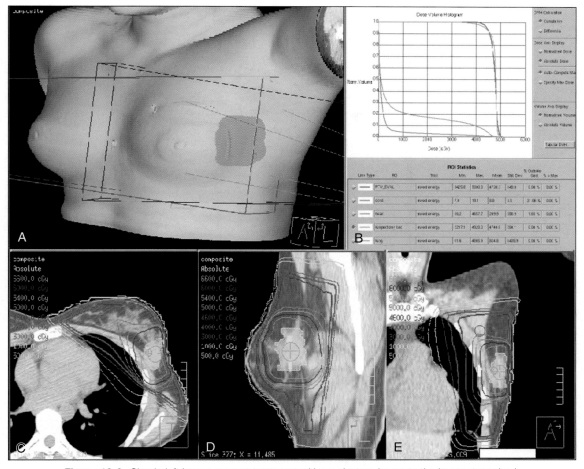

Figure 16-3. Simple left breast tangent treatment with an electron boost to the lumpectomy bed.

lymph nodes should be abandoned. Consequently, we offer PMXRT to all women with any number of positive axillary lymph nodes.

Factors associated with an increased risk of local failure after mastectomy include number/ratio of positive lymph nodes, tumor size, extent of axillary surgery, invasion of skin or pectoral fascia, and lymphovascular invasion. Other more putative risk factors include extracapsular extension and positive margins.[81]

Primary Chemotherapy (Neoadjuvant Chemotherapy) and Mastectomy

Risk of locoregional recurrence after mastectomy typically drives the recommendations for PMXRT. Conventionally, when a risk of locoregional failure is 15% to 20% or more, PMXRT is recommended. The estimate of locoregional failure was traditionally based on the pathologic and clinical factors at the time of surgery (e.g., number of positive lymph nodes, chest wall invasion), but before the administration of chemotherapy. Now with the advent of chemotherapy before surgery the estimate of locoregional failure determined only from clinical and pathologic factors at the time of surgery may no longer be accurate. One may need also to consider the risk of locoregional failure with respect to tumor response to neoadjuvant chemotherapy. Specifically, if a clinically node-positive patient has a pathologic complete response to neoadjuvant chemotherapy, does she still need PMXRT?

Owing to the novelty of neoadjuvant chemotherapy and the lack of large prospective or retrospective studies addressing PMXRT patients treated with neoadjuvant chemotherapy, controversy exists regarding when to recommend PMXRT. One may argue to use prechemotherapy

Table 16-3. Effect of Nodal Status on the Impact of PMRT on Overall Survival

Study	Year	1–3 Positive Nodes			≥4 Positive Nodes		
		% Survival with Chemotherapy Alone	% Survival with Chemotherapy + PMRT	% Absolute Improvement	% Survival with Chemotherapy Alone	% Survival with Chemotherapy + PMRT	% Absolute Improvement
Overgaard et al[18]*	1997	54	62	8	20	32	12
Overgaard et al[20]*	1999	44	55	11	17	24	7
Overgaard et al[78]†	2007	48	57	9	12	21	9
Ragaz et al[19]‡	2005	50	57	7	17	31	14

*10-year data in pre- and postmenopausal patients, in the 1997 and 1999 reports, respectively. Control arm was tamoxifen rather than chemotherapy for the postmenopausal patients. The P values for the overall groups, which also include a small number of patients (≤10% of the overall group) with T3N0 stage disease, were <.001 and .03 in the pre- and postmenopausal patients, respectively.

†15-year data in the subset of node-positive women with eight or more sampled axillary nodes pooled from the two prior reports (i.e., the 1997 report of premenopausal and the 1999 report of postmenopausal women). P = .03 for both subgroups.

‡20-year data. P = .03 for the overall population, and P > .05 in the subgroups with one to three and four or more positive nodes.

PMRT, postmastectomy radiation therapy.

From Marks LB, Zeng J, Prosnitz LR: One to three versus four or more positive nodes and postmastectomy radiotherapy: time to end the debate. J Clin Oncol 26:2075–2077 2008: Table 1.

pathologic and clinical information to recommend PMXRT, but, again, this does not address the potentially predictive information provided by tumor response to chemotherapy. Most of the recommendations concerning risks of locoregional failure come from NSABP B-18 and B-27 and retrospective studies from MD Anderson.[6,8,82] According to the NSABP trials, patients with any residual nodal disease after neoadjuvant chemotherapy have at least a 15% risk of locoregional failure after mastectomy alone. Retrospective studies report a greater than 20% risk of locoregional failure in patients with clinical stage III cancer who achieve a pathologic complete remission.[7,9,83–85] Alternatively, patients with clinical stage II disease and pathologic complete remission have locoregional failure of less than 10% and thus may not benefit from PMXRT. Given the limited data, it may be prudent to offer PMXRT to any patient with residual nodal disease after neoadjuvant chemotherapy and to patients presenting with stage III disease, regardless of their pathologic response.

PMXRT Technique

All three modern PMXRT trials showed a survival benefit associated with the addition of radiation. All three trials used similar radiation fields and similar biologically effective doses.[18–20] The treated fields include the chest wall and supraclavicular and internal mammary nodes. The axilla was included in all trials, although it may not have received full dose. Similar fields are recommended for women with positive axillary node disease who have had either a BCS or mastectomy.

The value of internal mammary lymph node (IMLN) radiation often generates vigorous debate. Some claim that a recurrence in an IMLN is sufficiently rare that routine treatment of this nodal group is not warranted.[86] We disagree. Basically, three lines of evidence justify treatment of the IMLN. First, these three PMXRT trials, all of which irradiated the IMLN, are the first to show a clear survival benefit with PMXRT. Second, two pathologic series, evaluating the incidence of IMLN metastases, revealed essentially the same result despite the fact that these studies are more than 20 years apart.[87–90] In these two series, there was a 9% to 13% risk of pathologically positive IMLNs in women who had a pathologically negative axilla. However,

this risk increased to 28% to 37% in women with a pathologically positive axilla. The third line of evidence comes from an accidental trial reported by Stemmer and colleagues. In this report, women in a bone marrow transplant trial received PMXRT, which included IMLN radiation via electrons.[91] Halfway through the trial, the researchers lost electron therapy capability and discontinued treatment of the IMLNs. When the authors reviewed the outcome of these patients, they found a statistically significant improvement in disease-free survival and a trend toward improved overall survival in favor of IMLN irradiation. Thus, based on the latter three arguments, we conclude that IMLN irradiation should be considered for patients receiving adjuvant nodal irradiation.

The dose of radiation in PMXRT is typically 46 to 50 Gy in 25–28 fractions to all fields. To the best of our knowledge there is no randomized trial supporting the role of additional radiation (boost) to the mastectomy scar. Consequently, a scar boost is at the physician's discretion. In addition, bolus or bolus equivalent material is placed on the chest wall during treatment. Bolus reduces skin-sparing and ensures that a therapeutic dose is delivered to the skin since it is at risk for recurrent disease. See Figure 16-4 for typical radiation treatment planning for postmastectomy radiation in a patient with breast reconstruction.

Radiation Toxicity

Acute Effects

Radiation therapy, though beneficial in improving both local control and survival, is not without social and physical costs. The social costs are lost time from loved ones and livelihood, whereas the physical costs may include rib, lung, nerve, and soft tissue damage. Note that the toxic effects of radiation can be affected by several treatment- and patient-related factors. Treatment factors include type and energy of radiation, area treated, dose, fraction size, immobilization devices, and dosimetric plans.[92,93] Patient-related factors associated with increased toxicity include obesity (high body mass index [BMI]), concurrent chemotherapy, and comorbidities (i.e., diabetes, connective tissue diseases, renal failure, smoking, previous radiation exposure).[94]

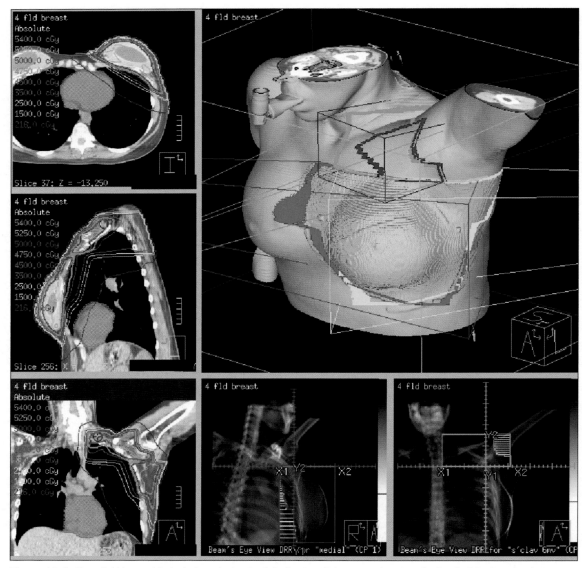

Figure 16-4. Four-field isocentric technique to treat a left chest wall. Isocenter is set at the level of the junction between the supraclavicular/axillary fields and the tangent chest wall fields.

Side effects or toxicities can be separated into two general categories; early and late (Box 16-2). Early or acute toxicities occur during the course of radiation, whereas late toxicities may occur 6 weeks to several years after radiation. The most common acute side effects from whole breast irradiation are fatigue and skin irritation. These side effects and all others vary greatly from patient to patient. The fatigue tends to be very mild such that many women are able to continue working full time during the course of treatment. Skin irritation, that is, radiation dermatitis, is also fairly common. In some reports, up to 90% of patients develop some form of radiation dermatitis.[95]

The deep layer of the epidermis contains basal stem cells. These stem cells are responsible for the cells that make up the cornified layer of the epidermis. Radiation damages the stem cells. As a consequence, there is dry desquamation (i.e., shedding of the cornified layer). The radiation also causes capillary dilatation, increased permeability, and an inflammatory response resulting in erythema and edema. There is also hyperpigmentation from migration of the melanocytes to the surface, epilation, and loss of

---

Box 16-2. Complications of Radiation Therapy of the Breast

Early
Fatigue
Skin changes
  Desquamation
  Necrosis
  Edema
  Hyperpigmentation
  Telangectasias
  Atrophy

Late
Skin toxicity
(?) Ischemic heart disease
Radiation pneumonitis
(?) Secondary non-breast malignancies
(?) Contralateral breast cancer
Lymphedema
Brachial plexopathy
Spontaneous rib fracture
Decreased shoulder range of motion

---

sweat and sebaceous glands, resulting in dry and pruritic skin. With continued loss of the basal cell layer, the dermis becomes exposed, resulting in moist desquamation. This may progress to frank ulceration. Healing entails re-epithelialization via repopulation of the residual basal cells or migration of basal cells from neighboring areas.[95,96]

A multitude of putative treatments are available for acute radiation-induced skin toxicity. Unfortunately, very few have proved to be more effective than the best supportive care in clinical trials. Putative therapies include washing with mild soap, application of aloe, barrier films, corticosteroids, antimicrobial creams (silver sulfadiazine), and trolamine (Biafine). Two therapies have been studied in a prospective fashion and found to be somewhat effective. In a randomized prospective trial, Calendula officinalis cream was found to significantly reduce skin toxicity when compared with trolamine.[97] Trolamine has been shown to be no better than best supportive care. When compared in a randomized prospective trial with placebo, hyaluronic acid cream was found to significantly delay the onset of severe skin toxicity.[98] Although ensuring a reduction in skin toxicity is a laudable goal given the lack of effective agents, one should provide supportive care at the minimum, including, if possible, pain relief.

Late Effects

Late breast side effects associated with whole breast irradiation may include breast shrinkage, fibrosis, edema, telangiectasias, hypo-/hyperpigmentation, and tenderness.[98,99] Because of their proximity to the treated breast, other organs/structures may suffer radiation-induced toxicities. One such toxicity is radiation pneumonitis (RP). Radiation pneumonitis is characterized by interstitial inflammation within the irradiated field, a nonproductive cough, and/or low-grade fever. The risk of developing radiation pneumonitis ranges from 1% to 29% and has been linked to patient and treatment factors such as age, body mass index, radiation dose/volume and treatment fields, chemotherapy, and hormonal therapy.[94,98,100–102] The literature supporting these putative predictive factors for radiation pneumonitis is mixed. For example, Taghian and colleagues and Burstein and associates reported an increase in the risk of radiation pneumonitis with concurrent and sequential taxane chemotherapy.[103,104] However, Ellerboek and coworkers and Allen and colleagues were not able to find a relation between standard-dose chemotherapy and radiation pneumonitis in women receiving radiation.[98,105] There is also some debate as to whether dose-volume histograms (DVH) metrics can accurately predict the risk of radiation pneumonitis.[94,98,100–102,106,107] Although there is some debate about predictive factors for radiation pneumonitis, one should always minimize the incidental lung exposure. Using modern radiation techniques and standard doses to treat the chest wall/breast and all regional nodal groups, the modern risk of symptomatic radiation pneumonitis appears to be closer to 1% to 7%.[19,94,96] A short course of corticosteroids followed by a slow taper has been used successfully to treat this condition.

Another very rare and unique lung complication is radiation-associated bronchiolitis obliterans organizing pneumonia (BOOP) associated with radiation. In the few papers describing this entity, the incidence appears to be 0.5% to 2%.[108,109] It is characterized by ground-glass opacities/interstitial changes extending beyond the irradiated lung, which appear to be migratory in nature. BOOP associated with radiation is seen most commonly in older patients and those receiving concurrent endocrine therapy. Treatment is typically a prolonged course of corticosteroids, which may last months to years.

Cardiotoxicity

With left breast/chest wall treatment, there is a risk of radiation exposure to the heart. Meta-analyses using studies with outdated radiation techniques have shown an increased rate of cardiac events in those who received radiation compared with those who did not.[75] This increase in cardiac events was not obvious until 15 years after therapy. However, with today's modern radiation machines and techniques, there is little evidence of a significant increase in cardiac morbidity with radiation. For example, in the three modern PMXRT trials in which the chest wall, supraclavicular, axillary, and internal mammary lymph nodes were treated, no statistically significant difference in cardiac morbidity was found between those who did and those who did not receive radiation.[19,110,111] Still, as the use of systemic chemotherapy increases, especially with agents known to be cardiotoxic such as anthracyclines and trastuzumab, it is necessary to remain vigilant both in avoiding and in assessing potential radiation-induced cardiac toxicity.

Some institutions use active breathing control or respiratory gating when treating left breasts to decrease the amount of heart that is irradiated.[112–114] With active breathing control, the patient is coached to hold the breath when the lung is expanded to 80% of its maximum volume. Radiation is delivered only during the breath hold. Chest expansion with breath hold increases the distance between the heart and the chest wall and therefore lowers the radiation exposure to the heart. Systems using respiratory gating track the breathing cycle with an external fiducial marker. The radiation is gated so that it activates only during the deep inspiration part of the breathing cycle when the heart is farthest from the chest wall.

Lymphedema

Lymphedema is abnormal swelling of the ipsilateral arm as a result of disrupted lymph flow and is perhaps one of the most feared late effects of radiation. The definition of clinically significant lymphedema varies greatly in the literature. Some define lymphedema as a greater than 2 cm difference in circumference between the affected arm and the nonaffected arm measured at 10 cm above and below the olecranon. Others define lymphedema as a cumulative difference of more than 10 cm between the arm measurements; still others look for a difference in volume measured by water displacement when the arm is placed in a water bath. In part, as a consequence of a non–universally accepted definition, reported rates of lymphedema vary greatly. The highest rates appear to be associated with a full axillary dissection (levels I–III) combined with axillary radiation.[115] Other factors have been associated with an increased risk of lymphedema, such as obesity, age, hypertension, infection, radiation fields and dose, number of nodes removed, and number of nodes containing metastatic disease.[116–120] Fortunately, rates appear to have dropped significantly with the advent of sentinel node biopsies, limited nodal dissection (levels I–II only), and judicial use of modern radiation techniques. In the PMXRT randomized trials, in which all regional nodal groups were irradiated, the incidence of lymphedema was 9% to 14%.[19,110]

Unfortunately, there is no cure for lymphedema. Intervention is motivated by the desire to palliate symptoms and reduce the risk of complications. Management of lymphedema includes massage, sequential compression, and compressive garments.[121] Patients are also instructed to avoid infections, blood draws, and blood pressure screening in the arm at risk. We recommend that the patient be seen by a lymphedema specialist at the earliest sign of swelling in the arm.

Second Non-Breast Malignancy

Another feared and often-mentioned potential side effect of radiation is the development of a second non-breast malignancy. Approximately 7% to 8% of women undergoing adjuvant radiation for breast cancer develop a second non-breast malignancy. However, when compared with that of similar patients who did not undergo radiation, a very small to insignificant difference in the rate of second non-breast malignancies appears to occur.[122,123] Although Obedian and associates and Woodward and colleagues found no overall significant difference in the rate of second malignancy in women who did and women who did not receive radiation for breast cancer, Galper and coworkers reported a 1% absolute increase in second non-breast malignancies associated with radiation.[124]

There have been mixed reports with respect to the possible increased risk of lung cancer in women who smoke and receive radiation for breast cancer. Harvey and Brinton reported an increase in lung cancer in women treated with radiation for breast cancer.[125] Zablotska and Neugut reported a statistically significant increase in lung cancer in women treated with PMXRT but not lumpectomy and radiation. In addition, this increased risk was not evident until 10 years after exposure.[126] Obedian and associates found no increased risk of new lung primaries in women treated with BCT compared with that in those treated with mastectomy alone. However, the authors did report a correlation between lung primaries and smoking. The 15-year risk of developing a lung cancer after BCT was 0.3%, 4.7%, and 6% for nonsmokers, previous smokers, and current smokers, respectively.[122] There is a report suggesting an increased risk of acute myelogenous leukemia associated with radiation for breast cancer. However, the authors were not able to show whether this was independent of chemotherapy.[127]

Second Breast Malignancy

Contralateral breast cancer (CBC) is the most common second primary malignancy in women diagnosed with breast cancer.[128] Although it is known that different breast/chest wall radiation treatment techniques may expose the contralateral breast to 0.5 to 7.1 Gy, the data showing a correlation between CBC risk and radiation are inconclusive. In a review of 134,501 women diagnosed with breast cancer between 1973 and 1996 in the SEER database, Gao and coworkers demonstrated an overall 4.25% incidence of CBC. On multivariate analysis, no correlation was found between radiation and CBC. However, on subset analysis, the authors report an absolute 1.6% increased risk of CBC at 20 years in women treated with radiation. The results of this study are uncertain, since the information is from a large centralized databank, which lacks treatment details. Some authors have shown a correlation between increased CBC risk and radiation but only in women younger than 45 years old, whereas others found no correlation in any subset of women.[122,129] On analysis of

EORTC trial 10853, which randomized women after lumpectomy for DCIS to radiation or no radiation, there was a small but significant increase in CBC in the irradiated group.[27] However, in NSABP B-17, an identical trial, no significant correlation was identified.[26] Nielsen and associates in a review of the Danish Breast Cancer Group PMXRT trials, found no significant increase in CBC in women who received radiation.[130] Obviously, the literature is inconsistent regarding the correlation between radiation and CBC. Nonetheless, one should use techniques that minimize radiation exposure to the contralateral breast.

Other late side effects of radiation with standard fractionation include brachial plexopathy (1%), spontaneous rib weakening or fracture (2–3%), decreased shoulder mobility (5%), and grade 2 breast fibrosis (4%).[98,100]

Primary Radiation Therapy

Surgical resection is crucial to the treatment of breast cancer; however, there are several rare and controversial circumstances in which radiation and/or chemotherapy can potentially be made use of without surgical intervention. These situations include the treatment of so-called "occult" breast cancer and potentially the treatment of axillary lymph nodes.

Occult Breast Cancer

Most patients with breast cancer present either with a palpable breast mass or with a mammographic abnormality. However, occasionally women present with palpable lymphadenopathy. Even more infrequently, subsequent imaging does not reveal the primary tumor in the breast, and these patients are diagnosed as having occult breast cancer. The incidence of occult breast cancer was originally reported in 1954 as 0.3%.[131] Although this figure is still quoted in the literature, the modern incidence is probably much lower because some subset of these patients would likely have radiographically evident breast cancer with modern imaging. A variety of treatment modalities have been recommended, ranging from right upper outer quadrant quadrantectomies (the most likely site of breast cancer), total mastectomies, and various combinations of chemotherapy and radiation therapy.[132] In a recent survey of breast surgeons, the plurality or

43% indicated they would treat with mastectomy, whereas 37% indicated they would treat with whole breast irradiation.[133] All the studies that have compared mastectomy alone against radiation alone have been small and retrospective, and the results are mixed. Some have claimed equivalent outcomes;[134] others have shown increased survival after mastectomy.[135] Given this uncertainty, treatment recommendations should be individualized with the patient's informed cooperation.

Conclusion

Radiation therapy has revolutionized the treatment of breast cancer. A disease that was once treated with invasive, radical surgery can now be treated minimally invasively when combined with radiation. Though not without complications, radiation therapy has made BCT in both invasive cancer and DCIS possible and has helped decrease local failure and increase survival in select patients. Radiation also can be used to palliate metastatic disease. The science of radiation therapy continues to change. As techniques are investigated to improve survival, decrease local recurrence, decrease complications, and improve patient access and satisfaction, it is likely that the indications for radiation will continue to increase.

References

1. Morrow M, White J, Moughan J, et al: Factors predicting the use of breast-conserving therapy in stage I and II breast carcinoma. J Clin Oncol 19(8):2254–2262, 2001.
2. McCarthy EP, Ngo LH, Roetzheim RG, et al: Disparities in breast cancer treatment and survival for women with disabilities. Ann Intern Med 145(9):637–645, 2006.
3. Cutuli B, Cottu PH, Guastalla JP, et al: A French national survey on infiltrating breast cancer: analysis of clinico-pathological features and treatment modalities in 1159 patients. Breast Cancer Res Treat 95(1):55–64, 2006.
4. Janz NK, Mujahid M, Lantz PM, et al: Population-based study of the relationship of treatment and sociodemographics on quality of life for early stage breast cancer. Qual Life Res 14(6):1467–1479, 2005.
5. Bellon JR, Come SE, Gelman RS, et al: Sequencing of chemotherapy and radiation therapy in early-stage breast cancer: updated results of a prospective randomized trial. J Clin Oncol 23(9):1934–1940, 2005.
6. Bear HD, Anderson S, Smith RE, et al: Sequential preoperative or postoperative docetaxel added to preoperative doxorubicin plus cyclophosphamide for operable breast cancer: National Surgical Adjuvant Breast and Bowel Project Protocol B-27. J Clin Oncol 24(13):2019–2027, 2006.
7. Buchholz TA, Hunt KK, Whitman GJ, et al: Neoadjuvant chemotherapy for breast carcinoma: multidisciplinary considerations of benefits and risks. Cancer 98(6):1150–1160, 2003.
8. Fisher B, Bryant J, Wolmark N, et al: Effect of preoperative chemotherapy on the outcome of women with operable breast cancer. J Clin Oncol 16(8):2672–2685, 1998.
9. Bafaloukos D: Neo-adjuvant therapy in breast cancer. Ann Oncol 16 Suppl 2:ii174–181, 2005.
10. Clarke M, Collins R, Darby S, et al: Effects of radiotherapy and of differences in the extent of surgery for early breast cancer on local recurrence and 15-year survival: an overview of the randomised trials. Lancet 366(9503):2087–2106, 2005.
11. Freedman GM, Fowble BL: Local recurrence after mastectomy or breast-conserving surgery and radiation. Oncology (Williston Park) 14(11):1561–1581; discussion 1581–1582, 1582–4, 2000.
12. Fisher ER, Sass R, Fisher B, et al: Pathologic findings from the National Surgical Adjuvant Breast Project (protocol 6). I. Intraductal carcinoma (DCIS). Cancer 57(2):197–208, 1986.
13. Clark RM, Whelan T, Levine M, et al: Randomized clinical trial of breast irradiation following lumpectomy and axillary dissection for node-negative breast cancer: an update. Ontario Clinical Oncology Group. J Natl Cancer Inst 88(22):1659–1664, 1996.
14. Veronesi U, Luini A, Del Vecchio M, et al: Radiotherapy after breast-preserving surgery in women with localized cancer of the breast. N Engl J Med 328(22):1587–1591, 1993.
15. Malmstrom P, Holmberg L, Anderson H, et al: Breast conservation surgery, with and without radiotherapy, in women with lymph node-negative breast cancer: a randomised clinical trial in a population with access to public mammography screening. Eur J Cancer 39(12):1690–1697, 2003.
16. Forrest AP, Stewart HJ, Everington D, et al: Randomised controlled trial of conservation therapy for breast cancer: 6-year analysis of the Scottish trial. Scottish Cancer Trials Breast Group. Lancet 348(9029):708–713, 1996.
17. NIH Consensus Conference on Treatment of Early Stage Breast Cancer. JAMA 265:391–395, 1991.
18. Overgaard M, Hansen PS, Overgaard J, et al: Postoperative radiotherapy in high-risk premenopausal women with breast cancer who receive adjuvant chemotherapy. Danish Breast Cancer Cooperative Group 82b trial. N Engl J Med 337(14):949–955, 1997.
19. Ragaz J, Olivotto IA, Spinelli JJ, et al: Locoregional radiation therapy in patients with high-risk breast cancer receiving adjuvant chemotherapy: 20-year results of the British Columbia randomized trial. J Natl Cancer Inst 97(2):116–126, 2005.
20. Overgaard M, Jensen MB, Overgaard J, et al: Postoperative radiotherapy in high-risk postmenopausal breast-cancer patients given adjuvant tamoxifen: Danish Breast Cancer Cooperative Group DBCG 82c randomised trial. Lancet 353(9165):1641–1648, 1999.
21. Fisher B, Anderson S, Bryant J, et al: Twenty-year follow-up of a randomized trial comparing total mastectomy, lumpectomy, and lumpectomy plus irradiation for the treatment of invasive breast cancer. N Engl J Med 347(16):1233–1241, 2002.
22. Mirza NQ, Vlastos G, Meric F, et al: Predictors of locoregional recurrence among patients with early-stage breast cancer treated with breast-conserving therapy. Ann Surg Oncol 9(3):256–265, 2002.
23. Voogd AC, Nielsen M, Peterse JL, et al: Differences in risk factors for local and distant recurrence after breast-conserving therapy or mastectomy for stage I and II breast cancer: pooled results of two large European randomized trials. J Clin Oncol 19(6):1688–1697, 2001.
24. van Dongen JA, Voogd AC, Fentiman IS, et al: Long-term results of a randomized trial comparing breast-conserving therapy with mastectomy: European Organization for Research and Treatment of Cancer 10801 trial. J Natl Cancer Inst 92(14):1143–1150, 2000.
25. Vinh-Hung V, Verschraegen C: Breast-conserving surgery with or without radiotherapy: pooled-analysis for risks of ipsilateral breast tumor recurrence and mortality. J Natl Cancer Inst 96(2):115–121, 2004.
26. Fisher B, Dignam J, Wolmark N, et al: Lumpectomy and radiation therapy for the treatment of intraductal breast cancer: findings from National Surgical Adjuvant Breast and Bowel Project B-17. J Clin Oncol 16(2):441–452, 1998.
27. EORTC Breast Cancer Cooperative Group, EORTC Radiotherapy Group, Bijker N, et al: Breast-conserving treatment with or without radiotherapy in ductal carcinoma-in-situ: ten-year results of European organisation for research and treatment of cancer randomized phase III trial 10853–a study by

the EORTC Breast Cancer Cooperative Group and EORTC radiotherapy group. J Clin Oncol 24(21):3381–3387, 2006.

28. Bland K, Copeland D (eds): The Breast: Comprehensive Management of Benign and Malignant Disorders, 3rd ed. St. Louis, MO, Saunders, 2004.

29. Fisher ER, Dignam J, Tan-Chiu E, et al: Pathologic findings from the National Surgical Adjuvant Breast Project (NSABP) eight-year update of protocol B-17: intraductal carcinoma. Cancer 86(3):429–438, 1999.

30. Komoike Y, Akiyama F, Iino Y, et al: Ipsilateral breast tumor recurrence (IBTR) after breast-conserving treatment for early breast cancer: risk factors and impact on distant metastases. Cancer 106(1):35–41, 2006.

31. Neri A, Marrelli D, Rossi S, et al: Breast cancer local recurrence: risk factors and prognostic relevance of early time to recurrence. World J Surg 31(1):36–45, 2007.

32. Zhou P, Gautam S, Recht A: Factors affecting outcome for young women with early stage invasive breast cancer treated with breast-conserving therapy. Breast Cancer Res Treat 101(1):51–57, 2007.

33. Wong JS, Kaelin CM, Troyan SL, et al: Prospective study of wide excision alone for ductal carcinoma in situ of the breast. J Clin Oncol 24(7):1031–1036, 2006.

34. Lim M, Bellon JR, Gelman R, et al: A prospective study of conservative surgery without radiation therapy in select patients with stage I breast cancer. Int J Radiat Oncol Biol Phys 65(4):1149–1154, 2006.

35. Hughes KS, Schnaper LA, Berry D, et al: Lumpectomy plus tamoxifen with or without irradiation in women 70 years of age or older with early breast cancer. N Engl J Med 351(10):971–977, 2004.

36. Fyles AW, McCready DR, Manchul LA, et al: Tamoxifen with or without breast irradiation in women 50 years of age or older with early breast cancer. N Engl J Med 351(10):963–970, 2004.

37. Benitez PR, Chen PY, Vicini FA, et al: Partial breast irradiation in breast conserving therapy by way of interstitial brachytherapy. Am J Surg 188(4):355–364, 2004.

38. Vicini FA, Remouchamps V, Wallace M, et al: Ongoing clinical experience utilizing 3D conformal external beam radiotherapy to deliver partial-breast irradiation in patients with early-stage breast cancer treated with breast-conserving therapy. Int J Radiat Oncol Biol Phys 57(5):1247–1253, 2003.

39. Fisher B, Bryant J, Dignam JJ, et al: Tamoxifen, radiation therapy, or both for prevention of ipsilateral breast tumor recurrence after lumpectomy in women with invasive breast cancers of one centimeter or less. J Clin Oncol 20(20):4141–4149, 2002.

40. Benitez PR, Streeter O, Vicini F, et al: Preliminary results and evaluation of MammoSite balloon brachytherapy for partial breast irradiation for pure ductal carcinoma in situ: a phase II clinical study. Am J Surg 192(4):427–433, 2006.

41. Chen PY, Vicini FA, Benitez P, et al: Long-term cosmetic results and toxicity after accelerated partial-breast irradiation: a method of radiation delivery by interstitial brachytherapy for the treatment of early-stage breast carcinoma. Cancer 106(5):991–999, 2006.

42. Orecchia R, Ciocca M, Lazzari R, et al: Intraoperative radiation therapy with electrons (ELIOT) in early-stage breast cancer. Breast 12(6):483–490, 2003.

43. Orecchia R, Luini A, Veronesi P, et al: Electron intraoperative treatment in patients with early-stage breast cancer: data update. Expert Rev Anticancer Ther 6(4):605–611, 2006.

44. Vaidya JS, Baum M, Tobias JS, et al: The novel technique of delivering targeted intraoperative radiotherapy (targit) for early breast cancer. Eur J Surg Oncol 28(4):447–454, 2002.

45. Zellars RC, Stearns V, Frassica D, et al: Feasibility trial of partial breast irradiation with concurrent dose-dense doxorubicin and cyclophosphamide in early-stage breast cancer. J Clin Oncol 27(17):2816–2822, 2009.

46. Formenti SC, Truong MT, Goldberg JD, et al: Prone accelerated partial breast irradiation after breast-conserving surgery: preliminary clinical results and dose-volume histogram analysis. Int J Radiat Oncol Biol Phys 60(2):493–504, 2004.

47. Silverstein MJ, Poller DN, Waisman JR, et al: Prognostic classification of breast ductal carcinoma-in-situ. Lancet 345(8958):1154–1157, 1995.

48. de Mascarel I, Bonichon F, MacGrogan G, et al: Application of the Van Nuys prognostic index in a retrospective series of 367

ductal carcinomas in situ of the breast examined by serial macroscopic sectioning: practical considerations. Breast Cancer Res Treat 61(2):151–159, 2000.

49. Hughes LL, Wang M, Page DL, et al: Local excision alone without irradiation for ductal carcinoma in situ of the breast: a trial of the Eastern Cooperative Oncology Group. J Clin Oncol 27(32):5319–5324, 2009.

50. Hughes LL, Wang M, Page DL, et al: Local excision alone without irradiation for ductal carcinoma in situ of the breast: a trial of the Eastern Cooperative Oncology Group. J Clin Oncol 27(32):5319–5324, 2009.

51. Fujishiro S, Mitsumori M, Kokubo M, et al: Cosmetic results and complications after breast conserving therapy for early breast cancer. Breast Cancer 7(1):57–63, 2000.

52. Johansen J, Overgaard J, Rose C, et al: Cosmetic outcome and breast morbidity in breast-conserving treatment: results from the Danish DBCG-82TM national randomized trial in breast cancer. Acta Oncol 41(4):369–380, 2002.

53. Lilla C, Ambrosone CB, Kropp S, et al: Predictive factors for late normal tissue complications following radiotherapy for breast cancer. Breast Cancer Res Treat 106(1):143–150, 2007.

54. Moro G, Stasi M, Borca VC: Does concomitant chemoradiotherapy influence cosmetic outcome in conservative treatment of breast cancer? Tumori 83(4):743–747, 1997.

55. Palazzi M, Tomatis S, Valli MC, et al: Impact of radiotherapy technique on the outcome of early breast cancer treated with conservative surgery: a multicenter observational study on 1,176 patients. Int J Radiat Oncol Biol Phys 65(5):1361–1367, 2006.

56. Sarin R, Dinshaw KA, Shrivastava SK, et al: Therapeutic factors influencing the cosmetic outcome and late complications in the conservative management of early breast cancer. Int J Radiat Oncol Biol Phys 27(2):285–292, 1993.

57. Taylor ME, Perez CA, Halverson KJ, et al: Factors influencing cosmetic results after conservation therapy for breast cancer. Int J Radiat Oncol Biol Phys 31(4):753–764, 1995.

58. Wolden SL, Hancock SL, Carlson RW, et al: Management of breast cancer after Hodgkin's disease. J Clin Oncol 18(4):765–772, 2000.

59. Deutsch M: Repeat high-dose external beam irradiation for in-breast tumor recurrence after previous lumpectomy and whole breast irradiation. Int J Radiat Oncol Biol Phys 53(3):687–691, 2002.

60. Niehoff P, Dietrich J, Ostertag H, et al: High-dose-rate (HDR) or pulsed-dose-rate (PDR) perioperative interstitial intensity-modulated brachytherapy (IMBT) for local recurrences of previously irradiated breast or thoracic wall following breast cancer. Strahlenther Onkol 182(2):102–107, 2006.

61. Chen AM, Obedian E, Haffty BG: Breast-conserving therapy in the setting of collagen vascular disease. Cancer J 7(6):480–491, 2001.

62. De Naeyer B, De Meerleer G, Braems S, et al: Collagen vascular diseases and radiation therapy: a critical review. Int J Radiat Oncol Biol Phys 44(5):975–980, 1999.

63. Ross JG, Hussey DH, Mayr NA, et al: Acute and late reactions to radiation therapy in patients with collagen vascular diseases. Cancer 71(11):3744–3752, 1993.

64. Bradley B, Fleck A, Osei EK: Normalized data for the estimation of fetal radiation dose from radiotherapy of the breast. Br J Radiol 79(946):818–827, 2006.

65. Mazonakis M, Varveris H, Damilakis J, et al: Radiation dose to conceptus resulting from tangential breast irradiation. Int J Radiat Oncol Biol Phys 55(2):386–391, 2003.

66. Woo JC, Yu T, Hurd TC: Breast cancer in pregnancy: a literature review. Arch Surg 138(1):91–98; discussion 99, 2003.

67. Wapnir IL, Anderson SJ, Mamounas EP, et al: Prognosis after ipsilateral breast tumor recurrence and locoregional recurrences in five National Surgical Adjuvant Breast and Bowel Project node-positive adjuvant breast cancer trials. J Clin Oncol 24(13):2028–2037, 2006.

68. Fowble B: Ipsilateral breast tumor recurrence following breast-conserving surgery for early-stage invasive cancer. Acta Oncol 38 Suppl 13:9–17, 1999.

69. Freedman GM, Hanlon AL, Fowble BL, et al: Recursive partitioning identifies patients at high and low risk for ipsilateral tumor recurrence after breast-conserving surgery and radiation. J Clin Oncol 20(19):4015–4021, 2002.

70. Kirova YM, Stoppa-Lyonnet D, Savignoni A, et al: Risk of breast cancer recurrence and contralateral breast cancer in

relation to BRCA1 and BRCA2 mutation status following breast-conserving surgery and radiotherapy. Eur J Cancer 41(15):2304–2311, 2005.

71. Harris EE, Hwang WT, Lee EA, et al: The impact of HER-2 status on local recurrence in women with stage I-II breast cancer treated with breast-conserving therapy. Breast J 12(5):431–436, 2006.

72. Matthews RH, McNeese MD, Montague ED, et al: Prognostic implications of age in breast cancer patients treated with tumorectomy and irradiation or with mastectomy. Int J Radiat Oncol Biol Phys 14(4):659–663, 1988.

73. Bartelink H, Horiot JC, Poortmans P, et al: Recurrence rates after treatment of breast cancer with standard radiotherapy with or without additional radiation. N Engl J Med 345(19):1378–1387, 2001.

74. Romestaing P, Lehingue Y, Carrie C, et al: Role of a 10-gy boost in the conservative treatment of early breast cancer: results of a randomized clinical trial in Lyon, France. J Clin Oncol 15(3):963–968, 1997.

75. Cuzick J, Stewart H, Rutqvist L, et al: Cause-specific mortality in long-term survivors of breast cancer who participated in trials of radiotherapy. J Clin Oncol 12(3):447–453, 1994.

76. Overgaard M: Overview of randomized trials in high risk breast cancer patients treated with adjuvant systemic therapy with or without postmastectomy irradiation. Semin Radiat Oncol 9(3):292–299, 1999.

77. Recht A, Gray R, Davidson NE, et al: Locoregional failure 10 years after mastectomy and adjuvant chemotherapy with or without tamoxifen without irradiation: experience of the Eastern Cooperative Oncology Group. J Clin Oncol 17(6):1689–1700, 1999.

78. Overgaard M, Nielsen HM, Overgaard J: Is the benefit of postmastectomy irradiation limited to patients with four or more positive nodes, as recommended in international consensus report? A subgroup analysis of the DBCG 82 b&c randomized trials. Radiother Oncol 82:244–253, 2007.

79. Zellars R: Post-mastectomy radiotherapy. Clin Adv Hematol Oncol 7(8):533–543, 2009.

80. McGale P, Darby S, Taylor C, et al: The 2006 worldwide overview of the effects of local treatments for early breast cancer on long term outcome. Int J Radiat Oncol Biol Phys 66(3):S2, 2006.

81. Pierce LJ: The use of radiotherapy after mastectomy: a review of the literature. J Clin Oncol 23(8):1706–1717, 2005.

82. Wolmark N, Wang J, Mamounas E, et al: Preoperative chemotherapy in patients with operable breast cancer: nine-year results from National Surgical Adjuvant Breast and Bowel Project B-18. J Natl Cancer Inst Monogr (30):96–102, 2001.

83. Buchholz TA, Lehman CD, Harris JR, et al: Statement of the science concerning locoregional treatments after preoperative chemotherapy for breast cancer: a National Cancer Institute conference. J Clin Oncol 26:791–797, 2008.

84. Garg AK, Oh JL, Oswald MJ, et al: Effect of postmastectomy radiotherapy in patients < 35 years old with stage II–III breast cancer treated with doxorubicin-based neoadjuvant chemotherapy and mastectomy. Int J Radiat Oncol Biol Phys 69:1478–1483, 2007.

85. McGuire SE, Gonzalez-Angulo AM, Huang EH, et al: Postmastectomy radiation improves the outcome of patients with locally advanced breast cancer who achieve a pathologic complete response to neoadjuvant chemotherapy. Int J Radiat Oncol Biol Phys 68:1004–1009, 2007.

86. Fowble B, Hanlon A, Freedman G, et al: Internal mammary node irradiation neither decreases distant metastases nor improves survival in stage I and II breast cancer. Int J Radiat Oncol Biol Phys 47(4):883–894, 2000.

87. Yu J, Li G, Li J, et al: The pattern of lymphatic metastasis of breast cancer and its influence on the delineation of radiation fields. Int J Radiat Oncol Biol Phys 61(3):874–878, 2005.

88. Veronesi U, Valagussa P: Inefficacy of internal mammary nodes dissection in breast cancer surgery. Cancer 47(1):170–175, 1981.

89. Veronesi U, Cascinelli N, Greco M, et al: Prognosis of breast cancer patients after mastectomy and dissection of internal mammary nodes. Ann Surg 202(6):702–707, 1985.

90. Veronesi U, Cascinelli N, Bufalino R, et al: Risk of internal mammary lymph node metastases and its relevance on prognosis of breast cancer patients. Ann Surg 198(6):681–684, 1983.

91. Stemmer SM, Rizel S, Hardan I, et al: The role of irradiation of the internal mammary lymph nodes in high-risk stage II to IIIA breast cancer patients after high-dose chemotherapy: a prospective sequential nonrandomized study. J Clin Oncol 21(14):2713–2718, 2003.

92. Altundag M, Altundag K, Cengiz M, et al: The field of radiation therapy may effect health-related quality of life in patients with operable breast cancer. J Clin Oncol 22(9):1765; author reply 1765–1766, 2004.

93. Hojris I, Andersen J, Overgaard M, et al: Late treatment-related morbidity in breast cancer patients randomized to postmastectomy radiotherapy and systemic treatment versus systemic treatment alone. Acta Oncol 39(3):355–372, 2000.

94. Allen AM, Prosnitz RG, Ten Haken RK, et al: Body mass index predicts the incidence of radiation pneumonitis in breast cancer patients. Cancer J 11(5):390–398, 2005

95. Porock D, Kristjanson L: Skin reactions during radiotherapy for breast cancer: the use and impact of topical agents and dressings. Eur J Cancer Care (Engl) 8(3):143–153, 1999.

96. McQuestion M: Evidence-based skin care management in radiation therapy. Semin Oncol Nurs 22(3):163–173, 2006.

97. Pommier P, Gomez F, Sunyach MP, et al: Phase III randomized trial of calendula officinalis compared with trolamine for the prevention of acute dermatitis during irradiation for breast cancer. J Clin Oncol 22(8):1447–1453, 2004.

98. Meric F, Buchholz TA, Mirza NQ, et al: Long-term complications associated with breast-conservation surgery and radiotherapy. Ann Surg Oncol 9(6):543–549, 2002.

99. Harper JL, Franklin LE, Jenrette JM, et al: Skin toxicity during breast irradiation: pathophysiology and management. South Med J 97(10):989–993, 2004.

100. Lind PA, Wennberg B, Gagliardi G, et al: ROC curves and evaluation of radiation-induced pulmonary toxicity in breast cancer. Int J Radiat Oncol Biol Phys 64(3):765–770, 2006.

101. Lind PA, Marks LB, Hardenbergh PH, et al: Technical factors associated with radiation pneumonitis after local +/- regional radiation therapy for breast cancer. Int J Radiat Oncol Biol Phys 52(1):137–143, 2002.

102. Minor GI, Yashar CM, Spanos WJ, Jr, et al: The relationship of radiation pneumonitis to treated lung volume in breast conservation therapy. Breast J 12(1):48–52, 2006.

103. Burstein HJ, Bellon JR, Galper S, et al: Prospective evaluation of concurrent paclitaxel and radiation therapy after adjuvant doxorubicin and cyclophosphamide chemotherapy for stage II or III breast cancer. Int J Radiat Oncol Biol Phys 64(2):496–504, 2006.

104. Taghian AG, Assaad SI, Niemierko A, et al: Is a reduction in radiation lung volume and dose necessary with paclitaxel chemotherapy for node-positive breast cancer? Int J Radiat Oncol Biol Phys 62(2):386–391, 2005.

105. Ellerbroek N, Martino S, Mautner B, et al: Breast-conserving therapy with adjuvant paclitaxel and radiation therapy: feasibility of concurrent treatment. Breast J 9(2):74–78, 2003.

106. Gagliardi G, Bjohle J, Lax I, et al: Radiation pneumonitis after breast cancer irradiation: analysis of the complication probability using the relative seriality model. Int J Radiat Oncol Biol Phys 46(2):373–381, 2000.

107. Tsujino K, Hirota S, Kotani Y, et al: Radiation pneumonitis following concurrent accelerated hyperfractionated radiotherapy and chemotherapy for limited-stage small-cell lung cancer: dose-volume histogram analysis and comparison with conventional chemoradiation. Int J Radiat Oncol Biol Phys 64(4):1100–1105, 2006.

108. Katayama N, Sato S, Katsui K, et al: Analysis of factors associated with radiation-induced bronchiolitis obliterans organizing pneumonia syndrome after breast-conserving therapy. Int J Radiat Oncol Biol Phys 73(4):1049–1054, 2009.

109. Ogo E, Komaki R, Fujimoto K, et al: A survey of radiation-induced bronchiolitis obliterans organizing pneumonia syndrome after breast-conserving therapy in Japan. Int J Radiat Oncol Biol Phys 71(1):123–131, 2008.

110. Hojris I, Andersen J, Overgaard M, et al: Late treatment-related morbidity in breast cancer patients randomized to postmastectomy radiotherapy and systemic treatment versus systemic treatment alone. Acta Oncol 39(3):355–372, 2000.

111. Hojris I, Overgaard M, Christensen JJ, et al: Morbidity and mortality of ischaemic heart disease in high-risk breast-cancer patients after adjuvant postmastectomy systemic treatment

with or without radiotherapy: analysis of DBCG 82b and 82c randomised trials. radiotherapy committee of the Danish Breast Cancer Cooperative Group. Lancet 354(9188):1425–1430, 1999.

112. Berson AM, Emery R, Rodriguez L, et al: Clinical experience using respiratory gated radiation therapy: comparison of free-breathing and breath-hold techniques. Int J Radiat Oncol Biol Phys 60(2):419–426, 2004.

113. Krauss DJ, Kestin LL, Raff G, et al: MRI-based volumetric assessment of cardiac anatomy and dose reduction via active breathing control during irradiation for left-sided breast cancer. Int J Radiat Oncol Biol Phys 61(4):1243–1250, 2005.

114. Jagsi R, Moran JM, Kessler ML, et al: Respiratory motion of the heart and positional reproducibility under active breathing control. Int J Radiat Oncol Biol Phys 68(1):253–258, 2007.

115. Coen JJ, Taghian AG, Kachnic LA, et al: Risk of lymphedema after regional nodal irradiation with breast conservation therapy. Int J Radiat Oncol Biol Phys 55(5):1209–1215, 2003.

116. Golshan M, Martin WJ, Dowlatshahi K: Sentinel lymph node biopsy lowers the rate of lymphedema when compared with standard axillary lymph node dissection. Am Surg 69(3):209–211; discussion 212, 2003.

117. Golshan M, Smith B: Prevention and management of arm lymphedema in the patient with breast cancer. J Support Oncol 4(8):381–386, 2006.

118. Hinrichs CS, Watroba NL, Rezaishiraz H, et al: Lymphedema secondary to postmastectomy radiation: incidence and risk factors. Ann Surg Oncol 11(6):573–580, 2004.

119. Silberman AW, McVay C, Cohen JS, et al: Comparative morbidity of axillary lymph node dissection and the sentinel lymph node technique: implications for patients with breast cancer. Ann Surg 240(1):1–6, 2004.

120. Kocak Z, Overgaard J: Risk factors of arm lymphedema in breast cancer patients. Acta Oncol 39(3):389–392, 2000.

121. Kligman L, Wong RK, Johnston M, et al: The treatment of lymphedema related to breast cancer: a systematic review and evidence summary. Support Care Cancer 12(6):421–431, 2004.

122. Obedian E, Fischer DB, Haffty BG: Second malignancies after treatment of early-stage breast cancer: lumpectomy and radiation therapy versus mastectomy. J Clin Oncol 18(12):2406–2412, 2000.

123. Woodward WA, Strom EA, McNeese MD, et al: Cardiovascular death and second non-breast cancer malignancy after postmastectomy radiation and doxorubicin-based chemotherapy. Int J Radiat Oncol Biol Phys 57(2):327–335, 2003.

124. Galper S, Gelman R, Recht A, et al: Second nonbreast malignancies after conservative surgery and radiation therapy for early-stage breast cancer. Int J Radiat Oncol Biol Phys 52(2):406–414, 2002.

125. Harvey EB, Brinton LA: Second cancer following cancer of the breast in Connecticut, 1935–1982. Natl Cancer Inst Monogr 68:99–112, 1985.

126. Zablotska LB, Neugut AI: Lung carcinoma after radiation therapy in women treated with lumpectomy or mastectomy for primary breast carcinoma. Cancer 97(6):1404–1411, 2003.

127. Renella R, Verkooijen HM, Fioretta G, et al: Increased risk of acute myeloid leukaemia after treatment for breast cancer. Breast 15(5):614–619, 2006.

128. Gao X, Fisher SG, Emami B: Risk of second primary cancer in the contralateral breast in women treated for early-stage breast cancer: a population-based study. Int J Radiat Oncol Biol Phys 56(4):1038–1045, 2003.

129. Boice JD, Jr, Harvey EB, Blettner M, et al: Cancer in the contralateral breast after radiotherapy for breast cancer. N Engl J Med 326(12):781–785, 1992.

130. Nielsen HM, Overgaard J, Grau C, et al: Audit of the radiotherapy in the DBCG 82 b&c trials: a validation study of the 1,538 patients randomised to postmastectomy radiotherapy. Radiother Oncol 76(3):285–292, 2005.

131. Owen HW, Dockerty MB, Gray HK: Occult carcinoma of the breast. Surg Gynecol Obstet 98:302–308, 1954.

132. Lloyd MS, Nash AG: 'Occult' breast cancer. Ann R Coll Surg Engl 83:420–424, 2001.

133. Khandelwal AK, Garguilo GA: Therapeutic options for occult breast cancer: a survey of the American Society of Breast Surgeons and review of the literature. Am J Surg 190:609–613, 2005.

134. Campana F, Fourquet A, Ashby MA, et al : Presentation of axillary lymphadenopathy without detectable breast primary. Radiotherp Oncol 15:321–325, 1989.

135. Blanchard DK, Farley DR: Retrospective study of women presenting with axillary metastases from occult breast carcinoma. W J Surg 28:535–539, 2004.

Neoadjuvant Therapy

17

Susanne Briest and Vered Stearns

KEY POINTS

- Neoadjuvant or preoperative or primary systemic chemotherapy became widely accepted in the treatment of patients with inoperable locally advanced disease, improving their surgical options.
- In women with primary operable breast cancer, no survival differences could be found in multiple trials that compared the same adjuvant and neoadjuvant chemotherapy regimens, establishing that neoadjuvant chemotherapy is equivalent to the postoperative therapy in terms of efficacy.
- Although a large difference in survival was not seen between women who received adjuvant and those who received neoadjuvant therapy, women who achieved pathologic complete response after neoadjuvant therapy had improved outcomes.
- Neoadjuvant endocrine treatment and chemotherapy enhance the chances of breast conservation.
- When preoperative endocrine therapy is considered in postmenopausal women with endocrine-responsive disease to enhance breast conservation or to improve surgical options, aromatase inhibitors should be favored.
- Generally, anthracycline- and taxane-based regimens are recommended.
- The addition of trastuzumab to preoperative anthracycline- and taxane-containing regimens in HER2-positive disease is associated with an impressive improvement of the pathologic complete response.
- Early exposure to systemic therapy could theoretically minimize drug resistance.
- When breast conservation is considered, serial breast imaging is recommended. The highest sensitivity has

- been shown with serial MRI, followed by physical examination, ultrasound, and mammography.
- The optimal timing for sentinel lymph node biopsy for women with primary operable breast cancer and clinically negative axilla has not been established.
- Tumors shrink in different ways after neoadjuvant therapy. There are no standardized procedures to handle tissue specimens after neoadjuvant treatment. Tight cooperation among all disciplines involved in treatment of patients with neoadjuvant therapy is necessary.
- Whereas clinical practice guidelines concerning postmastectomy radiation without neoadjuvant therapy are fairly well established, there is not sufficient evidence to make recommendations for patients who have received preoperative chemotherapy.
- After neoadjuvant chemotherapy, the extent of local recurrence is highly associated with postchemotherapy pathologic primary tumor size and any category of positive lymph nodes.
- When a decision is made to administer neoadjuvant chemotherapy, current consensus reports support the use of all planned chemotherapy before surgery. Whether women with large residual disease should receive additional chemotherapy after the definitive surgery is not known.
- Another important goal that has emerged is to use the neoadjuvant therapy as an in vivo sensitivity marker of tumor response.
- The neoadjuvant approach has also become an important vehicle for the evaluation of new agents and the introduction and testing of surrogate markers for the prediction of tumor response and clinical outcome.

Historical Perspective

Development of Systemic Treatment

Historically, the treatment of choice for breast cancer was a surgical one. William Stewart Halsted,[1] at the time the head of surgery at the Johns Hopkins Hospital in Baltimore, suggested that breast cancer is a highly localized disease that can be cured by a radical local therapy. Unfortunately, radical surgeries did not prevent subsequent recurrences and breast cancer-related deaths. Schinzinger[2] and Sir George Beatson[3] proposed in the 19th century a relation between the removal of the ovaries and the

Chemotherapy Acronyms	
AC	doxorubicin (Adriamycin) and cyclophosphamide
CMF	cyclophosphamide, methotrexate, and 5-fluorouracil
CVAP	cyclophosphamide, vincristine, doxorubicin, and prednisone
FEC	5-fluorouracil, epirubicin, and cyclophosphamide
NX	vinorelbine and capecitabine
TAC	docetaxel, doxorubicin, and cyclophosphamide
VACP	vincristine, doxorubicin, cyclophosphamide, and prednisone
VbMF	vinblastine, methotrexate with calcium leucovorin rescue, and fluorouracil

regression of advanced breast cancer, suggesting a systemic component. Only decades later the idea of administration of systemic treatment during the early stages of the disease was introduced.[4] The paradigm of breast cancer as a systemic disease was pushed forward by Bernhard Fisher who proposed that breast cancer metastasizes unpredictably and would be best treated with conservative local treatment and systemic therapy. With his colleagues at the National Surgical Adjuvant Breast and Bowel Project (NSABP) he initiated innovative breast cancer trials starting in 1957.

Adjuvant systemic therapy is now administered to almost every woman with breast cancer and may include endocrine manipulations, chemotherapy, biologic therapy, or a combination. The most recent Oxford Overview of the Early Breast Cancer Trialists' Cooperative Group (EBCTCG), designed to summarize the benefits and toxicities of adjuvant chemotherapy was published in 2000 and included data from 102 clinical trials with 53,353 participants.[5] The addition of any type of adjuvant chemotherapy reduces the risk of breast cancer recurrence and mortality rate by 22% and 15%, respectively, and reduces all-cause mortality rate by 13%. Anthracycline-based regimens provide additional benefit compared with the traditional cyclophosphamide, methotrexate, and 5-fluorouracil (CMF)-containing regimens. Women who received anthracycline-based regimens had a reduction in annual odds of breast cancer recurrence by 11% and all-cause death by 15% compared with those who received CMF-like regimens. More recently, taxanes have been added to anthracycline-based therapy in combination or a sequential manner and have further improved disease-free and overall survival.[6]

Chemotherapy has been traditionally used after the completion of breast-conserving surgery or mastectomy. Neoadjuvant therapy, also designated preoperative or primary chemotherapy, has been used for more than three decades to treat women with locally advanced breast cancer. Based on the success of adjuvant chemotherapy and the promising experiences with neoadjuvant therapy in older women or those with advanced disease, the neoadjuvant approach reached the center of interest for women with primary operable breast cancer. In these women, the initial goal was to improve overall survival based on the hypothesis that the administration of chemotherapy prior to the locoregional therapy could eradicate micrometastasis. Local control was a secondary objective that was recognized as a result of impressive tumor regression in some cases.[7]

Indications for Systemic Therapy

Before recommending the administration of neoadjuvant chemotherapy to women with primary operable disease, it is crucial to determine that chemotherapy is indeed indicated. Several organizations and international panels, including the National Comprehensive Cancer Network (NCCN), and the expert panel of St. Gallen, Switzerland, have been convened to create consensus recommendations regarding adjuvant systemic treatment for early breast cancer. Risk groups for recurrence are defined using prognostic factors, such as tumor size, grade, vascular invasion or age, as well as estrogen receptor (ER) and HER2 status. In the most recent St. Gallen symposium, three large categories of breast tumors were proposed including highly endocrine responsive, endocrine-nonresponsive and incompletely endocrine-responsive. Whereas nonresponsive disease is characterized by the absence of steroid receptors, differentiation between endocrine-responsive (ideally highly ER and progesterone receptor [PR]-positive) and incompletely endocrine-responsive is defined by the degree of ER and PR positivity. Furthermore, three risk categories were defined in St. Gallen: low, intermediate, and high. Depending on the risk categories and the endocrine responsiveness, endocrine therapy or chemotherapy alone or in combination is recommended.[8] Overall, when a woman presents with clinical stage II or III breast cancer for which chemotherapy would be recommended as part of the multidisciplinary treatment, there may be advantages in the consideration of neoadjuvant chemotherapy in some cases.

Objectives of Neoadjuvant Treatment

The emphasis of neoadjuvant therapy was initially the improvement of surgical options to obtain better local control in patients with locally advanced breast cancer. The therapy was designated induction chemotherapy and prospective studies confirmed that patients with inoperable locally advanced breast cancer who responded to the therapy could subsequently have a mastectomy. Neoadjuvant chemotherapy in women with primary operable disease was first investigated to improve disease-free or overall survival. In contrast to the primary aim of preoperative therapy in patients with locally advanced disease, the goal of multidisciplinary treatment in patients with operable breast cancer is to obtain freedom from disease.[9]

Over a dozen studies compared the same chemotherapy in the adjuvant and neoadjuvant settings. Mauri and colleagues[10] performed a meta-analysis that included data from nine studies comparing adjuvant with neoadjuvant chemotherapy with a total of 3946 patients. The primary outcomes of the analysis were death, disease progression, distant disease recurrence, and locoregional disease recurrence. The investigators reported that neoadjuvant therapy was equivalent to adjuvant treatment in terms of survival and overall disease progression. The response to chemotherapy and the ability to perform breast conservation were prognostic indicators for 5-year disease-free survival and overall survival.[11]

Although neoadjuvant chemotherapy did not improve disease-free and overall survival compared with adjuvant treatment, the rate of breast-conserving therapy has been consistently superior.[12] In the Mauri meta-analysis, seven trials reported that neoadjuvant therapy was associated with a higher rate of breast conservation, whereas one trial was associated with a borderline difference, and three other studies revealed no difference.[10] However, there was a considerably high variability across these trials,

which enrolled patients between 1983 and 1999. The studies included different treatment regimens, and surgery was not mandated in all of the trials after neoadjuvant chemotherapy.

The first large preoperative trial was conducted by the NSABP. NSABP B-18 trial enrolled 1523 patients who were randomly assigned to four cycles of doxorubicin and cyclophosphamide (AC) every 3 weeks before or after the definitive surgery. Compared with the adjuvant treatment group, 12% more lumpectomies were performed in the preoperative group.[13] The European Cooperative Trial in Operable breast cancer (ECTO), randomized 1355 patients to four cycles of doxorubicin and paclitaxel followed by four cycles of CMF and found that breast preservation was feasible in 65% versus 34% ($P < .001$) for the administration of the therapy pre- and postoperatively, respectively.[14]

Other potential benefits of neoadjuvant chemotherapy have been proposed (Table 17-1). When chemotherapy is administered in the adjuvant setting, the effectiveness for an individual patient cannot be determined. In contrast, the response to neoadjuvant therapy may be appreciated after as few as one or two cycles. The early response to neoadjuvant chemotherapy can identify patients with a high probability of achieving a pathologic complete response (pCR)[15] and thus serve as a predictor for pCR. Indeed, achieving a pCR correlated with improved disease-free survival and overall survival compared with those experiencing a partial or no response to neoadjuvant chemotherapy.[16] Whereas overall survival (70% and 69%, respectively) and disease-free survival (55% and 53%, respectively) did not differ between the preoperative and the postoperative treatment group, a statistically significant improvement in survival rate occurred for patients who achieved a pCR compared with those with residual invasive tumor at the time of operation (85% versus 73% alive at 9 years).

The results of the NSABP B-18 trial concerning pCR were confirmed by NSABP B-27.[17] The NSABP B-27 trial was designed to evaluate the effects of adding docetaxel to AC preoperative treatment on response rate, disease-free survival, and overall survival. The 2411 participating patients were randomized to either AC followed by surgery (Group 1), AC followed by docetaxel and surgery (Group 2) or AC fol-

Table 17-1. Potential Advantages and Disadvantages of Neoadjuvant Therapy

Advantages

Clinical

Improve overall survival*
Improve disease-free survival*
Enhance breast-conserving surgery (BCS)
Individualize treatment: in vivo sensitivity
Gain prognostic information

Research

Predictive factors
    Imaging: Standard: Mammogram, Ultrasound
            Emerging: MRI, PET
    Tissue: IHC, gene array, proteomics
    Serum: Circulating markers, proteomics
Drug mechanism of action:
    Standard: Endocrine therapies, chemotherapy, anti
    HER2 agents
    Emerging: Novel targeted treatments

Disadvantages

Increased local recurrence after BCS
Loss of prognostic information
Overtreatment
What if large residual disease?

*Theoretical.
IHC, immunohistochemistry; MRI, magnetic resonance imaging; PET, positron emission tomography.

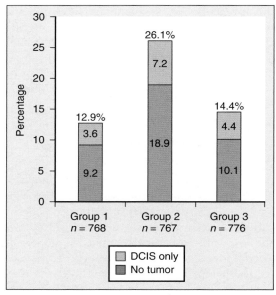

Figure 17-1. Pathologic tumor response at the time of surgery by treatment arm. $P < .0001$ for testing percentage of patients with pathologic complete response in group 2 (after doxorubicin and cyclophosphamide [AC] plus docetaxel) versus groups 1 and 3 combined (after AC), adjusted for age, clinical tumor size, and clinical nodal status. DCIS, ductal carcinoma in situ. (From Bear HD, Anderson S, Smith RE, et al: Sequential preoperative or postoperative docetaxel added to preoperative doxorubicin plus cyclophosphamide for operable breast cancer: National Surgical Adjuvant Breast and Bowel Project Protocol B-27. J Clin Oncol 24:2019–2027, 2006. Reprinted with permission from the American Society of Clinical Oncology.)

lowed by surgery and adjuvant docetaxel (Group 3). Although the addition of docetaxel had no statistically significant effect on disease-free survival and overall survival, the pCR rate increased from 13.7% to 26.1% ($P < .001$). Furthermore, the proportion of patients with negative nodes following neoadjuvant therapy was higher with the addition of docetaxel to AC compared with patients who received AC alone (50.8% versus 58.2%, respectively; $P < .001$). The B-27 trial results confirmed that response to chemotherapy is a significant predictive factor for disease-free survival and overall survival in individual patients. In addition, the rate of local relapses in this study was even lower when docetaxel was added to preoperative AC in the neoadjuvant group compared with relapse in the adjuvant group[17] (Figs. 17-1 and 17-2).

Another important goal is to use neoadjuvant therapy as an in vivo sensitivity marker for tumor response. Assessment of tumor response is directly possible by clinical means and imaging as well as by biochemical measurements. It has been suggested that the primary tumor can be used as a monitor for treatment of micrometastasis. pCR after neoadjuvant therapy could then

be a surrogate marker for the eradication of residual micrometastasis.[9] Another hypothesis is that drug resistance may be minimized with early exposure to systemic therapy.[18]

In recent years, the study of predictors of response to chemotherapy has become a new consideration for neoadjuvant treatment. In contrast to adjuvant trials, which require a large sample size and years of accrual and follow-up, the neoadjuvant treatment paradigm offers knowledge regarding outcomes much sooner and with considerably fewer participants. The neoadjuvant approach has thus become an important vehicle for the evaluation of new agents and the introduction and testing of surrogate markers for the prediction of tumor response and clinical outcome.

One model is to use early evaluation of response (e.g., following two cycles of neoadjuvant chemotherapy) to discriminate between patients with sensitive versus resistant tumors.

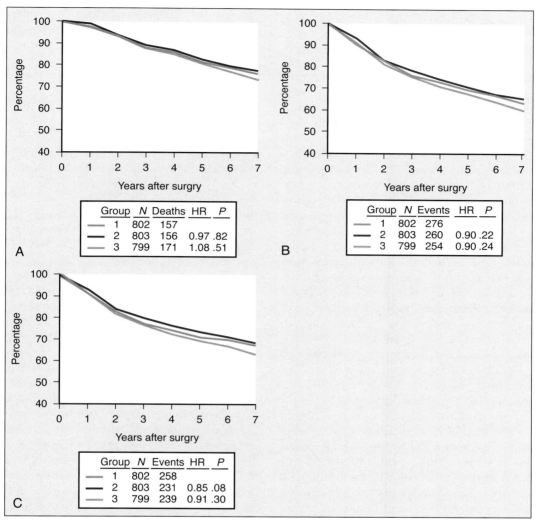

Figure 17-2. Overall (A), disease-free (B), and relapse-free (C) survival for groups 1, 2, and 3. Hazard ratios (HR) and *P* values shown are for comparisons of groups 2 or 3 with group 1. (From Bear HD, Anderson S, Smith RE, et al: Sequential preoperative or postoperative docetaxel added to preoperative doxorubicin plus cyclophosphamide for operable breast cancer: National Surgical Adjuvant Breast and Bowel Project Protocol B-27. J Clin Oncol 24:2019–2027, 2006. Reprinted with permission from the American Society of Clinical Oncology.)

The German Preoperative Adriamycin Docetaxel (GEPAR)TRIO trial randomized 2106 patients to two cycles of docetaxel, doxorubicin, and cyclophosphamide (TAC).[15] Patients whose tumors responded were treated with another four or six cycles of TAC. Those whose tumor did not respond to the initial two cycles of TAC received either four additional cycles of TAC or a non–cross-resistant chemotherapy regimen with vinorelbine and capecitabine (NX). Whereas the pCR rate was 17.9% overall, patients responding to TAC reached a pCR rate of 22.9% compared with nonresponders treated with TAC (pCR rate 7.3%) or NX (pCR rate 3.1%). It is not yet clear whether a change in regimen might provide a survival benefit, because the data of the phase III trial are not sufficiently mature.[19] However, an early response after two to three cycles of neoadjuvant chemotherapy was predictive of pCR, which is by itself an important indicator of long-term outcome in earlier studies.[20]

Another model uses the presurgical period for short-term administration of novel agents to evaluate biomarker modulation or to study mechanism of action. Finally, the use of new imaging methods and the ability to obtain serial tissue biopsies may assist in evaluating the treatment effects and make neoadjuvant therapy an attractive model to study mechanism of action of standard and novel therapies.

At the same time, the neoadjuvant approach may have potential disadvantages. One major concern was that an increased rate of breast conservation may be associated with higher locoregional recurrence rates. Particular attention must be given to women initially scheduled for mastectomy who were subsequently candidates for breast conservation following neoadjuvant chemotherapy. Indeed, it has been demonstrated in NSABP B-18 that ipsilateral breast tumor recurrence rate was higher in women who were downstaged to a lumpectomy (15.4%) compared with those who were candidates for a lumpectomy before chemotherapy (9.9%).[16]

In the GEPARDUO Trial, 913 patients were treated preoperatively with either 8-week dosedense doxorubicin and docetaxel or 24-week AC followed by docetaxel. The published details of the surgical procedures of 607 patients, including the retrospective collection and central review of surgical and pathologic reports, revealed that 70% of the patients were treated with breast conservation; however, 21.1% required reexcision (12.4%) or a mastectomy (8.7%).[21]

The Mauri meta-analysis reported a statistically significant higher risk for recurrence after neoadjuvant therapy.[10] However, this effect was greater in trials in which patients received only radiation therapy without surgical removal of the primary tumor following the neoadjuvant systemic treatment, a strategy that is not recommended. As in primary surgery, negative margins are critical after preoperative therapy.

Neoadjuvant Treatment

The potential benefits of preoperative chemotherapy together with the evidence supporting the use of adjuvant systemic treatment led to the implementation of neoadjuvant chemotherapy for the treatment of breast cancers in women with stage I and stage II disease. Neoadjuvant therapy is composed of the same components used in the adjuvant setting and may include chemotherapy, endocrine therapy, and targeted therapy.

Neoadjuvant Chemotherapy

Initial studies of neoadjuvant chemotherapy compared the same chemotherapy regimen given in the preoperative with that given in the postoperative setting. Although a difference in survival was not observed, these preoperative trials established that neoadjuvant chemotherapy is equivalent to the postoperative therapy in terms of efficacy.[9]

Early trials included CMF-like and anthracycline-based regimens and more recent trials have also included taxanes. The Aberdeen trial was the first study incorporating a taxane.[22] The 162 randomized patients received four cycles of an anthracycline-containing regimen (cyclophosphamide, vincristine, doxorubicin, and prednisone, CVAP) and were then—depending on their response to therapy—further stratified to either four cycles of docetaxel (nonresponder) or to another four cycles of CVAP versus four cycles of docetaxel (responder). The addition of docetaxel to the treatment of the responders was associated with an improved pCR rate of 34% compared with 16% with CVAP. With a 65-month follow-up, an impressive survival benefit could be demonstrated in the Aberdeen study in women who received a taxane in addition to anthracycline-based regimen.[23] The Aberdeen trial results suggested that the implementation of a non–cross-resistant agent might improve the outcome for patients regardless of response to the initial therapy. MD Anderson Cancer Center investigators performed a similar study that included 190 patients treated with three cycles of vincristine, doxorubicin, cyclophosphamide, and prednisone (VACP). After surgery, women were assigned according to the pathologic tumor size. Patients with a residual tumor smaller than 1 cm^3 received five additional cycles of the preoperative regimen, whereas patients with a residual tumor larger than 1 cm^3 were stratified to a non–cross-resistant therapy consisting of vinblastine, methotrexate with calcium leucovorin rescue, and fluorouracil (VbMF).[24] The pCR rate after VACP was relatively small (12.2%). The difference between the two postoperative treatment regimens in terms of relapse-free survival and overall survival did not reach statistical significance; however, the sample size was small. Given the small sample size in studies reported to date, it is too early to state whether responders or nonresponders have more benefit when crossing to a nonresistant regimen.[9] These observations provided inspiration to a number of large prospective trials, such as the GEPARTRIO trial.

The largest neoadjuvant trial that incorporated a taxane was the NSABP B-27, and its results were concordant with the results of the Aberdeen trial with a larger number of patients and a different anthracycline-containing regimen (AC.)[25] Different chemotherapy regimens have been administered in the neoadjuvant setting including sequential, concurrent, and both sequential and concurrent delivery of substances. The International Expert Panel reviewed the available data and recommended that, once a decision is made, all chemotherapy should be administered before surgery and that the preoperative regimen should include anthracyclines and taxanes[26] (Table 17-2).

Neoadjuvant Chemotherapy and/or Trastuzumab

Trastuzumab is an integral part of adjuvant therapy in women with high-risk primary breast tumors that overexpress or amplify HER2. Trastuzumab was evaluated in several small studies in the neoadjuvant setting. MD Anderson Cancer Center investigators conducted a study that compared paclitaxel followed by 5-fluorouracil, epirubicin, and cyclophosphamide (FEC) with or without trastuzumab. The authors noted a high proportion of pCR in the study participants, which led to an evaluation by the data safety monitoring board and to an early closure of the trial. Indeed, 66.7% of women who received the combination of trastuzumab and chemotherapy had a pCR compared with 25% who received chemotherapy alone.[27] In a recent update, the investigators reported that the pCR among a larger cohort of women treated with neoadjuvant chemotherapy plus trastuzumab was 60%.[28] Recently Gianni and associates[29] presented data of the Neoadjuvant Herceptin (NOAH) trial, a phase III trial, in which patients with HER2-positive tumors were randomized to three cycles of doxorubicin and paclitaxel, followed by four cycles of paclitaxel and three cycles of CMF with or without trastuzumab. The addition of trastuzumab improved both overall response rate (81% versus 73%; $P = .18$), and pCR rate (43% versus 23%; $P = .002$) (Table 17-3).

Interestingly, Baylor investigators reported a 20% response (0–60.4%) to trastuzumab alone administered for 3 weeks. These data suggest that single-agent trastuzumab may be an option for some women. Other studies are required to assess who may benefit from trastuzumab alone.[30] Several studies are evaluating different trastuzumab and other anti–HER2-based regimens. For example, the American College of Surgeons Oncology Group (ACOSOG) has recently initiated Trial Z1041, a phase III study comparing the sequence of fluorouracil, epirubicin, and cyclophosphamide (FEC) with trastuzumab followed by paclitaxel with trastuzumab versus paclitaxel with trastuzumab followed by FEC. As a result of the data available to date, an International Expert Panel recommended the addition of trastuzumab in combination with neoadjuvant chemotherapy in women with HER2-positive tumors.[26]

Neoadjuvant Endocrine Treatment

The idea of preoperative endocrine treatment was introduced many decades ago to avoid surgery in elderly women.[31] Despite a low toxicity profile, neoadjuvant endocrine treatment is not commonly used because chemotherapy is thought to be more active and the outcomes are better documented. Preoperative endocrine therapy is associated with fairly low pCR rates.[32] A comparison of preoperative endocrine therapy for patients with ER-positive tumors and preoperative chemotherapy for those who failed the endocrine therapy or were ER-negative revealed the same survival with a median follow-up of 7.5 years.[33] Semiglazov and colleagues[34] conducted a phase II study randomizing patients with hormone receptor-positive breast cancer to 3 months of the aromatase inhibitors anastrozole or exemestane versus four cycles of doxorubicin and paclitaxel. The overall response rate was similar, whereas the rate of breast-conserving therapy was slightly higher in the endocrine-treated women (33% versus 24%; $P = .058$).

These results suggest that predictive factors such as hormone receptor status may be used to select women for neoadjuvant endocrine treatment alone. Indeed, women with low-grade ER-positive tumors and those with infiltrating lobular tumors may not be good candidates for neoadjuvant chemotherapy.[26] Several trials compared 3 to 4 months of neoadjuvant treatment with aromatase inhibitor to tamoxifen (Table 17-4). In a trial that compared letrozole with tamoxifen, the overall objective response was

Table 17-2. Selected Randomized Trials Incorporating Neoadjuvant Chemotherapy with Taxanes

Trial	Author (Year)	Number of Patients	Treatment Arms	Definition of pCR	pCR	Rate of BCT	Local Recurrence Rate
Aberdeen Trial	Smith et al[22] (2002)	162	After 4×CVAP (1000/1.5/50/40) q3w further stratification to: Nonresponder Allocated to 4×Doc (100) q3w → OP vs Responder 4×CVAP (1000/1.5/50/40) q3w → OP vs 4×Doc (100) q3w → OP	No invasive cancer in breast	16% vs 34%*	48% vs 67%*	No data
NSABP B-27	Bear et al[25] (2003) Bear et al[17] (2006)	2411	4×AC (60/600) q3w → OP vs 4×AC (60/600) q3w → 4×Doc (100) q3w → OP vs 4×AC (60/600) q3w → OP → 4×Doc (100) q3w	No invasive cancer in breast	9.2% vs 18.9% vs 10.1%[†]	85.7% vs 90.7% vs 85.4%	8.5% vs 4.7% vs 5.5%
ECTO	Gianni et al[14] (2005)	1355	OP → 4×A (75) q3w → 4×CMF (600/40/600) q4w vs OP → 4×AP (60/200) q3w → 4×CMF (600/40/600) q4w vs 4×AP (60/200) q3w → 4×CMF (600/40/600) q4w → OP	No invasive cancer in breast	23%	34% vs 65% P < .001	3.6% vs 1.4% n.s.
GEPARDUO	von Minckwitz et al[20] (2005) Raab et al[69] (2005)	913	4×ADoc (60/75) q2w → OP vs 4×AC (60/600) q3w → 4×Doc (100) q3w → OP	No invasive cancer or DCIS in breast and nodes	7% vs 14.3 % P < .001	58.1% vs 63.4% P = .05	No data
	Evans et al[70] (2005)	363	4×ADoc (60/75) q2w → OP vs 4×AC (60/600) q3w → 4×Doc (100) q3w → OP	No invasive cancer or DCIS in breast	24% vs 21% n.s.	20% vs 20%	55 pts vs 45 pts n.s.

Group	Author (year)	N	Regimen	pCR definition	Result	Result 2	Result 3
MD Anderson	Green et al[71] (2005)	258	4×P (225) q3w vs N– 12×P (80) q1w N+ 12×P(175) q1w for 3 of 4 weeks followed by 4×FAC (500 d1+4/50/500) q3w → OP	No invasive cancer in breast and nodes	15.7% vs 28.2% P = .02	18.6% vs 23.6% P = .05	No data
AGO	Untch et al[72] (2002) (abstract)	678	3×E (150) q2w → 3×P (250) q2w vs 4×EP (90/175) q3w followed by → OP → 3×CMF (500/40/600) d1+8 q4w → OP	No invasive cancer or DCIS in breast and nodes	19% vs 10%	61% vs 50% P = .02	No data
MD Anderson	Thomas et al[24] (2004)	193	3×VACP q3w → OP If residual tumor ≤ 1 cm³: 5×VDCP q3w If residual tumor ≥ 1 cm³: randomization to 5×VACP q3w vs 5×VbMF q3w	No invasive cancer in breast	12.2%	5.3%	No data
GEPARTRIO	Von Minckwitz et al[19] (2006) (abstract)	2106	After 2×ACDoc (50/500/75) q3w further stratification to: Nonresponder 4×ACDoc (50/500/75) q3w → OP vs 4×NX (25 d1+8, 2000 d1-14) q3w → OP vs Responder 4×ACDoc (50/500/75) q3w → OP vs 6×ACDoc (50/500/75) q3w → OP	No invasive cancer or DCIS in breast and nodes	5.6% vs 25.2%‡	28.5 vs 40.7%†‡ P < .0001	No data

*CVAP versus docetaxel after 4 cycles of CVAP.
†pCR without DCIS.
‡Nonresponder versus responder.

A, doxorubicin; C, cyclophosphamide; Doc, docetaxel; E, epirubicin; F, 5-fluorouracil; M, methotrexate; N, vinorelbine; P, paclitaxel; V, vincristine; VACP preop, vincristine (1500), doxorubin (60/70/75), cyclophosphamide (600/700/750), prednisone (40 d1-5); VACP postop, postoperative: same doses as preoperative at the highest dosage level reached; VbMF, vinoblastine (1500 d1-3), methotrexate (120), fluorouracil (1000 d2); X, capecitabine. ( ), concentration in mg/m²; q1/2/3/4w: every 1/2/3/4 weeks; BCT, breast-conserving therapy; N+/–, nodal positive/negative; OP, operation; pCR, pathologic complete response; n.s., not significant. AGO, Arbeitsgemeinschaft Gynaekologische Onkologie; EORTC, European Organization for Research and Treatment of Cancer; ECTO, European Cooperative Trial in Operable breast cancer; GEPAR, German Preoperative Adriamycin Docetaxel; NSABP, National Surgical Adjuvant Breast and Bowel Project.

Table 17-3. Selected Randomized Trials Incorporating Neoadjuvant Trastuzumab

Trial	Author (Year)	Number of Patients	Treatment Arms	Definition of pCR	pCR
	Burstein et al[73] (2003)	40	4×P (175) q3w + T q1w/12 wk (4 mg/kg loading dose, then 2 mg/kg/wk) → OP → 4×AC (60/600)	No invasive cancer in breast	18%
	Buzdar et al[27] (2005) Buzdar et al[28] (2007)	64 (initially 42)	4×P (225) q3w → 4×FEC (500 d1+4/75/500) q3w → OP vs 4×P (225) q3w → 4×FEC (500 d1+4/75/500) q3w + T q1w/24 wk (4 mg/kg loading dose, then 2 mg/kg/wk) → OP	No invasive cancer in breast	25% vs 66.7% P = .02
TECHNO	Untch et al[74] (2005)	230	4×EC (90/600) q3w → 4×P (175)q3w + T q3w (8 mg/kg loading dose, then 6 mg/kg) → OP → T q3w/52 wk	No invasive cancer in breast	37%
	Mohesin et al[30] (2005)	35	T q1w/3 wk (4 mg/kg loading dose, then 2 mg/kg/wk) → 4×Doc (100) q3w + Tq1w → OP	No data	No data
	Chang et al[75] (2006)	48	4×DocCarbo(75/AUC6) q3w If HER2 positive: 4×DocCarbo(75/AUC6) q3w + T q1w/24 wk (4 mg/kg loading dose, then 2 mg/kg/wk) → OP vs 4×DocCarbo(75/AUC6) q3w → OP → T q3w/ 52 wk (8 mg/kg loading dose, then 6 mg/kg)	No data	29.7% (11 pts of 37 pts)*
NOAH	Gianni et al[29] (2007)	228	3×AP (60/150) q3w → 4×P (175) q3w → 3×CMF (600/40/600) q4w d1+8 → OP → T q3w/52 wk (8 mg/kg loading dose, then 6 mg/kg) vs 3×AP (60/150) q3w → 4×P (175) q3w → 3×CMF (600/40/600) q4w d1+8 + T q3w (8 mg/kg loading dose, then 6 mg/kg) → OP → T q3w/52 wk	No data	43% vs 23% P = .002

*With complete pathologic verification.
A, doxorubicin; C, cyclophosphamide; Carbo, carboplatin; Doc, docetaxel; E, epirubicin; F, 5-fluorouracil; M, methotrexate; P, paclitaxel; T, trastuzumab.
( ), concentration in mg/m²; q1/3w, every 1/3 weeks; HER2, human epithelial growth factor 2; OP, operation; pt/pts, patient/patients; pCR, pathologic complete response; po, by mouth.
NOAH, Neoadjuvant Herceptin; TECHNO, Taxol-Epirubicin-Cyclophosphamide-Herceptin Neoadjuvant.

Table 17-4. Overview of Published and Ongoing Trials Incorporating Aromatase Inhibitors in the Preoperative Setting in Postmenopausal Women with Hormone Receptor–Positive Breast Cancer

Trial	Author (Year)	Number of Patients	Treatment Arms	Duration of Treatment	Objective Response
	Cameron et al[34] (1997)	94	After 3 months of hormones Responder: further hormones Nonresponder: chemotherapy		
	Eiermann et al[33] (2001)	337	Letrozole vs tamoxifen	16 wk	55% vs 36% P < .001
IMPACT	Smith et al[37] (2005)	330	Tamoxifen vs anastrozole vs combination	12 wk	36% vs 37% vs 39% n.s.
	Semiglazov et al[35] (2005)	151	Exemestane vs tamoxifen	12 wk	76.3% vs 40% P = .05
PROACT	Cataliotti et al[39] (2006)	451	Anastrozole vs tamoxifen ± chemotherapy	12 wk	Numerically higher for anastrozole without reaching significance
ACOSOG Z1031	Ongoing	Target: 375	Anastrozole vs letrozole vs exemestane	16 wk	

n.s., not significant; ACOSOG, American College of Surgeons Oncology Group; IMPACT, Immediate Preoperative Anastrozole, Tamoxifen, or Combined with Tamoxifen; PROACT, Preoperative Arimidex Compared to Tamoxifen.

statistically significantly higher in the letrozole group (55% versus 36%; $P < .001$).[32] A subsequent hypothesis-generating analysis revealed that 60% of the patients with centrally confirmed ER- and/or PR-positive tumors treated with letrozole responded to the treatment compared with 41% of the tamoxifen-treated patients ($P = .004$). Tumors that overexpressed epidermal growth factor receptors (EGFR or ErbB or *HER*) 1 or 2, were associated with response rates of 88% versus 21% ($P = .0004$) in letrozole and tamoxifen, respectively.[35]

The Immediate Preoperative Anastrozole, Tamoxifen, or Combined with Tamoxifen (IMPACT) trial was designed to mirror the large adjuvant ATAC (Arimidex [anastrozole], Tamoxifen Alone or in Combination) trial. The investigators hypothesized that studies in the preoperative setting may provide similar conclusions as trials in the adjuvant setting but with a smaller number of patients and a shorter follow-up. The authors did not observe significant differences in the objective response among the three treatment groups. A trend favoring anastrozole was observed in the HER2-positive cancers (overall response 58% in anastrozole-treated compared with 22% in tamoxifen-treated women; $P = .18$), but the number of patients in this subgroup was very small ($n = 34$).[36] More recently, a retrospective analysis of the tumor blocks obtained from patients treated in the ATAC trial with either adjuvant anastrozole or tamoxifen alone could not confirm differences between the two agents in women with HER2-positive or -negative disease.[37]

In contrast to the IMPACT trial, the Preoperative "Arimidex" Compared to Tamoxifen (PROACT) trial assessed objective responses with anastrozole or tamoxifen in the neoadjuvant setting with or without chemotherapy. The authors demonstrated that preoperative treatment with anastrozole was at least as effective as tamoxifen in all patients and was perhaps more effective than tamoxifen in certain subgroups.[38]

The ACOSOG is currently comparing response and biomarker modulation with anastrozole, letrozole, and exemestane administered for 16 weeks in a neoadjuvant setting. This immediate comparison will provide valuable information regarding the responsiveness, side effects, and efficacy in relation to the expression of ER, PR, and HER2. Until further information is available, preoperative endocrine therapy should be used only in postmenopausal patients with endocrine-responsive disease to enhance breast conservation or to improve surgical options. Since response rates and breast conservation rates were higher in women treated with an aromatase inhibitor, the International Expert Panel recommended that an aromatase inhibitor should be favored over tamoxifen in this setting.[9]

Multidisciplinary Management of Patients Receiving Neoadjuvant Therapy

Although neoadjuvant therapy may provide some benefits to individuals, such as breast conservation and prognostic information, it may also be associated with some disadvantages (see Table 17-1). A careful selection of patients planned for neoadjuvant therapy and an experienced team are highly important to achieve the predefined treatment goal.

Selection of Patients

Several factors may predict an unfavorable outcome following neoadjuvant therapy. The hormone receptor status plays a crucial predictive role in the response to neoadjuvant chemotherapy. Results of the NSABP B-27 trial showed higher pCR rates for ER-negative (16.7% versus 8.3%; $P < .001$) compared with ER-positive tumors.[25] In a study aimed to identify predictive factors for the outcome of neoadjuvant chemotherapy, patients whose tumors lacked expression of ER and PR ($P < .0001$), or those with a nuclear grade 3 ($P = .001$) enjoyed high rates of pCR in the breast and lymph nodes following neoadjuvant chemotherapy. The investigators reported a pCR rate of 33.3% versus 7.5% for patients with ER-negative and ER-positive tumors, respectively. Furthermore, 42.9% of women with ER-negative tumors were node-negative at the time of surgery compared with 21.7% with ER-positive tumors. Despite these differences, disease-free survival was significantly worse for patients with ER-/PR-negative tumors (41% versus 74%; $P < .0001$), probably owing to the subsequent use of endocrine therapies administered to women with ER-/PR-positive disease.[39]

Since HER2 expression may be a predictive factor for taxane and anthracycline sensitivity, its role as predictor of response to neoadjuvant chemotherapy has been evaluated. An earlier review of patients treated with AC combined with or without docetaxel reported lower response rates for women with HER2-negative tumors compared to those with HER2-positive tumors (51% versus 75%; $P = .06$). The addition of docetaxel was associated with a higher response rate in patients with HER2-negative tumors[40] (Fig. 17-3). This may explain why the prospective central assessment of HER2 by fluorescence in situ hybridization (FISH) was not a predictive factor of pCR in the GEPARTRIO trial.[41] In contrast, the expression of HER2 mRNA in gene expression analysis of patients treated in the GEPARTRIO trial was predictive for pCR ($P = .017$) and overall response ($P = .037$).[42] Indeed, a recent study demonstrated that gene expression profiles might be predictive for the outcomes of neoadjuvant chemotherapy. A multigene assay with 74 markers had a 78% positive predictive accuracy for pCR in patients treated with paclitaxel, followed by fluorouracil, doxorubicin, and cyclophosphamide.[43]

Age may also be a predictive factor of response. Young patients have a better response to neoadjuvant chemotherapy compared with patients older than 35 years. However, their long-term outcome is worse, an observation that may be confounded by hormone receptor status.[44]

Finally, the tumor type is also an important predictive factor. The Austrian Breast and Colorectal Study Group (ABCSG) 24 trial revealed that patients who presented with an invasive lobular carcinoma ($n = 37$) were less likely to respond to neoadjuvant therapy compared with those with an invasive ductal carcinoma ($n = 124$). Compared with invasive ductal tumors, invasive lobular carcinomas are more likely to be ER-positive (86% versus 52%; $P < .0001$), HER2-negative (69% versus 84%), and have a low grade (nuclear grade 3: 16% versus 46%; $P < .001$). The pCR rate was 3% in women with invasive lobular carcinomas compared with 20% for those with invasive ductal tumors ($P < .009$). Rate of breast conserving therapy was 51% versus 79% in women with invasive lobular and invasive ductal carcinomas, respectively.[45] Given these data, and an expected low rate of breast conservation, preoperative chemotherapy is not generally recommended to women with infiltrating lobular cancer.[26]

Accuracy of Pretreatment Staging and Prediction of Tumor Response

A crucial part of neoadjuvant therapy is establishing the diagnosis before treatment to prevent overtreatment. The identification of markers for

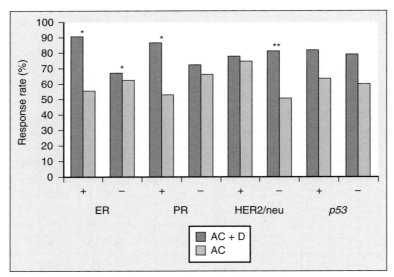

Figure 17-3. The percentages of clinically positive responses are illustrated by pretreatment prognostic factor status and treatment group. AC, doxorubicin and cyclophosphamide; D, docetaxel; ER, estrogen receptor; PR, progesterone receptor; −, negative; +, positive. Single asterisks indicate P values <.05 (on univariate analysis only), and double asterisks indicate P values <.05 (on both univariate and multivariate analysis). (From Learn PA, Yeh IT, McNutt M, et al: HER2/neu expression as a predictor of response to neoadjuvant docetaxel in patients with operable breast carcinoma. Cancer 103:2252–2260, 2005.)

response during the therapy and the extent of residual disease are important to guide the surgical therapy. The standard of care today is a diagnostic core biopsy to obtain histopathologic features that are crucial to characterize the tumor. Whenever possible, a metal clip should be placed at the time of diagnostic biopsy to allow a proper localization of the tumor bed.

Different methods are available to establish the tumor size and axillary involvement. Whereas a thorough clinical examination is mandatory, an appropriate imaging modality should be considered to obtain objective information before, during, and after neoadjuvant treatment, especially if breast conservation is desired. Bilateral mammography and affected breast ultrasound should be requested as a minimum. A retrospective study with 189 patients revealed a moderate correlation of physical examination and imaging with mammography and ultrasound with the residual pathologic tumor size after neoadjuvant treatment. An accuracy ±1 cm was found in 66% of the patients for physical examination, 75% for ultrasound, and 70% for mammography.[46] In a published phase III study from a single center with 162 patients, the accordance between predicted and pathologic response was 53% for physical examination, 67% for mammography and ultrasound, and 63% for the combination of all methods. Sensitivity for the prediction of pCR for mammography and ultrasound was 78.6%, with a specificity of 92.5%.[47] If the results of the imaging are not consistent with the clinical examination or in case of multicentricity and invasive lobular tumors, additional methods should be used.

Other imaging techniques such as magnetic resonance imaging (MRI) and positron emission tomography (PET) are under investigation and may provide additional information regarding tumor response. For example, blood flow and metabolic parameters may predict response to therapy and possibly pCR.[48] MRI provides the highest sensitivity for the determination of response, followed by physical examination, ultrasound, and mammography.[49] In one study, sensitivity, specificity, and the negative predictive value for the [^{18}F]fluorodeoxyglucose (FDG)-PET during neoadjuvant treatment were 61%, 96%, and 68% after one course of chemotherapy, 89%, 95%, and 85% after two courses, and 88%, 73%, and 83% after three courses, respectively. The same parameters with ultrasound and mammography were 64%, 43%, and 55%, and 31%, 56%, and 45%, respectively.[50] Tissue and circulating biomarkers are also under extensive investigations and may enable us to predict tumor response.

Surgical Management of the Breast

One of the main advantages of neoadjuvant therapy is increasing the rate of breast conservation. A concern, however, is the potential increase in local recurrence rate. Initial studies have proven higher rates for breast conservation with neoadjuvant chemotherapy yet without a statistically significant increased risk for local relapse.[16,51] Some studies suggested a further reduction of local recurrence rate by the addition of taxanes to preoperative therapy.[17] Overall, for properly selected patients and with adequate margins, local recurrence rate is not higher after neoadjuvant chemotherapy compared with primary surgical approach.

The NSABP B-18 trial investigators reported an inverse relationship between conversion from a mastectomy planned before initiating chemotherapy to breast conservation following neoadjuvant therapy and overall survival. The European Organization for Research and Treatment of Cancer (EORTC) 10902 trial investigators reported similar findings. It has been suggested that patients scheduled to have a mastectomy but who subsequently underwent breast-conserving surgery after neoadjuvant treatment had a less favorable outcome.[51] However, this investigation was not from a prospective randomized comparison and may also reflect a more advanced stage at diagnosis. A French study evaluated retrospectively 257 patients who were treated with neoadjuvant chemotherapy followed by breast-conserving surgery for predictors of breast cancer recurrence. The investigators reported a local recurrence rate of 16% and 21% after 5 and 10 years of follow-up, respectively. Factors supporting a less favorable outcome included age under 40 years, close margins (distance between tumor and margin of 2 mm), clinical tumor size greater than 2 cm at the time of surgery and S-phase-fraction greater than 4%.[52]

These recent reports support a careful selection of women who would be appropriate candidates for breast conservation following neoadjuvant chemotherapy.

Surgical Management of the Axilla

The axillary node evaluation is an integral part of surgery for women with breast cancer. The procedure is performed for diagnostic and therapeutic reasons. Depending on the results, further decisions concerning the adjuvant treatment in terms of systemic therapy and radiation are made. Studies, such as the EORTC 10902 trial, showed that 25% of women with positive nodes in the axilla before the initiation of treatment estimated by palpation and mammography were node-negative after therapy.[51]

Until recently, axillary lymph node dissection (ALND) represented standard of care; however, sentinel lymph node biopsy (SLNB) has replaced ALND for women with a clinically negative axilla undergoing primary surgery due to fewer adverse effects.[53] In 2005, the American Society of Clinical Oncology (ASCO) suggested in their guidelines that SLNB is an appropriate initial alternative to ALND for patients with early breast cancer with clinically negative axillary nodes.[54]

The value of SLNB after a preoperative therapy raises some concerns. First, identification of the sentinel lymph node may be inaccurate with large primary tumors. Second, there may be an increase in the false-negative rate with large primary tumors. Finally, it is difficult to predict the pattern of shrinkage of micrometastases in the lymph nodes. If the tumor disappears in the sentinel lymph node, it is not known with certainty whether tumor is present in the nonsentinel lymph nodes. Several studies evaluated the identification rate and accuracy of sentinel node biopsy following neoadjuvant therapy. Unfortunately, these studies included often small numbers of patients, the techniques of the SLNB varied among institutions, and there was no standardized pathology procedure. Although these studies reported acceptable identification and false-negative rates, prospective studies comparing ALND with SLNB after preoperative chemotherapy have not been reported. The largest retrospective data set was published by Mamounas and colleagues[55] as part of NSABP B-27. SLNB was performed in 428 patients. The rate of lymph node identification was 84.8% overall and slightly higher with the use of a radioisotope (87.6% to 88.9%) compared with that with lymphazurin alone (78.1%; $P = .03$). SLNB followed by ALND was conducted in 343 patients. The false-negative rate for the nonsentinel node was 10.7%. The authors did not describe significant differences in false-negative rates according to patient and tumor characteristics, method of lymphatic mapping, or breast tumor response to chemotherapy and reasoned that the SLNB after a preoperative therapy should be considered.[55] A meta-analysis, published by Xing and colleagues[56] in 2006, included 21 studies and 1273 patients treated with SLNB and subsequent ALND after neoadjuvant chemotherapy. The authors found an identification rate of 90% (ranging from 72% to 100%) and a sensitivity of 88% (67% to 100%).

MD Anderson Cancer Center investigators evaluated the role of SLNB after neoadjuvant chemotherapy in women with a known fine-needle aspiration–positive node.[57] In 69 patients, axillary metastases were identified before neoadjuvant treatment by ultrasound-guided fine-needle aspiration. The patients underwent SLNB after chemotherapy except for eight patients who underwent ALND. The false-negative rate was 25%. The authors concluded, that SLNB is feasible after neoadjuvant chemotherapy, even if proven metastasis is present in the axilla at initial diagnosis, but that the false-negative rate is much higher in this group of patients compared with those with clinically negative nodes. Thus, the sentinel lymph node status after neoadjuvant chemotherapy cannot be used as an indicator for residual disease.[57]

Only a few reports documented SLNB evaluation before neoadjuvant therapy. In one report, 25 patients with T2N0 tumors underwent SLNB. The 11 patients who had involved nodes were treated with ALND, and 4 had additional positive nonsentinel lymph nodes in the complete lymph node dissection. There were no axillary recurrences in the 15 other patients with negative sentinel lymph nodes and SLNB only after a median follow-up of 18 months. These data suggest that SLNB in T2N0 tumors before neoadjuvant therapy is feasible and safe.[58] Another group compared 52 patients who underwent a SLNB before systemic therapy with a retrospective analysis of 36 patients who underwent SLNB after chemotherapy at the same institution. The identification rate before and after neoadjuvant chemotherapy was 100% versus 80.6%, respectively. Only 64% of the patients who presented with clinically negative nodes at diagnosis were truly negative at the time of SLNB after neoadjuvant treatment. The authors reported a false-negative rate of 11% and thus recommended SLNB prior to neoadjuvant therapy.[59] SLNB before preoperative treatment may also improve the staging accuracy and may enable the acquisition of standard markers and biomarkers. Furthermore, the complete pathologic axillary response can be used as a prognostic factor.[60]

In summary, SLNB is feasible after preoperative therapy in a clinically negative axilla. It is not clear, however, whether negative results in the axilla after preoperative therapy have an impact on prognosis or survival. Whereas the ASCO panel in 2005 did not recommend an optimal timing,[54] data available to date suggest that it is reasonable to consider histologic evaluation of the axilla before or after the initiation of preoperative chemotherapy.

Pathologic Evaluation

One critical problem when trying to compare results of different neoadjuvant trials is the variation in the definition of pCR. Whereas the NSABP defines pCR as the absence of invasive tumor in the breast,[25,61] the criteria are more stringent in other studies. Most of the European studies consider a pCR if neither residual invasive tumor nor ductal carcinoma in situ (DCIS) is found in the breast and the axillary lymph nodes.[20,51] The International Expert Consensus Panel agreed that pCR should be designated when there are no residual invasive and noninvasive tumor cells in the breast and axillary lymph nodes. To define a pCR, an extensive examination of the histologic specimen should be conducted, characteristic changes in the tumor bed after neoadjuvant chemotherapy should be documented, and the ypTNM (pathologic) classification should be used[9] (Fig. 17-4). Furthermore, there is no standard system for evaluating regression of disease after neoadjuvant therapy.[62,63] If possible, a regression score should be indicated in the pathology report.[26]

The proper determination of margins is mandatory and raises additional concern. Tumors shrink in different ways after neoadjuvant therapy[64] (Fig. 17-5). Although most tumors shrink concentrically, other tumors respond in a patchy or random form, resulting in nests of tumor cells embedded in normal breast tissue. This microscopic residual disease can be situated in the area of the original volume as well as in a smaller area corresponding to the new dimension of the tumor. Whereas the first pattern can allow for excision with clear margins, the latter form

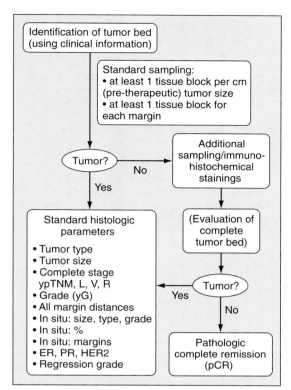

Figure 17-4. Standardized histopathologic approach to the assessment of breast cancer specimen from neoadjuvant chemotherapy. ER, estrogen receptor; pCR, pathologic complete response; PR, progesterone receptor; ypTNM, pathologic TNM classification. (From Kaufmann M, von Minckwitz G, Bear HD, et al: Recommendations from an international expert panel on the use of neoadjuvant (primary) systemic treatment of operable breast cancer: new perspectives 2006. Annals Oncol 18:1927–1934, 2007.)

may require several excisions and ultimately may not allow for breast conservation. Otherwise, conservation in this group may result in an unacceptable local recurrence rate.[16]

These observations support the need for a close communication among the different subspecialties treating patients with neoadjuvant therapy and a certain degree of experience to achieve the best possible outcome for the patient. One of the most important requirements is very tight cooperation between the surgeon and the pathologist.[64]

Postoperative Radiation

Radiation therapy following breast-conserving therapy is an integral part of the local therapy of breast cancer.[65] Use of radiation therapy to

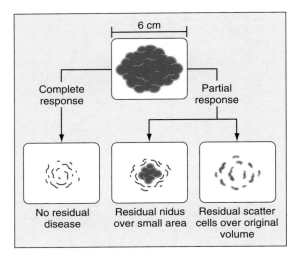

Figure 17-5. Examples of the various pathologic responses observed after neoadjuvant chemotherapy. In some instances, malignant cells are clustered around a residual nidus after disease response. In other cases, residual tumor cells are scattered over the residual volume of disease. A breast-conserving surgical procedure directed toward a central nidus may leave different volumes of residual disease in these two clinical scenarios. (From Buchholz TA, Hunt KK, Whitman GJ, et al: Neoadjuvant chemotherapy for breast carcinoma: multidisciplinary considerations of benefits and risks. Cancer 98:1150–1160, 2003.)

the axilla after breast-conserving therapy and the radiation of the chest wall, locoregional nodes, and the axilla after mastectomy depends mostly on lymph node involvement. ASCO's practice guidelines concerning postmastectomy radiation in women who did not receive preoperative therapy are clear and include patients with more than four involved lymph nodes and tumors larger than 5 cm or locally advanced.[66] It remains controversial whether patients with one to three positive lymph nodes should receive locoregional and axillary radiation. Furthermore, data were not sufficient to make recommendations for patients receiving preoperative chemotherapy.[67] One concern is that preoperative chemotherapy may result in downstaging the axilla. ALND or SLNB after preoperative chemotherapy could thus lead to an undertreatment of patients. Buchholz and colleagues[64] reported that the extent of local recurrence was highly associated with any postchemotherapy pathologic primary tumor size and any category of positive lymph nodes. Even following a pCR, the local recurrence rate without postmastec-

tomy radiation was 19% after a median follow-up of 4.1 years.

Postmastectomy radiation is suggested for patients presenting with T3 and T4 tumors before neoadjuvant chemotherapy because of a high local recurrence rate in this group regardless of response.[68] Since the extent of involved nodes is altered by neoadjuvant therapy, radiation may be considered for patients with clinically negative nodes at the time of diagnosis, without a histologic staging before systemic treatment.

What If Neoadjuvant Therapy Doesn't Work?

One of the greatest concerns raised by patients and their doctors when neoadjuvant therapy is administered is that this approach may not be effective. Large studies show that the percentage of patients with progression while receiving therapy is extremely low. Only 1% of patients developed progressive disease while on neoadjuvant therapy in the ECTO trial,[14] compared with 4% in the NSABP B-18 trial.[13] The addition of taxanes in the preoperative setting revealed an even larger overall clinical response rate when compared with an anthracycline-based regimen, as shown in the NSABP B-27 (preoperative AC versus AC followed by docetaxel 85.7% versus 90.7%).[25] Disease progression has occurred in 3.5% of patients in the GEPARDUO study with no difference between the doxorubicin/docetaxel and the AC plus docetaxel arms.[20]

Several studies revealed that even patients who did not respond to one chemotherapy regimen can derive a more favorable outcome when sequenced to a non–cross-resistant regimen.[20,24,25] By achieving pCR through switching, overall survival may improve. The ability to switch patients to a non–cross-resistant regimen is only possible in the neoadjuvant setting, since the tumor may serve as an in vivo marker for response. When progression or lack of response is observed, it may also be reasonable to discontinue the preoperative treatment and proceed with immediate surgery.

Recommendations for Neoadjuvant Therapy

The neoadjuvant approach is as efficacious as adjuvant therapy for properly selected patients.

Neoadjuvant chemotherapy may be offered to women who are expected to be candidates for adjuvant systemic therapy. Compared with adjuvant therapy, neoadjuvant chemotherapy does not adversely affect disease-free or overall survival, but it may enhance breast conservation. The response to neoadjuvant chemotherapy measured as pCR is a surrogate marker for disease-free and overall survival for individuals. The doxorubicin-taxane–based regimens are the most effective chemotherapies and should be recommended. Neoadjuvant endocrine treatment may be recommended for postmenopausal women with ER-positive tumors. Aromatase inhibitors should be preferred to tamoxifen because of the higher response rates. Women with cancers that overexpress or amplify HER2 should receive trastuzumab-based therapy. The optimal duration of neoadjuvant treatment needs to be defined.[9]

Open Questions and Ongoing Studies

Despite the reduction in breast cancer-related recurrence and death, many women suffer a breast cancer relapse or present with new metastatic disease. Metastatic breast cancer may be controlled or treated for many years, but remains largely incurable. Therefore, the optimization of early-stage cancer treatment for individual women remains a major goal. It is hoped that with our growing knowledge of the different features of breast tumors and host factors, future treatment will become much more individualized and targeted.

Although it is expected that most women will benefit from systemic therapy, many will suffer recurrence despite treatment, emphasizing the need for studies to evaluate drug resistance and mechanism of action. An exciting area of investigation is the implementation of new agents, antibodies, and small molecules into the treatment of breast cancer. The neoadjuvant approach offers opportunities to understand drug mechanism of action and may be an important tool to test drug sensitivity and a model to incorporate novel agents while minimizing the risks for patients not responding to the initial therapy.

References

1. Halsted WS: The results of operations for the cure of cancer of the breast performed at Johns Hopkins Hospital from June 1889 to January 1894. Johns Hopkins Hospital Bulletin 4:497–555, 1894.
2. Schinzinger A: Ueber carcinoma mammae. Verh Dtsch Ges Chir 18:28–29, 1889.
3. Beatson G: On the treatment of inoperable cases of carcinoma of the mamma: suggestions for a new method of treatment with illustrative cases. Lancet 2:104–107, 1896.
4. Cole MP: The place of radiotherapy in the management of early breast cancer: a report of two clinical trials. Br J Surg 51:216–220, 1964.
5. Effects of chemotherapy and hormonal therapy for early breast cancer on recurrence and 15-year survival: an overview of the randomised trials. Lancet 365:1687–1717, 2005.
6. Berry DA, Cronin KA, Plevritis SK, et al: Effect of screening and adjuvant therapy on mortality from breast cancer. N Engl J Med 353:1784–1792, 2005.
7. Harris LN, Kaelin CM, Bellon JR, et al: Preoperative therapy for operable breast cancer. In Harris LN, Kaelin CM, Bellon JR, et al (eds): Diseases of the Breast. Philadelphia: Lippincott Williams & Wilkins, 2004, pp 929–943.
8. Goldhirsch A, Wood W, Gelber R, et al: Progress and promise: highlights of the international expert consensus on the primary therapy of early breast cancer 2007. Ann Oncol 18:1133–1144, 2007.
9. Kaufmann M, Hortobagyi GN, Goldhirsch A, et al: Recommendations from an international expert panel on the use of neoadjuvant (primary) systemic treatment of operable breast cancer: an update. J Clin Oncol 24:1940–1949, 2006.
10. Mauri D, Pavlidis N, Ioannidis JP: Neoadjuvant versus adjuvant systemic treatment in breast cancer: a meta-analysis. J Natl Cancer Inst 97:188–194, 2005.
11. Schwartz GF, Birchansky CA, Komarnicky LT, et al: Induction chemotherapy followed by breast conservation for locally advanced carcinoma of the breast. Cancer 73:362–369, 1994.
12. Chen AM, Meric-Bernstam F, Hunt KK, et al: Breast conservation after neoadjuvant chemotherapy. Cancer 103:689–695, 2005.
13. Fisher B, Brown A, Mamounas E, et al: Effect of preoperative chemotherapy on local-regional disease in women with operable breast cancer: findings from National Surgical Adjuvant Breast and Bowel Project B-18. J Clin Oncol 15:2483–2493, 1997.
14. Gianni L, Baselga J, Eiermann W, et al: Feasibility and tolerability of sequential doxorubicin/paclitaxel followed by cyclophosphamide, methotrexate, and fluorouracil and its effects on tumor response as preoperative therapy. Clin Cancer Res 11:8715–8721, 2005.
15. von Minckwitz G, Blohmer JU, Raab G, et al: In vivo chemosensitivity-adapted preoperative chemotherapy in patients with early-stage breast cancer: the GEPARTRIO pilot study. Ann Oncol 16:56–63, 2005.
16. Wolmark N, Wang J, Mamounas E, et al: Preoperative chemotherapy in patients with operable breast cancer: nine-year results from National Surgical Adjuvant Breast and Bowel Project B-18. J Natl Cancer Inst Monogr 30:96–102, 2001.
17. Bear HD, Anderson S, Smith RE, et al: Sequential preoperative or postoperative docetaxel added to preoperative doxorubicin plus cyclophosphamide for operable breast cancer: National Surgical Adjuvant Breast and Bowel Project Protocol B-27. J Clin Oncol 24:2019–2027, 2006.
18. Wolff AC, Davidson NE: Primary systemic therapy in operable breast cancer. J Clin Oncol 18:1558–1569, 2000.
19. von Minckwitz G, Kuemmel S, du Bois A, et al: Individualized treatment strategies according to in vivo-chemosensitivity assessed by response after 2 cycles of neoadjuvant chemotherapy. Final results of the GEPARTRIO study of the German Breast Group [abstract]. Breast Cancer Res Treat 100:42, 2006.
20. von Minckwitz G, Raab G, Caputo A, et al: Doxorubicin with cyclophosphamide followed by docetaxel every 21 days compared with doxorubicin and docetaxel every 14 days as preoperative treatment in operable breast cancer: the GEPARDUO study of the German Breast Group. J Clin Oncol 23:2676–2685, 2005.
21. Loibl S, von Minckwitz G, Raab G, et al: Surgical procedures after neoadjuvant chemotherapy in operable breast cancer: results of the GEPARDUO trial. Ann Surg Oncol 13:1434–1442, 2006.
22. Smith IC, Heys SD, Hutcheon AW, et al: Neoadjuvant chemotherapy in breast cancer: significantly enhanced response with docetaxel. J Clin Oncol 20:1456–1466, 2002.

23. Heys SD, Sarkar T, Hutcheon AW: Primary docetaxel chemotherapy in patients with breast cancer: impact on response and survival. Breast Cancer Res Treat 90:169–185, 2005.

24. Thomas E, Holmes FA, Smith TL, et al: The use of alternate, non-cross-resistant adjuvant chemotherapy on the basis of pathologic response to a neoadjuvant doxorubicin-based regimen in women with operable breast cancer: long-term results from a prospective randomized trial. J Clin Oncol 22:2294–2302, 2004.

25. Bear HD, Anderson S, Brown A, et al: The effect on tumor response of adding sequential preoperative docetaxel to preoperative doxorubicin and cyclophosphamide: preliminary results from National Surgical Adjuvant Breast and Bowel Project Protocol B-27. J Clin Oncol 21:4165–4174, 2003.

26. Kaufmann M, von Minckwitz G, Bear HD, et al: Recommendations from an international expert panel on the use of neoadjuvant (primary) systemic treatment of operable breast cancer: new perspectives 2006. Ann Oncol 18:1927–1934, 2007.

27. Buzdar AU, Ibrahim NK, Francis D, et al: Significantly higher pathologic complete remission rate after neoadjuvant therapy with trastuzumab, paclitaxel, and epirubicin chemotherapy: results of a randomized trial in human epidermal growth factor receptor 2-positive operable breast cancer. J Clin Oncol 23: 3676–3685, 2005.

28. Buzdar AU, Valero V, Ibrahim NK, et al: Neoadjuvant therapy with paclitaxel followed by 5-fluorouracil, epirubicin, and cyclophosphamide chemotherapy and concurrent trastuzumab in human epidermal growth factor receptor 2-positive operable breast cancer: an update of the initial randomized study population and data of additional patients treated with the same regimen. Clin Cancer Res 13:228–233, 2007.

29. Gianni L, Semiglazov V, Manikhas GM, et al: Neoadjuvant trastuzumab in locally advanced breast cancer (NOAH): antitumour and safety analysis [Meeting Abstracts]. J Clin Oncol 25: abstract 532, 2007.

30. Mohsin SK, Weiss HL, Gutierrez MC, et al: Neoadjuvant trastuzumab induces apoptosis in primary breast cancers. J Clin Oncol 23:2460–2468, 2005.

31. Preece PE, Wood RA, Mackie CR, et al: Tamoxifen as initial sole treatment of localised breast cancer in elderly women: a pilot study. Br Med J (Clin Res Ed) 284:869–870, 1982.

32. Eiermann W, Paepke S, Appfelstaedt J, et al: Preoperative treatment of postmenopausal breast cancer patients with letrozole: a randomized double-blind multicenter study. Ann Oncol 12:1527–1532, 2001.

33. Cameron DA, Anderson ED, Levack P, et al: Primary systemic therapy for operable breast cancer—10-year survival data after chemotherapy and hormone therapy. Br J Cancer 76: 1099–1105, 1997.

34. Semiglazov V, Kletsel A, Semiglazov V, et al: Exemestane (e) vs tamoxifen (t) as neoadjuvant endocrine therapy for postmenopausal women with ER+ breast cancer (T2N1-2, T3N0-1, T4N0M0) [Meeting Abstracts]. J Clin Oncol 23:abstract 530, 2005.

35. Ellis MJ, Coop A, Singh B, et al: Letrozole is more effective neoadjuvant endocrine therapy than tamoxifen for ERBB-1- and/or ERBB-2-positive, estrogen receptor-positive primary breast cancer: evidence from a phase III randomized trial. J Clin Oncol 19:3808–3816, 2001.

36. Smith IE, Dowsett M, Ebbs SR, et al: Neoadjuvant treatment of postmenopausal breast cancer with anastrozole, tamoxifen, or both in combination: the immediate preoperative anastrozole, tamoxifen, or combined with tamoxifen (impact) multicenter double-blind randomized trial. J Clin Oncol 23:5108–5116, 2005.

37. Dowsett M, Allred C, Knox J, et al: Relationship between quantitative estrogen and progesterone receptor expression and human epidermal growth factor receptor 2 (her-2) status with recurrence in the Arimidex, tamoxifen, alone or in combination trial. J Clin Oncol 26:1059–1065, 2008.

38. Cataliotti L, Buzdar AU, Noguchi S, et al: Comparison of anastrozole versus tamoxifen as preoperative therapy in postmenopausal women with hormone receptor-positive breast cancer: the Pre-operative "Arimidex" Compared to Tamoxifen (PROACT) trial. Cancer 106:2095–2103, 2006.

39. Colleoni M, Viale G, Zahrieh D, et al: Chemotherapy is more effective in patients with breast cancer not expressing steroid hormone receptors: a study of preoperative treatment. Clin Cancer Res 10:6622–6628, 2004.

40. Learn PA, Yeh IT, McNutt M, et al: Her-2/neu expression as a predictor of response to neoadjuvant docetaxel in patients with operable breast carcinoma. Cancer 103:2252–2260, 2005.

41. Loibl S, Blohmer JU, Raab G, et al: Prospective central assessment of HER-2 status by FISH is not a predictive factor for pathologic complete response (pCR) in 648 breast cancer patients treated preoperatively with an anthracycline/taxane based regimen in the multicenter GeparTrio trial [abstract]. Breast Cancer Res Treat 94:1023, 2005.

42. Rody A, Karn T, Gatje R, et al: Gene expression profiling of breast cancer patients treated with docetaxel, doxorubicin, and cyclophosphamide within the GEPARTRIO trial: HER-2, but not topoisomerase II alpha and microtubule-associated protein tau, is highly predictive of tumor response. Breast 16:86–93, 2007.

43. Ayers M, Symmans WF, Stec J, et al: Gene expression profiles predict complete pathologic response to neoadjuvant paclitaxel and fluorouracil, doxorubicin, and cyclophosphamide chemotherapy in breast cancer. J Clin Oncol 22:2284–2293, 2004.

44. Braud AC, Asselain B, Scholl S, et al: Neoadjuvant chemotherapy in young breast cancer patients: correlation between response and relapse? Eur J Cancer 35:392–397, 1999.

45. Wenzel C, Bartsch R, Hussian D, et al: Invasive ductal carcinoma and invasive lobular carcinoma of breast differ in response following neoadjuvant therapy with epidoxorubicin and docetaxel + g-CSF. Breast Cancer Res Treat 104:109–114, 2007.

46. Chagpar AB, Middleton LP, Sahin AA, et al: Accuracy of physical examination, ultrasonography, and mammography in predicting residual pathologic tumor size in patients treated with neoadjuvant chemotherapy. Ann Surg 243:257–264, 2006.

47. Peintinger F, Kuerer HM, Anderson K, et al: Accuracy of the combination of mammography and sonography in predicting tumor response in breast cancer patients after neoadjuvant chemotherapy. Ann Surg Oncol 13:1443–1449, 2006.

48. Mankoff DA, Dunnwald LK, Gralow JR, et al: Changes in blood flow and metabolism in locally advanced breast cancer treated with neoadjuvant chemotherapy. J Nucl Med 44:1806–1814, 2003.

49. Ollivier L, Balu-Maestro C, Leclere J: Imaging in evaluation of response to neoadjuvant breast cancer treatment. Cancer imaging: the official publication of the International Cancer Imaging Society 5:27–31, 2005.

50. Rousseau C, Devillers A, Sagan C, et al: Monitoring of early response to neoadjuvant chemotherapy in stage II and III breast cancer by [18f]fluorodeoxyglucose positron emission tomography. J Clin Oncol 24:5366–5372, 2006.

51. van der Hage JA, van de Velde CJ, Julien JP, et al: Preoperative chemotherapy in primary operable breast cancer: results from the European Organization for Research and Treatment of Cancer Trial 10902. J Clin Oncol 19:4224–4237, 2001.

52. Rouzier R, Extra JM, Carton M, et al: Primary chemotherapy for operable breast cancer: incidence and prognostic significance of ipsilateral breast tumor recurrence after breast-conserving surgery. J Clin Oncol 19:3828–3835, 2001.

53. Kim T, Giuliano AE, Lyman GH: Lymphatic mapping and sentinel lymph node biopsy in early-stage breast carcinoma: a meta-analysis. Cancer 106:4–16, 2006.

54. Lyman GH, Giuliano AE, Somerfield MR, et al: American Society of Clinical Oncology guideline recommendations for sentinel lymph node biopsy in early-stage breast cancer. J Clin Oncol 23:7703–7720, 2005.

55. Mamounas EP, Brown A, Anderson S, et al: Sentinel node biopsy after neoadjuvant chemotherapy in breast cancer: results from National Surgical Adjuvant Breast and Bowel Project Protocol B-27. J Clin Oncol 23:2694–2702, 2005.

56. Xing Y, Foy M, Cox DD, et al: Meta-analysis of sentinel lymph node biopsy after preoperative chemotherapy in patients with breast cancer. Br J Surg 93:539–546, 2006.

57. Shen J, Gilcrease MZ, Babiera GV, et al: Feasibility and accuracy of sentinel lymph node biopsy after preoperative chemotherapy in breast cancer patients with documented axillary metastases. Cancer 109:1255–1263, 2007.

58. van Rijk MC, Nieweg OE, Rutgers EJ, et al: Sentinel node biopsy before neoadjuvant chemotherapy spares breast cancer patients axillary lymph node dissection. Ann Surg Oncol 13:475–479, 2006.

59. Jones JL, Zabicki K, Christian RL, et al: A comparison of sentinel node biopsy before and after neoadjuvant chemotherapy: timing is important. Am J Surg 190:517–520, 2005.

60. Cox CE, Cox JM, White LB, et al: Sentinel node biopsy before neoadjuvant chemotherapy for determining axillary status and treatment prognosis in locally advanced breast cancer. Ann Surg Oncol 13:483–490, 2006.

61. Fisher B, Bryant J, Wolmark N, et al: Effect of preoperative chemotherapy on the outcome of women with operable breast cancer. J Clin Oncol 16:2672–2685, 1998.

62. Sinn HP, Schmid H, Junkermann H, et al: [Histologic regression of breast cancer after primary (neoadjuvant) chemotherapy]. Geburtshilfe Frauenheilkd 54:552–558, 1994.

63. Chevallier B: [Inflammatory breast cancer]. Bull Cancer 80:1024–1034, 1993.

64. Buchholz TA, Hunt KK, Whitman GJ, et al: Neoadjuvant chemotherapy for breast carcinoma: multidisciplinary considerations of benefits and risks. Cancer 98:1150–1160, 2003.

65. Fisher B, Bauer M, Margolese R, et al: Five-year results of a randomized clinical trial comparing total mastectomy and segmental mastectomy with or without radiation in the treatment of breast cancer. N Engl J Med 312:665–673, 1985.

66. Recht A, Edge SB, Solin LJ, et al: Postmastectomy radiotherapy: Clinical practice guidelines of the American Society of Clinical Oncology. J Clin Oncol 19:1539–1569, 2001.

67. Recht A, Edge SB: Evidence-based indications for postmastectomy irradiation. Surg Clin North Am 83:995–1013, 2003.

68. Huang EH, Tucker SL, Strom EA, et al: Postmastectomy radiation improves local-regional control and survival for selected patients with locally advanced breast cancer treated with neoadjuvant chemotherapy and mastectomy. J Clin Oncol 22:4691–4699, 2004.

69. Raab G, Kaufmann M, Schuette M, et al: Preoperative doxorubicin/cyclophosphamide followed by docetaxel (AC-DOC) versus dose-dense doxorubicin and docetaxel (ADOC) as preoperative treatment in operable breast cancer: first analysis of the event-free survival of the GEPARDUO-study [abstract]. Breast Cancer Res Treat 94:5047, 2004.

70. Evans TR, Yellowlees A, Foster E, et al: Phase III randomized trial of doxorubicin and docetaxel versus doxorubicin and cyclophosphamide as primary medical therapy in women with breast cancer: an Anglo-Celtic Cooperative Oncology Group Study. J Clin Oncol 23:2988–2995, 2005.

71. Green MC, Buzdar AU, Smith T, et al: Weekly paclitaxel improves pathologic complete remission in operable breast cancer when compared with paclitaxel once every 3 weeks. J Clin Oncol 23:5983–5992, 2005.

72. Untch M, Konecny GE, Ditsch N, et al: Dose-dense sequential epirubicin-paclitaxel as preoperative treatment of breast cancer: results of a randomised AGO study. Proc Am Soc Clin Oncol 21: abstract 133, 2002.

73. Burstein HJ, Harris LN, Gelman R, et al: Preoperative therapy with trastuzumab and paclitaxel followed by sequential adjuvant doxorubicin/cyclophosphamide for her2 overexpressing stage II or III breast cancer: a pilot study. J Clin Oncol 21:46–53, 2003.

74. Untch M, Stoeckl D, Konecny G, et al: A multicenter phase II study of preoperative epirubicin, cyclophosphamide (EC) followed by paclitaxel (P) plus trastuzumab (T) in her2 positive primary breast cancer. Breast Cancer Res Treat 94: abstract 1064, 2005.

75. Chang HR, Slamon D, Prati R, et al: A phase II study of neoadjuvant docetaxel/carboplatin with or without trastuzumab in locally advanced breast cancer: response and cardiotoxicity [Meeting Abstracts]. J Clin Oncol 24: abstract 10515, 2006.

18 Cost-Effective Staging of Breast Cancer

Virginia F. Borges and Lara Hardesty

KEY POINTS

- A cost-effective analysis provides a calculation of the cost-per-unit benefit that an intervention incurs. It does not conclude whether that result is worthy of subsequently using or withholding the intervention.
- Cost-effective breast cancer staging integrates accurate determination of the extent of disease in the breast, involvement of the local regional nodes, and determination of the presence of distant metastasis with minimization of procedures and risks—thereby minimization of costs.
- Advances in radiologic imaging have made a significant impact on the ability to stage breast cancer, but studies evaluating the cost-effectiveness of these modalities are limited.
- Local staging of the breast and axilla may be improved by the addition of radiologic studies decided on a case-by-case basis, such as magnetic resonance imaging (MRI) or fluorodeoxyglucose-positron emission tomography (FDG-PET), but these studies are not warranted in all newly diagnosed cases outside of a research protocol.
- Systemic staging for distant metastasis in the asymptomatic patient is most useful only in stages IIB and III patients.
- The optimal cost-effective staging modalities for identification of metastatic disease remain to be defined.
- Treatment recommendations should not change based on results of nonstandard radiologic imaging without histologic confirmation to confirm upstaging results.

Overview

At diagnosis, significant effort is invested to accurately determine the stage of the breast cancer to both inform prognosis and guide therapeutic interventions. Breast cancer staging follows the traditional TNM classification. Recent revisions to the classification schema have delineated greater detail of tumor presentations and extent of pathologic nodal involvement (Table 18-1).

Conversely, as the staging system has provided more delineation of degree of pathologic staging, medical oncology recommendations for adjuvant therapy are moving away from the traditional TNM classification. The number of nodes is no longer used for chemotherapy decision making. Without nodal involvement, tumor size is now balanced against the biologic characteristics of the cancer. Enhanced understanding of the biologic prognostic features of breast cancer, such as estrogen receptor status, progesterone receptor status, *HER2/neu* gene overexpression, and the recent addition of tumor genomic profiling are changing the landscape of prognosis and adjuvant treatment recommendations. Metastasis detectable at the time of breast cancer diagnosis, however, is the remaining aspect of staging that most significantly affects therapeutic choices and prognosis. With advances in radiologic imaging, we are potentially upstaging more patients than in the past. The resultant dilemma of the best treatment approach for oligometastatic disease remains a research question.

The technologic advances that have made all the aforementioned improvements possible come with an increased expense to the overall breast cancer cost burden. Increasingly, countries outside the United States are requiring cost-effectiveness data at the time of submission for funding/reimbursement of a new diagnostic modality within its socialized or third-party payer system. However, in the United States, new modalities for staging are frequently available and potentially reimbursed before data availability or in spite of negative data for cost-effectiveness. In fact, cost-effectiveness is

Table 18-1. Overview of the Tumor, Nodal, and Metastasis Staging Schema for Invasive Breast Cancer

	T		N		M
T1mic	0.1 cm or less	N0 (i−)	No lymph node mets, negative IHC	M0	No distant mets
T1a	>0.1 cm–0.5 cm	N0(i+)	Malignant cells no greater than 0.2 mm by IHC or H&E, including ITC	cM0(i+)	Deposits of mol or micro detected tumor cells in blood, BM or non-regional nodal tissue ≤0.2 mm without sx
T1b	>0.5 cm–1 cm	N0(mol−)	Negative RT-PCR	M1	Distant mets
T1c	>1 cm–2 cm	N0(mol+)	Positive RT-PCR only		
T2	>2 cm–5 cm	N1mic	>0.2 mm and/or 200 cells, but none > 2 mm		
T3	>5 cm–10 cm	N1a	1–3 nodes, at least one >2.0 mm		
T4a	Involves chest wall or skin (ulcerated or skin nodules)	N1b	Internal mammary nodes with micro or macro mets not clinically detected		
T4b	Edema, ulceration or ipsilateral satellite skin nodules, including peau d'orange not at T4d extent	N1c	Both N1a and N1b		
T4c	Both T4a and T4b	N2a	4–9 nodes (>2 mm)		
T4d	Inflammatory	N2b	Clinically apparent IM nodes without axillary nodes		
		N3a	>10 nodes or infraclavicular node (>2 mm)		
		N3b	Clinically apparent IM nodes with axillary nodes or IM micro or macro mets found by biopsy with >3 axillary nodes		
		N3c	Ipsilateral supraclavicular node		

The revisions of the American Joint Committee on Cancer (6th and 7th editions) broadened the categories of pathologic nodal staging with emphasis on the numbers of nodes involved and the defining microscopic and cytologic levels of nodal metastasis.
BM, bone marrow; IHC, immunohistochemistry; IM, internal mammary node; H&E, hemotoxylin and eosin staining; RT-PCR, reverse transcriptase polymerization chain reaction; sx, signs or symptoms.
Adapted from AJCC Cancer Staging Manual, 7th ed. New York: Springer, 2010, pp 439–442.

specifically not used by the Health Care Financing Administration (HCFA) for making decisions about what new technologies will be eligible for Medicare reimbursement.[1] Thus, the level of rational decision making for appropriate and (hopefully) cost-effective staging often remains with the health care providers and the patient.

A cost-effective analysis calculates the cost-per-unit benefit of an intervention. It provides a numerical result without passing judgment as to the value of that result or whether we should interpret the result as being worthy. In contrast, a cost-benefit analysis quantifies cost and benefit in the same units, and it queries which is greater—the cost or the benefit. Efficacy of an intervention is the value that an intervention

offers when performed under ideal conditions. Conversely, effectiveness is the value of the intervention under routine conditions. Because of the very nature of advanced technologic staging techniques, these issues are of paramount importance for maintaining clarity for data interpretation and decision making.[2]

Cost-effectiveness can be determined in several ways. Prospective and retrospective observational studies of changes in clinical management and their outcomes constitute a common method. However, these studies are expensive, require lengthy follow-up, and can be so large that they are impractical to conduct. Alternatively, more sophisticated theoretical modeling can be used. One form of modeling focuses on groups with similar characteristics

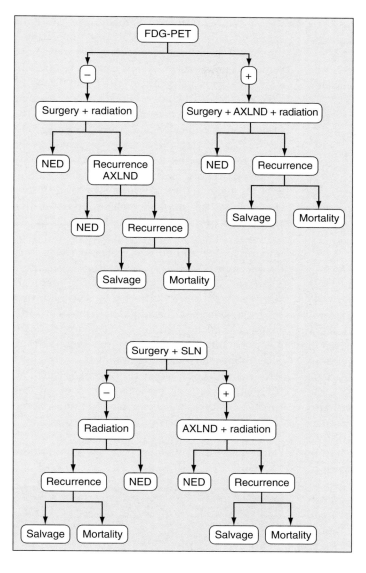

Figure 18-1. Decision tree analysis comparison of two methods of assessment of lymph node metastasis. The decision node or decision tree analysis modeling framework allows comparison between two interventions. The figure is an example of a model comparing surgical axillary nodal sampling (AXLND) with utilization of radiologic imaging to guide the need for surgical intervention. Numbers estimating the probability of a patient or situation following a particular branch would be entered, and the outcomes are based on assumptions entered into the model based on review of known literature or clinical experience. AXLND, axillary lymph node dissection; NED, no evidence of disease; SLN, sentinel lymph node dissection.

and uses the "decision tree analysis" or Markov modeling to compare interventions. This useful methodology is limited by requiring knowledge or making assumptions for procedural costs, sensitivity, and specificity of the techniques being compared, as well as the prevalence of outcome being investigated (i.e., nodal metastasis) to drive the model. Outcomes of costs versus survival, disease-free survival, or other desired endpoints are generated, thus enabling comparison among the modalities (Fig. 18-1). Alternatively, microsimulation models can be used to represent the history of disease in an individual and assess cost-effectiveness of one intervention over another, allowing for adaptation of the model to the results of the intervention on the individual. Micro-models are considered more robust and more capable of imitating the data obtained from observational studies[3] (Table 18-2).

The ultimate goal of a cost-wise breast cancer staging plan is to use the least number of interventions with the lowest possible risk to the patient that provides the highest degree of accuracy with the least cost to the system. Incorporation of new technology into this goal remains a struggle. This chapter reviews the current options and common practices of local and systemic staging of newly diagnosed breast cancer, the data for incorporating newer radiologic modalities into breast cancer staging, and the known data on the cost-effectiveness thereof.

Table 18-2. Comparison of Results of Macro- and Micro-Modeling for Cost-Effectiveness in Breast Cancer

Cited Reference	Modeling Method	Cost-Effectiveness
Rosenquist and Lindfors[4] (1998)	Decision tree within Markov model	$18,800–$16,100
Salzmann et al[5] (1997)	Markov model with Monte Carlo sensitivity analysis	$105,000

The input of different assumptions into a mathematical model and the robustness of the model used can greatly impact the results. Two modeling studies of mammograms for women aged 40–49 registered very different results.

Local Staging of Newly Diagnosed Breast Cancer

Breast cancer in the United States most commonly manifests as an abnormal finding on screening mammogram or a physical change apparent in the breast. Evaluation with diagnostic mammograms and ultrasound followed by a pathologic sampling via fine-needle aspirate, core needle biopsy, or excisional biopsy is the standard approach. When a malignancy is certain, completion of the local staging with determination of tumor size and status of local regional lymph nodes is required. Definitive surgical removal of the tumor is both diagnostic and therapeutic. Surgical evaluation of the axillary bed with sentinel lymph node sampling and/or axillary node dissection is diagnostic and potentially therapeutic, although this remains incompletely resolved. The development of breast-specific magnetic resonance imaging (MRI) and nuclear imaging with positron emission tomography using fluorodeoxyglucose (FDG-PET) has introduced additional and potentially alternative means of determining in-breast tumor extent and nodal status. Already widely used in many centers across the United States, the cost-effectiveness of these additional imaging modalities has not been proved.

In-Breast Staging

Accurate methods for determining the extent of carcinoma in the affected breast are important for guiding treatment choices. Surgical management is enhanced by the avoidance of multiple surgeries to obtain clear margins and preservation of cosmesis. In addition, appropriate guidance for the implementation of neoadjuvant systemic therapy can be obtained. MRI has emerged as a highly sensitive tool for staging the breast, but remains encumbered by low specificity, lack of standardization, and uncertain generalizability. The role of MRI and other advanced imaging techniques in the screening for breast cancer, the evaluation of clinically concerning breast lesions, and its cost-efficiency in those settings is addressed under Evaluating for Distant Metastasis.

Several reports published in the 1990s demonstrated the ability of breast MRI to improve the accuracy of radiologic imaging to determine the extent of cancer in the affected breast.[6–10] Whereas mammography and ultrasound may underestimate tumor size, particularly in very dense breasts, MRI is associated with more accurate correlation with final pathologic size.[9,11,12] Histologic differences within breast cancer may impact the added usefulness of MRI. Invasive lobular carcinoma (ILC) is notorious for being occult with standard imaging. MRI is reported to enhance detection of ILC from 34% with mammogram alone to 96% with MRI and to change surgical management 50% of the time.[10,13] However, these same studies noted that ultrasound improved detection up to 86% and MRI did not add to detection in a statistically significant manner (Fig. 18-2). A more

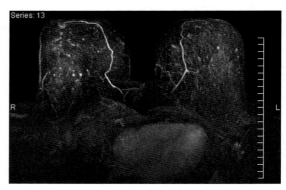

Figure 18-2. MRI imaging does not add significantly to in-breast staging for all newly diagnosed breast cancers. A woman presents with a screening mammogram showing an 18-mm new spiculated mass with pleomorphic calcifications surrounding it, overall area of suspicious measured 50 × 10 × 10 mm in the far posteriorly 10 o'clock left breast. The mammogram questioned pectoral involvement. Ultrasound was negative. Stereotactic biopsy of the mass demonstrated invasive ductal carcinoma with extensive in situ component. MRI was performed to evaluate extent of disease, specifically to evaluate pectoral involvement. MRI showed no suspicious enhancement in either breast even in area of biopsy-proven invasive cancer.

recent study has correlated histologic grade with MRI-enhanced tumor staging in the breast. High-grade tumors correlated with pathologic tumor size; however, low-grade tumors had significantly poorer correlation with pathologic size and were overestimated in their extent in 13% of cases.[12]

In addition to evaluation of tumor size, MRI of the affected breast can improve preoperative detection of mammographic and clinically occult tumor foci distinct from the index lesion. Multifocality and multicentricity have been reported in 16% to 37% of cases in which preoperative MRI was added to conventional radiologic studies, with the MRI result changing surgical management in 11% to 14%.[8,14,15] Moreover, MRI is a very useful tool for identifying occult primary lesions in the setting of axillary nodal metastasis, potentially permitting breast conservation in lieu of the prior standard of mastectomy and chest wall radiation therapy.[16–18]

MRI as an in-breast staging tool for newly diagnosed breast cancer is limited by the lack of specificity it offers and the limitation of readily available MR-guided localization and biopsy of detected areas of enhancement. Benign lesions and normal breast tissue may enhance in a manner that is concerning for the presence of additional foci. Second-look ultrasound may identify the lesion and clarify the nature of the enhancement, however, not in all cases. The ability to perform subsequent MR-guided biopsy with technical expertise is limited at present, resulting in a diagnostic dilemma for the patient. MRI specificity ranges from 30% to 99% in the literature, and positive predictive value is reported at 30% to 74%.[8,10,19] Overestimation of the extent of disease of the primary lesion has been reported to be 21% when used alone. Interpretation of the MRI in the context of the mammogram and clinical examination were more sensitive than any one test or combination of other tests, and it lowered the overestimation of disease to 6%.[10] With these uncertainties about MRI breast staging, it is critical that histologic determination of areas of uncertainty be performed before surgical decision making ensues and that MRI findings alone should not guide recommendation for mastectomy in a clinical scenario otherwise acceptable for breast conservation (Fig. 18-3).

Overall, reported results on the role of MRI in the staging of newly diagnosed breast cancer have been relatively small single-institution studies done almost exclusively at major aca-

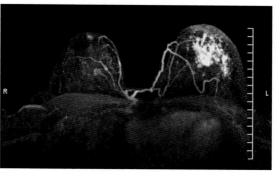

Figure 18-3. MRI provides clarity of tumor extent but cannot guide surgical recommendations without histologic correlation. A woman presenting with palpable left breast fullness for 5 months has a mammogram with vague architectural distortion and 28-mm shadowing an irregular solid mass on ultrasound. Guided core biopsy reveals invasive lobular carcinoma. MRI for extent of disease preoperatively showed enhancement of left breast consistent with known cancer measuring 47 × 47 × 35 mm (note significantly larger than ultrasound measurements). MRI also showed two enhancing oval masses in the right breast that required post-MRI second-look right breast ultrasound, which identified two solid masses. Ultrasound-guided core biopsies of both right breast masses were benign. Therefore, the right breast MRI findings were false-positives and added cost, but the left MRI better showed the size of the invasive lobular cancer than did ultrasound or mammography.

demic centers with advanced breast imaging centers. The results of these studies are promising, but must be taken in the context of the variability inherent in current MR imaging. Issues such as the best Tesla strength magnet, the best breast coil and compression, the specific dose of gadolinium, the imaging protocol itself, and finally the interpretation of the images with determination of what is clinically significant enhancement raise concern over the generalizability of the results of these studies. Results of ongoing large multi-institutional trials are awaited to clarify the role of MRI for in-breast staging. Finally, whether the intervention of MRI is more cost-effective than conventional breast staging remains unreported at this time. The clinical implications of detecting small occult tumors in breasts that would be treated with radiation and also potentially impacted with antiendocrine therapy are unknown. Therefore, MRI as a breast-staging tool in newly diagnosed cancers cannot be recommended for all cases. Individual situations exist for which MRI may have important decision-making impact. However, careful shared decision making among the multidisciplinary breast team and the patient is required to determine the goals, possible results, and anticipated decisions that the MRI will add before initiating the study.

The Ipsilateral Axilla

Metastatic involvement with breast cancer in the ipsilateral axillary nodes remains an important prognostic feature that strongly influences adjuvant therapy recommendations. Until our understanding of the primary tumor obviates our need for knowing the nodal status, surgical sampling is required. The current standard is to offer the sentinel node procedure to women with no clinical evidence of nodal spread at diagnosis. Despite the reduced extent of surgery, adverse effects such as with paresthesia, lymphedema, and shoulder complications may still occur. Intensive pathologic examination of the sentinel node has resulted in upstaging and in the detection of microscopic, single cell, and immunohistochemical staining only of levels of metastatic involvement, as emphasized in the most recent American Joint Committee on Cancer (AJCC) staging system (see Table 18–1). Clinical relevance of these categories remains under investigation. Among women with breast tumors smaller than 2.1 cm, less than 20% of these women will have nodal involvement. For women with a positive sentinel node, subsequent completion axillary dissection of levels I and II nodes is a standard approach. If an imaging modality could convincingly predict the presence or absence of clinically relevant nodal involvement, it would spare the sentinel node procedure from the node-negative and eliminate it as a step ahead of axillary dissection for the node-positive. Given the cost of a sentinel node procedure and the cost of medical interventions for the axillary complications that can ensue, a cost-effective analysis would be expected to demonstrate monetary saving for the imaging modality.

FDG-PET has been studied as a means of identifying axillary nodal metastasis at the time of initial breast cancer diagnosis to predict which patients can safely forgo axillary sampling. Most prospective analysis comparing axillary detection with axillary lymph node dissection have reported a sensitivity range of 80% to 100%.[20–23] Three studies had lower results with 37% in one recent study, 33% in one of pT1 tumors, and 61% for a relatively larger (N = 360) multi-

center U.S. study.[24–26] In studies comparing FDG-PET with the sentinel node procedure with its more detailed level of analysis, the sensitivity declined to 20% to 84%. Conversely, the specificity and positive predictive value were higher at 96% and 88%, respectively.[27] If it is accepted that a positive sentinel lymph node requires a completion axillary dissection, then a positive FDG-PET could obviate the need for sentinel lymph node procedure. FDG-PET for detection of breast primary tumors mirrors the results with MRI, that is, less sensitive for detection of tumors smaller than 1 cm or those of low histologic grade.[28] Therefore, the results compared with sentinel lymph node sampling are not surprising with the low tumor burden found in many patients.

At present, the identification of an imaging modality to replace routine axillary surgical sampling in all cases of invasive breast cancer remains a research agenda. Clarity regarding the level of nodal involvement remains clinically relevant at present. However, the improved ability to detect for distant metastasis with primary tumor characteristics alone may permit using an imaging modality alone and accepting a degree of axillary downstaging in cases at low risk for nodal involvement.

Two groups have shown via modeling that FDG-PET would be cost-effective as axillary staging if clinicians and patients were accepting of forgoing axillary surgery in lower-risk populations.[29,30] One group acknowledged that follow-up scans would potentially be considered as monitoring in the population, which if more than one follow-up scan were planned, the cost-effectiveness was lost.[29]

Evaluating for Distant Metastasis

The diagnosis of stage IV breast cancer at presentation of disease significantly alters the prognosis and potentially the management of the situation. Determining which newly diagnosed cases of breast cancer merit systemic staging entails eliciting symptoms and performing a complete physical examination and laboratory analysis with particular attention to alkaline phosphatase and liver functions. When there are no concerning findings from these measures, the clinician is left with the stage of the cancer based on T and N staging to determine whether the risk of M1 disease is high enough to merit further evaluation. Of the major breast cancer guidelines, only the National Comprehensive Cancer Network (NCCN) and the European Society of Medical Oncology (ESMO) incorporates recommendations as to when and what radiologic studies could be considered for otherwise stage I–III breast cancer.[31,32] According to the NCCN guidelines, for asymptomatic patients without laboratory abnormalities, chest imaging is recommended in all newly diagnosed stage I–III patients. Abdominal imaging is considered indicated in stage IIB (T3N1) disease and optional for stage IIA and IIB (T2N1 or T3N0) disease. Bone scans are recommended as optional, though considered indicated for stage IIB (T3N1) disease. Despite these guidelines and the significant body of literature that supports the withholding of systemic staging in earlier stage disease, practice patterns, particularly in the United States, have evolved to include not only systemic staging in some stage I and most stage II patients, but to utilize more recent technologies to perform the staging, thus adding to the expenses generated.

Both the available guidelines and many clinical study entrance criteria call for chest imaging. Chest x-rays alone or in combination with liver ultrasound and/or bone scans have been extensively studied for the ability to detect otherwise asymptomatic, occult pulmonary metastasis. The detection rates of pulmonary metastasis via chest x-ray for stage I–III disease range from 0.099% to 1.2%. Similarly, imaging of the abdomen, with focus on the liver, is recommended by NCCN guidelines and the available literature for stage IIB (T3N1) or if clinically indicated, and optional for stage IIA, IIB (T2N1 and T3N0) disease. Liver ultrasound as a staging modality is associated with low rates of cancer detection (0.51% to 3.3%).[33,34] Concerning findings on either a chest x-ray or liver ultrasound would predict for subsequent evaluation by additional imaging studies, such as a contrast-enhanced diagnostic computed tomography scan (CT), or FDG-PET. Therefore, these modalities are of limited usefulness in the modern staging evaluation of asymptomatic newly diagnosed breast cancer.

A common approach among oncologists in the United States in the last 10 years has been to obtain a CT and nuclear bone scintigraphy scan (bone scan) as staging evaluation to rule out metastatic disease at diagnosis. Currently, a CT of the body entails three separate studies: chest, abdomen, and pelvis, which are billed and require patient medical insurance copayments for three separate tests. The usefulness of inclusion of the pelvis in breast cancer staging has been specifically analyzed in large series of breast cancer patients not isolated to new diagnosis, with only 0.5% detection of breast cancer metastasis isolated to the pelvis. However, indeterminate findings on CT prompted 254 additional examinations and 50 subsequent surgeries with only three gynecologic malignancies detected.[35] The authors conclude that inclusion of the pelvis on CT imaging infrequently yields information that would change patient management. Furthermore, abdominal imaging by CT also yields indeterminate findings, particularly with liver lesions under 1.5 cm, with reported incidence rates of 29.4% to 35%.[36,37] These results often generate follow-up or additional scanning with MRI. Imaging with subsequent CT showed no correlation between indeterminate lesions at initial CT and subsequent development of liver metastasis. Likewise, MRI for further characterization of CT lesions was of marginal benefit, with only 2 of 38 cases proving metastasis in one study.[38] These data suggest that the absence of overt evidence of liver metastasis at initial staging is not further defined with additional imaging in the absence of clinical findings.

Bone scans constitute an area in which higher detection rates in otherwise asymptomatic early-stage breast cancer have been reported. The prevalence of bone metastasis across stage I–III disease has been reported in up to 6.3% of patients with stage I and stage II, having equal detection rates of 5%, and stage III disease at 14% in a recent study.[34] Older literature presented ranges of 0.5% to 11% with a distinct trend to the majority detection being in stage III patients. Bone scan detects degenerative changes, which can be difficult to distinguish from metastasis, although additional single-photon emission computed tomography (SPECT) imaging may be helpful. For cost-effectiveness analysis, bone scans have been lumped with chest x-ray and liver ultrasound as a baseline staging plan. One study estimated a savings of $259,367.68 in 2003 and prevention of 528 "impaired quality of life months" (528 patients living for 1 month with anxiety while awaiting confirmation or exclusion of metastasis) through abandonment of perioperative staging in asymptomatic stage I–II newly diagnosed breast cancer.[39]

The role of FDG-PET or FDG-PET/CT in the initial staging of newly diagnosed breast cancer remains investigational with no published cost-effectiveness data currently found for the use of FDG-PET or CT with or without bone scan as initial investigation in asymptomatic breast cancer. One retrospective study has reported on FDG-PET/CT for the combined ability to screen for axillary metastasis and metastatic disease in 21 newly diagnosed cases. FDG-PET/CT detected metastatic disease in six patients, with 100% sensitivity and 90% specificity. Pathologic sampling or follow-up imaging results were used as confirmation in all cases.[40] Details of these cases, including the presence or absence of other features that might have suggested metastasis, are not available. A prospective study comparing FDG-PET for in-breast and systemic staging with chest x-ray, liver ultrasound, mammography, and bone scan noted a greater sensitivity of FDG-PET in in-breast staging for detecting malignant lesions, in detecting multifocality, and in correctly identifying metastatic disease in seven patients, with no false-positives or false-negatives found in 117 cases.[41] However, as previously noted, the comparison studies in this trial would not be considered routine practice in the United States at this time. One study compared modern staging with CT and bone scan with FDG-PET for newly diagnosed patients. Appropriately, the study was limited to a high-risk population (50% IIA, 26% IIIA, 9% occult primary, and 15% locoregional recurrence). FDG-PET detected disease in four patients (5%; three with supraclavicular nodes and one with ipsilateral new primary) that changed management over conventional staging. For detection of metastatic disease, both modalities performed equally. Combination of conventional studies with PET has the highest true-positive and lowest false-positive results. The authors plan a cost-effectiveness analysis of their data.[42]

A disadvantage of FDG-PET in breast cancer diagnosis that limits its usefulness is the rate of false-negative results. The ability of FDG-PET to accurately identify primary breast cancer correlates with tumor size over 1 cm, higher-grade tumors, and variably sized tumors with nonlobular histology. Other prognostic features, including hormone receptor status, *HER2/neu* gene status, age, menopausal status, and p53 did not correlate.[28,43]

Several investigators have shown that FDG-PET and PET/CT are useful in the confirmation of metastasis in patients undergoing restaging due to clinical suspicion, including elevated serum tumor markers, abnormal findings on other radiologic studies, and symptom manifestations. For systemic metastasis, FDG-PET has been reviewed in a meta-analysis, with sensitivity and specificity ranging from 80% to 97% and 75% to 94%, respectively.[44] For patients with rising tumor markers, FDG-PET sensitivity was 94%. When analyzed to specifically investigate the ability of FDG-PET versus CT to identify mediastinal or internal mammary nodal metastasis at the time of locoregional recurrence, FDG-PET outperformed CT, with sensitivity and specificity of 85% versus 50% and 90% versus 83%.[45] Comparisons between FDG-PET with FDG-PET/CT and FDG-PET/CT with CT for restaging in breast cancer have been performed in modest-sized, single-institution studies. Both comparisons have reported a small-to-modest benefit of FDG-PET/CT over either FDG-PET or CT alone for accurately detecting breast cancer metastasis.[46,47] Cited reasons for incorrect FDG-PET findings were breast cancers with only mild hypermetabolic activity, benign inflammatory lesions, and physiologic variants.[48]

One area in which FDG-PET has been identified as potentially lacking compared with more traditional imaging is in the detection of bone lesions compared with bone scan. Equal rates of detection are seen for osteolytic lesions, but osteoblastic lesions are significantly less detectable by FDG-PET than by bone scan.[49] However, this study classified lesions by CT scan criteria; therefore, the remaining question of CT and bone scan versus FDG-PET/CT, including diagnostic contrast-enhanced CT fused with FDG-PET imaging, as the preferable restaging option remains unanswered. Invariably, as imaging techniques are refined, other options may supersede these current modalities, with FDG-PET for bone imaging and whole body MRI as potential candidates.[50]

Summary

The current options for staging to rule out metastatic disease at the time of breast cancer diagnosis or with suspicion for recurrence offer several modalities with varying degrees of evidence to support or refute their use. Clearly, limiting staging investigations in the asymptomatic patient has an important impact on the overall cost burden of breast cancer care. Newly diagnosed stage III disease merits staging studies using available modern imaging techniques. Similarly, with clinical suspicion for metastatic disease at or subsequent to initial diagnosis, a combination of CT, bone scan, or FDG-PET/FDG-PET/CT is indicated. Cost analysis and impact on clinical outcomes for these various investigations are not available in the published literature at this time. Therefore, the treating clinician determines the level of clinical suspicion for recurrence and determines which test would most likely and completely reveal metastasis in a given scenario.

References

1. Vladek BC: Governmental policies on health management with special attention to radiology: USA. Eur Radiol 10(Suppl 3): S395–S396, 2000.
2. Lipton MJ, Metz CE: Cost-effectiveness in radiology. Eur Radiol 10(Suppl 3): S390–S392, 2000.
3. Sullivan DC: NIH and cost-effectiveness studies for imaging. Eur Radiol 10(Suppl 3):S408–S410, 2000.
4. Rosenquist CJ, Lindfors KK: Screening mammography beginning at age 40 years. Cancer 82:2235–2240, 1998.
5. Salzmann P, Kerlikowske K, Phillips K: Cost-effectiveness of extending screening mammography guidelines to women age 40–49 years of age. Ann Intern Med 127:955–965, 1997.
6. Esserman L, Hylton N, Yassa L, et al: Utility of magnetic resonance imaging in the management of breast cancer: evidence for improved preoperative staging. J Clin Oncol 17:110–119, 1999.
7. Fisher U, Kopka L, Grabbe E: Breast carcinoma: effect of preoperative contrast-enhanced MR imaging on the therapeutic approach. Radiology 213:881–888, 1999.
8. Mumtaz H, Hall-Craggs MA, Davidson T, et al: Staging of symptomatic primary breast cancer with MR imaging. Am J Roentgenol 169:417–424, 1997.
9. Boetes C, Mus RD, Holland R, et al: Breast tumors: comparative accuracy of MR imaging relative to mammography and US for demonstrating extent. Radiology 197:43–47, 1995.
10. Rodenko GN, Harris SE, Pruneda JM, et al: MR imaging in the management before surgery of lobular carcinoma of the breast: correlation with pathology. Am J Roentgenol 167:1415–1419, 1996.
11. Berg WA, Gutierrez L, NessAiver MS, et al: Diagnostic accuracy of mammography, clinical examination US and MR imaging in preoperative assessment of breast cancer. Radiology 223(3): 830–849, 2004.
12. Blair S, McElroy M, Middleton MS, et al: The efficacy of predicting breast conservation therapy. J Surg Oncol 94:220–225, 2006.
13. Weinstein SP, Orel SG, Heller R, et al: MR imaging of the breast in patients with invasive lobular carcinoma. Am J Roentgenol 176:399–406, 2001.
14. Harms SE, Flamig DP, Hensley KL, et al: MR imaging of the breast with rotating delivery of excitation off resonance: clinical experience with pathologic correlation. Radiology 187:493–501, 1993.
15. Orel SG, Schnall MD, Powell CM, et al: Staging of suspected breast cancer: effect of MR and MR guided biopsy. Radiology 196:115–122, 1995.
16. Orel SG, Weinstein SP, Schnall MD, et al: Breast MR imaging in patients with axillary node metastasis and unknown primary malignancy. Radiology 212:543–549, 1999.
17. Tilanus-Linthhorst MM, Obdeijn AI, Bontenbal M, et al: MRI in patients with axillary metastasis of occult breast carcinoma. Breast Cancer Res Treat 44:179–182, 1997.
18. Schorn C, Fischer U, Luftner N, et al: MRI of the breast in patients with metastatic disease of unknown primary. Eur Radiol 9:470–473, 1999.
19. Orel S, Schnall M: MR imaging of the breast for the detection, diagnosis and staging of breast cancer. Radiology 220(1):13–30, 2001.
20. Crowe JP, Adler LP, Shenk RR, et al: Positron emission tomography and breast masses: comparison with clinical, mammographic and pathological findings. Ann Surg Oncol 1:132–140, 1994.
21. Smith IC, Ogston KN, Whitford P, et al: Staging of the axilla in breast cancer: accurate in vivo assessment using positron emission tomography with 2 (fluotine-18)-fluoro-2-deoxy-D-glucose. Ann Surg 228:220–227, 1998.
22. Scheidhauer K, Scharl A, Pietrzyk U: Qualitative [18F] FDG positron emission tomography in primary breast cancer: clinical relevance and practicability. Eur J Nucl Med 23:618–623, 1996.
23. Reiber A, Schirrmeister H, Gabelmann A, et al: Pre-operative staging of invasive breast cancer with MR mammography and/or PET: boon or bunk? Br J Radiol 75:789–798, 2002.
24. Veronesi U, De Cicco C, Galimberti VE, et al: A comparative study on the value of FDG-PET and sentinel node biopsy to identify occult axillary mestastases. Ann Oncol 18:473–478, 2007.
25. Avril N, Dose J, Janicke F, et al: Assessment of axillary lymph node involvement in breast cancer patients with positron emission tomography using radiolabeled 2-(fluorine-18)-fluoro-2-deoxy-D-glucose. J Natl Cancer Inst 88:1204–1209, 1996.
26. Whal RL, Siegel BA, Coleman RE: PET Study Group. Prospective multicenter study of axillary nodal staging by positron emission tomography in breast cancer: a report of the staging breast cancer with PET Study Group. J Clin Oncol 22:277–285, 2004.
27. Crippa F, Gerali A, Alessi A, et al: FDG-PET for axillary lymph node staging in primary breast cancer. Eur J Nucl Med Mol Imaging 31(Suppl 1):S97–S102, 2004.
28. Kumar R, Chauhan A, Zhuang H, et al: Clinicopathologic factors associated with false negative FDG-PET in primary breast cancer. Breast Cancer Res Treat 98:267–274, 2006.
29. Sloka JS, Hollett PD, et al: Cost-effectiveness of positron emission tomography in breast cancer. Mol Imaging Biol 7:351–360, 2005.
30. Miles KA: An approach to demonstrating cost-effectiveness of diagnostic imaging modalities in Australia illustrated by positron emission tomography. Australas Radiol 45:9–18, 2001.
31. National Comprehensive Cancer Network Practice Guidelines in Oncology, vol. 2, 2007. Available at *www.nccn.org*.
32. Pestalozzi BC, Luporsi-Gely E, Jost LM, et al: ESMO Guidelines Task Force. ESMO minimum clinical recommendations for diagnosis, adjuvant treatment and follow-up of primary breast cancer. Ann Oncol 16 (Suppl 1):i7–i9, 2005.
33. Ravaioli A, Pasini G, Polselli A, et al: Staging of breast cancer: new recommended standard procedure. Breast Cancer Res Treat 72:53–60, 2002.
34. Puglisi F, Follador A, Minisini AM, et al: Baseline staging tests after a new diagnosis of breast cancer: further evidence of their limited indications. Ann Oncol 16:263–266, 2005.
35. Drotman MB, Machnicki SC, Schwartz LH, et al: Breast cancer: assessing the use of routine pelvic CT in patient evaluation. Am J Roentgenol 176:1433–1436, 2001.
36. Krakora GA, Coakley FV, Williams G, et al: Small hypoattenuating hepatic lesions at contrast enhanced CT: prognostic importance in patients with breast cancer. Radiology 233(3):667–673, 2004.
37. Khalil HI, Patterson SA, Panichek DM: Hepatic lesions deemed too small to characterize at CT: prevalence and importance in women with breast cancer. Radiology 235:872–878, 2005.
38. Patterson SA, Khalil HI, Panichek DM: MRI evaluation of small hepatic lesions in women with breast cancer. Am J Roentgenol 187:307–311, 2006.
39. Gerber B, Seitz E, Muller H, et al: Perioperative screening for metastatic disease is not indicated in patients with primary breast cancer and no clinical signs of tumor spread. Breast Cancer Res Treat 82:29–37, 2003.
40. Iagaru A, Masamed R, Keesara S, et al: Breast MRI and 18F FDG PET/CT in the management of breast cancer. Ann Nucl Med 21(1):33–38, 2007.

41. Schirrmeister H, Kühn T, Guhlmann A, et al: Fluorine 18 2-deoxy-2-fluoro-D-glucose PET in the preoperative staging of breast cancer: comparison with the standard staging procedures. Eur J Nucl Med 28(3):351–358.

42. Port ER, Yeung H, Gonen M, et al: 18F-2-fluoro-2-deoxy-D-glucose positron emission tomography scanning affects surgical management in selected patients with high-risk, operable breast carcinoma. Ann Surg Oncol 13(5):677–684, 2006.

43. Avril BN, Rose CA, Schelling M, et al: Breast imaging with positron emission tomography and fluorine-18 fluorodeoxyglucose: use and limitations. J Clin Oncol 18:3495–3502, 2000.

44. Isasi CR, Moadel RM, Blaufox MD: A meta-analysis of FDG-PET for the evaluation of breast cancer recurrence and metastasis. Breast Cancer Res Treat 90(2):105–112, 2005.

45. Eubank WB, Mankoff DA, Takasugi J, et al: 18 Fluorodeoxyglucose positron emission tomography to detect mediastinal or internal mammary metastasis in breast cancer. J Clin Oncol 19(15):3516–3523, 2001.

46. Piperkova E, Raphael B, Altinyay ME, et al: Impact of PET–CT in comparison with same day contrast enhanced CT in breast cancer management. Clin Nucl Med 32(6):429434.

47. Veit-Haibach P, Antoch G, Beyer T, et al: FDG-PET/CT in restaging of patients with recurrent breast cancer: possible impact on staging and therapy. Br J Radiol 10:1–8, 2007.

48. Fueger BJ, Weber WA, Quon A, et al: Performance of 2-deoxy-2-[f-18] fluoro-D-glucose positron emission tomography and integrated PET/CT in restaged breast cancer patients. Mol Imaging Biol 7:369–376, 2005.

49. Nakai T, Okuyama C, Kuboto T: Pitfalls of FDG-PET for the diagnosis of osteoblastic bone metastasis in patients with breast cancer. Eur J Nucl Med Mol Imaging 32(11):1253–1258, 2005.

50. Kuehl H, Veit P, Rosenbaum SJ, et al: Can PET/CT replace separate diagnostic CT for cancer imaging? Optimizing CT protocols for imaging cancer of the chest and abdomen. J Nucl Med 48:45S–57S, 2007.

19

Adjuvant Systemic Therapy

Anthony D. Elias, Daniel Bowles, and Peter Kabos

KEY POINTS

- The most common subtypes of breast cancer are the estrogen receptor (ER)-positive, HER2-amplified, and the triple-negative phenotypes.
- By gene expression arrays and other methods, these tumor types appear to have distinct biologic characteristics and natural histories and are treated differently.
- The statistical risk for metastatic relapse and mortality can be determined by traditional clinical parameters such as breast cancer subtype, nodal status, and tumor size, but more recent molecular characterizations may be more useful for the individual patient.
- Adjuvant chemotherapy statistically can benefit most women with local-regional breast cancer, but the absolute benefit of chemotherapy must be balanced against the absolute risks of treatment to determine whether this intervention is worthwhile.
- Antiestrogen therapy is the mainstay of treatment for ER-positive breast cancer. The benefits of chemotherapy can be estimated from the residual risk of relapse after accounting for the benefits of endocrine therapy.
- Trastuzumab is approved for use in the United States for node-positive HER2-positive breast cancer in conjunction with chemotherapy, although it is frequently used for higher-risk node–negative, HER2-positive tumors.

Types of Breast Cancer

The recognized histologic subtypes of breast cancer are reviewed in Chapter 2. Invasive cancers can be divided into biologically diverse histologies, although within most histologies biologic aggressiveness ranges from indolent to aggressive and is traditionally expressed as histologic grade (grades 1–3) and proliferative thrust (e.g., S-phase fraction, Ki-67, or MIB-1). Certain histologies such as tubular, "typical" medullary, papillary (non-micro type), and mucinous carcinomas are usually low-grade cancers. Breast cancer is also divided into three general biologic subsets, as defined by estrogen receptors (ER) and progesterone receptors (PR) and HER2 expression (HER2): (1) ER-positive or PR-positive; (2) HER2-positive; and (3) triple-negative (negative for ER, PR, and HER2).

Molecular Subtypes of Breast Cancer

Perou, Sorlie, and colleagues[1] set off a paradigm shift in our thinking about breast cancer in their seminal paper describing the molecular portraits of breast cancer by gene expression array. Subsequent papers using both similar and dissimilar techniques have generally confirmed that there appear to be a limited number of biologically distinct subtypes of breast cancer—the most common of which are ER-positive low proliferation (luminal A), ER-positive high proliferation (luminal B), HER2-positive, and triple negative (basal). This chapter is organized with recognition of the interplay between the molecular and clinical classifications. A discussion of adjuvant therapy must balance the risks of tumor recurrence and subsequent mortality with the benefits and risks of the various therapies that can be offered.

Risk of Breast Cancer Recurrence and Mortality

The size of the primary tumor (T), nodal involvement (N), and presence of metastases (M) are the three main clinical criteria for determining stage and prognosis of breast cancer. Other factors contribute to prognosis to a lesser degree. Tumor grade clearly influences prognosis: grade

1 tumors exhibit less propensity for regional and disseminated metastases compared with grade 3 tumors. Unfortunately, pathologists have only about a 40% to 60% agreement when assigning grade. Proliferative thrust as measured by Ki-67 or other nuclear protein markers inversely correlates with outcome. Lymphovascular invasion also predicts increased rates of local-regional recurrence, nodal involvement, and distant metastasis, although limited sampling of the tumor specimen may lead to underestimation of the usefulness of this marker. Untreated, ER-positive and ER-negative tumors have similar 10-year rates of recurrence, although ER-positive tumors tend to be more indolent in their natural history. HER2-positive as well as PR low-proliferation tumors are more aggressive biologically and tend to have a shorter time to recurrence and a greater rate of recurrence.

Not infrequently, the constellation of traditional prognostic factors provides a mixed message. Several newer methods attempt to integrate biology with stage in an effort to improve prognostication. Adjuvant! Online is a Web-based computerized modeling program developed by Dr. Peter Ravdin. It integrates stage (T and N), ER status, and grade to provide estimates for recurrence risk and mortality in patients who are untreated and/or treated with different types of chemotherapy regimens and/or hormonal therapies.[2] This program has proved to be a useful aid for many oncologists during the discussion of adjuvant therapy with newly diagnosed patients. One of its beneficial features is the recognition that patients at various ages have different competing risks for mortality. These considerations may be particularly relevant for older persons who are trying to decide whether a potentially toxic intervention might be worth pursuing. It has proved to be quite accurate in predicting outcomes of a population of patients,[3] but it has been less accurate in predicting the outcome of individual patients.[4] The current version does not yet account for HER2 status or treatment with trastuzumab.

Recently, two methods of evaluating multigene expression have been approved by the Food and Drug Administration (FDA) for use in early-stage breast cancer. The more mature test is the Oncotype Dx assay. It has been approved for use in newly diagnosed patients presenting with ER-positive node-negative breast cancer.[5,6] The other test, Mammaprint, has been approved as a prognostic test for a more diverse population of node-negative, early-stage breast cancers.[4,7] Oncotype Dx is a commercial assay measuring mRNA levels using quantitative reverse transcription-polymerase chain reaction (RT-PCR) from paraffin-embedded formalin-fixed tissues. Sixteen cancer-related genes, including ER, HER2, proliferation genes, and invasion signaling genes, are measured along with five housekeeping genes that serve to normalize the raw data. Validation is extensive and the reproducibility of the assay appears to be excellent. Based on the National Surgical Breast and Bowel Project (NSABP) B-14 and B-20 studies, the recurrence score is a continuous variable ranging from 1 to 100 and provides a prediction for the residual risk of recurrence at 10 years' follow-up, assuming that the patient will have taken 5 years of tamoxifen.[5,6] The level of ER mRNA expression appears to correlate well with the degree of benefit from tamoxifen, and the level of PR mRNA expression appears to correlate inversely with the biologic aggressiveness of the breast cancer. Size remains a weak independent prognostic factor, not accounted for in the recurrence score. HER2-positive tumors are underrepresented in the sample. The test has not yet been validated in node-positive breast cancers. Mammaprint measures the mRNA of 70 genes using fresh tissue and a cDNA chip platform. It dichotomizes the breast cancer population into "good risk" and "poor risk." This assay has been validated in a more heterogeneous set of patients and treatments than Oncotype Dx has and thus does not provide specific prognostic or predictive information (e.g., response to therapy). Both of these assays are integrated into large ongoing clinical trials that are reviewed later in this chapter.

Adjuvant Chemotherapy

Principles and Overview

With over 20 years of follow-up, adjuvant chemotherapy for breast cancer has been shown to reduce the risk of metastatic recurrence and to increase overall survival. With the gradual evolution of clinical trials from small to large, from broad eligibility to more narrowly defined disease processes, and from aggressive biology to more indolent tumors, the incremental benefits of adjuvant chemotherapy have been demonstrated in essentially all types and stages of breast cancer. It is clear from individual studies and from the Early Breast Cancer Trialists' Collaborative Group (EBCTCG) meta-analyses[8] that combination therapy is more effective than single-agent therapy, that anthracycline-based chemotherapy appears superior to non-anthracycline regimens, that taxanes appear to add to anthracycline-based therapies, that maintenance chemotherapy beyond six or eight cycles does not increase survival, and that the targeted therapies (antiestrogen and anti-HER2) add significantly to chemotherapy when the targets are present in the tumor.

As a first approximation, chemotherapy's relative risk reduction (e.g., the proportion of overall risk of tumor recurrence over time) appears to be constant across tumor biology and stage. That is, adjuvant CMF (cyclophosphamide, methotrexate, and 5-fluorouracil) or AC (cyclophosphamide and doxorubicin) chemotherapy may, on average, reduce the risk of recurrence by 25% for all breast cancers over 10 years. However, patients with high-risk tumors (large, node-positive) have a greater absolute improvement in both recurrence risk and mortality risk with a given chemotherapy regimen compared with a person with a low-risk tumor because these tumors have a higher absolute risk of recurring. The absolute benefits of a given treatment must be counterbalanced with the absolute risks of a given treatment in order to decide whether that intervention is worthwhile.

Weighing this therapeutic index ratio is the focus of one of the raging controversies in the adjuvant treatment of breast cancer. In the United States, chemotherapy is used much more often than in Europe for a given tumor stage and biology. Some practitioners in the United States also use the most aggressive chemotherapy for all patients, arguing that these regimens provide the greatest risk reduction and that most, if not all, toxicities are generally reversible. Other practitioners, who often include the more conservative academic oncologists, use risk-adjusted chemotherapy. They are more likely to use aggressive regimens for poor-risk tumors and less aggressive therapies for better-risk tumors. The facts regarding toxicities and benefits are agreed to, but the differences

in practice represent cultural differences in patient and physician expectations and in the physician-patient relationship.

At present, there is a paradigm shift away from the thinking that the benefits of chemotherapy or a given chemotherapy agent will be uniform across stage and tumor biology. Increasingly, trials are being tailored to address specific biologic subtypes of breast cancer, and many trials are attempting to identify which patients do not need chemotherapy at all.

Standards of Care

There are two general classes of adjuvant chemotherapy regimens: low aggressive and high aggressive. As a rule, the low-aggressive regimens are associated with lower potential toxicities and may be shorter in duration. Adjuvant! Online classifies these two classes as first- and third-generation regimens, respectively.

Low-Aggressive Regimens

CMF (cyclophosphamide, methotrexate, and 5-fluorouracil) was one of the first regimens developed and is still in use. There are many variations of this regimen, but the most effective version is oral cyclophosphamide for 14 days with intravenous methotrexate and 5-fluorouracil on day 1 and day 8. One cycle lasts 28 days, and a full course of therapy is given over 6 months.

In the United States, AC (doxorubicin and cyclophosphamide) given intravenously every 3 weeks for four cycles largely supplanted CMF therapy after two NSABP trials demonstrated its equivalence to CMF. Most medical oncologists and patients opted for the shorter AC course. Elsewhere in the world, FEC (5-fluorouracil, epirubicin, and cyclophosphamide) has been the typical standard of care using either the Canadian MA.5 or, more typically, the French regimen.[9,10]

Recently, Jones and colleagues[11] reported the 5-year results of a randomized trial comparing the standard AC regimen with TC (docetaxel, cyclophosphamide) for four cycles. This trial demonstrated clear superiority of the TC regimen regarding progression-free survival and overall survival, with a 33% reduction in risk of recurrence (Fig. 19-1). Notably, TC therapy had greater neuropathy and low-grade docetaxel-associated toxicities, but did not have associated

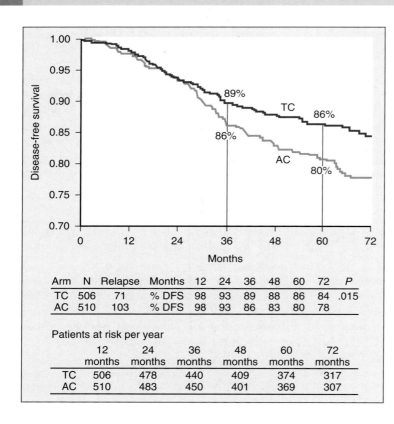

Figure 19-1. Low-aggressive regimens. Chart illustrates disease-free survival (DFS) in AC (doxorubicin and cyclophosphamide) versus TC (docetaxel and cyclophosphamide). (From Jones SE, Savin MA, Holmes FA, et al: Phase III trial comparing doxorubicin plus cyclophosphamide with docetaxel plus cyclophosphamide as adjuvant therapy for operable breast cancer. J Clin Oncol 24:5381–5387, 2006. Erratum in: J Clin Oncol 25(13):1819, 2007.)

Arm	N	Relapse	Months	12	24	36	48	60	72	P
TC	506	71	% DFS	98	93	89	88	86	84	.015
AC	510	103	% DFS	98	93	86	83	80	78	

Patients at risk per year

	12 months	24 months	36 months	48 months	60 months	72 months
TC	506	478	440	409	374	317
AC	510	483	450	401	369	307

cardiac toxicity nor (to date) significant leukemic risks.

High-Aggressive Regimens

In a paper summarizing the 20-year sequence of adjuvant trials in the Cancer and Leukemia Group B (CALGB) for node-positive breast cancer, Berry and colleagues[12] highlight the incremental benefits accrued from dose optimization of (F)AC, the addition of paclitaxel to AC, and the impact of dose density on three-drug regimens. Allowing for cross-trial comparisons and historical controls, the sum total resulted in a doubling of progression-free survival in a similar population of patients. Through such sequences of randomized controlled trials, current standards of care such as adjuvant dose-dense AC → T have been established.

High-aggressive regimens have been supported by several studies. TAC (docetaxel, doxorubicin, and cyclophosphamide) given for six cycles once every 3 weeks became one of the options for node-positive breast cancer after it was associated with a 17% reduction in risk of recurrence compared with FAC in the Breast Cancer International Research Group (BCIRG) 001 trial[13] (Fig. 19-2). The PACS 01 (phosphofurin acidic cluster sorting protein 1) trial compared six cycles of FEC chemotherapy with three cycles of FEC followed by three cycles of docetaxel.[14] The cross-over arm with docetaxel showed a 14% reduction in risk of recurrence compared with FEC alone. The benefit of docetaxel was also confirmed in the neoadjuvant trial NSABP B-27, although no survival advantage has yet been documented in this study.

In summary, the addition of docetaxel given every 3 weeks or dose-dense paclitaxel given every 2 weeks has resulted in consistent improvements in progression-free survival and, in several studies, overall survival advantages. Given the superiority of TC over AC in a head-to-head comparison, a legitimate question that must be raised is how much and in which patients does doxorubicin significantly reduce relapse.

Chemotherapy Integration with Antiendocrine Therapy

Tamoxifen is used sequentially both with chemotherapy and radiation. The sequential treat-

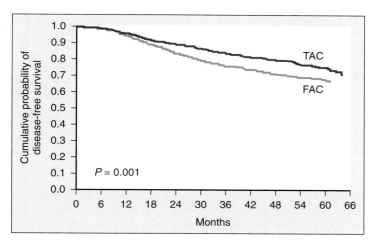

Figure 19-2. High-aggressive regimens. Chart illustrates disease-free survival in TAC (docetaxel plus doxorubicin and cyclophosphamide) versus FAC (fluorouracil plus doxorubicin and cyclophosphamide). (From Martin M, Pienkowski T, Mackey J, et al: Adjuvant docetaxel for node-positive breast cancer. N Engl J Med 352:2302–2313, 2005.)

Table 19-1. Impact of Adding Chemotherapy to Tamoxifen for Postmenopausal Women with ER-Positive, Node-Positive Breast Cancer According to the Oncotype DX Recurrence Score

	10-Year Disease-Free Survival Estimates (%)	
	Tamoxifen ($n = 148$)	CAF $\rightarrow$ Tamoxifen ($n = 219$)
Low recurrence score (<18)	60	64
Intermediate recurrence score (18–30)	49	63
High recurrence score (≥31)	43	55

From Albain K et al. Prognostic value of the Oncotype DX assay in the chemotherapy-based arms of SWOG-8814. Breast Cancer Update 2, 2008. Available at www.breastcancerupdate.com/medonc/2008/2/albain.asp.
CAF, cyclophosphamide, doxorubicin, and 5-fluorouracil; ER, estrogen receptor.

ment is largely based on in vitro studies, showing a decrease in sensitivity of cultured breast cancer cells to radiation when concurrently treated with tamoxifen. It is further supported by clinical observations of increased pulmonary toxicity with the concurrent approach.[15] Chemotherapy integration with antiendocrine therapy has been examined in the SWOG (Southwest Oncology Group) S8814 trial[16] (Table 19-1). In this trial, postmenopausal women with ER-positive node-positive breast cancer were randomized to tamoxifen alone (T); cyclophosphamide, doxorubicin, and 5-fluorouracil (CAF) chemotherapy concurrent with tamoxifen (CAFT); or CAF chemotherapy followed by tamoxifen (CAF $\rightarrow$ T). Although only available in abstract form at this point, the finding that chemotherapy improved survival compared with tamoxifen alone in this population of patients has been influential. Even more important has been the finding that sequential therapy with CAF followed by tamoxifen was superior to the other two groups. A definitive report of this trial will

be published shortly in a major journal (Albain KS et al). The mechanism of sub-additive efficacy when combining tamoxifen with CAF is unknown. One possibility is that the reduction of proliferative thrust by reducing estrogenic signaling could reduce chemosensitivity. If so, then concurrent administration of aromatase inhibitors or other endocrine therapies with chemotherapy should not be done, although this hypothesis has not been tested adequately.

Future Directions

Predictors of Response/Benefit to Particular Chemotherapy Agents

Using biologic markers to determine who will benefit from certain agents is an area of significant interest. For example, knowing who will benefit most from anthracyclines is of clinical importance. The presence of the topoisomerase II enzyme (topo II) is required for topoisomerase II inhibitors (e.g., anthracyclines) to be effective. Recent studies reported by the National Cancer Institute of Canada (NCIC) suggest that the high nuclear staining for topo II seen in approximately 25% to 30% of breast cancers predicts a better response to anthracyclines.[17] Less convincing are reports examining elevated topo II mRNA levels or topo II gene amplification. Topo II gene is amplified in up to 35% of HER2-amplified breast cancers, but it is relatively rare in the HER2-negative breast cancers. The presence of HER2 amplification appears to be associated with a greater benefit to anthracycline-containing regimens, but this is not as clearly explained by topo II changes.

A number of predictors of sensitivity and resistance to taxanes have been published using a battery of immunohistochemistry probes or gene expression arrays.[18,19] These have been variably validated in neoadjuvant chemotherapy trials, but have not yet been tested in definitive prospective trials. New taxanes and taxoids, such as nab-paclitaxel and the epotheliones, will be or are already being tested in the adjuvant setting.

Several large clinical trials have completed accrual evaluating the role of capecitabine (US Oncology) or gemcitabine (NSABP B-38) in combination with the anthracycline-taxane–containing regimens and should be reporting interim results over the next 2 to 3 years.

Advances in pharmacogenomics and the ability to measure global expression of single nucleotide polymorphisms (SNPs) will contribute to personalized medicine. Ambrosone and colleagues[20] recently reported that the presence of SNPs associated with high levels of myeloperoxidase, and thus heightened ability to form free radicals and oxidative reactive intermediates, appears to be associated with a greater benefit from cyclophosphamide-containing chemotherapy. Along similar lines, population heterogeneity with respect to SNPs for genes regulating tamoxifen metabolism and activation may play a significant role in determining benefit from tamoxifen. These studies cannot be performed without rigorous and comprehensive tissue banking of suitable specimens.

Chemotherapy integration with biologic therapies will be well represented in the next wave of adjuvant clinical trials. The antiangiogenic agent bevacizumab (Avastin) will be combined with chemotherapy to evaluate its role in changing progression-free and overall survival for stage II breast cancer. Specific questions that will be addressed include whether bevacizumab should be given concurrently with chemotherapy, after chemotherapy as maintenance, or in both ways. The significant cost and lack of specific predictors to response and/or resistance to bevacizumab will limit our ability to use this agent in much of the world. Many other biologic agents are in earlier phases of testing (e.g., in metastatic disease) but will undoubtedly make it to testing in the adjuvant setting.

One of the more exciting areas of progress is in the identification of molecular subtypes of breast cancer and the elucidation of therapeutic targets in each of these subtypes. We have long separated the ER-positive from the ER-negative and the HER2-positive from the HER2-negative. This very separation forms the basis of how this chapter is organized. So far, we know that chemotherapy consisting of DNA-damaging agents and antitubulins appears to be more active in the HER2-positive and triple-negative types of breast cancer compared with the ER-positive breast cancers. Whether this is primarily related to the increased proliferative thrust of the first two types or whether there are other better predictors for benefit remains to be seen. In ER-positive breast cancers, we get a much better idea about who will respond to chemotherapy based on the ongoing TAILORx (Trial Assigning IndividuaLized Options for Treatment [Rx]) and MINDACT (Microarray in Node-Negative Disease May Avoid ChemoTherapy) studies.

The TAILORx trial will enroll 11,000 women with ER-positive node-negative breast cancers and categorize them according to Oncotype Dx recurrence score.[21] Approximately 30% are expected to have low recurrence scores (less than 11) and to have antiestrogen therapy alone. The approximately 20% expected to have high recurrence scores (more than 25) will receive chemotherapy followed by endocrine therapy. The remainder with intermediate recurrence scores will be randomized to receive antiestrogen therapy with or without chemotherapy. By measuring progression-free survival, it is hoped that up to 50% of women with intermediate recurrence scores will be found not to require chemotherapy.

The MINDACT study, based on the Mammaprint assay, will assign about 8000 women with stage I node-negative disease (including ER-negative) to good or bad prognosis by both standard clinical features and by gene expression profiling.[22] Those with discordance between the clinical prognosis and the gene expression prognosis will be randomized to receive therapy based on either the clinical prognosis or the gene expression prognosis. This will help determine whether the gene expression profile predicts biologic behavior and response to therapy better than standard clinical parameters.

Within the triple-negative phenogenotype, there are identifiable sub-subtypes of breast cancer. For example, a group of these are either the *BRCA1* mutated tumors or tumors with loss of *BRCA1* protein expression. These tumors appear to be exquisitely sensitive to alkylating agents and radiation therapy because of defects in DNA repair pathways.[23] Poly (ADP-ribose) polymerase (PARP) inhibition may increase this sensitivity.[24] Others appear to have increased activation of the androgen receptor pathway genes.[25] It remains to be seen whether anti-androgen receptor therapy will have activity in some triple-negative tumors. Undoubtedly, other sub-subtypes will be identified on the basis of increased epidermal growth factor receptor (EGFR) expression, sensitivity to Src or c-Met inhibition, or other characteristics. Once confirmed in metastatic disease trials, these concepts will rapidly disseminate to adjuvant and/or neoadjuvant settings.

Another concept that may become a standard of care in the future is the use of bisphosphonates as adjuvant therapy for breast cancer. The bisphosphonates inhibit osteoclast function and are widely used for the treatment and prevention of osteoporosis. They have also proved to decrease the rate of progression of breast and other cancers involving bone and to decrease rates of fracture and pain from metastases. In model systems, breast cancer cells home to bone marrow spaces, activate osteoclasts through parathyroid hormone-related protein (PTHrP) and other mechanisms. Osteoclasts, in turn, release various cytokines such as interleukin-6 (IL-6) and tumor growth factor-β (TGF-β) from bone matrix, which then support breast cancer cell growth and survival. Interruption of these pathways can make bone a less friendly environment for breast cancer cells to grow.[26]

Three clodronate adjuvant trials have been reported; two demonstrated a small survival advantage with 10-year follow-up.[27-30] A fourth trial (NSABP B-34) has completed accrual, but

has not reached maturity. The AZURE trial, comparing zoledronate with placebo, has likewise completed accrual. SWOG S0307 is an intergroup trial randomizing patients to three different bisphosphonates for 3 years. This trial is asking the question whether more potent aminobisphosphonates (ibandronate and zoledronate) would be more effective than clodronate (a weak bisphosphonate).

Adjuvant Hormone Therapy

Principles and Overview

In the 19th century, Beatson[30a] observed an improvement in the prognosis of women with advanced breast cancer who underwent oophorectomy. This was the first step in recognizing the estrogen-dependent nature of breast cancer and the therapeutic importance of hormone deprivation.

Two estrogen receptors (ERα and ERβ) have been described. Estrogen receptors belong to a family of nuclear steroid receptors that includes thyroid hormone, vitamin D, and retinoids. The ERα and ERβ proteins are coded on chromosomes 6 and 14. ERβ is expressed broadly in a variety of tissues, whereas ERα has a more restricted expression pattern (breast, ovary, uterus, and endometrium). Clinically, ERα is used as a measure of ER positivity in breast cancer. There are no clinically available assays for ERβ.

Between 70% and 80% of all breast cancers express ER. ER expression correlates with slower tumor growth, better differentiation, and a longer natural history. Lack of both ER and PR is, on the other hand, associated with poor prognosis and a decrease in overall survival. Response to hormone therapy correlates with higher levels of hormone expression at the protein and at the mRNA level.[31] For example, 60% of women who are ER-positive/PR-positive respond to treatment, 30% of ER-positive/PR-negative or ER-negative/PR-positive respond, and less than 10% of women who are ER-negative/PR-negative respond. The ER and PR status can also change over the natural course of the disease, in addition to being a result of hormone treatment.[32]

Our understanding of the biology of steroid hormone receptors (HRs) led to the development of treatments based on estrogen and its

Table 19-2. Therapeutic Agents That Target Estrogen or Its Receptor

Therapeutic Agent	Pathway	Example
Selective estrogen-receptor modulators (SERMs)	Bind the ER receptor and modulate downstream gene transcription and function as partial ER-agonists and antagonists	Tamoxifen
Aromatase inhibitors (AIs)	Block the peripheral conversion of adrenal androgens into estrogen; thus, only successful in women without ovarian function	Anastrozole, letrozole, and exemestane
Steroidal 7*-alkylamide analogues	Bind to the ER receptor and lead to its degradation	Fulvestrant

receptors. Three major classes of therapeutic agents target estrogen or its receptor in clinical use today (Table 19-2). First, selective estrogen receptor modulators (SERMs) bind the ER receptor and modulate downstream gene transcription and function as partial ER agonists and antagonists. Tamoxifen is the best-known example. Second, aromatase inhibitors (AIs) block the peripheral conversion of adrenal androgens into estrogen.[33,34] Thus, they are successful only in women without ovarian function. Examples of AIs are anastrozole, letrozole, and exemestane. Third, there are agents that bind to the ER receptor and lead to its degradation. The only currently clinically available agent in this class is fulvestrant.

Hormone manipulations have become an integral part of breast cancer treatment since their discovery over a century ago. However, we are still learning how to optimize and sequence endocrine therapy in breast cancer. The following sections discuss the current standards in the use of hormone therapy in breast cancer.

Menopausal Breast Cancer Patients

The selection of hormone therapy for HR-positive breast cancer depends largely on the patient's menopausal status. Debate is ongoing regarding the definition of menopause in breast cancer patients, since amenorrhea is a well-described side effect of chemotherapy.[35] Moreover, ovarian function and estradiol levels can be partially preserved despite chemotherapy-induced amenorrhea. In general, younger patients require more chemotherapy to achieve amenorrhea. More than 80% of women age 40 and older achieve menopause after six cycles of CMF (cyclophosphamide, methotrexate, and 5-fluorouracil), compared with less than 50% of

women age 40 and younger. Less amenorrhea is also seen with the AC (cyclophosphamide and doxorubicin) and AC → T (cyclophosphamide and doxorubicin plus tamoxifen) regimens when compared with CMF.

A more accurate definition of menopause became increasingly important when multiple clinical studies demonstrated superiority of AIs over tamoxifen in the treatment of breast cancer. AIs, however, cannot be used in the pre- or perimenopausal patient as monotherapy. As previously described, AIs inhibit the peripheral conversion of androgens to estrogens. They do not block estrogen synthesis within a functioning ovary. Thus, women with preserved ovarian function who are taking AIs still produce estrogen. In fact, one study showed that 27% of women with chemotherapy-induced amenorrhea regained ovarian function within a median of 12 months after starting therapy with an AI.[36] Furthermore, AIs may lead to a rise in gonadotropins, and for this reason letrozole has been used for induction of ovulation in infertility.[37]

The standards for defining menopause still vary among clinical trials. Most clinicians consider more than 12 months of amenorrhea together with postmenopausal levels of estrogen and follicle-stimulating hormone as sufficient proof of menopause.

Premenopausal Breast Cancer Patients

Tamoxifen was the first selective estrogen receptor modulator used to treat breast cancer and has been the cornerstone of hormone therapy for more than 30 years. It competes with estrogen for ER binding sites and has both estrogenic and antiestrogenic actions. The agonist activity is responsible for some of its beneficial effects such as prevention of osteoporosis. On the other hand, it increases thromboembolic events from about 1% to 2% and endometrial carcinomas from about 4 in 1000 to 8 in 1000.[38] More common side effects are hot flashes and vaginal discharge.

The question of tamoxifen's benefit in younger patients has been answered by the EBCTCG overview analysis demonstrating a survival benefit with tamoxifen use in the adjuvant setting, regardless of patient age.[39] The analysis further shows a 41% decrease in the annual risk of relapse and a 34% decrease in the annual risk of death among ER-positive women with breast cancer.[38] Proportional risk benefits are similar in different age groups and independent of their node status. However, women with node-positive disease have a larger absolute benefit (16%). Tamoxifen's benefit appears to be independent of chemotherapy use. Treatment with tamoxifen also reduces the relative risk of developing contralateral breast cancer by 55%.[40]

A period of 5 years of tamoxifen therapy is considered standard of care based on multiple trials demonstrating superiority of a 5-year regimen over 2 years of treatment.[41,42] However, both the NSABP and the Scottish trials demonstrated that 10 years of tamoxifen was slightly less effective than 5 years.[43,44] Both trials included a majority of women with node-negative disease. These results are thought to be partly due to the development of tamoxifen resistance during the course of treatment. In fact, in preclinical studies, long-term exposure to tamoxifen can lead to tamoxifen-dependent breast cancer cell lines.

Ovarian Suppression

In addition to the previously described hormone therapies, there is evidence that oophorectomy is of benefit to premenopausal women with breast cancer. This observation led to the question of whether chemical ovarian suppression with a GnRH agonist may be of benefit. A recent meta-analysis tried to answer this question using individual patient data from 16 trials[45] (Fig. 19-3). As expected, the GnRH agonists are not effective in HR-negative patients. In ER-positive disease, the addition of GnRH agonists to tamoxifen, chemotherapy, or both reduces the absolute risk of recurrent disease by 12.7% and the risk of death following recurrence by 15.1%.

The optimal length of treatment with GnRH agonists is not known. The absolute benefit of oophorectomy or ovarian suppression when combined with tamoxifen is also unclear.

Two protocols by IBCSG (International Breast Cancer Study Group) have been designed to better define the role of ovarian suppression in premenopausal women with breast cancer. The SOFT trial (Suppression of Ovarian Function Trial) randomizes premenopausal women with ER-positive breast cancer to tamoxifen or ovarian suppression (GnRH agonist or surgical or ovarian irradiation) combined with tamoxifen or exemestane. The TEXT (Tamoxifen and Exemestane Trial) trial randomizes the same group of patients to therapies similar to the latter two arms of the SOFT trial. The TEXT trial is attempting to mimic the success of AIs in postmenopausal women and is nearing its accrual goal.

Postmenopausal Breast Cancer Patients

The development of AIs changes the standard of care for postmenopausal women with breast cancer. To date each study that has compared an AI with tamoxifen has demonstrated AI superiority. AIs have been tested as up-front therapy in place of tamoxifen after 2 to 3 years of tamoxifen and also after completion of 5 years of tamoxifen. As previously mentioned, AIs can be used only in women who lack ovarian function because of their mechanism of action.

Two large studies compared an AI head-to-head regimen with tamoxifen. The ATAC trial[46] used anastrozole and the BIG (Breast International Group) 1–98 trial letrozole.[47] Both trials showed a greater improvement in disease-free survival and time to progression in the AI arms. There was a trend in improvement of overall survival that is expected to reach statistical significance on further analyses. Use of AI was associated with fewer thromboembolic events and endometrial cancers, but it caused more osteoporosis. Tamoxifen was associated with lower cholesterol levels.

Another study that compared a continuation of tamoxifen after 2 years of therapy with a change to exemestane also showed an improvement in disease-free survival in the AI arm. The absolute benefit was 4.7% after only 3 years.[48] Similar benefits were documented in the ITA (Italian Tamoxifen Arimidex), ARNO

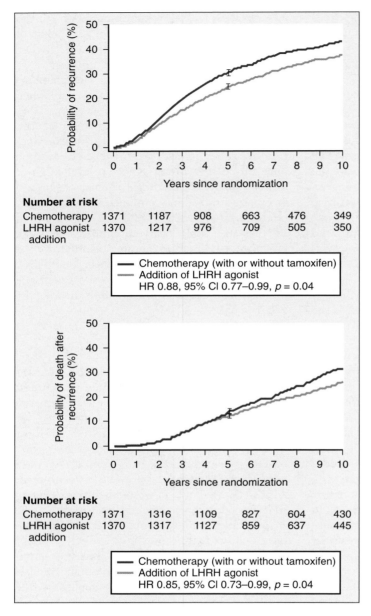

Figure 19-3. Ovarian suppression.
Chart illustrates the addition of luteinizing hormone-releasing hormone (LHRH/GnRH) agonist to chemotherapy with or without tamoxifen. (From Cuzick J, Ambroisine L, Davidson N, et al: Use of luteinising-hormone-releasing hormone agonists as adjuvant treatment in premenopausal patients with hormone-receptor-positive breast cancer: a meta-analysis of individual patient data from randomised adjuvant trials. Lancet 369:1711–1723, 2007.)

(Arimidex-Nolvadex), and ABCSG (Austrian Breast and Colorectal Cancer Study Group) 08 trials when crossing over to anastrozole after 2 years of tamoxifen.[49,50]

A combined analysis of the latter two large trials showed a 40% decrease in the risk of an event in the AI group (hazard ratio 0.60). Confirming results from other studies, AI (anastrozole in this case) was associated with a statistically significant increase in fractures and a decrease in thromboses. Since most of the recurrences in women receiving tamoxifen are found after 5 years of therapy (rate of 1.5% to 2% per year), the MA.17 trial was designed to test continued hormone therapy with an AI following tamoxifen.[51] It was stopped early after an interim analysis as a result of an improvement in disease-free survival (4.6% absolute reduction) after a median follow-up of 2.4 years. After maturing, the MA.17 is also the first trial to show an overall survival benefit for an AI (Table 19-3).

According to the most recent American Society of Clinical Oncology (ASCO) guidelines, AIs are to be used in postmenopausal

Table 19-3. Summary of Adjuvant Aromatase Inhibitor (AI) Trials

	ATAC	BIG	IES	ABCSG/ARNO	MA.17
Number treated	6241	8010	4724	3224	5187
EFS/DFS HR	0.87	0.81	0.67	0.60	0.58
OS HR	0.97	0.86	0.83	0.73	0.82*
Contralateral reduction in HR	0.58	—	0.44	—	0.50
3 years EFS AI	90%	94%	91.5%	96%	95%
Tamoxifen	88.5%	92%	86.8%	93%	90%

*Overall survival statistically significant for node-positive patients.
DFS, disease-free survival; EFS, event-free survival; HR, hormone resistance; OS, overall survival.

women with HR-positive breast cancer, if tamoxifen is contraindicated. For all other women, a decision should be made between 5 years of an AI and 2 to 3 years of tamoxifen followed by an AI.

Based on the currently available data. it is clear that the addition of an AI to adjuvant therapy in HR-positive women with breast cancer is beneficial. The question of sequencing of tamoxifen and AIs, both its necessity as well as its length of treatment, remain unanswered. Although we do have statistical models hinting at the benefit of sequencing, these results are hypothesis generating, and only further randomized trials will be able to clarify this issue. Results from a second randomization of patients from the MA.17 study to continued treatment versus placebo, as well as a comparison of AI alone versus crossover from tamoxifen are needed to come to a definitive conclusion.

Mechanisms of Hormone Resistance

Hormone resistance is a well-recognized problem in patients with breast cancer, and it can occur de novo or it can be acquired during therapy. There are many proposed mechanisms of resistance including the loss of ER in tumor cells, change in the binding of antiestrogens to tumor cells, and crosstalk between ER and other receptor pathways.[52] Estrogen classically exerts its action via ER, activating transcription of target genes in the nucleus. It is, however, the nongenomic hypothesis of crosstalk with growth factor pathways and their direct activation that is thought to play a crucial role in hormone resistance. Multiple pathways including HER2/neu, an insulin-like growth factor-I receptor (IGF-IR), an epidermal growth factor receptor

(EGFR) and cyclooxygenase (COX)-2 have been implicated.[53-55] Lapatinib, an EGFR and HER2 oral tyrosine kinase inhibitor (TKI), is being evaluated to reverse resistance to various hormone therapies. Another strategy that may need testing in the adjuvant setting is SWOG S0226, a randomized study of anastrozole with or without fulvestrant in ER-positive metastatic breast cancer. Since fulvestrant competes with estradiol for binding to ER, removal of the ligand with an AI may allow greater fulvestrant activity. Fulvestrant may also reduce ligand-independent ER signaling.

Adjuvant HER2-Targeted Therapies

In addition to chemotherapeutic and antiestrogen agents, the adjuvant role of trastuzumab (Herceptin), a monoclonal antibody targeted against HER2, has been evaluated. In general, it is effective in the adjuvant setting and has become the standard of care for patients with HER2-positive tumors.

Clinical Efficacy of Trastuzumab

Five randomized controlled trials have been investigating the role of trastuzumab as adjuvant therapy for breast cancer. The first two trials were the NSABP B-31 and the North Central Cancer Treatment Group-Coordinated Intergroup trial N9831.[56] Originally designed as parallel trials, their results were combined for publication with approval of the National Cancer Institute. NSABP B-31 enrolled 2043 women with HER2-positive, node-positive breast cancer to receive four cycles of AC (doxorubicin and cyclophosphamide) followed by paclitaxel (T) every 3 weeks (AC → T) versus the same regimen plus 52 weeks of weekly trastuzumab (AC → TH). N9831 randomized 2614 women with HER2-positive, node-positive, or high-risk node-negative disease (ER-positive/PR-positive and greater than 2 cm or ER-negative/PR-negative and greater than 1 cm) to receive four cycles of AC, then either 12 weeks of weekly paclitaxel (AC → T), weekly paclitaxel followed by 52 weeks of trastuzumab (AC → T → H), or concurrent paclitaxel and trastuzumab followed by 40 weeks of trastuzumab alone (AC → TH). Enrollment for both studies required HER2 gene amplification by fluorescence in situ hybridization (FISH) or 3+ or greater staining by immunohistochemistry. Mean follow-up was 18 months.

The results for the combined studies were striking. There was a hazard ratio of 0.48 for disease-free survival at 3 years between the concurrent trastuzumab group and the no-trastuzumab group. The absolute risk reduction was 12%, yielding a number needed to treat (NNT) of only 8. Despite short follow-up, for overall survival the hazard ratio was 0.67 with an absolute risk reduction of 2.6% (NNT 38). In a preliminary analysis of the N9831 arms, concurrent trastuzumab and paclitaxel seemed superior to sequential treatments, with a 2-year disease-free survival hazard ratio of 0.64 ($P = .114$) and an overall survival hazard ratio of 0.74 ($P = .26$) between concurrent and sequential therapy.[57] Toxicity seemed greater with concurrent therapy in both trials.

The results of the combined NSABP B-31/Intergroup N9831 trial were corroborated by the Herceptin Adjuvant (HERA) trial.[58] Patients with HER2-positive tumors by 3+ immunostaining or gene amplification ($N = 5081$) were randomized to receive none, 1 year, or 2 years of trastuzumab after surgery, chemotherapy, and radiation of their primary oncologist's choosing (chemo → obs versus chemo → H). Compared with patients enrolled in NSABP B-31 and N9831, fewer patients received a taxane (26% versus 100%), and more had node-negative disease (33% versus 5.7%). They were not divided into T1cN0 or T1a/bN0. The initial results at a median follow-up of 12 months revealed a 2-year disease-free survival hazard ratio of 0.52 with an absolute risk reduction of 8.4% (NNT 12). There was no statistical difference in overall survival rate. Follow-up to this original report shows more encouraging results.

With a median follow-up of 23.5 months, there was a 36% reduction in disease recurrence at 3 years (hazard ratio 0.64, absolute risk reduction 6.3%, NNT 16). Analysis at this point showed a 2.7% absolute survival benefit (hazard ratio 0.66, NNT 37).[59] The data for patients treated with 2 years of trastuzumab are not yet available.

The role of adjuvant trastuzumab combined with either an anthracycline or non–anthracycline-containing regimen is also being investigated. BCIRG trial 006 assigned 3222 women with HER2-positive, node-positive or high-risk node-negative disease (tumor size larger than 2 cm, ER- and PR-negative, histologic and/or nuclear grade 2–3, or age under 35 years) to receive AC followed by docetaxel (AC → T), AC-docetaxel and 1 year of trastuzumab starting during docetaxel administration (AC → TH), or docetaxel plus carboplatin and 1 year of trastuzumab (TCbH).[60] In the second interim analysis presented at the 2006 San Antonio Breast Symposium, the absolute disease-free survival benefit from years 2 to 4 was 6% for AC → TH versus AC → T (hazard ratio 0.61, NNT 17) and 5% for TCbH versus AC-T (hazard ratio 0.67, NNT 20) at a median follow-up of 36 months. The absolute overall survival benefit at four years was 6% for AC → TH (hazard ratio 0.59, NNT 17) and 5% for TCbH (hazard ratio 0.66, NNT 20). The safety profile may be better in the TCbH group than AC → TH.

Finally, one small European trial looked at the effect of short course adjuvant trastuzumab. In the FinHer trial, 232 women with HER2-positive breast cancer by gene amplification were randomized to docetaxel followed by 5-fluorouracil, epirubicin, and cyclophosphamide (T → FEC), T plus FEC and 9 weekly infusions of trastuzumab (TH → FEC), vinorelbine plus FEC (V → FEC), or V plus FEC and trastuzumab (VH → FEC).[61] At a median follow-up of 36 months, disease-free survival was significantly improved in women receiving adjuvant trastuzumab (hazard ratio 0.42, absolute risk reduction 11.7, NNT 9). Overall survival was also improved in the trastuzumab arms (hazard ratio 0.41, absolute risk reduction 6.6, NNT 15). These results are similar to regimens using 1 year of trastuzumab in both disease-free survival and overall survival and may provide significant cost savings. Furthermore, the short-course regimen seems to have less associated toxicity than longer courses. Docetaxel was also superior to vinorelbine in the larger trial.

Adverse Events and Cardiac Toxicity

Although the five studies have shown marked benefit of adjuvant trastuzumab, significant cardiac toxicity is associated with this therapy. In the B-31 study, 4.1% of patients developed New York Heart Association class III or IV heart failure compared with 0.8% receiving observation. Fourteen percent of patients had to stop taking trastuzumab because of asymptomatic decreases in left ventricular ejection fraction (LVEF) of more than 15%. In the Intergroup N9831 study, a similar number of women developed heart failure in the concurrent (3.3%) and sequential (2.2%) groups compared with the observation group (0%). There were also significantly more cases of asymptomatic decreases in LVEF.[57] The HERA study confirmed an increase in heart failure (1.7%) and diminished LVEF (7.1%) in patients treated with trastuzumab compared with the observation group (0.06% and 2.2%, respectively). Again, these trends are confirmed in the second interim analysis BCIRG 006. Patients receiving trastuzumab had an increased risk of developing heart failure and decreased LVEF, particularly when co-administered with an anthracycline. These data are summarized in Table 19-4. It is an interesting point that the FinHer study did not find increased cardiotoxicity with the short regimen of trastuzumab. Indeed, it appears that 1 year

of trastuzumab may increase cardiac dysfunction in the adjuvant setting, but that short-term dosing may not.

Cost-Effectiveness

Trastuzumab and other biologic agents are very expensive, and frequent use of this agent could cause significant financial burden to society. To evaluate the cost-effectiveness of adjuvant trastuzumab, Kurian and colleagues[62] compared conventional chemotherapy without trastuzumab, anthracycline-based regimens with trastuzumab, and the non-anthracycline regimen used in B-31/N9831, HERA, and BCIRG 006. They found that adjuvant therapy without trastuzumab yields 9.35 quality-adjusted life years (QALYs) at a cost of $133,429 compared with 10.77 QALYs for $190,092 with an anthracycline-based regimen and 10.61 QALYs for $206,561 with the non-anthracycline regimen. The anthracycline-based regimen had an incremental cost-effectiveness ratio of $39,892/QALY compared with adjuvant therapy without trastuzumab. It was superior to the non–anthracycline-based regimens. Liberato and colleagues[63] analyzed B-31/N9831 and a meta-analysis by the Early Breast Cancer Trialists' Collaborative Group and found that adjuvant trastuzumab cost $18,970 per QALY saved. Both groups concluded that the benefits of adjuvant trastuzumab justify its significant cost.

Future Directions

A new agent for treating HER2-positive tumors is lapatinib, a combined inhibitor of EGFR and HER2. A study comparing capecitabine alone versus lapatinib with capecitabine in women who progressed on trastuzumab found a hazard ratio of 0.49 ($P < .001$) for combined therapy.[64] A new international adjuvant trial comparing trastuzumab, lapatinib, the sequence, or the combination of the two when integrated with chemotherapy is about to be activated.

Summary

Several randomized controlled studies have confirmed a greater than 50% improvement in disease-free survival for women receiving concurrent trastuzumab and a less robust improvement in disease-free survival for women receiving

Table 19-4. Summary of Cardiac Toxicity and Trastuzumab in the Adjuvant Setting

Study	Regimen	Decrease in LVEF >10% (%)	Heart Failure (%)
HERA	Chemo → obs	2.2	0.06
HERA	Chemo → H	7.1	1.7
N9831	AC → T	6.7*	0
BCIRG 006	AC → T	10	0.4
B31	AC → TH	14*	4.1
N9831	AC → TH	16.7*	3.3
BCIRG 006	AC → TH	18	1.9
N9831	AC → T → H	14.2*	2.2
BCIRG 006	TCbH	8.6	0.4

*Decrease in left ventricular ejection fraction of more than 15%.
AC, cyclophosphamide and doxorubicin; LVEF, left ventricular ejection fraction; obs, observation; T, docetaxel; TCbH, docetaxel, carboplatin, trastuzumab; TH, Taxol, trastuzumab.

sequential trastuzumab. The disease-free survival is similar in patients treated with AC-taxane and 1 year of trastuzumab regimens and in those receiving short courses of trastuzumab. Overall survival data seem to trend with disease-free survival, but the studies are still too immature to prove definitive. Non-anthracycline regimens such as TCbH (docetaxel, carboplatin, and trastuzumab) appear to be only moderately less efficacious but are associated with less toxicity and higher cost. There is an increased risk of cardiac dysfunction in patients treated with adjuvant trastuzumab, but the long-term harmful effects are not yet known.

The FDA has recently approved adjuvant trastuzumab in conjunction with chemotherapy for HER2-positive, node-positive breast cancers. Many to most oncologists would also recommend trastuzumab for high-risk node-negative breast cancers, although there is substantial uncertainty over what constitutes a high enough risk to warrant administration of chemotherapy plus trastuzumab and its potential toxicity.

Conclusion

Systemic adjuvant therapy substantially reduces the risk of recurrence. Steady incremental improvements in survival have been achieved throughout the last 10 to 15 years. The usual sequence after surgery is chemotherapy followed by radiation therapy and/or antiestrogen therapy if indicated. If trastuzumab is indicated, it is typically started with a taxane during the chemotherapy phase, continued through radiation therapy if given, and continued to complete 1 year total.

Biology directs therapy, both in terms of risk assessment and prediction of which therapies will provide benefit and which therapies are not worthwhile. Current and future clinical trials will define patient populations with indolent tumor biology that will not need standard chemotherapy and will define tumor and patient populations who will benefit from specific targeted approaches.

References

1. Perou CM, Sorlie T, Eisen MB, et al: Molecular portraits of human breast tumours. Nature 406:747–752, 2000.
2. www.adjuvantonline.com/
3. Olivotto IA, Bajdik CD, Ravdin PM, et al: Population-based validation of the prognostic model ADJUVANT! for early breast cancer. J Clin Oncol 23:2716–2725, 2005.
4. Buyse M, Loi S, van't Veer L, et al: Validation and clinical utility of a 70-gene prognostic signature for women with node-negative breast cancer. J Natl Cancer Inst 98:1183–1192, 2006.
5. Paik S, Tang G, Shak S, et al: Gene expression and benefit of chemotherapy in women with node-negative, estrogen receptor-positive breast cancer. J Clin Oncol 24:3726–3734, 2006.
6. Paik S, Shak S, Tang G, et al: A multigene assay to predict recurrence of tamoxifen-treated, node-negative breast cancer. N Engl J Med 351:2817–2826, 2004.
7. van de Vijver MJ, He YD, van't Veer LJ, et al: A gene-expression signature as a predictor of survival in breast cancer. N Engl J Med 347:1999–2009, 2002.
8. Early Breast Cancer Trialists' Collaborative Group (EBCTCG): Effects of chemotherapy and hormonal therapy for early breast cancer on recurrence and 15-year survival: an overview of the randomised trials. Lancet 365:1687–1717, 2005.
9. Parulekar WR, Day AG, Ottaway JA, et al: Incidence and prognostic impact of amenorrhea during adjuvant therapy in high-risk premenopausal breast cancer: analysis of a National Cancer Institute of Canada Clinical Trials Group Study—NCIC CTG MA.5. J Clin Oncol 23:6002–6005, 2005.
10. French Adjuvant Study Group: Benefit of a high-dose epirubicin regimen in adjuvant chemotherapy for node-positive breast cancer patients with poor prognostic factors: 5-year follow-up results of French Adjuvant Study Group 05 randomized trial. J Clin Oncol 19:602–611, 2001.
11. Jones SE, Savin MA, Holmes FA, et al: Phase III trial comparing doxorubicin plus cyclophosphamide with docetaxel plus cyclophosphamide as adjuvant therapy for operable breast cancer. J Clin Oncol 24:5381–5387, 2006. Erratum in: J Clin Oncol 25(13):819, 2007.
12. Berry DA, Cirrincione C, Henderson IC, et al: Estrogen-receptor status and outcomes of modern chemotherapy for patients with node-positive breast cancer. JAMA 295:1658–1667, 2006.
13. Martin M, Pienkowski T, Mackey J, et al: Adjuvant docetaxel for node-positive breast cancer. N Engl J Med 352:2302–2313, 2005.
14. Roche H, Fumoleau P, Spielmann M, et al: Sequential adjuvant epirubicin-based and docetaxel chemotherapy for node-positive breast cancer patients: the FNCLCC PACS 01 Trial. J Clin Oncol 24:5664–5671, 2006.
15. Bentzen SM, Skoczylas J, Overgaard M, et al: Radiotherapy-related lung fibrosis enhanced by tamoxifen. J Natl Cancer Inst 88:918–922, 1996.
16. Albain KS, Green SJ, Ravdin PM, et al: Adjuvant chemohormonal therapy for primary breast cancer should be sequential instead of concurrent: initial results from intergroup trial 0100 (SWOG-8814) [abstract 143]. Proc Am Soc Clin Oncol 21: A37, 2002.
17. O'Malley FP, Chia S, Tu D, et al: Prognostic and predictive value of topoisomerase II alpha in a randomized trial comparing CMF to CEF in premenopausal women with node positive breast cancer (NCIC CTG MA.5) [abstract 533]. Proc ASCO 24:11s, 2006.
18. Rouzier R, Rajan R, Wagner P, et al: Microtubule-associated protein tau: a marker of paclitaxel sensitivity in breast cancer. Proc Natl Acad Sci USA 102:8315–8320, 2005.
19. Chang JC, Wooten EC, Tsimelzon A, et al: Gene expression profiling for the prediction of therapeutic response to docetaxel in patients with breast cancer. Lancet 362:362–369, 2003.
20. Ambrosone CB, Barlow W, Yeh I-T, et al: Pharmacogenetics and breast cancer treatment outcomes: results on oxidative stress-related genotypes (MPO, MnSOD) from a Southwest Oncology Group Intergroup Trial (INT-0102) [abstract 37]. San Antonio Breast Cancer Symposium, 2006.
21. Sparano JA: TAILORx: trial assigning individualized options for treatment (Rx). Clin Breast Cancer 7:347–350, 2006.
22. Bogaerts J, Cardoso F, Buyse M, et al: Gene signature evaluation as a prognostic tool: challenges in the design of the MINDACT trial. Nat Clin Pract Oncol 10:540–551, 2006.
23. Garber JE, Richardson A, Harris LN, et al: Neo-adjuvant cisplatin (CDDP) in triple-negative breast cancer (BC) [abstract 3074]. San Antonio Breast Cancer Symposium, 2006.
24. Yap TA, Boss DS, Fong PC, et al: First in human phase I pharmacokinetic and pharmacodynamic study of KU-0059436, a small molecule inhibitor of poly ADP-ribose polymerase (PARP) in cancer patients, including BRCA 1/2 mutation carriers. Proc ASCO 25:145s (A-3529), 2007.

25. Doane AS, Danso M, Lal P, et al: An estrogen receptor-negative breast cancer subset characterized by a hormonally regulated transcriptional program and response to androgen. Oncogene 25:3994–4008, 2006.

26. Powles T, McCroskey E, Paterson A: Oral bisphosphonates as adjuvant therapy for operable breast cancer. Clin Cancer Res 12(20 Pt 2):6301s–6304s, 2006.

27. Powles TJ, Paterson A, McCloskey E, et al: Reduction in bone relapse and improved survival with oral clodronate for adjuvant treatment of operable breast cancer. Breast Cancer Res 8:R13, 2006.

28. Saarto T, Vehmanen L, Blomqvist C, Elomaa I: Ten-year follow-up of a randomized controlled trial of adjuvant clodronate treatment in node-positive breast cancer patients. Proc Am Soc Clin Oncol 23:8, 2004.

29. Diel IJ, Solomayer EF, Costa SD, et al: Reduction in new metastases in breast cancer with adjuvant clodronate treatment. N Engl J Med 339:357–363, 1998.

30. Jaschke A, Bastert G, Solomayer EF, et al: Adjuvant clodronate treatment improves the overall survival of primary breast cancer patients with micrometastases to the bone marrow-long term follow up [abstract 529]. Am Soc Clin Oncol 22:9s, 2004.

30a. Beatson GT: On the treatment of inoperable cases of carcinoma of the mammary: suggestions for a new method of treatment with illustrative cases. Lancet 2:104–107, 162–165, 1896.

31. Osborne CK, Yochmowitz MG, Knight WA, et al: The value of estrogen and progesterone receptors in the treatment of breast cancer. Cancer 46(12 Suppl):2884–2888, 1980.

32. Anderson WF, Chu KC, Chatterjee N, et al: Tumor variants by hormone receptor expression in white patients with node-negative breast cancer from the surveillance, epidemiology, and end results database. J Clin Oncol 19:18–27, 2001.

33. Goldhirsch A, Gelber RD: Endocrine therapies of breast cancer. Semin Oncol 23:494–505, 1996.

34. Dowsett M, Jones A, Johnston SR, et al: In vivo measurement of aromatase inhibition by letrozole (CGS 20267) in postmenopausal patients with breast cancer. Clin Cancer Res 1: 1511–1515, 1995.

35. Bines J, Oleske DM, Cobleigh MA: Ovarian function in premenopausal women treated with adjuvant chemotherapy for breast cancer. J Clin Oncol 14:1718–1729, 1996.

36. Oktay K, Buyuk E, Libertella N, et al: Fertility preservation in breast cancer patients: a prospective controlled comparison of ovarian stimulation with tamoxifen and letrozole for embryo cryopreservation. J Clin Oncol 23:4347–4353, 2005.

37. Smith I, Dowsett M, Yap TS, et al: Adjuvant aromatase inhibitors for early breast cancer after chemotherapy-induced amenorrhea: caution and suggested guidelines. J Clin Oncol 24:2444–2447, 2006.

38. EBCTCG: Effects of chemotherapy and hormonal therapy for early breast cancer on recurrence and 15-year survival: an overview of the randomised trials. Lancet 365:1687–1717, 2005.

39. Tamoxifen for early breast cancer: an overview of the randomised trials. Early Breast Cancer Trialists' Collaborative Group. Lancet 351:1451–1467, 1998.

40. Fisher B, Bryant J, Dignam JJ, et al: Tamoxifen, radiation therapy, or both for prevention of ipsilateral breast tumor recurrence after lumpectomy in women with invasive breast cancers of one centimeter or less. J Clin Oncol 20:4141–4149, 2002.

41. Stewart H, Prescott R, Forrest A: Scottish adjuvant tamoxifen trial: a randomized study updated to 15 years. J Natl Cancer Inst 93:456–462, 2001.

42. Swedish Breast Cancer Cooperative Group: Randomized trial of two versus five years of adjuvant tamoxifen for postmenopausal early stage breast cancer. J Natl Cancer Inst 88:1543–1549, 1996.

43. Fisher B, Bryant J, Dignam JJ, et al: Five versus more than five years of tamoxifen for lymph node-negative breast cancer: updated findings from the National Surgical Adjuvant Breast and Bowel Project B-14 randomized trial. J Natl Cancer Inst 93: 684–690, 2001.

44. Stewart HJ, Forrest A, Everington D, et al: Randomised comparison of 5 years of adjuvant tamoxifen with continuous therapy for operable breast cancer. The Scottish Cancer Trials Breast Group. Br J Cancer 74:297–299, 1996.

45. Cuzick J, Ambroisine L, Davidson N, et al: Use of luteinising-hormone-releasing hormone agonists as adjuvant treatment in premenopausal patients with hormone-receptor-positive breast cancer: a meta-analysis of individual patient data from randomised adjuvant trials. Lancet 369:1711–1723, 2007.

46. Howell A, Cuzick J, Baum M, et al: Results of the ATAC (Arimidex, Tamoxifen, alone or in combination) trial after completion of 5 years' adjuvant treatment for breast cancer. Lancet 365:60–62, 2005.

47. Thurlimann B, Keshaviah A, Coates AS, et al: A comparison of letrozole and tamoxifen in postmenopausal women with early breast cancer. N Engl J Med 353:2747–2757, 2005.

48. Coombes RC, Hall E, Gibson LJ et al: A randomized trial of exemestane after two to three years of tamoxifen therapy in postmenopausal women with primary breast cancer. N Engl J Med 350:1081–1092, 2004

49. Boccardo F, Rubagotti A, Puntoni M, et al: Switching to anastrozole versus continued tamoxifen treatment of early breast cancer: preliminary results of the Italian Tamoxifen Anastrozole Trial. J Clin Oncol 23:5138–5147, 2005.

50. Jakesz R, Jonat W, Gnant M, et al: Switching of postmenopausal women with endocrine-responsive early breast cancer to anastrozole after 2 years' adjuvant tamoxifen: combined results of ABCSG trial 8 and ARNO 95 trial. Lancet 366:455–462, 2005.

51. Goss PE, Ingle JN, Martino S, et al: Randomized trial of letrozole following tamoxifen as extended adjuvant therapy in receptor-positive breast cancer: updated findings from NCIC CTG MA.17. J Natl Cancer Inst 97:1262–1271, 2005.

52. Milano A, Dal Lago L, Sotiriou C, et al: What clinicians need to know about antioestrogen resistance in breast cancer therapy. Eur J Cancer 42:2692–2705, 2006.

53. Massarweh S, Schiff R: Unraveling the mechanisms of endocrine resistance in breast cancer: new therapeutic opportunities. Clin Cancer Res 13:1950–1954, 2007.

54. Benz CC, Scott GK, Sarup JC, et al: Estrogen-dependent, tamoxifen-resistant tumorigenic growth of MCF-7 cells transfected with HER2/neu. Breast Cancer Res Treat 24:85–95, 1992.

55. Borg A, Baldetorp B, Ferno M, et al: ERBB2 amplification is associated with tamoxifen resistance in steroid-receptor positive breast cancer. Cancer Lett 81:137–144, 1994.

56. Romond EH, Perez EA, Bryant J, et al: Trastuzumab plus adjuvant chemotherapy for operable HER2-positive breast cancer. N Engl J Med 353:1673–1684, 2005.

57. Perez EA, Suman VJ, Davidson NE, et al: www.roche.com.br/NR/rdonlyres/D0C0F72A-595E-4CFC-A915-46BBB183106E/1032/ASCO_Presentation__N9832.pdf. Accessed June 24, 2007.

58. Piccart-Gebhart M, Proctre M, Leyland-Jones B, et al: Trastuzumab after adjuvant chemotherapy in HER2-positive breast cancer. N Engl J Med 353, 1659–1672, 2005.

59. Smith I, Procter M, Gelber RD, et al: 2-year follow-up of trastuzumab after adjuvant chemotherapy in HER2-positive breast cancer: a randomised controlled trial. Lancet 369:29–36, 2007.

60. Slamon D, Eiermann W, Robert N, et al: Phase III Trial Comparing AC-T with AC-TH and with TCBH in the Adjuvant Treatment of HER2 positive Early Breast Cancer Patients: Second Interim Efficacy Analysis. Data presented at the 29th Annual San Antonio Breast Cancer Symposium, San Antonio, TX, December 14, 2006. www.bcirg.org. Accessed May 1, 2007.

61. Joensuu H, Kellokumpu-Lehtinen PL, Bono P, et al: Adjuvant docetaxel or vinorelbine with or without trastuzumab for breast cancer. N Engl J Med 354:809–820, 2006.

62. Kurian AW, Thompson RN, Gaw AF, et al: A cost-effectiveness analysis of adjuvant trastuzumab regimens in early HER2/neu-positive breast cancer. J Clin Oncol 25:634–641, 2007.

63. Liberato NL, Marchetti M, Barosi G: Cost effectiveness of adjuvant trastuzumab in human epidermal growth factor receptor 2-positive breast cancer. J Clin Oncol 25:625–633, 2007.

64. Geyer CE, Forster J, Lindquist D, et al: Lapatinib plus capecitabine for HER2-positive advanced breast cancer. N Engl J Med 355:2733–2743, 2006. Erratum in: N Engl J Med 356:1487, 2007.

Surveillance and Detection of Recurrence of Breast Cancer

20

Peter Kabos and Virginia F. Borges

KEY POINTS

- Surveillance of breast cancer survivors forms an integral part of their care, and its importance is growing with the increasing number of breast cancer survivors.
- Current standard of care for surveillance in patients with treated breast cancer constitutes scheduled history, physical examination, yearly mammograms, and breast self-exams.
- There is no good evidence supporting routine systemic imaging or laboratory testing (including tumor marker levels) in breast cancer survivors.
- Any additional workup should be symptom-directed.
- Breast cancer survivors should follow a care plan that includes the patient's surgeon, radiation and medical oncologists, as well as the primary care provider.

Introduction

The diagnosis and treatment of early stage breast cancer have improved dramatically over the last two decades, resulting in declining breast cancer mortality[1] (Fig. 20-1). Currently, there are over 2 million breast cancer survivors in the United States, accounting for 23% of all cancer survivors, which increases the importance of continued care and surveillance. Here we discuss the current recommendations and evidence for post-treatment surveillance in breast cancer survivors.

Although surveillance during the first 5 years after cancer diagnosis and treatment in solid tumors is considered crucial because it is the time with the highest risk for recurrent disease, this timeline does not fit well in breast oncology. Depending on the biologic characteristics of the primary tumor, the peak incidence of recurrence varies, and in all settings late recurrences can occur. There is a clear difference in the relapse pattern between estrogen receptor (ER)-

positive and ER-negative disease. In ER-negative cancer, the relapse pattern more closely follows the pattern of other solid tumors, with peak annual incidence of recurrence between 18 and 24 months. On the other hand, the Early Breast Cancer Trialists' Collaborative Group meta-analysis of hormone receptor-positive breast cancer treated with tamoxifen demonstrated a delay in recurrences, with rates three times higher at 15 years post-treatment when compared with 5 years[2] (Fig. 20-2).

Overall, the main goal of surveillance in breast oncology is early recognition of curable disease, presented as either local recurrence or a second primary breast cancer. Screening during physician follow-up should also focus on the early recognition of treatment-related complications, such as neuropathy, cardiac or hematologic adverse effects, and symptoms that could herald metastatic dissemination.

The Evidence Behind Current Surveillance Guidelines in Breast Cancer

Comprehensive guidelines for post-treatment surveillance in breast cancer have been published and updated in 2006 by the American Society of Clinical Oncology (ASCO).[3,4] Several other groups have published evidence-based recommendations, which are largely similar to the ASCO guidelines. Characteristic of all the recommendations is a paucity of prospective randomized data supporting a given surveillance protocol. However, a minimum follow-up requirement comparable to other solid organ tumors has been established. Scheduled history, physical examination, yearly mammograms, and breast self-examinations form the basis of sur-

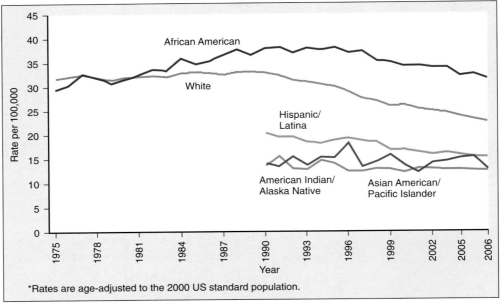

Figure 20-1. Trends in female breast cancer death rates* by race and ethnicity, United States, 1975–2006.
(From American Cancer Society, *Breast Cancer Facts and Figures* 2009–2010, Figure 4b, p. 6. Atlanta: American Cancer Society, Inc. Data source: National Center for Health Statistics, Centers for Disease Control and Prevention, 2009. For Hispanics, information is included for all states except Connecticut, Louisiana, Maine, Maryland, Minnesota, New Hampshire, New York, North Dakota, Oklahoma, Vermont, and Virginia and the District of Columbia.)

veillance in breast cancer and are considered the standard of care in the United States. The best interval for these measures was decided empirically (Table 20-1).

Despite recommended guidelines, actual surveillance practices differ considerably among practitioners as documented by a recent study by Keating and colleagues.[5] In this study, 50% of breast cancer survivors saw a medical oncologist in the first year, but only 27% of patients saw an oncologist yearly for the first 3 years. The patients who were seen by an oncologist were more likely to have tumor markers checked and computed tomography (CT) scans and chest x-rays performed compared with patients seen by primary care practitioners. The rate of testing has declined with time in all patients in this study. However, adherence of clinicians to the proposed surveillance guidelines has also been shown to lead to significant savings in health care costs and should be encouraged[6] (Box 20-1).

Detecting Locoregional Recurrences

In-breast tumor recurrences after breast-conserving surgery and radiation therapy occur

at a rate of 1% to 2% per year. Postoperative scarring makes it difficult to interpret mammograms at the lumpectomy site. Further compounding the problem is local scarring, which often continues for years after surgery. With mammography, 25% to 45% of ipsilateral recurrences can be detected. The sensitivity of mammograms increases in the presence of microcalcifications.[7] In the case of a palpable suspicious local lesion, a needle biopsy may offer

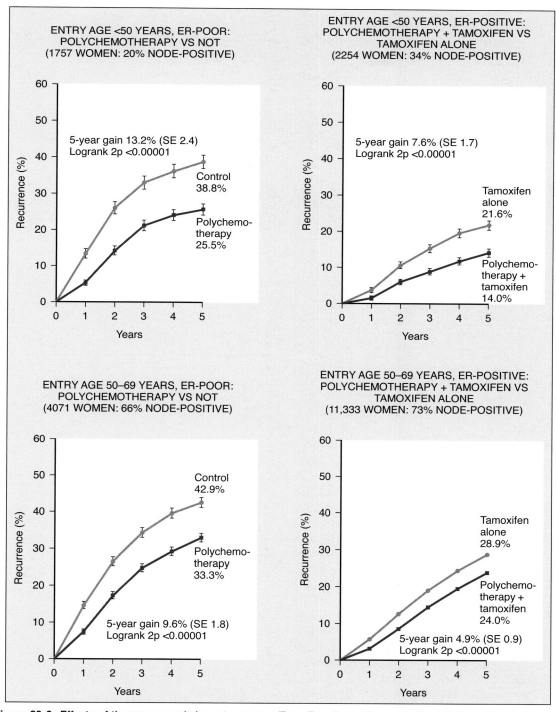

Figure 20-2. Effects of therapy on early breast cancer. (From Early Breast Cancer Trialists' Collaborative group: Effects of chemotherapy and hormonal therapy for early breast cancer on recurrence and 15-year survival: an overview of the randomised trials. Lancet 365(9472):1687, 2005.)

Table 20-1. ASCO Guidelines for Post-treatment Surveillance

Follow-Up Care Test	Recommendation
Medical history and physical examination	Visit your doctor every 3–6 months for the first 3 years after the first treatment, every 6–12 months for years 4 and 5, and every year thereafter.
Post-treatment mammography	Schedule a mammogram 1 year after first mammogram that led to diagnosis, but no less than 6 months after radiation therapy. Obtain a mammogram every 6–12 months thereafter.
Breast self-examination	Perform a breast self-examination every month. This procedure is not a substitute for a mammogram.
Pelvic examination	Continue to visit a gynecologist regularly. Women taking tamoxifen should report any vaginal bleeding to their doctor.
Coordination of care	About 1 year after diagnosis, continue to visit your oncologist or transfer care to primary care doctor. Women receiving hormone therapy should talk with their oncologist about how often to schedule follow-up visits for reevaluation of their treatment.
Genetic counseling referral	Tell your doctor if there is a history of cancer in your family. The following risk factors may indicate that breast cancer could run in the family: • Ashkenazi Jewish heritage • Personal or family history of ovarian cancer • Any first-degree relative (mother, sister, daughter) diagnosed with breast cancer before age 50 • Two or more first-degree or second-degree relatives (grandparent, aunt, uncle) diagnosed with breast cancer • Personal or family history of breast cancer in both breasts • History of breast cancer in a male relative

From http://www.cancer.net/patient/ASCO+Resources/Patient+Guides/ASCO+Patient+Guide%3A+Follow-Up+Care+for+Breast+Cancer

the most cost-effective method of diagnosing a breast cancer recurrence, thus preventing extensive imaging workup, which in the end may be inconclusive. Ultrasound evaluation of any palpable mass is considered routine as well, similar to its role in primary breast cancer detection.

One of the important questions in surveillance for locoregional disease is who is the one who detects the recurrence—the patient or the physician. A recent meta-analysis of 12 studies involving 5045 patients showed that 40% of patients with locoregional recurrences were diagnosed during routine clinic visits or routine testing, whereas the remaining 60% of patients developed symptomatic recurrences before their scheduled visits with clinicians.[8] Therefore, a monthly breast self-examination is part of the ASCO recommendations, although it has not been prospectively evaluated in breast cancer survivors (Fig. 20-3). In previously unaffected women, many randomized trials and a meta-analysis[9] showed no benefit in mortality for breast self-exams. The largest of these evaluated more than 250,000 Chinese women who were not routinely screened with yearly mammo-

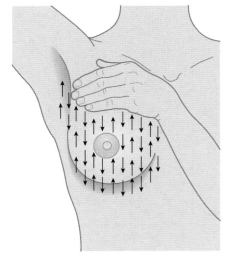

Figure 20-3. Breast self-examination. Breast self-examination is important for early detection of a local recurrence after breast cancer treatment. The recommended method is to examine up to the collarbone, out to the armpit, in to the middle of the chest, and down to the rib cage. (From American Cancer Society, *How to Perform a Breast Self Examination.* http://www.cancer.org/docroot/CRI/content/CRI_2_6x_How_to_perform_a_breast_self_exam_5.asp?sitearea=.)

grams. In this population, a breast self-exam did not offer a survival benefit.[10] Meta-analysis of published data on breast self-exams in patients without a personal history of breast cancer did not show an improvement in overall survival or an improvement in quality of life. Moreover, the specificity and sensitivity of clinician breast exams in the post-treatment period are also not known.

Currently, insufficient evidence exists to support additional radiologic studies for locoregional surveillance of the asymptomatic breast beyond the recommended clinician exams, self-exams, and annual mammograms. The role of magnetic resonance imaging (MRI) in surveillance of the asymptomatic treated breast has not been determined, although MRI has demonstrated enhanced breast cancer detection in unaffected women whose lifetime risk is 20% or greater.[11] These data suggest that affected women with this same risk profile may benefit from an MRI in addition to mammogram for secondary surveillance. In the setting of suspected locoregional recurrence, additional radiologic studies can be considered with some evidence for them. [18]Fluorodeoxyglucose-positron emission tomography (FDG-PET) has been compared primarily with MRI in the evaluation of locoregional recurrences, including lymph node metastases. In a small case series by Hathaway and coworkers,[12] nine patients with regional recurrence were evaluated. MRI detected recurrent disease in five cases and was indeterminate in four. PET scan identified all nine patients. In a larger study of 32 patients, MRI had a sensitivity of 79% and specificity of 94% compared with 100% and 72% for PET scan, respectively.[13]

Early detection of local recurrence of breast cancer is anticipated to enhance the survival of the patient by reducing dissemination and progression to metastatic disease. The site of locoregional recurrence influences survival as well. The 5-year overall survival rate with a locoregional recurrence confined to the breast parenchyma or skin of the ipsilateral breast was 60% compared with 24% for recurrence involving regional nodes or recurrence in the non-breast skin of the ipsilateral chest wall.[14] Therefore, even without clear evidence-based efficacy measures to detect locoregional disease, breast self-examination, clinician examination, and mammographic screening have been adopted into post-treatment surveillance guidelines.

Detecting Asymptomatic Systemic Metastases

For continued surveillance of cancer survivors, one has to take into account the pattern of recurrence. In breast cancer, bone, subcutaneous tissue, lung, liver, and brain are most commonly targeted. A thorough review of systems during surveillance visits should include these organ systems in detail to rule out concerning symptoms. In the truly asymptomatic setting, the increase in diagnostic modalities available to clinicians makes it increasingly important to address the extent and intensity of radiologic and laboratory surveillance that would benefit the patient, without causing unnecessary testing or anxiety. In a prospective randomized trial of the GIVIO (Interdisciplinary Group for Cancer Care Evaluation [Italy]) investigators in Italy, over 1300 patients were assigned either to intensive follow-up that included bone scans, liver ultrasounds, chest x-rays, and laboratory studies at predefined intervals or to history, physical examinations, and yearly mammograms performed with the same frequency.[15] At a median follow-up of 71 months, the investigators found no difference in the overall survival rate or in the quality of life between the two groups. In a similar study, Roselli Del Turco and colleagues[16] compared standard follow-up with the addition of chest x-ray and bone scan every 6 months for 5 years. A difference in detection of bone and thoracic metastases was seen between the two groups as would be expected, but again no difference in overall mortality was seen. In both studies, authors did not recommend intensive follow-up in breast cancer surveillance. Ten-year update of the GIVIO group's study confirmed the lack of survival advantage with intensive follow-up protocol.[17]

Historically, minimal emphasis has been placed on the early detection of asymptomatic metastatic recurrence owing to the lack of curative options for this setting. However, with increasingly improved therapeutic options, including biologic agents whose potency may be impacted by overall disease burden, it remains a research imperative to investigate whether oligometastatic disease can be identified by a more intensive screening protocol with resultant improved survival outcomes. This could be seen as a theoretical B0 state similar to prostate cancer (disease detected by elevation of prostate-specific antigen only according to the Whitmore-

Box 20-2. ASCO Patient Guide: Follow-up Care for Breast Cancer

The following tests are currently *not* recommended by ASCO for regular follow-up care because they have not been shown to lengthen the life of a person with breast cancer:

Compete blood count (CBC) test and liver and kidney function tests

Chest x-ray

Bone scan

Liver ultrasound

Computed tomography (CT) scan

[18]Fluorodeoxyglucose-positron-emission tomography (FDG-PET) scan

Breast magnetic resonance imaging (MRI)

Breast cancer tumor markers, such as CA15-3, CA27.29, and carcinoembryonic antigen (CEA)

From http://www.cancer.net/patient/ASCO+Resources/Patient+Guides/ASCO+Patient+Guide%3A+Follow-Up+Care+for+Breast+Cancer

Jewett staging system), equivalent to success with early intervention in advanced prostate cancer. Given the lack of current evidence, however, intensive radiologic screening cannot be justified or recommended (Box 20-2).

Symptom-Directed Workup

Once the suspicion of recurrent disease is raised, based on either physical examination or symptoms, multiple modalities are available to the clinician for further investigation (Table 20-2). Usually, the initial workup includes routine laboratory evaluation including tumor markers. Imaging should be symptom-guided and can include x-ray, ultrasound, CT or PET/CT, and MRI. Selection of the sequence of studies is largely clinician-dependent and with limited evidence for guidance. In all cases symptoms indicating possible recurrence are of particular concern to patients and their clinicians, and timely evaluation with appropriate diagnostic studies is essential.

Newer modalities such as FDG-PET scan and MRI offer some advantages in the workup of recurrent breast cancer, and we discuss their integration into the current clinical algorithm. FDG-PET has been assessed in the settings of evaluation of primary lesions, staging, treatment follow-up, and surveillance in breast cancer in an effort to find the optimal use for this powerful diagnostic modality. After initial studies, it is clear that FDG-PET has a low sensitivity and only moderate specificity in the initial staging of breast cancer. Moreover, the ability of this modality to detect breast cancer is dependent on the biologic subtype of the breast cancer—most accurate with high-grade tumors but less so with nonproliferative/low-grade lesions. In fact, in the initial workup of breast cancer, FDG-PET scan has been shown to have a lower sensitivity than MRI for evaluation of the primary lesion.[18] When screening for recurrent disease, however, it offers many advantages. First, FDG-PET allows whole body imaging in one test and, when combined with a CT scan, specificity is considerably improved, since it allows for better anatomic correlation. The reported average sensitivity in the setting of recurrent disease is 96%; specificity is 77%.[19] Second, FDG-PET adds the dimension of metabolic evaluation. Changes at the functional level precede anatomic changes in size and tissue density. On the down side, FDG-PET can introduce additional error based on glucose uptake or inflammation. FDG-PET scan is clearly superior to other modalities in detecting lymph node involvement in the axilla and internal mammary lymph nodes.[13]

One of the well-recognized drawbacks of FDG-PET is its low individual lesion-based

Table 20-2. Signs and Symptoms That Might Herald a Breast Cancer Recurrence

Symptom/Clinical Finding	Appropriate Diagnostic Studies
Breast lump	Mammogram, ultrasound
Bone pain	Bone scan
Chest pain	Chest x-ray, chest CT, bone scan
Abdominal pain	Liver function tests, ultrasound, abdominal CT
Shortness of breath or persistent cough	Chest x-ray, chest CT
Persistent headaches	Brain MRI
Rash on skin of breast	Mammogram, skin biopsy
Nipple discharge	Mammogram, ultrasound, ductogram

specificity, as opposed to overall specificity for presence versus absence of disease. This stems primarily from the inaccuracy in visualizing sclerotic and mixed osteoblastic/osteolytic bone lesions. In a study by Moon and associates,[20] 57 patients with suspicion of recurrent disease were retrospectively analyzed. The patient-based sensitivity of FDG-PET scan was 93%, similar to the results of other studies, whereas the lesion-based sensitivity was only 85%. Low sensitivity for detection of bone metastases has not been reported in all published studies; for example in a study of 75 patients by Bender and associates,[21] bone metastases were detected in all 15 patients.

Combining screening modalities can further increase the sensitivity and positive predictive value of FDG-PET scans. Suarez and colleagues[22] evaluated FDG-PET in patients with increased tumor markers and no other evidence of recurrent disease. The sensitivity in this study of 45 patients was 92%, and the positive predictive value 89%. As the availability and cost-effectiveness of new imaging modalities improve, whole body imaging may find a more widespread use in clinical practice. In a recent study by Schmidt and colleagues,[23] whole body MRI was compared with FDG-PET in 33 breast cancer patients and those with suspicion of recurrent disease (Fig. 20-4). As with prior studies evaluating these imaging techniques, FDG-PET scan was found to be more accurate in detecting lymph node metastases, whereas MRI was found to be more sensitive in detecting distant meta-

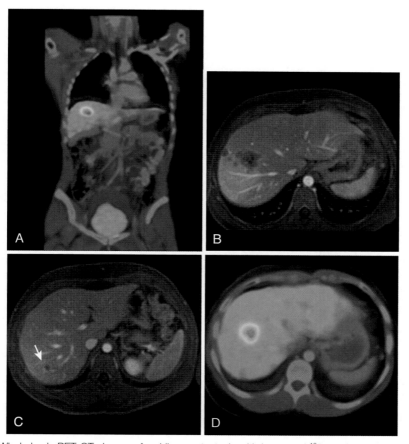

Figure 20-4. A, Whole body PET-CT shows a focal liver metastasis with increased [18]fluorodeoxyglucose (FDG) uptake. **B,** 3D-VIBE (volumetric interpolated breath-hold sequence)-MRI (1.5 T) of the liver in portal venous phase confirms a large liver metastasis and shows additional multiple small satellite lesions. **C,** Another focal liver metastasis (8 mm) is found in a different liver segment (*arrow*). **D,** Only the large metastasis shows FDG uptake in PET-CT (positron-emission tomography-computed tomography); the small satellite lesions are masked by physiologic background uptake of the liver. (From Schmidt GP, Baur-Melnyk A, Haug A: Comprehensive imaging of tumor recurrence in breast cancer patients using whole-body MRI at 1.5 and 3 T compared to FDG-PET-CT. Eur J Radiol 65:47, 2008.)

static disease. The overall sensitivity of whole body MRI in this study was 93%; its specificity was 86%.

Long-Term Complications of Adjuvant Chemotherapy for Breast Cancer

Adjuvant chemotherapy prolongs disease-free and overall survival in appropriately selected patients with breast cancer. However, as with any other treatment, chemotherapy poses both short-term and long-term risks to the patient. Short-term toxicities are usually easily recognizable and manageable. The long-term sequelae are much less prevalent, but when they occur the impact on a patient's quality of life and survival is significant. Cardiac toxicity, myelotoxicity, and cognitive dysfunction following chemotherapy are the most important long-term complications; these will be discussed in greater detail.

Cardiac Toxicity

The common use of anthracyclines and more recently trastuzumab in adjuvant therapy has brought cardiac toxicity to the forefront of our attention and monitoring. Anthracyclines are believed to cause immediate myocardial damage with the generation of free radicals, which can lead to acute toxicity such as arrhythmias, myocarditis, pericarditis, or decreased left ventricular function (LVEF).[24] In most cases, however, it may take months or even years for the damage to become clinically apparent. The risk of cardiotoxicity with an anthracycline-containing regimen is dose dependent and estimated to develop in up to 1% of patients receiving standard cumulative doses of 240–300 mg/m^2 of adriamycin.[25] Equimolar doses of epirubicin are considered less cardiotoxic than adriamycin.[26] Risk factors predisposing patients to heart failure secondary to the use of anthracyclines are the presence of pre-existing cardiac conditions, high cumulative doses of the drug (above 400 mg/m^2 of adriamycin), and chest wall radiation in the pre-CAT scan simulation era.[27] Because of the low prevalence of heart failure and other cardiotoxicities with anthracyclines, routine quantitative monitoring of cardiac function during therapy is not warranted. Screening for signs and symptoms of cardiac dysfunction should, however, be a part of the routine history and physical exam performed during each follow-up visit.

In contrast to anthracyclines, the use of trastuzumab alone and especially in combination with anthracyclines mandates routine quantitative monitoring of heart function. The reported incidence of severe congestive heart failure in adjuvant trials using trastuzumab was as high as 4.1%.[28] An even larger portion of patients treated adjuvantly with trastuzumab experienced asymptomatic decrease in their LVEF (up to 17%). ErbB2, the target of trastuzumab, is expressed on adult cardiomyocytes and is thought to play a role in the cardiac response to stress. Inhibition of downstream signaling of ErbB2 is thought to form the basis of the cardiac toxicity of trastuzumab.[29] Patients receiving trastuzumab should be monitored for changes in their LVEF using the same guidelines that were used in the North American randomized adjuvant trastuzumab studies, NSABP B-31 and Intergroup 9831, if an anthracycline regimen is used, or as per the BCIRG 006 study if the docetaxel, carboplatin, and trastuzumab regimen is chosen. In general, assessing baseline LVEF, reassessing after the anthracycline component if included, and reassessing again at the end of the chemotherapy component before single agent trastuzumab is continued for the full 12 months' duration is considered the minimum monitoring for standard of care. Any significant decline in LVEF requires additional testing and longer follow-up. Signs and symptoms of reduced cardiac function should prompt immediate reevaluation outside of this framework. The choice of modality for LVEF monitoring (radionucleotide ventriculography, echocardiogram) is largely based on physician preference and availability of a given test. It is, however, recommended that the same modality for LVEF monitoring be continued throughout treatment to allow for accurate comparison. A 15% decrease in absolute LVEF or LVEF that falls below the lower limit of normal for an institution should lead to withholding of the drug until recovery of LVEF is documented. Beta blockers and angiotensin-converting enzyme inhibitors form the basis for treatment of symptomatic heart failure.

Bone Marrow Toxicity

Both myelodysplasia and secondary leukemias are well-recognized side effects of adjuvant chemotherapy. Development of late myelotoxicity is largely dependent on the type of drug administered, cumulative dose, and treatment duration.[25] Two distinct leukemic syndromes have been described. The first is a leukemic transformation that is usually preceded by myelodysplasia. This is most commonly associated with alkylating agents such as cyclophosphamide. The time frame prior to onset of this syndrome is usually 5 to 7 years following completion of treatment. It is often associated with abnormalities in chromosomes 5 and 7.[30,31]

The second syndrome involves the onset of secondary leukemias, which develop more rapidly with a median time to onset of 24 to 36 months from treatment.[32] These present more commonly following the use of topoisomerase II inhibitors including anthracyclines. These leukemias are characterized by balanced translocations in the *MLL* gene found on chromosome 11. There may also be a small increase in the risk of developing secondary leukemia with the supportive use of G-CSF. This is based on retrospective observations from adjuvant breast cancer trials,[30] with varying degrees of risk reported in the literature depending on the age at which patients are included in the review. The overall risk of developing secondary long-term marrow toxicity with current standard adjuvant regimens ranges from 0.5% to 1.5% in the current literature,[30,33] with prospective data lacking. In general, chemotherapy-induced secondary myelodysplasia and leukemias do not respond well to treatment, and the prognosis for these patients is poor. No specific monitoring after adjuvant chemotherapy is recommended other than the usual routine blood work, for which no supportive data are offered in the literature. However, any evidence of cytopenias in a breast cancer survivor merits investigation to rule out a secondary malignancy.

Cognitive Dysfunction

Patients undergoing treatment for breast cancer report problems with cognition. The neurocognitive effects are most significant in patients who receive chemotherapy, though they have also been documented immediately after diagnosis and before any cancer-directed interventions have occurred. The most common symptoms include difficulty focusing and maintaining concentration, loss of short-term memory, and a generalized "fogginess." Initial surveys of neurocognitive function demonstrated the presence of cognitive impairment in up to 40% of patients.[34,35] Longitudinal studies that followed patients over a 1- to 2-year period have shown a gradual improvement, with an eventual return of cognition to baseline.[36]

The early studies of cognition in breast cancer patients have been criticized for a multitude of methodologic flaws. Many of the studies included only a small number of patients. Often no baseline evaluation prior to initiation of chemotherapy was included. Most importantly, the trials did not control for other factors, such as chemotherapy-induced menopause or preexisting medical and psychological conditions as well as antihormonal therapies, making the interpretation of these results difficult. Newer studies have addressed these shortcomings and have found a higher degree of cognitive impairment. These newer studies also confirmed the gradual resolution of symptoms over time, though some residual sequelae are common.[37]

Currently, it is well recognized that patients undergoing treatment for newly diagnosed breast cancer can develop a degree of cognitive impairment that is most likely multifactorial.[38] The etiology of this impairment, the comorbities or confounders that may influence its development, and, most importantly, interventions to prevent or treat it are the subjects of ongoing research. The results of these studies are eagerly awaited to provide better guidance for treating clinicians and their patients who require chemotherapy as part of their risk reduction against metastatic recurrence. At present, one guideline (the Canadian Clinical Practice Guidelines) recommends periodic cognitive testing in breast cancer survivors.[39] However, except in a clinical trial, this recommendation cannot practically be incorporated into routine practice in a validated manner.

Coordinating Medical Care

It is important to develop a care plan for cancer survivors. Patients with ER-positive breast cancer continue with adjuvant hormonal therapy and are routinely followed by their medical oncologists. It is prudent, however, to divide the follow-up among the medical oncologist and radiation oncologist, the surgeon, and the primary care physician. This approach is supported by a large Canadian trial that compared primary care with specialist follow-up in women with treated early-stage breast cancer.[40] The trial included 968 patients with early-stage breast cancer between 9 and 15 months after diagnosis who were randomized to follow-up by a specialist or by a family practitioner. There was no difference in recurrence-related serious clinical events between the two groups.

In patients with early breast cancer and a high probability of cure, the non–breast cancer-related health maintenance is equally important in continued cancer surveillance. Earle and colleagues[41] investigated health maintenance in breast cancer survivors and matched controls. In their large population study, the investigators show that breast cancer survivors are more likely to receive influenza vaccinations, lipid testing, cervical and colon cancer screening, and bone densitometry compared with age-matched controls.

The long-term adverse effects of therapy are becoming a greater health concern as more patients successfully complete therapy and are living longer (Box 20-3). The use of radiation therapy and cardiotoxic chemotherapeutic agents increases the importance of general internal medicine follow-up in breast cancer survivors. Many studies have shown an increase in the risk of cardiovascular complications in patients with breast cancer. For example, Hooning and colleagues[42] examined long-term cardiovascular risk in 10-year breast cancer survivors. They followed over 4000 breast cancer survivors (median follow-up 18 years) and showed an increased risk in myocardial infarctions and heart failure as well as valvular disease in patients receiving adjuvant therapy. Patients who received adjuvant chemotherapy in addition to radiation therapy had a further increase in cardiovascular risk. With the recent incorporation of trastuzumab into the adjuvant setting for the 25% of breast cancer patients with the *HER2/neu* gene amplification, the long-term cardiac risks and ideal follow-up remain unknown, and understanding of these risks and uncertainties as part of the survivorship care plan is crucial. Finally, yearly pelvic examinations are a part of the routine health maintenance for women and should be especially emphasized in patients receiving tamoxifen, which increases the incidence of uterine cancer in women over 50 at drug initiation.

The ASCO guidelines propose the option of completely transferring care to the primary care physician in patients with early-stage breast cancer after 1 year.[4] Personal preferences of the patient as well as of the physician have to be taken into account in the decision-making process. One also has to keep in mind the evolving standard of care in breast cancer. For example, the duration of hormonal therapy after the diagnosis of ER-positive breast cancer is still being investigated, as is the role of bisphosphonates in the prevention of bone metastasis as well as bone health maintenance in the setting of antiendocrine therapy. Recent advances in the field have also included lifestyle modifications, with emphasis on the importance of preventing and reducing weight gain in the treatment and post-treatment period and on the role of a low-fat diet and regular exercise in preventing recurrence.[43] Periodic connection with a member of the oncologic treatment team should help ensure timely communication of these advances.

Conclusions

From the available evidence, it is clear that no significant survival benefit or improvement in quality of life is associated with a more intensive surveillance routine following the diagnosis and treatment of breast cancer when compared with the currently recommended schedule. History, physical examination, breast self-examination, and yearly mammograms are presently considered the standard of care for post-treatment surveillance in patients with breast cancer in the United States. The major goals of surveillance are early detection of local recurrence, detection of a second primary breast cancer, as well as the detection of treatment-related complications

---

Box 20-3. Post-treatment Health Maintenance Screening and Intervention for Conditions Possibly Related to Breast Cancer Therapy

Cardiovascular health
Bone density
Cervical/endometrial cancer screening
Exercise
Weight loss
Sexual dysfunction
Fatigue
Cognitive dysfunction

and identification of metastatic disease before serious complications occur. Symptom-based and individually tailored evaluation remains very important in the follow-up of breast cancer survivors when there is an increased suspicion of recurrence on the basis of the initial screening. The sequence of studies used for detection of recurrent disease is largely clinician-dependent. Increasing evidence supports the integration of newer modalities such as MRI and PET/CT into the workup algorithm. Additional research is needed to determine whether alternative surveillance measures will improve the ability to detect and intervene in a clinically meaningful way for metastatic disease.

References

1. American Cancer Society 2007–2008 http://www.cancer.org/docroot/STT/content/STT_1x_Breast_Cancer_Facts_Figures_2007-2008.asp
2. Early Breast Cancer Trialists' Collaborative group: Effects of chemotherapy and hormonal therapy for early breast cancer on recurrence and 15-year survival: an overview of the randomised trials. Lancet 365(9472):1687–1717, 2005.
3. Khatcheressian JL, Wolff AC, Smith TJ, et al: American Society of Clinical Oncology 2006 update of the breast cancer follow-up and management guidelines in the adjuvant setting. J Clin Onc 24(31):5091–5097, 2006.
4. ASCO Patient Guide: follow-up care for breast cancer. http://www.cancer.net/patient/ASCO+Resources/Patient+Guides/ASCO+Patient+Guide%3A+Follow-Up+Care+for+Breast+Cancer
5. Keating NL, Landrum MB, Guadagnoli E, et al: Surveillance testing among survivors of early-stage breast cancer. J Clin Oncol 25:1074–1081, 2007.
6. Mille D, Roy T, Carrere MO, et al: Economic impact of harmonizing medical practices: compliance with clinical practice guidelines in the follow-up of breast cancer in a French Comprehensive Cancer Center. J Clin Oncol 18(8):1718–1724, 2000.
7. Bartella L, Smith CS, Dershaw DD, Liberman L: Imaging breast cancer. Radiol Clin N Am 45:45–67, 2007.
8. de Bock GH, Bonnema J, van Der Hage J, et al: Effectiveness of routine visits and routine tests in detecting isolated locoregional recurrences after treatment for early-stage invasive breast cancer. A meta-analysis and systematic review. J Clin Oncol 22:4010–4018, 2004.
9. Hackshaw AK, Paul EA: Breast self-examination and death from breast cancer: a meta-analysis. Br J Cancer 88(7):1047–1053, 2003.
10. Thomas DB, Gao DL, Ray RM, et al: Randomized trial of breast self-examination in Shanghai: final results. J Natl Cancer Inst 94(19):1445–1457, 2002.
11. Saslow D, Boetes C, Burke W, et al: American Cancer Society guidelines for breast screening with MRI as an adjunct to mammography. CA Cancer J Clin 57(2):75–89, 2007.
12. Hathaway PB, Mankoff DA, Maravilla KR, et al: Value of combined FDG PET and MR imaging in the evaluation of suspected recurrent local-regional breast cancer: preliminary experience. Radiology 210:807–814, 1999.
13. Goerres GW, Michel SC, Fehr MK, et al: Follow-up of women with breast cancer: comparison between MRI and FDG PET. Eur Radiol 13:1635–1644, 2003.
14. Wapnir IL, Anderson SJ, Mamounas EP, et al: Prognosis after ipsilateral breast tumor recurrence and locoregional recurrences in five National Surgical Adjuvant Breast and Bowel Project node-positive adjuvant breast cancer trials. J Clin Oncol 24:2028–2037, 2006.
15. Impact of follow-up testing on survival and health-related quality of life of breast cancer patients: a multicenter random-
16. ized controlled trial. The GIVIO Investigators. JAMA 271:1587–1592, 1994.
17. Rosselli Del Turco M, Palli D, Cariddi A, et al: Intensive diagnostic follow-up after treatment of primary breast cancer. A randomized trial. National Research Council Project on Breast Cancer follow-up. JAMA 271:1593–1597, 1994.
18. Intensive vs clinical follow-up after treatment of primary breast cancer: 10-year update of a randomized trial. JAMA 281:1586–1592, 1999.
19. Rousseau C, Campion L, Curtet C, et al: Lymphoscintigraphy in the sentinel lymph node technique for breast tumor: value of early and late images for the learning curve. Breast 12:17–22, 2003.
20. Siggelkow W, Rath W, Buell U, Zimny M: FDG PET and tumour markers in the diagnosis of recurrent and metastatic breast cancer. E J Nucl Med Mol Imaging 31:S118–124, 2004.
21. Moon DH, Maddahi J, Silverman DHS, et al: Accuracy of whole-body fluorine-18-FDG PET for the detection of recurrent or metastatic breast carcinoma. J Nucl Med 39:431–435, 1998.
22. Bender H, Kirst J, Palmedo H, et al: Value of 18-fluoro-deoxyglucose positron emission tomography in the staging of recurrent breast carcinoma. Anticancer Res 17:1687–1692, 1997.
23. Suarez M, Perez-Castejon MJ, Jimenez A, et al: Early diagnosis of recurrent breast cancer with FDG-PET in patients with progressive elevation of serum tumor markers. Q J Nucl Med 46:113–121, 2002.
24. Schmidt GP, Baur-Melnyk A, Haug A: Comprehensive imaging of tumor recurrence in breast cancer patients using whole-body MRI at 1.5 and 3 T compared to FDG-PET-CT. Eur J Radiol 65:47–58, 2008.
25. Healey Bird B, Swain SM: Cardiac toxicity in breast cancer survivors: review of potential cardiac problems. Clin Cancer Res 14:14–24, 2008.
26. Hortobagyi G: Adjuvant therapy for breast cancer. Annu Rev Med 51:377, 2000.
27. Minotti G, Menna P, Licata S, et al: Anthracycline metabolism and toxicity in human myocardium: comparisons between doxorubicin, epirubicin, and a novel disaccharide analogue with a reduced level of formation and [4-4S] reactivity of its secondary alcohol metabolite. Chem Res Toxicol 13:1336–1341, 2000.
28. Shan K, Lincoff AM, Young JB: Anthracycline-induced cardiotoxicity. Ann Intern Med 125:47, 1996.
29. Telli ML, Hunt SA, Carlson RW, Guardino AE: Trastuzumab-related cardiotoxicity: calling into question the concept of reversibility. J Clin Oncol 25:3525–3533, 2007.
30. Chien KR: Herceptin and the heart: a molecular modifier of cardiac failure. N Engl J Med 354:789–790, 2006.
31. Smith RE, Bryant J, DeCillis A, Andersen S: Acute myeloid leukemia and myelodysplastic syndrome after doxorubicin-cyclophosphamide adjuvant therapy for operable breast cancer: the national surgical adjuvant breast and bowel project experience. J Clin Oncol 21:1995, 2003.
32. Pedersen-Bjergaard J, Rowley JD: The balanced and the unbalanced chromosome aberrations of acute myeloid leukemia may develop in different ways and may contribute differently to malignant transformation. Blood 83:2780, 1994.
33. Pui CH, Relling MV: Topoisomerase II inhibitor-related acute myeloid leukaemia. Br J Haematol 109:13, 2000.
34. Weldon CB, Jaffe BM, Kahn MJ: Therapy-induced leukemias and myelodysplastic syndromes after breast cancer treatment: an underemphasized clinical problem. Ann Surg Oncol 9:738–744, 2002.
35. Van Dam FS, Schagen SB, Muller MJ, et al: Impairment of cognitive function in women receiving adjuvant treatment for high-risk breast cancer: high-dose versus standard-dose chemotherapy. J Natl Cancer Inst 90:210–218, 1998.
36. Wienke MHJ, Dienst ER: Neuropsychological assessment of cognitive functioning following chemotherapy for breast cancer. Psychooncology 4:61–66, 1995.
37. Mar Fan HG, Houede-Tchen N, Yi QL, et al: Fatigue, menopausal symptoms and cognitive function in women after adjuvant chemotherapy for breast cancer: 1- and 2-year follow-up of a prospective controlled study. J Clin Oncol 23:8025–8032, 2005.
38. Wagner LI, Sweet JJ, Butt J, et al: Trajectory of cognitive impairment during breast cancer treatment: a prospective analysis. J Clin Oncol 24(18S) abstract 8500, 2006.

38. Burstein HJ: Cognitive side-effects of adjuvant treatments. The Breast 16:166–168, 2007.
39. Grunfeld E, Dhesy-Thind S, Levine M: Clinical practice guidelines for the care and treatment of breast cancer: follow up after treatment for breast cancer (summary of the 2005 update). CMAJ 172:1319, 2009.
40. Grunfeld E, Levine MN, Julian JA, et al: Randomized trial of long-term follow-up for early-stage breast cancer: a comparison of family physician versus specialist care. J Clin Oncol 24(6): 848–855, 2006.
41. Earle CC, Burstein HJ, Winer EP, et al: Quality of non-breast cancer health maintenance among elderly breast cancer survivors. J Clin Oncol 21:1447–1451, 2003.
42. Hooning MJ, Botma A, Aleman BMP, et al: Long-term risk of cardiovascular disease in 10-year survivors of breast cancer. J Natl Cancer Inst 99:365–375, 2007.
43. Alfano CM, Day JM, Katz ML: Exercise and dietary change after diagnosis and cancer-related symptoms in long-term survivors of breast cancer: CALGB 79804. Psychooncology 18:128–133, 2008 [Epub ahead of print].

21 The Use of Molecular Profiles in the Management of Breast Cancer

Anthony D. Elias

KEY POINTS

- Biologic subtypes of breast cancer are currently defined by the presence of estrogen receptors and progesterone receptors and the level of expression of HER2/neu protein.
- Additional biomarkers and gene expression assays can further stratify breast tumor characteristics.
- Assays using these molecular profiles can be used to predict tumor prognosis as well as the patient's response to therapy.
- Assays that focus on response to therapy can guide appropriate therapy recommendations and prevent both under- and overtreatment of breast cancer.

Introduction

Types of Breast Cancer

The three major biologic subtypes of breast cancer are defined by estrogen (ER) and progesterone receptors (PR) and HER2 expression (HER2): (1) ER- or PR-positive, (2) HER2-positive, and (3) triple negative (negative for ER, PR, and HER2). These tissue biomarkers are used because they are validated to describe differences in prognosis and, above all, are predictive of the benefit of specific treatments. These biomarkers thereby guide and direct therapeutic choices.

Biomarkers

Biomarkers can serve multiple purposes, depending on the context of disease being evaluated. Prognostic markers can distinguish between good and poor risk, aggressive and indolent disease. Usually, this is in the context of patients receiving no therapy (i.e., the natural history of the tumor) or patients receiving a relatively homogeneous standard of care. These markers can be measured directly in tumor tissue as well as systemically in serum or urine. When measured in serum or urine rather than tumor tissue, they may reflect overall tumor burden. Predictive markers can identify host or tumor characteristics that differentiate a group that is likely to benefit or not from a specific treatment. These markers, which can be single or multiple, are integrated into a composite measure. Biomarkers can be both prognostic and predictive. Putative biomarkers may be causally related to the biologic behavior and/or the mechanism of action of the therapy given or can be "innocent bystanders," which just track reasonably closely with these biologic behaviors, but are not directly involved with driving that phenotype or mechanism of action.

Biomarkers are verified when their presence has been confirmed by more than one methodology. Validation of an assay, however, requires more stringency. A test is said to be validated when it is reproducible in the initial laboratory developing the assay, when it has been demonstrated to correlate with outcomes in an independently derived dataset with no overall relation to the original discovery set, and when it has been tested for its correlation to outcomes (either prognostic or predictive) in the population of patients, tumors, and treatments for the question being addressed. For example, the OncotypeDx assay has been extensively validated for a relatively narrow and homogeneous subset of breast cancers (ER-positive, node-negative, and largely HER2-negative), providing an assessment of residual risk of distant relapse after assuming the patient had taken 5 years of tamoxifen. This test can therefore be used to guide treatment choices in this subset of patients, but not in those with a different subtype of breast cancer.

On the other hand, the other commercially available multigene assay, Mammaprint, was initially developed as a prognosticator in a heterogeneous population of patients—with different tumor types, and variable treatments, including no treatment. Thus, this assay is now undergoing validation in the MINDACT (Microarray in Node-Negative Disease May Avoid Chemotherapy) trial to ask whether chemotherapy should be given to early-stage patients. In my opinion, there is no level 1 evidence to use these multiplex biomarkers to guide treatment choice yet; however, these tests are in widespread clinical use outside of clinical trials.

It is outside the scope of this review to provide a comprehensive and detailed explanation and critique of each technique used to detect biomarkers. Rather, a short summary is provided. Biomarkers include DNA (native, methylated, mutated, amplified, and deleted), various forms of RNA (mRNA, miRNA), proteins (native, modified [phosphorylated, glycosylated, acetylated, mutated, fixed]). Compared with RNA or protein, DNA tends to be the most stable and resistant to degradation during routine tissue handling and storage. Moreover, genetic changes tend to be characteristic of the tumor and drive its biologic behavior. On the other hand, the presence of DNA does not directly correlate with protein expression and therefore protein activity. mRNA is hardy to tissue handling and tends to correlate better with the level of protein. Assays of DNA and mRNA appear to be quantitative over a large dynamic range. On the other hand, proteins are the effectors of cell function. Levels of mRNA do not necessarily correlate strongly with protein concentration, nor with the vast array of post-translational modifications that proteins undergo during regulation of cellular processes. Thus, most biomarkers are still protein markers. Unfortunately, proteins are much less resistant to degradation during tissue handling and to proteases that remain active until the tissue is in deep freeze. Significant but variable loss of phosphorylation occurs within minutes of loss of blood supply. Another limitation in protein biomarkers is that most assays are linear over a narrow dynamic range and become nonlinear in clinically important concentrations.

Tumor tissue is most often queried with immunohistochemistry (IHC) and fluorescence in situ hybridization (FISH). Traditional markers by IHC include ER, PR, *HER2*, Ki67 or MIB-1 (markers of proliferation), and p63 (to determine invasiveness if uncertain) (Fig. 21-1). *HER2* is the only marker currently ascertained routinely by FISH, although topoisomerase II amplification in *HER2*-positive breast cancer may become useful if validated (Fig. 21-2). IHC and FISH have the advantages of being cheap, reproducible in multiple laboratories, and able to demonstrate tumor heterogeneity. They also have the most long-term clinical usage and are well validated. IHC typically measures proteins (presumably the business end of gene expression), and FISH measures gene copy number (a

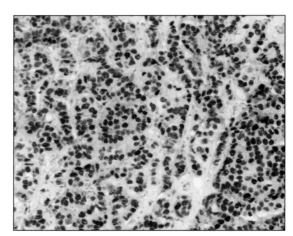

Figure 21-1. Immunohistochemistry for estrogen receptor. (From www.nibib.nih.gov/nibib/Image/Eadvances/scannerERbiopsy2.jpg.)

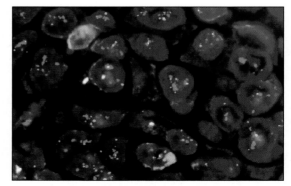

Figure 21-2. Fluorescence in situ hybridization for HER2/neu overamplification. (From Digital Atlas of Breast Pathology, Meenakshi Singh, MD, www.hsc.stonybrook.edu/gyn-atlas/breast-atlas/atlasrcp.htm)

more remote endpoint relative to protein function). Disadvantages of these techniques are that quality assurance among laboratories is poor or fair, they can interrogate only a few molecular pathways, and the intensity of IHC at least is linear only over a small range. Newer techniques use RT-PCR (reverse transcriptase polymerase chain reaction) or cDNA arrays to measure mRNA levels of various genes.

By giving more sophisticated individualized information, tumor profiling can supplement the conventional prognostic methods in use (e.g., Adjuvant Online, AJCC staging, and Nottingham Prognostic Index) and provide potential predictive information to minimize overtreatment and reduce undertreatment in the adjuvant setting.

Prognostic Profiles

The Intrinsic Subtype Assay

As discussed in Chapter 19, Perou and colleagues[1-3] first described molecular profiles of subtypes of breast cancer, generally concordant with clinical thinking. The intrinsic subtype assay requires fresh frozen tissue, although newer assays depending on RT-PCR or antibody panels in fixed tissues are being developed (Table 21-1). Luminal A assays are ER-positive, generally low grade with low proliferative thrust, and HER2-negative. Luminal B assays are ER-positive, high grade with high proliferative thrust, and occasionally HER2-positive. Frequently, they may be PR-low. HER2-positive breast cancers are driven by the characteristic HER2 gene amplification and are biologically aggressive with high grade and proliferation indices. These may be ER-negative or -positive. Basaloid or triple-negative breast cancers are characterized by the lack of HER2, ER, and PR, but are heterogeneous in other respects. They have high grade and proliferation. Sub-subtypes can be identified, although to date, none of these

patterns is validated nor carries clear therapeutic implications. This represents a fertile area for target and drug discovery. It is possible that a gene signature associated with *BRCA1* dysfunction may become an important subtype given the provocative data generated in the PARP inhibitor trials.

The OncotypeDx Recurrence Score

The OncotypeDx assay (Genomic Health, Inc, Redwood City, California) is a multiplex RT-PCR measurement of mRNA levels for 21 genes: 16 breast cancer–related and five housekeeping genes to normalize the data (Fig. 21-3). Fixed tissue is used. The expression levels of these 16 cancer genes were placed into an algorithm correlated with distant disease-free survival at 10 years in 447 patients. This assay was subsequently validated in ER-positive node-negative breast cancer tissues obtained from the National Surgical Adjuvant Breast and Bowel Project (NSABP) B-14 and B-20 trials.[4,5] The recurrence score (RS) as a continuous variable correlates with the distant disease-free survival (DDFS) at 10 years, assuming that the patient has taken tamoxifen for 5 years (Fig. 21-4).

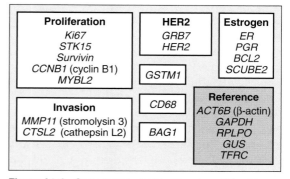

Figure 21-3. Gene panel used in OncotypeDX. (From Paik S, Shak S, Tang G, et al: A multigene assay to predict recurrence of tamoxifen-treated, node-negative breast cancer. N Engl J Med 351:2817–2826, 2004, Fig. 1.)

Table 21-1. Breast Cancer Intrinsic Subtypes Assay

Subtype	Estrogen Receptor	Grade	Her2/Neu
Luminal A	Positive	Low	Negative
Luminal B	Positive	High	Mostly negative, occasionally positive
Basaloid Triple negative	Negative	High	Negative
HER2-positive	Positive or negative	High	Positive

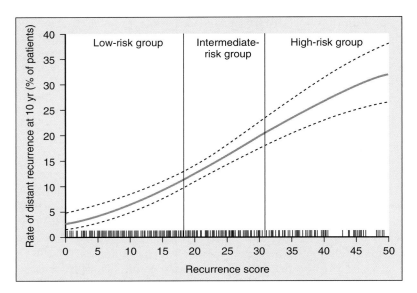

Figure 21-4. Rate of distant recurrence as a continuous function of the recurrence score. (From Paik S, Shak S, Tang G, et al: A multigene assay to predict recurrence of tamoxifen-treated, node-negative breast cancer. N Engl J Med 351:2817–2826, 2004, Fig. 4.)

More recent work suggests that the RS also will correlate with outcome in node-positive breast cancers.[6,7] As highlighted in Chapter 19, this assay is being prospectively validated in the TAILORx trial (Trial Assigning IndividuaLized Options for Treatment) and is used extensively in clinical decision making.[8]

The MammaPrint 70-Gene Profile

This gene expression cDNA profile (Agendia BV, The Netherlands) was generated on frozen tissue by comparing patients with negative lymph nodes, both ER-positive and -negative, having had a relapse within 5 years or not. It has been validated in two cohorts to divide patients into groups with good and bad prognosis.[9,10] Treatment for these validation sets was not controlled. The MINDACT trial is planning to compare clinical decision making (using the Nottingham Prognostic Index and Adjuvant Online) with the 70-gene profile to determine use of adjuvant chemotherapy in 6000 patients with newly diagnosed node-negative breast cancer (more fully described in Chapter 19).[11]

The Rotterdam 76-Gene Signature

This assay (Veridex, LLC, Warren, New Jersey) was initially developed in patients with node-negative disease.[12] Separate marker sets were developed for ER-positive and for ER-negative tumors, and then combined into this gene set. This assay has also been validated using indepen-dent sets of patients, and it can distinguish cohorts with good or poor prognosis (10-year DDFS of 94% versus 65–73%).[13,14] The assay provided additional information over the standard clinical factors and over Adjuvant! Online predictions.

Mammostrat

Mammostrat, another commercially available immunohistochemistry test (Applied Genomics, Inc, Huntsville, Alabama), uses a five-antibody panel to distinguish patients with a high risk or low risk of recurrence.[15] In multivariate analyses, prognostic significance was achieved in patients with ER-positive tumors, but not with ER-negative tumors. It, too, has had validation in the NSABP B-14 and B-20 studies.[16]

Grade, Wound Response, Rotterdam 76-Gene Set

Several other prognostic panels have been developed, but are not currently commercialized. By examining the genes altered by activation of fibroblasts, mimicking wound response, a gene expression array was constructed that did separate patients into poor or good prognosis (i.e., wound response signature present or absent).[17]

A gene expression array that distinguished grade 1 from grade 3 tumors was able to show that grade 2 tumors could be parsed into either grade 1 or 3 and correlated with clinical outcomes.[18] Numerous other gene sets have been examined. Validation is limited by tissue sets with heterogeneous biology, treatment, and follow-up.

Predictive Profiles

The Intrinsic Subtype Assay

Consistent with the extensive clinical data obtained with traditional biomarkers of grade, ER, PR, HER2, and Ki67, the intrinsic subtype assay provides broad predictive information.[2,3,19] Clinical outcome data are retrospective but suggest that luminal A subtypes are relatively indolent and respond very well to antiestrogen therapy. The HER2 and the basaloid tumors grow quickly but respond well to chemotherapy. The former also can respond to anti-HER2 therapy. This assay is currently being mined to discover new targets and new predictive biomarkers.

Predictors of Response to Endocrine Therapy

The OncotypeDx RS appears to predict the degree of benefit from tamoxifen within the ER-positive subset. In the subset analysis from the NSABP B-14 trial comparing tamoxifen with placebo, patients with low RS (<18) derived high degrees of benefit, whereas those with high RS (>31) appeared to have none.[4] Those with intermediate scores had intermediate benefit. This observation has been corroborated with anastrozole in the TransATAC trial.[20] Analysis of single gene levels in the GHI (Genomic Health, Inc.) database, ER mRNA levels, and to a lesser extent ER IHC was strongly predictive of benefit from tamoxifen, whereas PR mRNA levels appeared to have an inverse correlation with prognosis.[21] Similar findings have been reported when quantitating ER by IHC or by ligand assay.[22]

The two-gene ratio of HOXB13/IL17BR quantitated by RT-PCR has correlated with disease-free survival in patients with early-stage ER-positive breast cancer treated with tamoxifen.[23] This assay has been commercialized (AviaraDx, Carlsbad, California). Several groups have developed predictive gene sets by either examining tumors differentially responsive to tamoxifen[24] or by selecting genes that are activated by estrogen.[25,26]

HER2 amplification or overexpression appears to predict for relative resistance to tamoxifen. Preliminary results of a recent phase III trial comparing letrozole with or without lapatinib for patients with ER-positive metastatic disease in first-line therapy were reported.[27] Most tumors were HER-negative. The hypothesis was that resistance to endocrine therapy was in part mediated by upregulation of HER2 and epidermal growth factor receptor (EGFR) pathways; therefore, the addition of lapatinib would be expected to increase the overall response rates and increase the duration of response. Overall, no such effects were seen. However, in the subset of patients who had recently progressed on adjuvant tamoxifen, significant benefit was observed. This would suggest that upregulation of EGFR and HER2 pathways might be important for tamoxifen-resistant tumor cells, but may not be dominant mechanisms in resistance to estrogen depletion.

Predictors of Response/Benefit to Chemotherapy and to Particular Chemotherapy Agents

Subset analysis of numerous adjuvant chemotherapy trials suggests that benefit from chemotherapy is inversely related to ER status. For example, analysis of numerous Cancer and Leukemia Group B (CALGB) trials uniformly show that the ER-positive subsets do not appear to have as much benefit from increasing the dose intensity and dose density of adjuvant chemotherapy[28] and that very little benefit at all is found for the ER-positive HER2-negative subset.[29] One explanation for a reduced absolute benefit would be that after accounting for the benefit of antiestrogen therapy, there is less residual risk for the ER-positive subset when matching tumor characteristics. However, reduced response rates and pathologic complete response rates are seen in preoperative chemotherapy trials in the ER-positive subset, suggesting partial resistance to chemotherapy. Data from the NSABP B-20 trial (tamoxifen ± chemotherapy with MF or CMF [cyclosphosphamide, methotrexate, 5-fluorouracil]) demonstrates that the low RS group derived no obvious benefit from chemotherapy, yet the high RS group enjoyed substantial improvement[5] (Fig. 21-5). This was confirmed in the SWOG S8814 analysis reported by Albain and colleagues[7] for node-positive ER-positive breast

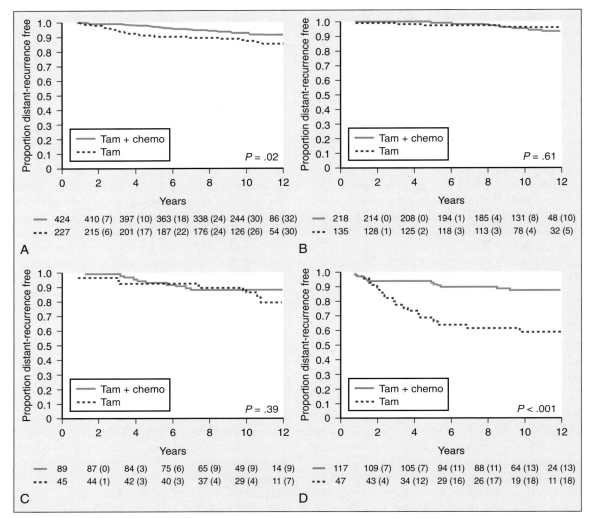

Figure 21-5. Kaplan-Meier plots for distant recurrence comparing treatment with tamoxifen (Tam) alone versus treatment with tamoxifen plus chemotherapy (Tam + chemo). (**A**) All patients. (**B**) Low-risk patients (recurrence score [RS] < 18). (**C**) Intermediate-risk patients (RS 18–30). (**D**) High-risk patients (RS ≥ 31). The number of patients at risk and the number of distant recurrences (in parentheses) are provided beneath each part of the figure. (From Paik S, Tang G, Shak S, et al: Gene expression and benefit of chemotherapy in women with node-negative, estrogen receptor-positive breast cancer. J Clin Oncol 24:3726–3734, 2006, Fig. 2.)

cancer. The Luminal A subtype appears to correspond to low RS ER-positive tumors. The Luminal B subtype appears to have higher proliferative thrust and greater responsiveness to chemotherapy. Other gene expression profiles have been published but not yet validated sufficiently for clinical use.[30]

Overexpression of HER2 also correlates with a higher likelihood of response to chemotherapy, and in particular to anthracyclines.[29,31] Fewer data are yet available to predict which HER2-positive tumors would benefit most from anti-HER2 therapy. In both the B-31 and the HERA trials, the HER2 gene copy number and the

amplification ratio did not correlate with clinical outcome.[32,33] A provocative preliminary result comparing lapatinib with trastuzumab resistance suggested differential response to these two agents, depending on the PI3K mutation and the PTEN loss status.[34]

Other biomarkers for predicting resistance or sensitivity to individual agents are as yet not clearly useful clinically. Topoisomerase II overexpression or amplification may correlate with sensitivity to anthracyclines. A commercial FISH assay (Dako, Glostrup, Denmark) is available. Mutations in β-tubulin or alterations in tubulin isoform expressions have been associated with taxane resistance. Upregulated m-Tau has been associated with resistance to paclitaxel, but not docetaxel or vinorelbine.[35-37] A 92-gene set has been identified for predicting sensitivity and/or resistance to docetaxel,[38] but it is not yet clinically applicable.

Conclusion

Much progress has been made in biomarker development and validation for refining prognosis and defining which tumors may be most sensitive or resistant to particular forms of therapy. We can now minimize overtreatment of patients with excellent prognosis and reduce undertreatment for those with biologically more aggressive tumors. Selection of specific agents for treatment remains an art, because the biomarker development has not been as robust. Challenges in biomarker validation include the heterogeneity of the patient populations included in the studies, limitations in the types of tumors collected for tissue banking, the adequacy of clinical follow-up, and the heterogeneity of clinical treatment.

Moreover, we know that the tumors themselves can change over time, in part because of selection pressure, but also in part because they are uniformly heterogeneous to any given biomarker. About 20% of ER-positive tumors can revert to ER-negative status across time, perhaps 10% to 15% of ER-negative tumors can become ER-positive, and HER2 status (even though a genetic marker) can change in 10% to 15% of cases. IHC staining and other in situ techniques definitively show heterogeneity of biomarkers. FISH for HER2 can demonstrate clones within primary tumors. Lymph node and other sites of metastases are different from the primary tumor and from each other. Most of the examples of gene profiles use population-averaging techniques in that the signal is extracted from a myriad of tumor cells, and thus the predominant signal is elicited. An elegant study by Allred and colleagues[39] demonstrated that different intrinsic subtypes of breast cancer coexist in a single specimen of ductal carcinoma in situ (DCIS) and found that the most such specimens were heterogeneous. Prostate pathologists recognize this problem by using the Gleason score, which accounts for two predominant histologies.

Another limitation of target discovery is the possibility that only a small percentage of tumor cells may be capable of propagating tumor indefinitely (tumor stem/progenitor cells). Thus, most tumor cells represent differentiated cells that are destined for cell death. The gene expression profile therefore will be generated from these differentiated cells. It may reflect the type of stem/progenitor cell that is present and the differentiation program available to that cell, but it may not pick out the relevant genes driving and supporting the stem/progenitor cell.

Pharmacogenomics, the study of the host-drug interaction, is another face of the die. There is growing evidence that drug delivery and drug metabolism vary among patients, which will affect clinical response and outcome.

Nonetheless, great strides have been made in the direction of personalized medicine. The technology has already made an impact on the standard care of breast cancer patients and is being expanded for many other tumor types. The clinician needs to understand their use and their limitations.[40]

References

1. Perou CM, Sorlie T, Eisen MB, et al: Molecular portraits of human breast tumours. Nature 406:747–752, 2000.
2. Sorlie T, Tibshirani R, Parker J, et al: Repeated observation of breast tumor subtypes in independent gene expression data sets. Proc Natl Acad Sci USA 100:8418–8423, 2003.
3. Sotirou C, Neo SY, McShane LM, et al: Breast cancer classification and prognosis based on gene expression profiles from a population-based study. Proc Natl Acad Sci USA 100: 10393–10398, 2003.
4. Paik S, Shak S, Tang G, et al: A multigene assay to predict recurrence of tamoxifen-treated, node-negative breast cancer. N Engl J Med 351:2817–2826, 2004.
5. Paik S, Tang G, Shak S, et al: Gene expression and benefit of chemotherapy in women with node-negative, estrogen receptor-positive breast cancer. J Clin Oncol 24:3726–3734, 2006.
6. Goldstein LJ, Gray R, Badve S, et al: Prognostic utility of the 21-gene assay in hormone receptor-positive operable breast cancer compared with classical clinicopathologic features. J Clin Oncol 26:4063–4071, 2008.
7. Albain K, Barlow W, Shak S, et al: Prognostic and predictive value of the 21-gene recurrence score assay in postmenopausal, node-positive, ER-positive breast cancer (S8814, INT0100). San Antonio Breast Cancer Symposium 2007; abstract 10.
8. Sparano JA: TAILORx: trial assigning individualized options for treatment (Rx). Clin Breast Cancer 7:347–350, 2006.
9. van de Vijver MJ, He YD, van't Veer LJ, et al: A gene-expression signature as a predictor of survival in breast cancer. N Engl J Med 347:1999–2009, 2002.
10. Buyse M, Loi S, van't Veer L, et al: Validation and clinical utility of a 70-gene prognostic signature for women with node-negative breast cancer. J Natl Cancer Inst 98:1183–1192, 2006.
11. Bogaerts J, Cardoso F, Buyse M, et al: Gene signature evaluation as a prognostic tool: challenges in the design of the MINDACT trial. Nat Clin Pract Oncol 10:540–551, 2000.
12. Wang Y, Klijn JG, Zhang Y, et al: Gene-expression profiles to predict distant metastasis of lymph-node negative primary breast cancer. Lancet 365:671–679, 2005.
13. Foekens JA. Atkins D, Zhang Y, et al: Multicenter validation of a gene expression-based prognostic signature in lymph node-

negative primary breast cancer. J Clin Oncol 24:1665–1671, 2006.

14. Desmedt C, Piette F, Loi S, et al: Strong time dependence of the 76-gene prognostic signature for node-negative breast cancer patients in the TRANSBIG multicenter independent validation series. Clin Cancer Res 13:3207–3214, 2007.

15. Ring BA, Seitz RS, Beck R, et al: Novel prognostic immunohistochemical biomarker panel for estrogen receptor-positive breast cancer. J Clin Oncol 24:3039–3047, 2006.

16. Ross DT, Kim CY, Tang G, et al: Chemosensitivity and stratification by a five monoclonal antibody immunohistochemistry test in the NSABP B14 and B20 trials. Clin Cancer Res 14:6602–6609, 2008.

17. Chang HY, Nuyten DS, Sneddon JB, et al: Robustness, scalability, and integration of a wound-response gene expression signature in predicting breast cancer survival. Proc Natl Acad Sci USA 102:3738–3743, 2005.

18. Sotiriou C, Wirapati P, Loi S, et al: Gene expression profiling in breast cancer: understanding the molecular basis of histologic grade to improve prognosis. J Natl Cancer Inst 98:262–272, 2006.

19. Rouzier R, Perou CM, Symmans WF, et al: Breast cancer molecular subtypes respond differently to preoperative chemotherapy. Clin Cancer Res 11:5678–5685, 2005.

20. Dowsett M, Cuzick J, Wales C, et al: Risk of distant recurrence using oncotype DX in postmenopausal primary breast cancer patients treated with anastrozole or tamoxifen: a TransATAC study. SABCS 2008; abstract 53.

21. Baehner FL, Habel LA, Quesenberry CP, et al: Quantitative RT-PCR analysis of ER and PR by Oncotype DX indicates distinct and different associations with prognosis and prediction of tamoxifen benefit. San Antonio Breast Cancer Symposium 2006; abstract 45.

22. Harvey JM, Clark GM, Osborne CK, et al: Estrogen receptor status by immunohistochemistry is superior to the ligand-binding assay for predicting response to adjuvant endocrine therapy in breast cancer. J Clin Oncol 17:1474–1481, 1999.

23. Ma XJ, Wang Z, Ryan PD, et al: A two-gene expression ratio predicts clinical outcome in breast cancer patients treated with tamoxifen. Cancer Cell 5:607–616, 2004.

24. Jansen MP, Foekens JA, van Staveren IL et al: Molecular classification of tamoxifen-resistant breast carcinomas by gene expression profiling. J Clin Oncol 23:732–740, 2005.

25. Oh DS, Troester MA, Usary J, et al: Estrogen-regulated genes predict survival in hormone receptor-positive breast cancers. J Clin Oncol 24:1656–1664, 2006.

26. Symmans WF, Hatzis C, Sotirou C, et al: Ability of a 200-gene endocrine sensitivity index (SET) to predict survival for patients who receive adjuvant endocrine therapy or for untreated patients. San Antonio Breast Cancer Symposium 2007; abstract 25.

27. Johnston S, Pegram M, Press M, et al: Lapatinib combined with letrozole vs. letrozole alone for front line postmenopausal hormone receptor positive (HR+) metastatic breast cancer (MBC): first results from the EGF30008 trial. San Antonio Breast Cancer Symposium 2008; abstract 46.

28. Berry DA, Cirrincione C, Henderson IC, et al: Estrogen-receptor status and outcomes of modern chemotherapy for patients with node-positive breast cancer. JAMA 295:1658–1667, 2006.

29. Hayes DF, Thor AD, Dressler LG, et al: HER2 and response to paclitaxel in node-positive breast cancer. N Engl J Med 357:1496–1506, 2007.

30. Hess KR, Anderson K, Symmans WF, et al: Pharmacogenomic predictor of sensitivity to preoperative chemotherapy with paclitaxel and fluorouracil, doxorubicin, and cyclophosphamide in breast cancer. J Clin Oncol 24:4236–4244, 2006.

31. Pritchard KI, Shepherd LE, O'Malley FP, et al: HER2 and responsiveness of breast cancer to adjuvant chemotherapy. N Engl J Med 354:2103–2111, 2006.

32. McCaskill-Stevens W, Procter M, Goodbrand J, et al: Disease-free survival according to local immunohistochemistry for Her 2 and central fluorescence in situ hybridization for patients treated with adjuvant chemotherapy with and without trastuzumab in the HERA (BIG 01-01) trial. Breast Cancer Res Treat [abstract 71]. 106(Suppl 1):S18, 2007.

33. Paik S, Kim C, Jeong J, et al: Benefit from adjuvant trastuzumab may not be confined to patients with IHC 3+ and/or FISH-positive tumors: central testing results from NSABP B-31. Proc ASCO 2007; abstract 511.

34. Migliaccio I, Gutierrez MC, Wu M-F, et al: PI3 kinase activation and response to trastuzumab or lapatinib in Her-2 overexpressing locally advanced breast cancer. San Antonio Breast Cancer Symposium 2008; abstract 34.

35. Andre F, Hatzis C, Anderson K, et al: Microtubule-associated protein-tau is a bifunctional predictor of endocrine sensitivity and chemotherapy resistance in estrogen receptor-positive breast cancer. Clin Cancer Res 13:2061–2067, 2007.

36. Rouzier R, Rajan R, Wagner P, et al: Microtubule-associated protein tau: a marker of paclitaxel sensitivity in breast cancer. Proc Natl Acad Sci USA 102:8315–8320, 2005.

37. Gralow JR, Barlow WE, Gown AM, et al: Expression of the microtubule-associated protein, tau, predicts improved survival, but not response, to a combination of docetaxel and vinorelbine in HER-2 negative metastatic breast cancer. San Antonio Breast Cancer Symposium 2007; abstract 2015.

38. Chang JC, Wooten EC, Tsimelzon A, et al: Gene expression profiling for the prediction of therapeutic response to docetaxel in patients with breast cancer. Lancet 362:362–369, 2003.

39. Allred DC, Wu Y, Mao S, et al: Ductal carcinoma in situ (DCIS) and the emergence of diversity during breast cancer evolution. ASCO Breast Cancer Symposium 2007; abstract 2.

40. Pusztai L: Current status of prognostic profiling in breast cancer. The Oncologist 13:350–360, 2008.

Partial Breast Irradiation

22

Rachel Rabinovitch

KEY POINTS

- Partial breast irradiation (PBI) was developed primarily to shorten treatment time when compared with whole breast irradiation (WBI).
- There are three techniques for delivering PBI: multicatheter interstitial brachytherapy, intracavitary brachytherapy, and external-beam radiation therapy (EBRT).
- WBI provides excellent tumor control and cosmesis and is the standard against which PBI outcomes must be compared.
- Suitable patient characteristics for PBI have not been clearly identified and are not necessarily comparable to whole breast radiation candidates.
- Randomized controlled trials comparing partial breast with whole breast techniques are ongoing, but mature data will not be available for many years.

No topic is more hotly debated and no treatment approach is more patient-driven in breast cancer therapy than partial breast irradiation (PBI). The following discussion focuses on treatment techniques delivered postoperatively, allowing for confirmation of pathologic staging and margin status. Intraoperative PBI techniques are therefore not discussed here.

Background

Accelerated PBI addresses two unrelated issues simultaneously: an oncologic hypothesis and a radiobiologic hypothesis. Namely, (1) can irradiation of *only* the tissue immediately surrounding the lumpectomy cavity render breast cancer control rates equivalent to traditional whole breast irradiation (WBI), and (2) can accelerated treatment (using significantly increased doses per fraction over shorter treatment times) render tumor control, toxicity, and cosmesis rates comparable to traditional therapy.

Challenging Whole Organ Therapy

The oncologic hypothesis questioning the value of whole organ (i.e., whole breast) irradiation is a timely one in the sequential evolution of local breast cancer management. Localized treatment approaches have previously addressed the entire organ, either through surgery alone (mastectomy) or a combination of surgery and radiation therapy (lumpectomy and whole breast radiation therapy). Surgery for early-stage disease has progressed over the last 30 years from surgical removal of the entire breast with underlying musculature (radical mastectomy), to mastectomy techniques that maintain integrity of the pectoralis muscles (modified radical mastectomy), to breast preservation consisting of removal of the tumor alone with varying but limited amounts of contiguous adjacent breast tissue (quadrantectomy, tylectomy, and lumpectomy). Breast-conserving surgery for breast cancer, which by definition does not resect the entire breast, is always followed by WBI. Trials comparing WBI versus observation after breast-conserving surgery consistently demonstrate that radiation therapy significantly reduces ipsilateral breast tumor recurrence rates compared with breast-conserving surgery alone.[1-4]

For the majority of solid organ tumors, whole organ treatment renders no additional curative benefit over localized therapy. This is primarily due to the relatively recent appreciation that solid organ malignancies are initiated through a localized malignant transformation on a cellular level, and spread of these clonogens occurs either by local cell division and direct contiguous invasion of adjacent tissue or via lymphatic and hematogenous routes. The latter modalities of spread are best addressed with either systemic therapy or local therapies directed at adjacent lymphatic drainage stations. Lung, esophagus, pancreas, kidney, rectum, and colon cancers are merely some of the common malignancies for which these oncologic principles apply; curative local therapies (i.e., surgery and/or radiation therapy) focus on the location of the tumor itself with a limited amount of surrounding tissue and not on the entire organ. Exceptions to this rule are primarily organs so small that an attempt to achieve both tumor excision and organ preservation is technically impossible, or that treatment of the tumor with margin essentially results in whole organ therapy by default. Cancers of the prostate, cervix, and tonsil are examples of the latter category.

The localized approach to treating the index lesion or gross disease, considered standard in most other solid malignancies, is only now being evaluated for cancer of the breast. Though ripe for investigation, this approach in early breast cancer is associated with several issues unique to this disease and to the patient population. Early-stage breast cancer is curable in most women, and death rates from breast cancer have significantly decreased compared with prior decades.[5] *Second* breast cancers in the decades following initial treatment are a recognized and significant health risk, realized increasingly because of successful control of local and distant disease after treatment of the first breast cancer. Reported rates of such tumors range consistently from 0.5% to 1% per year,[6] a seemingly tiny rate in any given year. However, with treatments resulting in increasing cure rates and with overall increasing life expectancy of the population, the probability of such events reaches a meaningful magnitude. For the average woman diagnosed at the age of 60 and expected to live to 80, risk of a second breast cancer is 10% to 20% (without adjuvant/preventive therapies). This cumulative risk only increases for a given patient as the age of diagnosis decreases and life expectancy increases. This is not the case for most other solid organ tumors, in which the lethality rate due to the initial diagnosis is very high or the likelihood of additional remote tumors in the same organ is unusual.

Second cancers are defined both as any tumor in the contralateral breast or as noncontiguous tumors in remote portions of the same breast; however, only the latter is relevant to consideration of the appropriateness of partial breast treatment. Put another way, the key question can be phrased as: Is the "normal" tissue in the ipsilateral breast any different from tissue in the contralateral breast? If not, then from a medical standpoint both should be managed similarly. All molecular and genetic evidence suggests that the malignant potential of uninvolved ipsilateral tissue is the same as that of contralateral breast tissue, and this is supported by the clinical observation that second malignancy rates in the ipsilateral breast are similar to contralateral breast cancer diagnosis rates after WBI.[7] Further supporting the idea that "elsewhere" failures in the breast are *new* primary tumors that develop over time and do not benefit from treatment with WBI is the observation that the incidence of elsewhere failure in the ipsilateral breast is minimally affected by whether WBI is delivered after lumpectomy.[8,9] These randomized trials from Canada and Italy document remarkably similar patterns of failure: 0.6% to 0.9% elsewhere failures after WBI and 2.8% to 3.5% elsewhere failures without WBI. Just as there is no indication for treatment of the contralateral normal breast in a woman with early-stage breast cancer, the hypothesis behind PBI states that tissue beyond the index tumor within the breast is no less normal and therefore ought not to require treatment. Randomized trials comparing WBI with PBI are attempting to verify this concept clinically.

The Case for WBI

This perspective is counterbalanced by pathologic data (though predating modern screening and treatment techniques) demonstrating that breast cancer cells can be detected in regions of the breast distant from the index tumor.[10,11] With these data in mind, the role of WBI is not only to treat the residual tumor cells immediately surrounding the lumpectomy bed, but also to eradicate microscopic clonogens in remote portions of the breast or in tissue more than 1 to 2 cm from the cavity. Further challenging the field of PBI is the track record of WBI in which excellent local control rates are achieved with minimal acute or long-term morbidity and excellent long-term cosmesis. Therefore, the question arises: What is being accomplished with

PBI? Are there any toxicity, cosmesis, or tumor control benefits? If not, then this treatment approach will be beneficial only in that it will be timesaving for the treated patient. The bar for PBI to overcome is therefore set quite high.

Several trials have recently been presented or updated using accelerated WBI fractionation schemas.[12–14] These approaches use 13 to 16 fractions delivered over 3 to 5 weeks. The equivalent and excellent tumor control outcomes with these accelerated approaches, accomplished without cosmesis deficits, further chip away at the potential benefit that PBI offers for a patient. Breast-conserving therapy for a woman with early-stage breast cancer no longer requires 5 to 6 weeks of daily radiation therapy. Treatment with WBI can be completed with 13 to 16 treatments delivered over 3 weeks, thus lessening the relative advantage of a 1-week PBI treatment option.

Patient Selection

The rationale for PBI supports the notion that any patient who is an appropriate candidate for breast conservation (unifocal resected tumor 5 cm or less with any pathologic nodal status) ought to be an appropriate candidate for PBI. Unfortunately, the available published experience and most of the clinical trials do not address this full range of patient presentations. As a result, the evidence to support (or refute) the

appropriateness of PBI for all subtypes of patient presentations will not be available for a long time. Furthermore, the features of enrolled patients in nearly all the PBI publications are more favorable than the actual eligibility criteria. Some of the published reports describe eligibility criteria for treatment/trial participation, but do not provide details of patient/tumor characteristics of patients actually treated. This lack of information renders analysis of the published data more difficult to interpret.

The clustering of enrolled patients around the most favorable eligibility criteria indicates a hesitancy of treating physicians to enroll younger patients with larger tumors in PBI studies. This was most dramatic in the enrollment of patients in NSABP B39/RTOG 0413 (National Surgical Adjuvant Breast and Bowel Project B 39/Radiation Therapy Oncology Group 0413), the randomized trial comparing PBI with WBI in North America.[15] An interim analysis of the patients rapidly enrolled in the first 2 years demonstrated that these included a far greater proportion of node-negative, postmenopausal, and estrogen receptor (ER)-positive patients than anticipated. The protocol was therefore amended to exclude further enrollment of postmenopausal node-negative and ER-positive patients or ER-positive ductal carcinoma in situ patients as of January 2007.

Table 22-1 summarizes the eligibility criteria for selected larger PBI series.[16–24] Most publica-

Series	Technique	N	Stage	Median Eligible Age	Margins
Polgár[16] Hungary[17]	Multicatheter	88	T1 N0-1 mi	Any	1 cm macroscopic
Vicini[20,21] Beaumont	Multicatheter	199	T1-2 (≤3 cm) N0	≥40	≥2 mm
Ott[18] Germany	Multicatheter	274	T1-2 (≤3 cm) N0	≥35	≥2 mm
Arthur[19] RTOG 95-17	Multicatheter	99	T1-2 (≤3 cm) N0-1	≥18	Negative
ASBS[20,25]	MammoSite	1449	T1-2 (≤3 cm) N0	≥40	Negative
Beaumont	EBRT 3D	91	T1-2 (≤3 cm) N0	≥50	Negative
Formenti[22]	EBRT IMRT	91	T1-2 (≤3 cm) N0-1	Any	Negative
Leonard[23]	EBRT IMRT	55	T0-1 N0	>40	≥2 mm
RTOG 0413[24]	Multicath/MammoSite/3D	Target accrual 4300	T1-2 (≤3 cm) N0-1	≥18	Negative

Table 22-1. Eligibility Criteria for PBI in Selected Series

ASBS, American Society of Breast Surgeons; EBRT, external-beam radiation therapy; IMRT, intensity-modulated radiation therapy; PBI, partial breast irradiation.

tions describe eligibility criteria for PBI as tumors of 3 cm or less, with invasive or in situ histologies and negative surgical margins (no tumor on ink) and negative axillary lymph nodes, as documented by either sentinel lymph node biopsy or axillary dissection. The RTOG studies have included the widest range of eligibility: tumors up to 3 cm, invasive or noninvasive disease, ductal or lobular invasive histologies, and node-positive tumors (up to three positive lymph nodes). NSABP B39/ RTOG 0413, which is currently accruing patients, will help identify the appropriateness of PBI for patients across the broader spectrum of breast-conserving therapy, addressing T2, node-positive, ER-negative disease, including presentations in premenopausal women.

There are several consensus documents defining patient selection parameters for PBI[25–29] (Table 22-2). They are based on the limited available published experience that addresses primarily postmenopausal women with T1N0 disease—patients with an extremely low risk for systemic and local relapse. Patients with higher rates of local and distant relapse are excluded, despite the fact that no data suggest that these patients have higher rates of ipsilateral breast tumor recurrence with PBI than lower-risk patients treated with PBI. In other words, patients not described in these definitions are not *ineligible*, but have not been evaluated yet in the clinical setting. The best that can be done at this point is to summarize the available clinical experience and encourage trial design and enrollment that will scientifically address these issues in the future.

The issues related to limiting tumor size for PBI consideration relates not only to a concern for increased breast cancer recurrence, but to technical factors as well. As the resection volume increases, the surface of the resection cavity and the amount of tissue requiring irradiation with PBI significantly increase as well. Researchers have made an effort to limit the proportion of treated normal breast tissue to ensure that the treatment is truly "partial" breast irradiation. For node-positive patients, an added consideration is whether or not regional nodal irradiation is an important component of therapy. For patients with node-positive disease who have undergone standard axillary dissection, regional nodal relapse is extremely rare.[30] Treatment with PBI without regional nodal irradiation is therefore a reasonable consideration and is being investigated.

Impact of Technologic Advances and Techniques

WBI was developed primarily as a replacement for whole organ surgical therapy—to allow for breast conservation. It also matured during an era when imaging and treatment planning technologies were comparatively crude. The trials of WBI were conducted in the 1970s and early 1980s when two-dimensional treatment planning was the norm; computed tomography (CT) was in its infancy as a diagnostic tool and not yet integrated into radiation therapy treatment planning systems. When these imaging and treatment planning technologies matured and were ultimately paired together, conformal or three-dimensional (3D) radiation therapy became possible. The ability to identify a target on multiple CT images, visualize it in 3D space, and relate the target to treatment parameters and dosime-

Table 22-2. Consensus Statements of PBI Eligibility

Source	Date	Histology	T	N	Age	Margins
American Society of Breast Surgeons[25]	2005	Invasive or noninvasive ductal	≤3 cm	0	>45	Negative
American Brachytherapy Society Breast Brachytherapy Task Group[26]	2007	Invasive ductal	≤3 cm	0	≥50	N/C
RTOG 9517, 0319, 0413[15,24,27,28]		Invasive	≤3 cm	0-3 + LNs		Negative
American College of Radiology Appropriateness Criteria Conservative Surgery and Radiation—Stage I–II Breast Carcinoma[29]	2008	No consensus for standard of care for PBI outside of protocol participation				

PBI, partial breast irradiation.

try set the stage for feasibility of a PBI approach. Stated another way: the ability to deliver PBI with any reproducible accuracy wasn't possible until the last decade, when imaging and treatment planning software became adequately sophisticated. All modern marketed software programs allow for 3D treatment plan design, whether with external-beam radiation therapy (EBRT) or brachytherapy. Although PBI has been attempted in past decades, it is no coincidence that the explosion of interest and delivery of PBI has occurred during this unique era in technologic development of the radiation therapy field.

PBI can now be delivered in a multitude of ways (Table 22-3), and can be best categorized into three distinct techniques: interstitial brachytherapy, intracavitary brachytherapy, and EBRT. Multicatheter interstitial brachytherapy is the technique with the longest track record in the modern era. Intracavitary brachytherapy (primarily with the MammoSite device) was the next to come into clinical practice. The newest approach with the shortest follow-up and experience is EBRT. All these approaches deliver radiation therapy to the 1 to 2 cm of tissue surrounding the lumpectomy cavity.

Commercial corporations have invested significant dollars into research and development of new devices made specifically for intracavitary breast brachytherapy. The proprietary nature of these commercially manufactured breast brachytherapy devices has led to significant marketing efforts, successfully publicizing the availability of this treatment approach to both patients and clinicians. Unique to brachytherapy are the marketing programs directed specifically to surgeons, who reap a financial benefit in placing an intracavitary brachytherapy device. This little-discussed "incentive" contributed to the promotion of brachytherapy PBI treatment approaches to patients.

At the same time, directed marketing and education of surgical specialists fostered a wide-based clinical support for this novel treatment approach, recognizing that all breast cancer patients are initially diagnosed by and referred from surgeons. Hence, acceptance of new treatment initiatives by the specialists who first interact with the breast cancer patient has had an important impact on the acceptance and implementation of these new treatment options. It is worth noting that patients treated with EBRT (WBI or PBI) or multicatheter PBI typically do not require billable support by surgical specialists and do not require purchase of marketed devices. As a result, there is far less publicity for these alternative PBI techniques, for which there is no financial incentive by any company to market them.

Interstitial Multicatheter Brachytherapy

Interstitial multicatheter brachytherapy was pioneered and promoted in the United States by Dr. Robert Kuske from the Ochsner Clinic in the early 1990s. His initial experience[31] led to numerous other single institution experiences, and ultimately to a phase II cooperative group study investigating this approach (RTOG 9517).[32] These implants were typically designed in two planes situated on the superficial and deep aspects of the lumpectomy cavity (Fig. 22-1). Templates were subsequently developed to allow for more even distribution of catheters, coverage of the target volume, and ease in catheter placement. This approach generally requires 15 to 20 catheters that traverse through the breast, resulting in excellent conformal coverage of the target volume (Fig. 22-2). The drawbacks of multicatheter brachytherapy are that the radiation oncologist must be comfortable with both invasive procedures and sophisticated brachytherapy treatment planning with appropriate physics support. These requirements are generally referenced as limiting this technique's popularity. Supporting this limitation is the observation that only 10 centers enrolled patients in RTOG 9517.

Because of the number of catheters required, interstitial multicatheter brachytherapy is the

Table 22-3. Partial Breast Irradiation Techniques

Multicatheter interstitial brachytherapy
   Low-dose rate (LDR)
   High-dose rate (HDR)
Intracavitary brachytherapy (always HDR)
   Balloon brachytherapy
     • MammoSite
     • Contura
   SAVI
   ClearPath
External-beam radiation therapy
   3D Conformal
   Intensity-modulated radiation therapy

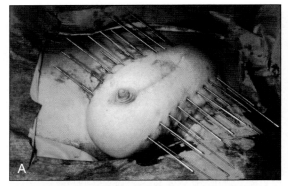

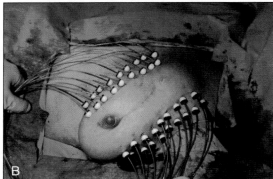

Figure 22-1. A, Placement of trochars to guide brachytherapy catheters in closed cavity technique. Ultrasound is used to guide trochars in two-plane implant at superior and inferior aspects of lumpectomy cavity. Once catheters are threaded, trochars are removed and fastening buttons are placed. **B,** Appearance at completion of catheter placement.

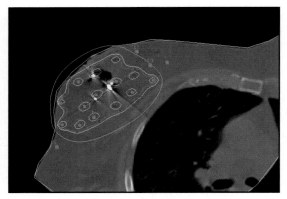

Figure 22-2. Example of treatment plan for multicatheter partial breast irradiation demonstrating good conformality.

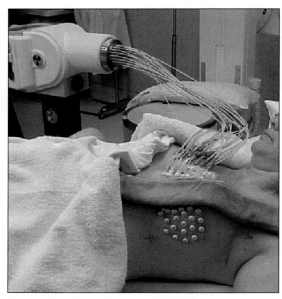

Figure 22-3. High-dose-rate (HDR) breast cancer treatment position in patient with implant using template technique.   Note large amount of breast tissue through which catheters traverse. Breast catheters are connected to connecting catheters, which in turn are affixed to appropriate channels in HDR machine. (Photo courtesy of Dr. Robert Kuske.)

most invasive of all PBI techniques (Fig. 22-3). Scarring at catheter entrance and exit sites can significantly affect the long-term cosmesis and acceptability of this treatment approach. This technique allowed for both low-dose-rate and high-dose-rate treatment.

MammoSite Radiation Therapy System

Capitalizing on the concept of PBI and recognizing the limitations of interstitial brachytherapy because of its complexity, Cytyc Corporation (Mountainview, California) developed an elegant and simple brachytherapy device. This device, the MammoSite Radiation Therapy System, consists of a balloon surrounding a double-lumen catheter: one lumen for insertion of a saline/contrast mixture into the balloon for uniform spherical expansion and the other lumen for insertion of the high-dose-rate brachytherapy source (Fig. 22-4). This novel

design, paired with marketing to both the surgical and radiation oncology community eliminated most of the obstacles associated with multicatheter brachytherapy. The single-catheter MammoSite device could now be easily placed by the radiation oncologist or the referring surgeon. Sophisticated physics support was no longer necessary, since the balloons were designed to have a single high-dose-rate

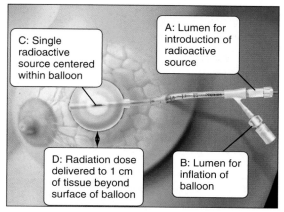

C: Single radioactive source centered within balloon

A: Lumen for introduction of radioactive source

D: Radiation dose delivered to 1 cm of tissue beyond surface of balloon

B: Lumen for inflation of balloon

Figure 22-4. Schematic of MammoSite balloon brachytherapy. (Courtesy of Hologic, Inc.)

source dwell position. Treatment was designed to deliver the prescription dose at a distance of 1 cm beyond the balloon surface.

The simplicity of the device, paired with aggressive marketing, resulted in rapid acceptance of this technique. Despite the lack of randomized data for PBI, use of the MammoSite for delivery of PBI in the community setting has been rapid. Over 38,000 MammoSite catheters have been sold as of December 2007.[33] The device was initially tested in 43 patients in a preliminary phase I/II trial between 2000 and 2001.[34] As a result of the acceptable early results, the FDA cleared the device for use in May 2002. As a condition for clearance, the FDA required Proxima Therapeutics to include a black box warning in the product labeling that the "safety and effectiveness of MammoSite as a replacement for whole breast irradiation to treat breast cancer has not been established." The American Society of Breast Surgeons (ASBS) partnered with MammoSite and supported data collection for a registry trial of treated patients. This experience comprises the largest collection of patients treated with PBI, regardless of technique (1440 patients), which to date has been published with a median follow-up of 30.1 months.[35] Despite the large number of MammoSite catheters sold, only a tiny minority of patients are included in any prospective evaluation. Although many single and pooled institution series describe outcomes of MammoSite treatment, there is significant overlap among these patients and those entered into the ASBS registry trial. The total number of patients treated with MammoSite

evaluable in the literature is therefore difficult to assess, but it is clearly less than 5% of all women treated.

The limitations of the MammoSite system include significant fluid or air around the balloon, distortion of the balloon's symmetry, and less than 5 to 7 mm of breast tissue between balloon surface and skin—any of which can render treatment with the device unacceptable. Implantation of external devices also places patients at risk for experiencing pain, infection, and late symptomatic seroma formation. With only a single catheter exiting the breast skin, the MammoSite system is far more attractive to both patients and clinicians than multicatheter brachytherapy, although it still involves placement of the device for 6 to 10 days, depending on practice patterns.

Other Intracavitary Devices

Other devices have been developed to improve upon the success of the MammoSite and overcome its specific limitations. The Contura Multi-Lumen Balloon, marketed by SenoRx, is essentially a modification of the MammoSite. It, too, is a balloon brachytherapy device, but has five treatment lumens rather than only one, which allows for shaping of dose away from critical structures such as skin (Figs. 22-5 and 22-6). This feature eliminates the constraints of balloon symmetry and minimal skin to balloon distance associated with the MammoSite. The Contura also has a vacuum port feature for extraction of fluid and air surrounding the balloon if needed, with extraction ports at both the near and distal aspects of the balloon. There is no patient experience published with this device to date. The criticisms of this device include the significantly larger diameter of the catheter and the concern that rotation of the balloon within the implanted cavity will render the initially designed treatment plan nonreproducible.

A device very similar to the MammoSite has also been designed for compatibility with electronic brachytherapy systems (Xoft Inc, Fremont, California). The Axxent balloon applicator (Fig. 22-7) uses the same planning and treatment principles as a MammoSite; however, instead of radioactive iridium, a kilovoltage source is used. This approach has lesser shielding requirements owing to the lower treat-

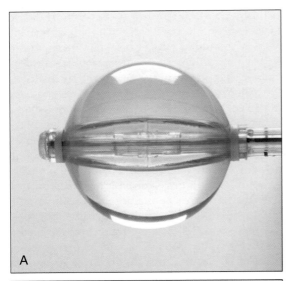

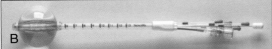

Figure 22-5. Contura multilumen balloon device.
This device is a modification of the MammoSite with five catheter options for loading (**A**) as well as inflation and vacuum ports (**B**).

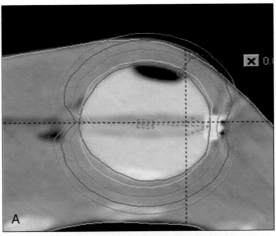

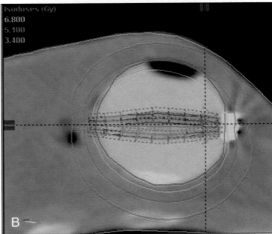

Figure 22-6. Example of dosimetry for cavity with minimal skin-balloon surface distance. A, Excessive skin dosing results with classic MammoSite loading (single dwell position in center of balloon). **B,** With the ability to use multiple lumens in the Contura device, skin dose is greatly decreased.

ment energy and lack of a radioactive source. No clinical data are as yet available on treated patients.

Two other multilumen intracavitary brachytherapy devices are commercially available that are not balloon devices: the SAVI (Strut Adjusted Volume Implant) multichannel device (BioLucent Corporation, Aliso Viejo, California) (Fig. 22-8) and the ClearPath multichannel device (North American Scientific Corporation, Chatsworth, California). These devices allow for added flexibility in treatment planning because of their multilumen design packaged within a convenient single device. Because breast tissue would come into direct contact with the individual catheters, this technique is more akin to multicatheter brachytherapy than the balloon devices. Dose gradients in breast tissue are significantly higher with these two devices, the significance of which is unknown.

External-Beam Radiation Therapy

The sophistication of modern EBRT treatment planning lends itself well to the field of PBI. EBRT can be delivered with either 3D (Fig.

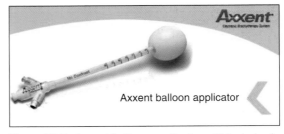

Figure 22-7. Axxent balloon applicator. This device is similar to the MammoSite but utilizes a kilovoltage source (Electronic Brachytherapy), not a true sealed radioactive source. (Courtesy of Xoft, Inc.)

22-9) or intensity-modulated radiation therapy (IMRT) technique. The significant advantage of any EBRT technique is that it is completely noninvasive. This is a significant advantage over all the brachytherapy techniques for which implantation of a device into the breast for 5 to 9 days is required, which is associated with sig-

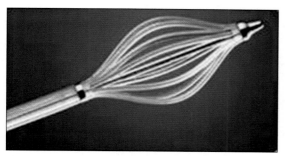

Figure 22-8. SAVI multichannel device. (Courtesy of BioLucent Corporation.)

nificant risks of pain, infection, and scarring. After initial experiences with 3D EBRT at William Beaumont Hospital, this technique was used in a small phase II study performed by the RTOG.[36] There are, however, no efficacy data published to date on the 58 patients enrolled in the study, although the treatment was documented to be technically feasible and reproducible in a cooperative group setting using exceptionally strict dosimetric criteria.[37]

For both 3D EBRT and IMRT, treatment design is nonstandardized with regard to dose constraints to both the target and organs at risk (i.e., normal tissues such as lung, heart, and ipsilateral breast). Although it is readily appreciated that IMRT can maximize targeted dosimetry, there are no data to document any clinical advantage of this incremental benefit over 3D EBRT. Furthermore, because of the lack of standardization, IMRT plans have the potential for

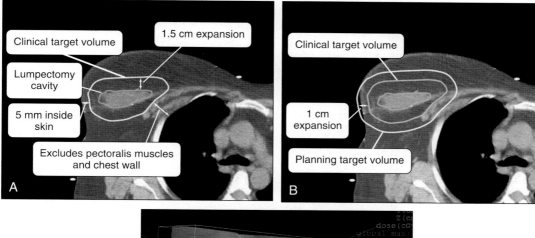

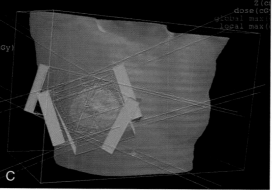

Figure 22-9. A, External-beam radiation therapy (EBRT) partial breast irradiation target delineation—lumpectomy cavity contoured. Clinical target volume (CTV) is defined as expansion of cavity by 1.5 cm, edited off pectoralis, and 5 mm from skin. **B,** Planning target volume (PTV) defined as expansion of CTV by 1.0 cm without editing. (Figs. 22-9A and B, courtesy of NSABP B-39/RTOG 0413, with permission). **C,** Once the target is defined, multiple beams are focused on PTV target creating 3D-conformal external-beam therapy arrangement, here with five treatment fields.

(Continued)

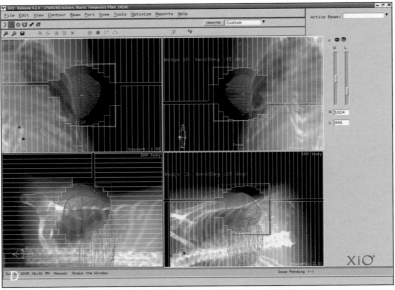

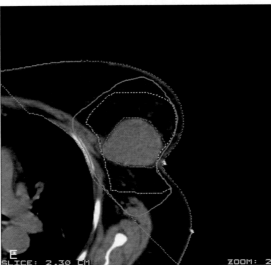

Figure 22-9, cont'd. D, Treatment fields from beam's eye view all encompassing lavender target. Note that the cardiac tissue is completely excluded from two of the treatment beams. **E,** Final dosimetry plan of a 3D EBRT case, demonstrating excellent conformality.

significant dose inhomogeneity and greater delivery of low radiation doses to normal tissues, depending on individual treatment techniques and dose constraints. Further complicating the issue is that insurance coverage of IMRT is nonuniform and varies by geographic location, resulting in significant barriers to treating patients with this more labor-intensive and technically sophisticated treatment approach. Numerous institutions have their own 3D or IMRT treatment protocols, and a modified version of the 3D technique used in RTOG

0319 is currently integrated into the randomized PBI trial (NSABP B39/RTOG 0413).

Fractionation

As previously described, one of the early pioneers of PBI is Dr. Robert Kuske. While at the Ochsner Clinic in New Orleans, a woman from South America with early-stage breast cancer following lumpectomy wanted breast irradiation, but was willing to stay in the United States for only 2 weeks. Dr. Kuske designed a multicatheter brachytherapy treatment for this patient, extrapolating from soft tissue sarcoma brachytherapy techniques, and completed her radiation therapy in less than 1 week. This vignette points to the primary benefit for most women seeking PBI—the time savings involved with the accelerated rate of treatment delivery (typically 5 consecutive weekdays rather than the traditional 25 to 33 days). The accelerated fractionation schema now firmly associated with PBI developed not as an answer to any oncologic question, but out of necessity. The initial techniques involved multicatheter brachytherapy that use invasive temporarily placed catheters, and dose design was loosely based on the extensive brachytherapy experience for soft tissue sarcomas after resection of gross disease. Shortened treatment times were therefore integral to this treatment approach. Fortunately, radiobiologic principles and clinical experience document that smaller tissue volumes can typically be treated more quickly with acceptable toxicity and that microscopic disease can be adequately treated with brachytherapy treatments delivered over 5 to 7 days.

Accelerated fractionation schedules for PBI vary greatly (Table 22-4) with regard to dose per fraction, total dose, and whether treatment is delivered once or twice daily. The twice-daily approach (typically delivered with a minimum of 6 hours between fractions) is used primarily to minimize total number of treatment days rather than to attain a radiobiologic advantage associated with twice-daily treatment. These varying fractionation techniques have been assessed by comparing their biologically effective dose values to each other and to standard WBI fractionation schemes.[38] Using these mathematical models, most PBI fractionation schedules are roughly equivalent to 50 Gy in standard fractionation, but have an inferior biologically effective dose compared with boost-containing regimens that deliver total doses of 60 to 66 Gy.

The most common fractionation regimens are 34 Gy delivered in 10 twice-daily fractions of 3.4 Gy each for all brachytherapy treatment techniques and 38.5 Gy delivered in 10 twice-daily fractions of 3.85 Gy for EBRT techniques. Long-term outcomes from clinical trials will determine the relative efficacy of the various fractionation schemes. The prescription doses for EBRT treatment are typically slightly higher than brachytherapy plans, since the former are capable of much greater dose homogeneity within the treated volume. Owing to the inverse square law associated with brachytherapy sources, the dose gradient in treated tissue is much greater, with tissue adjacent to the catheters or balloon surface receiving much larger doses than the prescription dose at the periphery of the target. There has been some speculation that the greater mean dose achieved with brachytherapy could yield a tumor control advantage, but this has yet to be proved in a prospective or randomized fashion.

Of note, much has been written describing the inconvenience of daily radiation therapy over 6 weeks and that this is so onerous that women choose not to follow through on this component of treatment or even opt for mastectomy to avoid this daily treatment. It is ironic that the least toxic of all breast cancer therapies is pinpointed as being unacceptably inconve-

	Dose/Fraction (Gy)	Total Fractions	Total Dose (Gy)	Fractions/Day	Total Days
Table 22-4. Fractionation Schedules					
HDR brachytherapy	4.0	8	32	2	4
	3.4	10	34	2	5
	3.85	10	38.5	2	5
	4.33	7	30.3		4
	5.2	7	36.4		5–7
LDR brachytherapy	Continuous	n/a	45	n/a	
	Continuous	n/a	50	n/a	5
EBRT	3.85	10	38.5	2	5
	3.4	10	34	2	5
	6.0	5	30	1	

EBRT, external-beam radiation therapy; HDR, high-dose-rate; LDR, low-dose-rate.

nient. On the other hand, the inconvenience of systemic therapy treatments is rarely commented on, which can now require up to 1 year of weekly or every-3-weekly intravenous infusions (trastuzumab [Herceptin]-containing regimens). These therapies are at least as inconvenient as breast radiation therapy.

Theoretically, external-beam PBI could be delivered in standard fractionation over 5 to 6 weeks just as WBI is delivered. This approach would address the oncologic hypothesis of partial breast treatment and eliminate the toxicity concerns associated with larger fraction sizes. However, this avenue of treatment delivery is not being investigated, since there is no clinical or research incentive to do so. Invasive techniques cannot be similarly administered over protracted time periods because of the indwelling nature of catheters and balloons with associated infection and pain rates. In addition, the experience with brachytherapy has rarely extended beyond 7 days for low-dose-rate brachytherapy in any disease site. Convenience issues typically dominate, and patients are therefore rarely treated with low-dose-rate brachytherapy.

Ipsilateral Breast Tumor Control

The most important function of PBI is tumor control. Compared with 10- and 20-year data available from randomized trials evaluating WBI,[1,7] the PBI experience is clearly in its infancy. There are few mature data to assess the efficacy of PBI techniques and no randomized data comparing one PBI technique with another. Most of the PBI experience has focused on very low-risk patients. The treatment technique with the longest follow-up is interstitial multicatheter brachytherapy followed by intracavitary balloon brachytherapy. The newest approach involves EBRT with either three dimensional or IMRT, and thus there is even less published experience with the shortest follow-up with this technique. The published ipsilateral breast tumor recurrence rates relevant to each of the three techniques are summarized in Tables 22-5 through 22-7.[21,23,39–44]

It is important to recognize that for many of the treated women in the PBI literature, ipsilateral breast tumor recurrence would be expected to be extremely low after treatment with lumpectomy and tamoxifen without any radiation therapy.[3,4] Furthermore, all phase II data and registry information are subject to cautionary conclusions since good patient selection can result in great outcomes. Only phase III data will truly identify the efficacy of PBI.

Despite these cautionary words, it is documented that local control rates in patients treated with PBI are uniformly good; ipsilateral breast tumor recurrence rates are roughly 1% per year or less, though with relatively short follow-up. The crude ipsilateral breast tumor recurrence rates are displayed in a scatter plot for comparison in Figure 22-10.

Table 22-5. Ipsilateral Breast Tumor Recurrence (IBTR) Rates in Multicatheter Brachytherapy Series

Source	Dose Rate	N	Median Follow-up	IBTR
Arthur[19] RTOG 95-17	HDR/LDR	66/33	6.1 years	6% crude 3%/6%
Ott[18] Germany		274	2.7 years	<1%
Polgar[16] Hungary	HDR	88	5.5 years	7% crude 4.7% (5-year actuarial)
Vicini Beaumont[17]	HDR/LDR	199	8.6 years	3% crude 1.6%/3.8% (5/10-year actuarial)
Lawenda[39] MGH	LDR	48	1.9 years	0
King Ochsner Clinic	HDR/LDR	51	6.2 years	2%
Wazer[40] 2002	HDR	32	2.8 years	3% crude 3% (4-year actuarial)

HDR, high-dose-rate; LDR, low-dose-rate.

Table 22-6. Ipsilateral Breast Tumor Recurrence (IBTR) Rates in MammoSite Brachytherapy Series

Source	Technique	Dose Rate	N	Follow-up (years)	IBTR
ASBS Vicini[20]	MammoSite	HDR	1449	2.5	1.6%
Cuttino[41]	MammoSite	HDR	483	2	1%
Beaumont[42]	MammoSite	HDR	80	1.8	2.5%
Benitez (DCIS)[43]	MammoSite	HDR	100	0.8	2%
Tsai[44] Kaiser	MammoSite	HDR	51	1.3	0%
Benitez FDA Trial	MammoSite	HDR	43	5.5	0%

ASBS, American Society of Breast Surgeons; HDR, high-dose-rate.

Table 22-7. Ipsilateral Breast Tumor Recurrence (IBTR) Rates in EBRT Partial Breast Irradiation Series

Source (Year)	Technique	N	Follow-up (years)	IBTR
Leonard[23] (2007)	IMRT	55	0.8	0
Vicini[21] (2007) Beaumont	3D	91	2	0
Formenti NYU (2004)	3D prone	47	1.5	0
Formenti NYU (2004)	IMRT	91	1	0

EBRT, external-beam radiation therapy; IMRT, intensity-modulated radiation therapy.

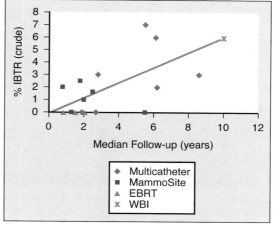

Figure 22-10. Scatter plot of published ipsilateral breast tumor recurrence rates (IBTR) from various partial breast irradiation techniques. Note that follow-up is longest for multicatheter brachytherapy and shortest for external-beam radiation therapy (EBRT). The aqua X is the IBTR rate associated with whole breast irradiation (WBI) alone, presented as reference. The 10-year IBTR with whole breast irradiation (WBI) alone in node-negative patients, 6%, presented as reference. (From Whelan T, Pignol JP, Julian J, et al: Long-term results of a randomized trial of accelerated hypofractionated whole breast irradiation following breast conserving surgery in women with node negative breast cancer [abstract]. Breast Cancer Res Treat 106(Supp 1):21, 2007.)

Toxicity and Complications

The toxicity profile of PBI varies with the treatment technique. Invasive brachytherapy techniques are clearly associated with the highest rates of infection, fat necrosis (Fig. 22-11), and symptomatic seroma formation. EBRT, on the other hand, is associated with the lowest rates of complications, but also has a shorter track record of experience. The complication rate of PBI, regardless of technique, must be compared with WBI, which has an excellent profile. Multicatheter brachytherapy is associated with symptomatic fat necrosis rates of 11% to 27%.[19,45] Fat necrosis was significantly associated with poorer overall cosmesis in the randomized trial from Hungary.[17] Among patients treated with MammoSite brachytherapy, symptomatic seroma formation developed in 10% to 12%, symptomatic fat necrosis in 1.2%, telangiectasias in 17%, pain in 16%, and infection in 9%.[13,46]

Cosmesis

Cosmesis is probably the outcome most difficult to assess because it is highly subjective and evaluated with numerous nonstandardized scoring tools. Factors that affect cosmesis include volume loss resulting from surgery and retraction of fibrotic breast tissue, skin pigment changes and development of telangiectasias, and "pockmarks" or scarring of catheter entrance

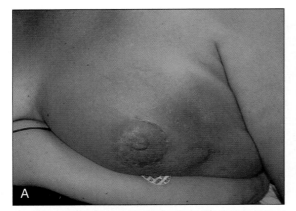

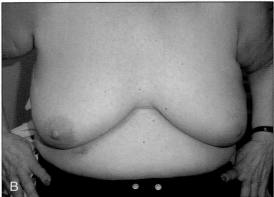

Figure 22-11. A, Symptomatic fat necrosis 1 month after MammoSite brachytherapy. **B,** Resolution of symptomatic fat necrosis 2 months later with good cosmesis.

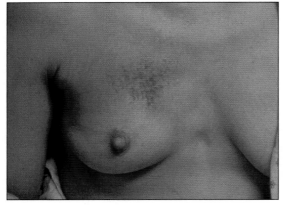

Figure 22-12. Scarring at catheter entrance sites and telangiectasias after multicatheter brachytherapy.

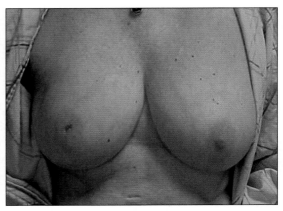

Figure 22-13. Good cosmesis after multicatheter brachytherapy.

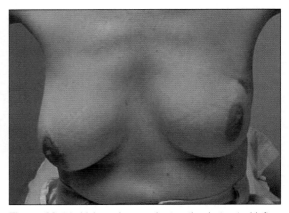

Figure 22-14. Volume loss and retraction in treated left breast with multicatheter brachytherapy.

and exit sites (Figs. 22-12 through 22-14). Furthermore, there is documented variation in perceived cosmesis between patient and clinician as well as between surgeons and radiation oncologists.[47] With a median follow-up of over 7 years, good to excellent 2-year cosmesis rates for multicatheter brachytherapy patients treated in the RTOG 9517 trial were 60% to 86%.[18] The ASBS analysis describes 1- and 4-year good-to-excellent cosmesis rates of 95% and 93% respectively,[13] and the cosmesis rates in the patients treated in the initial MammoSite clinical trial is 83%.[17] Figures 22-11 and 22-12 exemplify the range of cosmesis after PBI treatment. Cosmetic outcomes are improved with MammoSite brachytherapy with increased spacing between balloon and skin surfaces of more than 7 mm.[46]

Conclusions

PBI is an exciting evolving treatment approach with the intent of delivering effective adjuvant radiation therapy in a shortened time frame with minimal toxicity and acceptable cosmesis. Numerous techniques for PBI are in various stages of development, and only long-term randomized phase III outcome data will determine the role that this treatment approach will play in the future management of early-stage breast cancer.

References

1. Fisher B, Anderson S, Bryant J, et al: Twenty-year follow-up of a randomized trial comparing total mastectomy, lumpectomy, and lumpectomy plus irradiation for the treatment of invasive breast cancer. N Engl J Med 347(16):1233–1241, 2002.
2. Fisher B, Bryant J, Dignam JJ, et al: Tamoxifen, radiation therapy, or both for prevention of ipsilateral breast tumor recurrence after lumpectomy in women with invasive breast cancers of one centimeter or less. J Clin Oncol 20(20):4141–4149, 2002.
3. Fyles AW, McCready DR, Manchul LA, et al: Tamoxifen with or without breast irradiation in women 50 years of age or older with early breast cancer. N Engl J Med 351(10):963–970, 2004.
4. Hughes KS, Schnaper LA, Berry D, et al: Lumpectomy plus tamoxifen with or without irradiation in women 70 years of age or older with early breast cancer. N Engl J Med 351(10):971–977, 2004.
5. Cancer Facts and Figures 2008. American Cancer Society, www.cancer.org/docroot/stt/stt_0.asp, 3/2008
6. Gao X, Fisher SG, Emami B, et al: Risk of second primary cancer in the contralateral breast in women treated for early-stage breast cancer: a population-based study. Int J Radiat Oncol Biol Phys 56(4):1038–1045, 2003.
7. Veronesi U, Cascinelli N, Mariani L, et al: Twenty-year follow-up of a randomized study comparing breast-conserving surgery with radical mastectomy for early breast cancer. N Engl J Med 347(16):1227–1232, 2002.
8. Clark RM, McCulloch PB, Levine MN, et al: Randomized clinical trial to assess the effectiveness of breast irradiation following lumpectomy and axillary dissection for node-negative breast cancer. J Natl Cancer Inst 84(9):683–689, 1992.
9. Veronesi U, Marubini E, Mariani L, et al: Radiotherapy after breast-conserving surgery in small breast carcinoma: long-term results of a randomized trial. Ann Oncol 12(7):997–1003, 2001.
10. Holland R, Hendricks JH, Verbeek AL, et al: Extent, distribution, and mammographic/histologic correlations of breast ductal carcinoma in situ. Lancet 335:519–522, 1990.
11. Rosen PP, Fracchia AA, Urban JA, et al: "Residual" mammary carcinoma following simulated partial mastectomy. Cancer 35(3):739–747, 1975.
12. Whelan T, Pignol JP, Julian J, et al: Long-term results of a randomized trial of accelerated hypofractionated whole breast irradiation following breast conserving surgery in women with node negative breast cancer [abstract]. Breast Cancer Res Treat 106(Supp 1):21, 2007.
13. START Trialists' Group, Bentzen SM, Agrawal RK, Aird EG, et al: The UK Standardisation of Breast Radiotherapy (START) Trial B of radiotherapy hypofractionation for treatment of early breast cancer: a randomised trial. Lancet 371(9618):1098–1107, 2008. Epub 2008 Mar 19.
14. START Trialists' Group, Bentzen SM, Agrawal RK, Aird EG, et al: The UK Standardisation of Breast Radiotherapy (START) Trial A of radiotherapy hypofractionation for treatment of early breast cancer: a randomised trial. Lancet Oncol 9(4):331–341, 2008. Epub 2008 Mar 19
15. RTOG 0413: www.rtog.org/members/protocols/0413/0413.pdf
16. Polgár C, Fodor J, Major T, et al: Breast-conserving treatment with partial or whole breast irradiation for low-risk invasive breast carcinoma: 5-year results of a randomized trial. Int J Radiat Oncol Biol Phys 69(3):694–702, 2007.
17. Vicini F, Antonucci JV, Wallace M, et al: Long-term efficacy and patterns of failure after accelerated partial breast irradiation: a molecular assay-based clonality evaluation. Int J Radiat Oncol Biol Phys 68(2):341–346, 2007.
18. Ott OJ, Hildebrandt G, Potter R, et al: Accelerated partial breast irradiation with multi-catheter brachytherapy: local

control, side effects and cosmetic outcome for 274 patients. Results of the German-Austrian multi-centre trial. Radiother Oncol 82(3):281–286, 2007.
19. Arthur DW, Winter K, Kuske RR, et al: A phase II trial of brachytherapy alone after lumpectomy for select breast cancer: tumor control and survival outcomes of RTOG 95-17. Int J Radiat Oncol Biol Phys 72(2):467–473, 2008. [Epub ahead of print]
20. Vicini F, Beitsch PD, Quiet CA, et al: Three-year analysis of treatment efficacy, cosmesis, and toxicity by the American Society of Breast Surgeons MammoSite Breast Brachytherapy Registry Trial in patients treated with accelerated partial breast irradiation (APBI). Cancer 112(4):758–766, 2008.
21. Vicini FA, Chen P, Wallace M, et al: Interim cosmetic results and toxicity using 3D conformal external beam radiotherapy to deliver accelerated partial breast irradiation in patients with early-stage breast cancer treated with breast-conserving therapy. Int J Radiat Oncol Biol Phys 69(4):1124–1130, 2007.
22. Formenti SC, Gidea-Addeo D, Goldberg JD, et al: Phase I-II trial of prone accelerated intensity modulated radiation therapy to the breast to optimally spare normal tissue. J Clin Oncol 25(16):2236–2242, 2007.
23. Leonard C, Carter D, Kercher J, et al: Prospective trial of accelerated partial breast intensity-modulated radiotherapy. Int J Radiat Oncol Biol Phys 67(5):1291–1298, 2007.
24. RTOG 0413: www.rtog.org/members/protocols/0413/0413.pdf
25. American Society of Breast Surgeons Consensus Statement for Accelerated Partial Breast Irradiation. December 2005. www.breastsurgeons.org/apbi.shtml
26. Keisch M, Arthur D, Patel R, et al: American Brachytherapy Society Breast Brachytherapy Task Group, February, 2007. www.americanbrachytherapy.org/resources/abs_breast_brachytherapy_taskgroup.pdf
27. RTOG 9517: www.rtog.org/members/protocols/95-17/95-17.pdf. March 2008.
28. RTOG 0319: www.rtog.org/members/protocols/0319/0319.pdf
29. White JR, Halberg FE, Rabinovitch R, et al: American College of Radiology appropriateness criteria on conservative surgery and radiation: stages I and II breast carcinoma. J Am Coll Radiol 5(6):701–713, 2008.
30. Louis-Sylvestre C, Clough K, Asselain B, et al: Axillary treatment in conservative management of operable breast cancer: dissection or radiotherapy? Results of a randomized study with 15 years of follow-up. J Clin Oncol 22(1):97–101, 2004.
31. King TA, Bolton JS, Kuske RR, et al: Long-term results of wide-field brachytherapy as the sole method of radiation therapy after segmental mastectomy for T(is,1,2) breast cancer. Am J Surg 180(4):299–304, 2000.
32. Kuske RR, Winter K, Arthur D, et al: Phase II trial of brachytherapy alone after lumpectomy for select breast cancer: toxicity analysis of RTOG 95-17. Int J Radiat Oncol Biol Phys 65(1):45–51, 2006.
33. Personal communication, Hologic representative.
34. Benitez PR, Keisch ME, Vicini F, et al: Five-year results: the initial clinical trial of MammoSite balloon brachytherapy for partial breast irradiation in early-stage breast cancer. Am J Surg 194(4):456–462, 2007.
35. Vicini F, Beitsch PD, Quiet CA, et al: Three-year analysis of treatment efficacy, cosmesis, and toxicity by the American Society of Breast Surgeons MammoSite Breast Brachytherapy Registry Trial in patients treated with accelerated partial breast irradiation (APBI). Cancer 112(4):758–766, 2008.
36. RTOG 0319: a phase I/II trial to evaluate 3D conformal radiation therapy (3D-CRT) confined to the region of the lumpectomy cavity for stage I and II breast carcinoma. www.rtog.org/members/protocols/0319/0319.pdf. March 2008.
37. Vicini F, Winter K, Straube W, et al: A phase I/II trial to evaluate three-dimensional conformal radiation therapy confined to the region of the lumpectomy cavity for Stage I/II breast carcinoma: initial report of feasibility and reproducibility of Radiation Therapy Oncology Group (RTOG) Study 0319. Int J Radiat Oncol Biol Phys 63(5):1531–1537, 2005.
38. Rosenstein BS, Lymberis SC, Formenti SC: Biologic comparison of partial breast irradiation protocols. Int J Radiat Oncol Biol Phys 60(5):1393–1404, 2004.
39. Lawenda BD, Taghian AG, Kachnic LA, et al: Dose-volume analysis of radiotherapy for T1N0 invasive breast cancer treated

by local excision and partial breast irradiation by low-dose-rate interstitial implant. Int J Radiat Oncol Biol Phys 56(3):671–680, 2003.

40. Wazer DE, Kaufman S, Cuttino L, et al: Accelerated partial breast irradiation: an analysis of variables associated with late toxicity and long-term cosmetic outcome after high-dose-rate interstitial brachytherapy. Int J Radiat Oncol Biol Phys 64(2):489–495, 2006.

41. Cuttino LW, Keisch M, Jenrette JM, et al: Multi-institutional experience using the MammoSite radiation therapy system in the treatment of early-stage breast cancer: 2-year results. Int J Radiat Oncol Biol Phys 71(1):107–114, 2008. Epub 2007 Nov 26.

42. Chao KK, Vicini FA, Wallace M, et al: Analysis of treatment efficacy, cosmesis, and toxicity using the MammoSite breast brachytherapy catheter to deliver accelerated partial-breast irradiation: the William Beaumont Hospital experience. Int J Radiat Oncol Biol Phys 69(1):32–40, 2007. Epub 2007 Apr 30.

43. Benitez PR, Streeter O, Vicini F, et al: Preliminary results and evaluation of MammoSite balloon brachytherapy for partial breast irradiation for pure ductal carcinoma in situ: a phase II clinical study. Am J Surg 192(4):427–433, 2006.

44. Tsai PI, Ryan M, Meek K, et al: Accelerated partial breast irradiation using the MammoSite device: early technical experience and short-term clinical follow-up. Am Surg 72(10):929–934, 2006.

45. Lövey K, Fodor J, Major T, et al: Fat necrosis after partial-breast irradiation with brachytherapy or electron irradiation versus standard whole-breast radiotherapy—4-year results of a randomized trial. Int J Radiat Oncol Biol Phys 69(3):724–731, 2007.

46. Benitez PR, Keisch ME, Vicini F, et al: Five-year results: the initial clinical trial of MammoSite balloon brachytherapy for partial breast irradiation in early-stage breast cancer. Am J Surg 194(4):456–462, 2007.

47. Rabinovitch R, Winter K, Taylor M, et al: Toxicity and cosmesis from RTOG 95-17: a phase I/II trial to evaluate brachytherapy as the sole method of radiation therapy for stage I and II breast carcinoma [abstract]. Breast Cancer Res Treat 106(Supp 1): 4078, 2007.

23

Breast Cancer and Pregnancy

Scott W. McGee and Donald C. Doll

KEY POINTS

- Pregnancy-associated breast cancer (PABC) is defined as breast cancer occurring in pregnancy or within 1 year postpartum.
- The incidence of pregnancy-associated breast cancer is approximately 1 in 3000; however, the incidence is expected to rise as women delay childbearing.
- PABC most commonly presents as a painless mass.
- Staging and survival of PABC are similar to those of age-matched nonpregnant women.
- Mammography with abdominal shielding is safe in pregnancy. However, computed tomography (CT) scans should be avoided out of concern for potentially harmful radiation exposure to the developing fetus.
- Chemotherapy with doxorubicin-based regimens is safe if given during the second and/or third trimesters. FAC (fluorouracil, doxorubicin, cyclophosphamide) can be considered the regimen of choice.
- There are insufficient data to support the routine use of taxanes, trastuzumab, or tamoxifen in PABC.

Epidemiology

An estimated 192,500 cases of breast cancer were diagnosed in U.S. women in 2009.[1] Of these, an estimated 0.2% to 3.8% of breast cancers were in pregnant women,[2] which is approximately 1 in 3000 pregnancies.[3] Increasing age is a risk factor for breast cancer; thus the incidence of breast cancer during pregnancy is expected to increase as women delay childbearing. Data from the Centers for Disease Control and Prevention (CDC) show that the birth rate for older women continues to rise[4] (Fig. 23-1). The birth rate for women aged 35 to 39 years in 2004 was 45.4 per 1000 women, a 4% increase from the previous year. For women 40 to 44 years of age, the birth rate in 2004 was 8.9 per

1000 women, a 2% increase. For this same time period, the birth rate for women 15 to 34 decreased by 1%. Concomitant breast cancer and pregnancy may present difficulties for the medical team, since treatment of breast cancer may compromise the developing fetus, yet inadequate treatment of the breast cancer may portend a poor outcome for the mother.

Presentation

Pregnancy-associated breast cancer (PABC) is defined as breast cancer occurring in pregnancy or within 1 year postpartum. Breast cancer during pregnancy typically presents as a painless mass or thickening in the breast.[5] Series of pregnant women with breast cancer from the Mayo Clinic and from Britain showed that 60 of 63 (95%) and 146 of 178 (82%) women, respectively, presented with a painless mass.[6,7] A thorough breast examination early in pregnancy is critical. As pregnancy progresses, the breast tissue undergoes physiologic changes, including increasing firmness, nodularity, and hypertrophy, which may obscure a mass.[8] Combined with a low suspicion of malignancy in younger patients, these factors may lead to a delay in diagnosis and treatment, which recent studies estimate at 1 or 2 months.[9] For example, in a study from Memorial Sloan-Kettering Cancer Center, only 12 of 56 women with breast cancer during pregnancy were diagnosed before delivery.[10] This delay can lead to more advanced-stage disease at diagnosis. A 1-month delay in treatment of an early-stage breast cancer with a doubling time of 130 days increases the risk of axillary node metastases by 0.9%. A 3-month delay increases the risk by 2.6%, and a 6-month

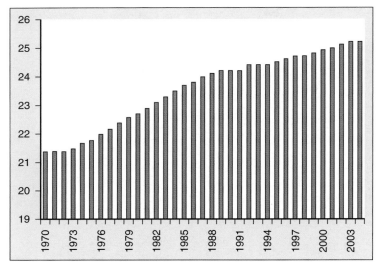

Figure 23-1. Mean age of mother at first birth, 1970–2003. (From National Center for Health Statistics Press Room Blog, April 19, 2007.)

delay by 5.1%. With a doubling time of 65 days, the risks are doubled.[11]

Pathology

Most cases of breast cancer in pregnant women are invasive ductal carcinoma, with invasive lobular carcinoma diagnosed infrequently. Most tumors are high grade, and lymphovascular invasion is common.[12] In one prospective study of 39 patients with breast cancer diagnosed during pregnancy, only 28% were estrogen receptor (ER)-positive and 24% were progesterone (PR)-receptor positive compared with 45% and 36%, respectively, of nonpregnant young women with breast cancer.[12] These results concur with the suggestion that hormone receptor–positive disease is age-related and is diagnosed more often in postmenopausal women. It has been hypothesized that high circulating levels of estrogens may even prevent ER-positive cancers.[13]

HER2/neu overexpression in PABC has been evaluated in a small number of case studies. In their study of PABC, Elledge and associates[14] noted that 7 of 12 patients (58%) overexpressed HER2/neu. A report by Middleton and associates[12] from M.D. Anderson did not find any difference in the HER2/neu expression rate (28%) in pregnant versus nonpregnant young women with breast cancer.

Recent reports seem to dispute the historical idea that inflammatory breast cancer was more common in pregnancy.[15] Indeed, data published since the 1960s have shown a similar incidence of inflammatory breast cancer in both pregnant and nonpregnant patients, ranging from 1.5% to 4.2%.[9]

Overall, these results suggest that the histopathologic and immunohistochemical properties of breast cancer in pregnant women are similar to those found in nonpregnant young women. It appears likely that age at diagnosis, rather than pregnancy, determines the biologic nature of the malignancy.[12]

Imaging

As in nonpregnant women, most breast masses detected during pregnancy are benign. However, a persistent or clinically suspicious mass in the breast and/or axilla should be imaged and biopsied, especially if imaging fails to suggest a benign etiology for the abnormality.[16]

Using modern equipment and shielding, mammography should pose little risk to the developing fetus. Standard bilateral mammography delivers a dose of 200 to 400 mGy. With appropriate shielding, the fetus is exposed to less than 50 mrad of radiation, which is well below the level of 10 rad (100 mGy) that increases the risk of fetal malformations by 1%

and is also less than the estimated environmental exposure of 2 mGy per week.[17]

Although it is considered safe, some controversy has surrounded the efficacy of mammography during pregnancy. As aforementioned, the breast undergoes physiologic changes during pregnancy, including increased density and nodularity, which may make interpretation of the mammogram difficult. In a review of cases by Max and Klamer[18] between 1970 and 1980, 6 of 8 pregnant women with breast cancer had normal mammograms. In contrast, a more recent study reported that 18 of 23 mammograms in patients with PABC were abnormal.[19] A 2003 report by Ahn and colleagues[20] evaluated the mammograms of 15 patients with breast cancer diagnosed during pregnancy. Despite all the patients having dense breasts, 13 had abnormal mammographic findings. In addition to identifying masses in eight patients, other abnormal findings included calcifications, axillary adenopathy, diffuse skin and trabecular thickening, and asymmetric densities. The authors concluded that even though increased breast density may obscure masses in a pregnant patient, there are other suspicious findings that can be identified.[20]

Ultrasonography is a safe and relatively sensitive method of imaging breast masses in pregnant patients. In a study by Liberman and colleagues,[19] 6 of 6 patients with PABC had a focal solid mass on ultrasound.[19] In their series, Ahn and colleagues[20] reported that 19 of 19 patients with PABC had a solid mass on ultrasound. It is interesting that the ultrasound findings in Ahn's report differed somewhat from ultrasound findings in non-PABC in that the investigators observed posterior acoustic enhancement and a marked cystic component in the PABC cases. Despite the disparity, they concluded that ultrasound is a highly useful imaging technique in PABC.[20]

The use of breast magnetic resonance imaging (MRI) in pregnant patients has not been thoroughly evaluated. Even though MRI has been used to evaluate fetal anomalies and appears safe in the second and third trimesters, it cannot be recommended in the first trimester because its effects on fetal organogenesis are unknown.[21] In addition, the use of gadolinium contrast is not recommended because it is known to cross the placenta and has been shown to cause developmental, skeletal, and visceral abnormalities in rats and because it is classified as a pregnancy category C drug.[21,22] Of interest, Talele and associates[23] reported a case of a lactating woman with a palpable breast mass in whom mammography and ultrasonography failed to reveal a mass. The patient then underwent MRI of the breast, which showed increased gadolinium uptake throughout the breasts, and in several areas the uptake was similar to that seen in cases of breast cancer. An excisional biopsy was performed and the pathology revealed benign changes consistent with lactation. The authors concluded that increased vascular permeability associated with lactation alters gadolinium uptake in the lactating breast and may mimic malignancy. Further study of the role of MRI in evaluating suspicious masses in the lactating breast was recommended.[23]

For the detection of metastatic disease, MRI is preferable to ultrasonography for imaging the liver if the patient is in the second or third trimester. MRI is also the safest and most sensitive method for imaging the brain.[24] CT scanning of the abdomen and pelvis is avoided during pregnancy because of the risk of fetal exposure to radiation. Bone scans can be done safely during pregnancy if there is adequate hydration and a urinary catheter is placed for 8 hours to avoid retention of radioactivity in the bladder.[25] For patients with no complaints suggestive of bony metastases outside the spine, a screening MRI of the thoracic and lumbosacral spine may be preferable.[26] Chest radiography is considered safe in pregnancy with estimated fetal exposure of 0 to 10 mrad. The exposure to the fetus is higher with portable x-ray films than with standard equipment.[9]

Biopsy

Pathologic diagnosis should be accomplished using the least invasive technique that will provide a definitive answer. In the setting of PABC, core needle biopsy has advantages over fine-needle aspiration (FNA) because it provides tissue for histopathologic study as well as determination of hormone receptor- and HER2/neu status. There has been concern over the development of a milk fistula as a complication of a core biopsy. However, this idea appears to have been overestimated with only one documented case reported in the literature.[27] Direct smears showing pregnancy-related changes in breast tissue versus primary breast cancer in pregnancy are shown in Figure 23-2.

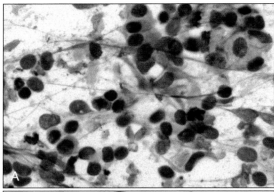

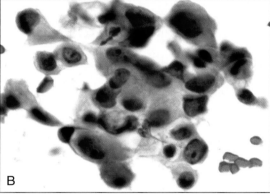

Figure 23-2. A, Direct smear of a pregnancy-associated change in the breast: dispersed cell pattern with enlarged cells, prominent nucleoli, granular debris in the background, and fraying of cytoplasmic borders. **B,** Direct smear of primary breast cancer in pregnancy: isolated and clusters of neoplastic epithelial cells with an intact cell membrane. (From Masood S: Breast. In Sidawy MK, Ali SZ: Fine Needle Aspiration Cytology. Philadelphia: Churchill Livingstone, 2007, Figs. 5–12 and 5–14.)

Staging

Since recommendations on therapy hinge on disease extent, accurate staging of PABC is crucial to the formulation of a reasonable treatment plan. Depending on the clinical stage at diagnosis, a complete staging evaluation should be undertaken, including chest x-ray with abdominal shielding, liver ultrasound, and screening noncontrast MRI of the spine to exclude bone metastases, if clinically indicated.[16] The use of CT scans should be discouraged.

Treatment

The optimal treatment for breast cancer includes a multimodality approach, including surgery, chemotherapy, and radiation (Fig. 23-3). For PABC, a similar strategy can be used, although radiation therapy is generally contraindicated in pregnancy owing to the putative risks to the fetus.

Surgery

As in the nonpregnant patient with breast cancer, surgical resection is the definitive treatment for PABC and should not be delayed because of pregnancy.[9] Nonobstetric surgery and anesthesia during pregnancy can be done without significant risk to the fetus.[28] Byrd and associates[29] performed breast biopsies on 134 pregnant women and reported only one miscarriage. Mazze and Kallen[30] found an increased risk of low and very-low-birth-weight infants in women who underwent surgery while pregnant, but the authors suggested that it was the underlying illness requiring surgery, rather than the surgery itself, that led to the low birth weights.

Mastectomy and axillary dissection are considered the optimal choice for stages I and II and some stage III tumors diagnosed in the first or second trimester when the patient desires to continue the pregnancy.[5] In nonpregnant patients, breast-conserving surgery (lumpectomy and axillary lymph node dissection) followed by radiation has been shown to be as effective as modified radical mastectomy for localized disease.[31] However, breast irradiation during pregnancy is relatively contraindicated because of concerns of excessive radiation exposure to the fetus, which could cause congenital abnormalities or an increased risk of malignancy in the child (Fig. 23-4). The estimated radiation dose to the fetus from breast radiation therapy depends on the stage of pregnancy[17] (Fig. 23-5). Mastectomy, which eliminates the need for postoperative radiation, is the recommended treatment.

Axillary dissection is preferred since the axillary nodal status has a significant impact on adjuvant therapy and because sentinel node evaluation poses an unknown risk. It has been suggested that sentinel node biopsy with a minimal dose of 500 to 600 μCi using double-filtered technetium-Tc99 (^{99m}Tc)-sulfur colloid is safe.[24] After a dose of 0.1 mCi of ^{99m}Tc-sulfur colloid for sentinel node mapping, Pandit-Taskar and associates[32] estimated a fetal absorption of 0.00014 cGy, an amount well below the National

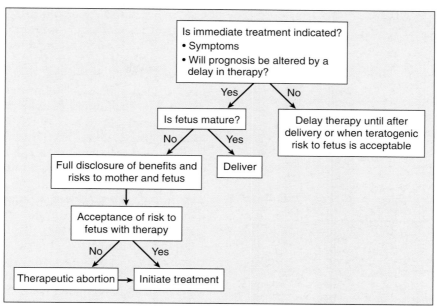

Figure 23-3. Cancer in pregnancy: approach to treatment. RT, radiation therapy. (From Wooldridge JE, Doll DC: Special issues in pregnancy. In Abeloff JO, Armitage JE, Niederhuber MB, et al (eds): Clinical Oncology, 3rd ed. Philadelphia: Elsevier, 2004, p 1336.)

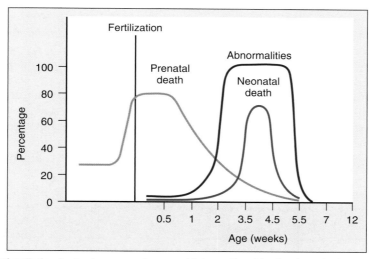

Figure 23-4. Risks of radiation to the human embryo and fetus. The risk of embryonic death is highest for radiation received at fertilization and for the first week. Neonatal abnormalities have a peak incidence between weeks 2 and 5. (From Brill AB, Forgotson EH: Radiation and congenital malformations. Am J Obstet Gynecol 90:1149, 1964.)

Council on Radiation Protection and Measurements limit for a pregnant woman. Mondi and associates[33] reported on nine pregnant women (three with breast cancer, six with melanoma) who underwent sentinel node mapping. There were no adverse reactions to the sentinel lymph node, and all patients had term deliveries of normal infants Although early reports suggest that sentinel node mapping in pregnant patients is safe, there are, however, no supporting studies for this procedure at this time.[9]

Chemotherapy

For node-positive patients and node-negative patients with tumors larger than 1 cm, adjuvant chemotherapy should be considered. Since almost all chemotherapy drugs used in breast

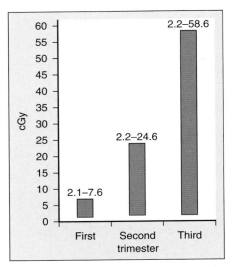

Figure 23-5. Total radiation dose to conceptus of a treatment course of 50 Gy to the breast with abdominal shielding to varying field sizes per trimester. (Data from Mazonakis M, Varveris H, Damilakis J, et al: Radiaton dose to conceptus resulting from tangential breast irradiation. Int J Radiat Oncol Biol Phys 55:386–391, 2003.)

cancer are pregnancy category D (teratogenic effects in humans have occurred), there is concern over giving these agents to pregnant patients (Box 23-1, Table 23-1). However, based on the literature, it appears that administering chemotherapy to pregnant patients is safe, particularly after the first trimester. A series of case reports demonstrates this principle[34-42] (Table 23-2). Data from the National

Cancer Institute's national registry contain 210 reports of chemotherapy use during pregnancy through 1985.[43] There were 52 associated birth defects, with all but two defects occurring in patients given chemotherapy during the first trimester. Doll and associates[44] reported a 16% risk of fetal malformations with first-trimester chemotherapy versus a 1.4% risk later in pregnancy (Tables 23-3 and 23-4). In another review, Williams and colleagues reported a 13% risk of birth defects in patients treated with alkylating agents in the first trimester; the risk was 4% later in pregnancy.[45] Based on these retrospective data, it appears that chemotherapy can be given safely to the pregnant patient, particularly after the first trimester. However, a variety of antineoplastic drugs are known to be secreted in breast milk, and breastfeeding during chemotherapy should be avoided (Box 23-2).

Currently, there is only one prospective clinical trial of chemotherapy in pregnant patients with breast cancer. Berry and associates[34] treated 24 patients with cyclophosphamide, doxorubicin, and fluorouracil. All patients were in the second or third trimester of pregnancy with the drugs being administered similar to nonpregnant patients. No congenital malformations were reported. Complications included one low birth weight, one case of hyaline membrane disease, three preterm deliveries, and two cases of transient tachypnea of the newborn. The only chemotherapy-specific complication was transient neutropenia in an infant delivered 2 days after the last chemotherapy cycle.[34]

Box 23-1. Food and Drug Administration Risk Categories for Drugs Administered During Pregnancy	
Category A	Controlled studies in women do not show risk to the fetus during first trimester, there is no evidence of risk in later trimesters, and possibility of fetal harm is remote.
Category B	Animal-reproduction studies have not shown a fetal risk, but there are not controlled studies in pregnant women; or animal-reproduction studies have shown an adverse effect (other than a decrease in fertility) but this has not been confirmed in controlled studies in women in first trimester (no evidence of a risk in later trimesters).
Category C	Studies in animals have revealed adverse effects on the fetus (teratogenic, embryocidal, or both) and there are no controlled studies in women, or studies in animals and women are unavailable. Drug should only be given if potential benefit justifies the risk to the fetus.
Category D	There is positive evidence of human fetal risk, but the benefits from use in pregnant women may be acceptable despite the risk (if the drug is needed in life-threatening situation for which other safer drugs are not available).
Category X	Studies in humans and animals have shown fetal malformations, there is evidence of fetal risk based on human experience, or both. The risk of use in a pregnant woman clearly outweighs any potential benefit. This drug is contraindicated in women who are or may become pregnant.

Reprinted from Federal Register 1980;44:37434-37467.

Table 23-1. Commonly Used Chemotherapeutic Agents and Their Pregnancy Risk Category

Drug	FDA Pregnancy Category
Methotrexate	X
Aminopterin	X
Cytosine arabinoside	D
5-Fluorouracil	D
6-Mercaptopurine	D
6-Thioguanine	D
Gemcitabine	D
Hydroxyurea	D
Chlorambucil	D
Cyclophosphamide	D
Ifosfamide	D
Melphalan	D
Thiotepa	D
Busulfan	D
Cisplatin	D
Carboplatin	D
Oxaliplatin	D
Dacarbazine	C
Procarbazine	D
Daunorubicin	D
Doxorubicin	D
Idarubicin	D
Epirubicin	D
Dactinomycin	C
Bleomycin	D
Mitoxantrone	D
Vinorelbine	D
Vincristine	D
Vinblastine	D
Paclitaxel	D
Docetaxel	D
Etoposide	D
Teniposide	D
Trauztamab	C
Imatinib	D
ATRA	D
Tamoxifen	D
Prednisone	B
Interferon α	C
Bevacuximab	C
Cetuximab	C
Rituximab	C
Erlotinib	D
Azacytidine	D
Thalidomide	X
Lenalidomide	X
Arsenic	D
Fludarabine	D
Cytarabine	D
Alemtuzumab	C
Gemtuzumab	D

FDA, U.S. Food and Drug Administration; ATRA, all-trans retinoic acid. From Shahab N, Doll DC: Chemotherapy in pregnancy. In Perry MC (ed): The Chemotherapy Source Book, 4th ed. Philadelphia: Lippincott Williams & Wilkins, 2008.

Many chemotherapy regimens for breast cancer have included methotrexate, which is strongly contraindicated in pregnancy. It is an abortifacient and the leading cause of chemotherapy-related birth defects.[43,46] In a retrospective case series of chemotherapy in pregnant patients from the United Kingdom, the only spontaneous abortion occurred in a woman given methotrexate during the first trimester.[47] Fluorouracil has been associated with one case of bone aplasia and hypoplasia, but in addition to receiving the drug during the first trimester, the mother had also been exposed to 0.5 cGy of radiation during diagnostic evaluation.[48]

Anthracyclines are also commonly incorporated into chemotherapy regimens for breast cancer. Grohard and colleagues[49] have reported a low rate of transplacental transfer of doxorubicin in vitro. Turchi and colleagues[36] reported on 28 pregnant women who received doxorubicin or daunorubicin after the first trimester for the treatment of acute myeloid leukemia, acute lymphoblastic leukemia, non-Hodgkin's lymphoma, sarcoma, or breast cancer. There were 24 normal infants, one terminated pregnancy, two miscarriages of physically normal fetuses, and one case of transient marrow hypoplasia. In the retrospective series of Ring and colleagues[47] from the United Kingdom, 16 patients received doxorubicin (11 patients) or epirubicin (5 patients) as adjuvant, neoadjuvant, or palliative therapy. There were no adverse fetal outcomes in these patients. Germann and associates[50] reported data on 160 patients who received anthracyclines while pregnant. Fetal outcome was normal in 73% of cases. Of the 5 cases with malformations, three occurred in women who received chemotherapy during the first trimester. Of 15 total fetal deaths, 6 were associated with maternal death. In this study 62% of patients received doxorubicin, and 31% were treated with daunorubicin. The authors reported an increase in fetal death associated with daunorubicin.[50]

A retrospective study from France by Giacalone and associates[51] reviewed the outcomes of 20 cases of breast cancer treated with chemotherapy during pregnancy. Ten of these patients received epirubicin as either adjuvant or neoadjuvant therapy. One fetus died after exposure to epirubicin and cyclophosphamide administered during the second trimester, one infant died on day 8 after third-trimester

Table 23-2. Congenital Anomalies after In Utero Exposure to Chemotherapy

Treatment	No. of Patients	Trimester	Results	Ref.
CAF	24	2,3	No anomaly	34
CMF, melphalan	2	1	2 spontaneous abortions	35
CAFV, tamoxifen	1	1	No anomaly	35
CAF, tamoxifen	1	3	No anomaly	35
CMF	1	3	No anomaly	35
CAMF	1	1	No anomaly	36
AC, radiation	1	1	Imperforate anus, rectovaginal fistula	37
CMF, melphalan	1	Unspecified	Spontaneous abortion	38
AV, prednisone	1	2	No anomaly	39
Tamoxifen	1	1,2,3	Goldenhar syndrome	40
Tamoxifen	1	1,2	Ambiguous genitalia	41
Tamoxifen, radiation	1	1,2,3	Preauricular skin tags	42

A, doxorubicin; C, cyclophosphamide; F, fluorouracil; M, methotrexate; V, vincristine.
From Shahin M, Sorosky J: The use of antineoplastic agents in pregnancy. In Yankowitz J, Niebyl J (eds): Drug Therapy in Pregnancy, 3rd ed. Philadelphia: Lippincott Williams & Wilkins, 2001.

Table 23-3. Chemotherapy During First Trimester of Pregnancy

Class	No. of Exposed Patients	No. of Fetal Malformations
Alkylating Agents		
Busulfan	24	2
Chlorambucil	6	1
Cyclophosphamide	7	3
Nitrogen mustard	6	0
Triethylenemelamine	4	0
Antimetabolites		
Aminopterin	52	10
Methotrexate	9	3
6-Mercaptopurine	20	0
Cytarabine	1	1
5-Fluorouracil	1	1
Hydroxyurea	3	0
Plant Alkaloids		
Vinblastine	14	1
Antibiotics		
Daunorubicin	1	0
Miscellaneous		
Procarbazine	1	1
Amsacrine	1	1
Cisplatin	1	0
Total	151	24 (15%)
Combination Chemotheray	54	9 (16%)

From Maghfoor I, Doll DC: Chemotherapy in pregnancy. In Perry MC (ed): The Chemotherapy Source Book, 3rd ed. Philadelphia: Lippincott Williams & Wilkins, 2001, p 537.

Table 23-4. Chemotherapy During Second and Third Trimesters of Pregnancy

Class	No. of Exposed Patients	No. of Fetal Malformations
Alkylating agents	26	1
Antimetabolites	38	0
Antibiotics	1	0
Plant alkaloids	6	0
Combinations	142	2
Total	213	3 (1.4%)

From Maghfoor I, Doll DC: Chemotherapy in pregnancy. In Perry MC (ed): The Chemotherapy Source Book, 3rd ed. Philadelphia: Lippincott Williams & Wilkins, 2001, p 537.

Box 23-2. Common Chemotherapy Drugs Found in Breast Milk

Cisplatin
Cyclophosphamide
Doxorubicin
Etoposide
Hydroxyurea
Interferon alfa
Methotrexate
Mitoxantrone

From Wooldridge JE, Doll DC: Special issues in pregnancy. In Abeloff MD, Armitage JO, Niederhuber JE, et al: Clinical Oncology, 3rd ed. Philadelphia: Elsevier, 2004, Table 68-4.

exposure, and one case each of anemia and transient leukopenia occurred in otherwise normal infants. Reynoso and Hueta[52] reported a case of fetal death 2 days after receiving idarubicin as consolidation therapy for acute myeloid leukemia. There are two additional case reports of transient dilated cardiomyopathy in infants exposed to idarubicin in utero.[53,54] Based on these reports, Cardonick and Iacobucci[55] concluded that in cases in which doxorubicin is as effective as the other anthracyclines, doxorubicin should be the preferred agent in pregnancy. Although Peccatori and colleagues[56] agreed that idarubicin should not be used in pregnancy, he disagreed concerning the use of epirubicin. Citing nine pregnant breast cancer patients that the authors treated with epirubicin, the only complication noted was a single case of vesiculoureteral reflux, which was successfully treated with antibiotics. The authors suggested that all patients given chemotherapy during pregnancy should be recorded in a registry to collect as much data as possible to aid in optimal decision making.

Taxanes are widely used in the treatment of node-positive breast cancer. The literature contains only five case reports on the use of taxanes in pregnant patients with breast cancer. Two of the cases were treated with paclitaxel, either alone[57] or in combination with epirubicin.[58] Chemotherapy was given during the second or third trimester. No congenital anomalies were reported. There are three case reports describing the use of docetaxel. One report details a case in which docetaxel was given during the third trimester to a pregnant patient with metastatic breast cancer.[59] The infant was born at 32 weeks and had no congenital anomalies. In the other two cases, docetaxel was given as a component of neoadjuvant therapy.[60] One infant was born with mild hydrocephalus, which resolved spontaneously; the other infant was healthy without malformations. Despite these favorable reports, there are insufficient data to support the routine use of taxanes in pregnant patients.[18]

Hormonal Therapy

Data from animal studies have shown an increased incidence of dysplastic and metaplastic changes in the epithelium of the uterus and reproductive tracts following exposure to tamoxifen in utero.[61-63] There are several case reports of tamoxifen use during human pregnancy. Cullins and associates[40] described a patient exposed to tamoxifen throughout pregnancy who gave birth to an infant with oculoauriculovertebral dysplasia (Goldenhar syndrome). However, the authors noted that the fetus had potentially been exposed to other potentially toxic agents (cocaine, marijuana, and a bone scan). Isaacs and colleagues[42] reported on a healthy male infant born to a mother who was treated with tamoxifen from the first trimester through delivery at 31 weeks. Noted in this infant was the presence of preauricular skin tags. Tewari and associates[41] reported a case in which the mother took tamoxifen for metastatic breast cancer until the 20th week of gestation. Because of deterioration of the mother's condition, the female infant was delivered at 29 weeks and displayed ambiguous genitalia. As of 2004, AstraZeneca had data regarding 50 pregnancies associated with tamoxifen. Eight pregnancies resulted in termination, 19 women had healthy babies, but 10 had fetal or neonatal disorders (two congenital craniofacial defects). In 13, the outcome was unknown.[64] Based on the limited clinical data and the experimental animal data, tamoxifen is not recommended as standard therapy for breast cancer associated with pregnancy.[18]

Trastuzumab

Trastuzumab (Herceptin) is a humanized monoclonal antibody of the IgG1 subclass that blocks the epidermal growth factor receptor, specifically the HER2/neu receptor. The U.S. Food and Drug Administration has labeled trastuzumab as pregnancy category B, based on studies in cynomolgus monkeys, which showed no harm to the fetus. Randomized trials have shown improvements in overall survival in patients with HER2/neu overexpressing metastatic breast cancer treated with trastuzumab and chemotherapy compared with chemotherapy alone.[65] There have also been promising results using trastuzumab in the adjuvant treatment of breast cancer.[66] However, experience using trastuzumab in pregnancy is limited to three case reports. Watson[67] described a patient treated with trastuzumab from conception through approximately 20 weeks gestation. An ultrasound done at 20 weeks showed anhydramnios, and no further trastuzumab was given. After drug cessation, the amniotic fluid index slowly increased, and the patient gave birth to a female infant at 37.5 weeks. The infant's renal function was normal, and there was no evidence of pulmonary hypoplasia. Waterston and Graham[68] reported a case of a woman who conceived 3 days after her second cycle of trastuzumab. The drug was discontinued and the baby was carried to term without sequelae. Bader and associates[69] described a third case of a woman exposed to 2 cycles of trastuzumab and paclitaxel for metastatic breast cancer. The drugs were given between 25 and 32 weeks gestation. During this time, the fetal abdominal circumference stopped increasing, the fetal kidneys were decreased below the fifth percentile, and anhydramnios developed. A male infant was delivered by cesarean section at 32 + 1 weeks and initially had a course complicated by hypotension, transient renal failure, and respiratory failure, possibly from sepsis. The infant recovered and development at 12 weeks was normal.

Summary

Breast cancer during pregnancy is an uncommon event, but its incidence is expected to increase as more women choose to delay childbearing. The most common presentation is a painless mass. Evaluation should include clinical examination, imaging, and biopsy. Mammography with shielding of the abdomen is safe, but the physiologic changes that occur in the breast during pregnancy may make the interpretation of these studies more difficult. Treatment planning for pregnant women with breast cancer is complex and must be individualized according to the trimester of pregnancy, the stage of disease, the wishes of the mother, and the potential risks to the developing fetus. Even though most of the available data on treatment come from case reports and retrospective series, it appears that doxorubicin-based regimens administered after the first trimester are safe and pose minimal risk to the fetus. Based on the only prospective study published to date, FAC (fluorouracil, doxorubicin, cyclophosphamide) given during the second and third trimesters can be considered the regimen of choice. Even though there are several case reports of taxanes and of tamoxifen used successfully during pregnancy, the data are insufficient at this time to recommend their routine use in this setting.

With the currently available data being very limited, the use of trastuzumab in pregnant women with HER2/neu overexpressing tumors cannot be recommended.

References

1. American Cancer Society. Cancer Facts & Figures 2009. Atlanta: American Cancer Society; 2009.
2. Wallack MK, Wolf JA, Bedwineck J, et al: Gestational carcinoma of the female breast. Curr Probl Cancer 7:1–58, 1983.
3. White TT: Prognosis of breast cancer for pregnant and nursing women. Surg Gynecol Obstet 100:661–666, 1955.
4. Martin JA, Hamilton BE, Sutton PD, et al: Births: final data for 2004. National vital statistics report. National Center for Health Statistics, vol. 55(1), 2004. www.cdc.gov/nchs/births.htm (accessed January 24, 2007).
5. Tobon H, Horowitz LF: Breast cancer during pregnancy. Breast Dis 6:127–134, 1993.
6. King RM, Welch JS, Martin JK, et al: Carcinoma of the breast associated with pregnancy. Surg Gynecol Obstet 160:228–232, 1985.
7. Ribeiro G, Jones D, Jones M: Carcinoma of the breast associated with pregnancy. Br J Surg 73:607–609, 1986.
8. Petrek JA: Breast cancer during pregnancy. Cancer 74:518–527, 1994.
9. Woo JC, Yu T, Hurd TC: Breast cancer in pregnancy. Arch Surg 138:91–98, 2003.
10. Petrek JA, Dukoff R, Rogatko A: Prognosis of pregnancy-associated breast cancer. Cancer 67:869–872, 1991.
11. Nettleton J, Long J, Kuban D, et al: Breast cancer during pregnancy: quantifying the risk of treatment delay. Obstet Gynecol 87:414–418, 1996.
12. Middleton LP, Amin M, Gwyn K, et al: Breast carcinoma in pregnant women: assessment of clinicopathologic and immunohistochemical features. Cancer 98:1055–1060, 2003.
13. Merkel D: Pregnancy and breast cancer. Semin Surg Oncol 12:370–375, 1996.
14. Elledge RM, Ciocca DR, Langone G, et al: Estrogen receptor, progesterone receptor, and HER-2/neu protein in breast cancers from pregnant patients. Cancer 71:2499–2506, 1993.
15. Gallenberg M, Loprinzi C: Breast cancer and pregnancy. Semin Oncol 16:369–376, 1989.
16. Loibl S, von Minckwitz G, Gwyn K, et al: Breast carcinoma during pregnancy: international recommendations from an expert panel. Cancer 106:237–246, 2006.
17. Mazonakis M, Varveris H, Damilakis J, et al: Radiaton dose to conceptus resulting from tangential breast irradiation. Int J Radiat Oncol Biol Phys 55:386–391, 2003.
18. Max MH, Klamer TW: Breast cancer in 120 women under 35 years old: a 10-year community wide survey. Am Surg 50:23–25, 1984.
19. Liberman L, Giess CS, Dershaw DD, et al: Imaging of pregnancy-associated breast cancer. Radiology 191:245–248, 1994.
20. Ahn BY, Kim HH, Moon WK, et al: Pregnancy- and lactation-associated breast cancer: mammographic and sonographic findings. J Ultrasound Med 22:491–497, 2003.
21. Huisman TAGM, Martin E, Kubik-Huch R, et al: Fetal magnetic resonance imaging of the brain: technical considerations and normal brain development. Eur Radiol 12:1941–1951, 2002.
22. Shellock FG, Kanal E: Safety of magnetic resonance imaging contrast agents. J Magn Reson Imaging 10:477–484, 1999.
23. Talele AC, Slanetz PJ, Edmister WB, et al: The lactating breast: MRI findings and literature review. Breast J 9:237–240, 2003.
24. Nicklas A, Baker M: Imaging strategies in pregnant cancer patients. Semin Oncol 27:623–632, 2000.
25. Baker J, Ali A, Grock MW, et al: Bone scanning in patients with breast carcinoma. Clin Nucl Med 67:519–524, 1987.
26. Gwyn K, Theriault R: Breast cancer during pregnancy. Oncology (Huntington) 15:39–46, 2001.
27. Schackmuth EM, Harlow CL, Norton LW: Milk fistula: a complication after core breast biopsy. AJR Am J Roentgenol 161:790–794, 1993.
28. Duncan PG, Pope WDB, Cohen MM, et al: Fetal risk of anesthesia and surgery during pregnancy. Anesthesiology 64:790–794, 1986.

29. Byrd BJ, Bayer D, Robertson J: Treatment of breast tumors associated with pregnancy and lactation. Ann Surg 155:940–947, 1962.

30. Mazze RI, Kallen B: Reproductive outcome after anesthesia and operation during pregnancy: a registry study of 5405 cases. Am J Obstet Gynecol 161:1178–1185, 1989.

31. Veronesi U, Paganelli G, Galimberti V, et al: Comparing radical mastectomy with quadrantectomy, axillary dissection, and radiotherapy in patients with small cancers of the breast. N Engl J Med 305:6–11, 1981.

32. Pandit-Taskar N, Dauer LT, Montgomery L, et al: Organ and fetal absorbed dose estimates from (99 m)Tc-sulfur colloid lymphoscintigraphy and sentinel node localization in breast cancer patients. J Nucl Med 47:1202–1208, 2006.

33. Mondi MM, Cuenca RE, Ollila DW, et al: Sentinel lymph node biopsy during pregnancy: initial clinical experience. Ann Surg Oncol 14:218–221, 2006.

34. Berry DL, Theriault RL, Holmes FA, et al: Management of breast cancer during pregnancy using a standardized protocol. J Clin Oncol 17:855–861, 1999.

35. Zemlickis D, Lishner M, Degendorfer P, et al: Fetal outcome after in utero exposure to cancer chemotherapy. Arch Intern Med 152:573–576, 1992.

36. Turchi J, Villasis C: Anthracyclines in the treatment of malignancy in pregnancy. Cancer 61:435–440, 1988.

37. Murray C, Reichert J, Anderson J, et al: Multimodal cancer therapy for breast cancer in the first trimester of pregnancy. JAMA 252:2607–2608, 1984.

38. Mulvihill J, McKeen E, Rosner F, et al: Pregnancy outcomes in cancer patients: experience in a large cooperative group. Cancer 60:1143–1150, 1987.

39. Tobias J, Bloom H: Doxorubicin in pregnancy (letter). Lancet 1:776, 1980.

40. Cullins SL, Pridjian G, Sutherland CM: Goldenhar's syndrome associated with tamoxifen given to the mother during gestation (letter). JAMA 271:1905–1906, 1994.

41. Tewari K, Bonebrake R, Asrat T, et al: Ambiguous genitalia in infant exposed to tamoxifen in utero (letter). Lancet 350:183, 1997.

42. Isaacs R, Hunter W, Clark K: Tamoxifen as systemic treatment of advanced breast cancer during pregnancy: case report and literature review. Gynecol Oncol 80:405–408, 2001.

43. Shahin M, Sorosky J: The use of antineoplastic agents in pregnancy. In Yankowitz J, Niebyl J (eds). Drug Therapy in Pregnancy, 3rd ed. Philadelphia: Lippincott Williams & Wilkins, 2001.

44. Doll D, Ringenberg Q, Yarbro J: Antineoplastic agents and pregnancy. Semin Oncol 16:337–346, 1989.

45. Williams S, Schilsky R: Antineoplastic drugs administered during pregnancy. Semin Oncol 27:618–622, 2000.

46. Ebert U, Loffler H, Kirch W: Cytotoxic therapy and pregnancy. Pharmacol Ther 74:207–220, 1997.

47. Ring AE, Smith IE, Jones A, et al: Chemotherapy for breast cancer during pregnancy: an 18-year experience from five London teaching hospitals. J Clin Oncol 23:4192–4197, 2005.

48. Stephens JD, Golbus MS, Miller TR, et al: Multiple congenital anomalies in a fetus exposed to 5-fluorouracil during the first trimester. Obstet Gynecol 137:747–749, 1980.

49. Grohard P, Akbaraly JP, Saux MC, et al: Transplacental passage of doxorubicin. J Gynecol Obstet Biol Reprod 18:595–600, 1989.

50. Germann N, Goffinet F, Goldwasser F: Anthracyclines during pregnancy: embryo-fetal outcomes in 160 patients. Ann Oncol 15:146–150, 2004.

51. Giacalone P-L, Laffargue F, Bénos P: Chemotherapy for breast carcinoma during pregnancy: a French National Survey. Cancer 86:2266–2272, 1999.

52. Reynoso EE, Hueta F: Acute leukemia and pregnancy—fatal fetal outcome after exposure to idarubicin during the second trimester. Acta Oncol 33:703–716, 1994.

53. Achtari C, Hohlfeld P: Cardiotoxic transplacental effect of idarubicin administered during the second trimester of pregnancy. Am J Obstet Gynecol 183:511–512, 2000.

54. Siu BL, Alonzo MR, Vargo TA, Fenrich AL: Transient dilated cardiomyopathy in a newborn exposed to idarubicin and all-trans-retinoic acid (ATRA) early in the second trimester of pregnancy. Int J Gynecol Cancer 12:399–402, 2002.

55. Cardonick E, Iacobucci A: Use of chemotherapy during human pregnancy. Lancet Oncol 5:283–291, 2004.

56. Peccatori F, Martinelli G, Gentilini O, Goldhirsch A: Chemotherapy during pregnancy: what is really safe? Lancet Oncol 5:398, 2004.

57. Gonzalez-Angulo AM, Walters RS, Carpeuter RJ, et al: Paclitaxel chemotherapy in a pregnant patient with bilateral breast cancer. Clin Breast Cancer 5:317–319, 2004.

58. Gadducci A, Cosio S, Fanucchi A, et al: Chemotherapy with epirubicin and paclitaxel for breast cancer during pregnancy: case report and review of the literature. Anticancer Res 23: 5225–5229, 2003.

59. De Santis M, Lucchese A, De Carolis S, et al: Metastatic breast cancer in pregnancy: first case of chemotherapy with docetaxel. Eur J Cancer Care 9:235–237, 2000.

60. Potluri V, Lewis D, Burton GV: Chemotherapy with taxanes in breast cancer during pregnancy: case report and review of the literature. Clin Breast Cancer 7:167–170, 2006.

61. Chamness GC, Bannayan LA, Landry JR, et al: Abnormal reproductive development in rats after neonatally administered antiestrogen (tamoxifen). Biol Reprod 21:1087–1090, 1979.

62. Iguchi T, Hirokawa M, Takasugi M: Occurrence of genital tract abnormalities and bladder hernia in female mice exposed neonatally to tamoxifen. Toxicology 42:1–11, 1986.

63. Diwan BA, Anderson LM, Ward JM: Proliferative lesions of oviduct and uterus in CD-1 mice exposed prenatally to tamoxifen. Carcinogenesis 18:2009–2014, 1997.

64. Barthelmes L, Gatelet CA: Tamoxifen and pregnancy. The Breast 13:446–451, 2004.

65. Slamon DJ, Leyland-Jones B, Shak S, et al: Use of chemotherapy plus a monoclonal antibody against HER2 for metastatic breast cancer that overexpresses HER2. N Engl J Med 344:783–792, 2001.

66. Romond EH, Perez EA, Bryant J, et al: Trastuzumab plus adjuvant chemotherapy for operable HER2-positive breast cancer. N Engl J Med 353:1673–1684, 2005.

67. Watson WJ: Herceptin (trastuzumab) therapy during pregnancy: association with reversible anhydramnios. Obstet Gynecol 105:642–643, 2005.

68. Waterston AM, Graham J: Effect of adjuvant trastuzumab on pregnancy. J Clin Oncol 24:321, 2006.

69. Bader AA, Schlembach D, Tamussino KF, et al: Anhydramnios associated with administration of trastuzumab and paclitaxel for metastatic breast cancer during pregnancy. Lancet Oncol 8: 79–81, 2007.

24

Mammary Ductoscopy

Edward R. Sauter

KEY POINTS

- Currently available breast cancer screening tools such as mammography and breast examination miss up to 40% of early breast cancers and are least effective in detecting cancer in young women, whose tumors are often more aggressive.
- Mammary ductoscopy (MD), or fiberoptic ductoscopy, allows one to visualize the breast ductal wall and sample the abnormal area for diagnostic purposes, and it provides specimens that are generally cellular.
- MD can identify intraductal lesions in most women with pathologic nipple discharge (PND) and is useful in directing therapy.
- Unlike galactography, MD can identify lesions that do not obstruct a duct and identify multiple lesions within the ductal system.
- With practice, cannulation of one or more nipple ducts can be successfully performed in the overwhelming majority of breasts that have not undergone prior surgery involving the nipple, areola, or central duct system.
- MD is limited by its ability to access and maneuver in breast ducts. These limitations are gradually diminishing.
- The depth to which one can introduce the scope is related to the diameter of the duct versus the diameter of the scope, whether prior breast surgery has been performed, and the pathology present within the breast.
- Although intraductal visual observations are related to pathology, a normal-appearing duct does not exclude breast cancer, either because the disease is beyond the reach of MD or because the duct cannulated is not the one containing disease.
- Prior surgical biopsy does not appear to hinder the ability of MD samples to contain abnormal cytology in women with ductal carcinoma in situ or invasive breast cancer.
- There is good evidence that ductoscopy is a useful tool to evaluate a subject with unilateral single duct nipple discharge to determine its etiology.
- The usefulness of MD in optimizing surgical therapy in women undergoing lumpectomy or partial mastectomy is under investigation, with conflicting results thus far.
- The feasibility of intraductal biopsy is technology limited, and will require improvements in technology before consistently adequate histologic specimens are obtained for diagnosis.
- The potential is great for using MD to screen patients at high risk for breast cancer because of an imaging abnormality, PND, or a strong family history of breast cancer.
- One concern with cytologic evaluation of MD specimens from women with PND is that the specimens can rarely be interpreted as malignant, when in fact they are benign. As such, atypical or malignant cytology in subjects with PND must be followed by a specimen allowing histologic review before definitive therapy.
- Intraductal delivery of therapeutic agents is currently possible by administration through the endoscope, but awaits improved microcatheters for injection into a specific ductal location.
- The feasibility of intraductal therapy to treat breast cancer has to be balanced against the concern that there could be disease outside the treated ductal system. On the other hand, intraductal therapy may be ideal for treating benign lesions such as papillomas, which cannot be completely removed through intraductal biopsy.

Introduction

Anatomically the breast comprises ducts and lobules, surrounded by supporting adipose and connective tissue (Fig. 24-1). The epithelial cells that line the ducts and lobules are at risk for malignant degeneration and are the origin of 99% of breast cancers.[1] There are three approaches to intraductal breast evaluation: nipple aspiration, ductal lavage (DL), and mammary or fiberoptic ductoscopy (MD). Although nipple aspiration has many strengths, a weakness is the relatively low number of epithelial cells in the specimens. Ductal lavage, which cannulates

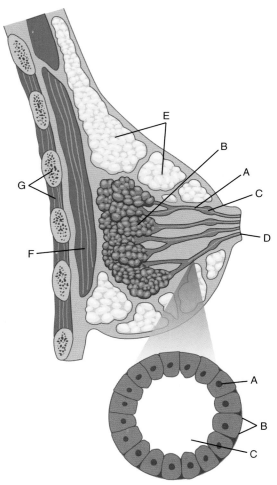

Figure 24-1. Cross-section anatomy of the normal breast (upper figure) and a normal breast duct (lower figure). **A,** Duct. **B,** Lobule (upper figure), basement membrane (lower figure). **C,** Duct lumen. **D,** Nipple. **E,** Fat. **F,** Pectoralis major muscle. **G,** Chest wall.

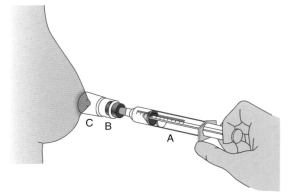

Figure 24-2. Nipple aspiration device. **A,** A 10-mL syringe; **B,** end of endotracheal tube; **C,** connector from endotracheal tube to respiratory machine.

one or more of the ducts through the nipple orifice, provides a sample with more cells than nipple aspirate fluid (NAF), but the location within the duct from which the cells were collected is unknown. MD allows one to visualize the breast ductal wall, sample the abnormal area for diagnostic purposes, and provides specimens which are generally cellular. Both ductal lavage and MD are usually preceded by nipple aspiration (Fig. 24-2), which identifies ducts containing breast fluid that can be cannulated. NAF distends the duct, making both procedures technically easier to perform. In addition, it has been demonstrated that breasts that provide NAF are at greater breast cancer risk than breasts that do

not, implying that NAF-producing ducts are more likely to contain disease.[2]

MD has been performed for over 10 years.[3,4] Direct visualization of the ductal lumen using MD provides a targeted approach to the diagnosis of disease arising in the ductal system, since the lesion can be visualized and samples can be taken through irrigation (lavage) with or without abrasion of the lesion to increase the cellularity of the specimen. Initial studies of MD evaluated women with spontaneous pathologic (unilateral single duct) nipple discharge (PND). MD currently offers a safe and perhaps better alternative to galactography in guiding breast surgery in the treatment of nipple discharge since MD can visualize lesions that do not obstruct the duct, can visualize multiple lesions, and can ensure that all the lesions have been removed.[3,5,6] This is especially important, for some women present with multiple intraductal lesions, one of which is benign and the other malignant. Since many of the malignant lesions form in the terminal duct-lobular unit, the malignant lesions tend to be farther from the nipple.[7] Some reports suggest that in breasts lacking PND, MD may be useful both in cancer assessment[8–12] and, when a preoperative cancer diagnosis has been secured, in determining the optimal margins of surgical resection.[8,13]

MD can be performed with topical or local infiltration anesthesia. A normal duct internal surface appears lustrous and smooth. Cancer in the duct wall appears white and elevated. Intraductal papillomas form solid nodules and are often yellow unless hemorrhage is present, when they are red (Fig. 24-3).

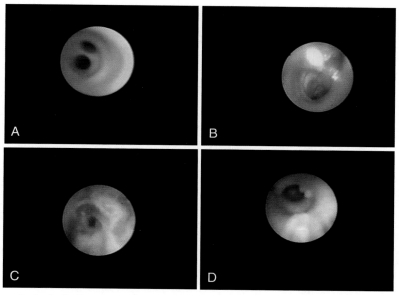

Figure 24-3. Histopathologic findings associated with intraductal views.   A, Normal. **B,** Papilloma. **C,** Hyperplasia without atypia. **D,** Ductal carcinoma in situ.

Technical Aspects of Performing MD

In women with PND, soilage on the bra or beading of fluid on the nipple from a single duct that brings a woman to seek medical attention generally reflects increased breast fluid production due to a disease process within the breast. The increased intraductal fluid distends the duct, allowing the scope to travel deeper into the breast compared with breasts without PND.[10]

Successful Cannulation and Maneuvering of the Scope within the Ducts

There is a learning curve for the performance of ductoscopic cannulation without perforation[11] (Fig. 24-4). Nonetheless, with practice cannulation of one or more nipple ducts can be successfully performed in the overwhelming majority of breasts that have not undergone prior surgery involving the nipple, areola, or central duct system. A recent report that evaluated breast duct anatomy in three dimensions found that seven ducts maintained a wide diameter to the nipple surface and drained approximately 75% of the breast; the remaining ducts (approximately 20) were too small to allow ductoscopic cannulation[14] (Fig. 24-5). For MD to maneuver

Figure 24-4. The mammary ductoscope.   The sheath is to the left. The scope contains a working channel to the right and irrigation and fiberoptic ports below.

within a duct that has been successfully cannulated, the duct must be of sufficient diameter to accept the endoscope. Thus, MD can in theory evaluate a large portion, but not all of the ductal anatomy of the breast.

The depth to which one can introduce the scope is related to (1) the diameter of the duct versus the diameter of the scope, (2) whether prior breast surgery has been performed, and (3) the pathology within the breast.[11] Specifically, the ability of the ductoscope to be introduced more than 10 cm—the length of the MD—before meeting a narrowing or obstruction that blocks further travel is related to the intraductal lesion pathology. One report found that the scope traveled more than 10 cm in 60% of breasts containing an atypical papilloma, in 36% with a papilloma without atypia, in 13% with hyperplastic lesions, and in 5% with invasive breast cancer (IBC).[11]

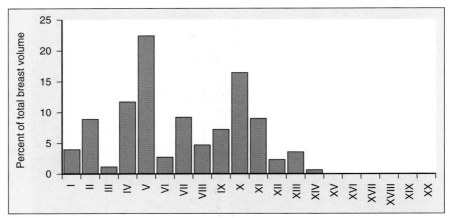

Figure 24-5. Duct system (lobe volumes as a percentage of total breast volume). One duct and its branches drained 23% of total breast volume (see V). The largest three systems drained 50.3%, and the largest six systems drained 75% of breast volume. At the other extreme, four collecting ducts ended blindly without branching, and four more together accounted for only 1.6% of total breast volume. (From Going JJ, Moffat DF: Escaping from Flatland: clinical and biological aspects of human mammary duct anatomy in three dimensions. J Pathol 203(1):538–544, 2004.)

Clinical Features with Use of MD

Association of Intraductal Visual Observations with Pathology

Intraductal visual observations are related to pathology.[11] The most common observation is an irregular duct wall, either due to scope trauma or disease or both. Intraductal scar is often observed in women who have undergone prior excisional biopsy. Extrinsic narrowing and abrupt ductal occlusion (in the absence of scar), as opposed to gradual duct narrowing, are generally observed only in cases of breast cancer. On the other hand, a normal-appearing duct does not exclude breast cancer, either because the disease is beyond the reach of MD or because the duct cannulated is not the one containing disease. In one report, in 83% of cases in which the duct appeared normal but the breast contained cancer, the histology was ductal carcinoma in situ (DCIS).[11] This is likely because with invasive disease, the ducts in the area of the breast where the lesion is located are compressed or occluded by a mass, whereas with DCIS if the disease is beyond the reach of the ductoscope or is in a different duct, the anatomy appears normal. Among women with PND, by far the most common lesion observed is a papilloma, with or without evidence of atypia. In women without PND, both papillomas and DCIS can present as an intraductal mass.

Association of MD Cytology with Pathology

Approximately two thirds of MD specimens contain sufficient epithelial cells to make a cytology diagnosis of benign, atypia, or malignancy.[11] The percentage of cytologically evaluable specimens is greater in ducts with disease, increasing from fewer than 50% of subjects with normal histology, to two thirds of subjects with hyperplasia/papilloma without atypia, to 70% to 90% of those with precancerous, DCIS, and invasive breast cancer. Cellularity can be increased by gently abrading the visualized lesion with the tip of the MD, or if a lesion is not observed, by abrading the duct wall.

The cytologic findings and their relation to histopathology results from one study are summarized as follows: mild atypia in 3 of 11 subjects (27%), 5 of 23 (22%), and 1 of 14 (7%) with normal, hyperplastic, and papilloma findings on histology, respectively, and in 0 of 5 subjects who did not undergo surgery.[11] Cytologic atypia was seen in 4 of 5 (80%) subjects with atypical papillomas. Atypical and malignant cells were found in 5 of 17 (29%) and 1 of 17 (6%) breasts with DCIS, respectively, and in 3 of 20 (15%) and 3 of 20 (15%) breasts with invasive breast cancer.

To the best of our knowledge, malignant MD cytology in breasts not presenting with PND has been found only in cancerous breasts. MD cytology from breasts with PND has rarely been found to be falsely interpreted as containing malignant cells,[10] owing to the fact that exfoliated cells from papillomas can appear abnormal when not viewed in the context of histologic architecture.

Influence of Prior Breast Surgery, Gross Intraductal Findings, and Depth of Endoscopy on MD Cytology

Because of the potential for prior excisional breast biopsy to cause scarring and prevent the ductoscope from reaching the tumor, the influence of this variable on the ability to detect breast cancer using ductoscopic cytology has been assessed. Despite this concern, prior excisional biopsy does not appear to hinder the ability of MD to identify samples that contain abnormal cytology in women with DCIS or invasive breast cancer.[11]

Methods of Increasing the Sensitivity of MD Sample Analysis

Incorporating Clinical Factors to Improve the Sensitivity of MD Cytology

Although cytologic evaluation of a breast specimen using needle aspiration is an accepted method of cancer diagnosis, cytologic evaluation of MD specimens has proved to be highly specific, but not highly sensitive in predicting whether a breast contains cancer[15] (Table 24-1). This deficiency does not eliminate the importance of cytologic review of MD specimens as an aid to breast cancer diagnosis and still has the advantage over other methods of detection, such as radiologic imaging studies and physical examination, of being able to provide a diagnosis sufficiently reliable, if positive, from which physicians can institute definitive therapy. The one caveat, as previously mentioned, is that cytologic review of MD specimen from a woman presenting with PND can rarely be falsely interpreted as malignant when the lesion is a papilloma.[10]

A model incorporating whether the subject had PND and MD cytology was 92% sensitive and 60% specific in predicting the presence of breast cancer.[10]

MD Findings in Women with and without PND

Because prior reports suggest that cytologic evaluation of PND may be falsely interpreted as containing malignancy, a prospective study was conducted to determine the differences in the role of MD in assessing whether a woman has breast cancer in breasts that do or do not present with PND.[10] Intraductal visual observations, MD cytology, pathologic findings in the resected specimen, and the quantity of epithelial cells appeared to be influenced by the presence or absence of PND. A model incorporating cytology and PND was 92% sensitive and 60% specific in predicting which women had breast cancer.

Indications for MD

Evaluation of PND

There is good evidence that ductoscopy is a useful tool to evaluate a subject with unilateral single-duct nipple discharge to determine its etiology. On the other hand, ductography (1) may

Table 24-1. Sensitivity and Specificity of Different Diagnostics for 17 Cases (Breasts) with Nipple Discharge Followed by Open Surgical Duct Excision

	Ultrasonography (%) (n = 17)	Nipple Smear (%) (n = 12)	Galactography (%) (n = 5)	Ductoscopy (%) (n = 16)
Sensitivity (true positive)	75.0	33.3	60.0	53.3
Specificity (true negative)	100.0	0.0	0.0	100.0
Efficiency (diagnostic value)	76.5	33.3	60.0	56.3
Positive predictive value (probability to predict abnormal result)	100.0	100.0	100.0	100.0
Negative predictive value (probability to rule out abnormal result)	20.0	0.0	0.0	12.5

From Grunwald S, Bojahr B, Schwesinger G, et al: Mammary ductoscopy for the evaluation of nipple discharge and comparison with standard diagnostic techniques. J Minim Invasive Gynecol 13(5):418–423, 2006.

miss lesions that do not obstruct a duct, (2) does not detect other lesions deeper within the same duct when a proximal lesion is obstructing, and (3) requires a separate surgical procedure to determine the etiology of the obstruction. In contrast, MD allows one to visualize the lesion, can often maneuver beyond an obstructing lesion to determine whether a second or third lesion exists, and allows targeted resection of the lesion.

Assessment of Occult Intraductal Pathology and Surgical Margins in Breast Cancer Patients

A preliminary report suggested that MD may be helpful in optimizing surgical therapy in women undergoing lumpectomy or partial mastectomy.[8] Specifically, in 38% of cases MD demonstrated more extensive intraluminal disease than anticipated, prompting a wider breast resection than planned and reducing the need for re-excision. This observation was followed by a larger study involving 201 subjects with biopsy-proven atypical ductal hyperplasia, DCIS, or invasive breast cancer. Seventy-five percent of the subjects had successful endoscopy. Additional lesions outside the anticipated resection margins of the lumpectomy site were identified in 41% of cases. Comparing the 150 women in whom MD was successfully performed with the 51 in whom it was not, the percentage of specimens with a positive margin was lower (5% versus 23.5%) in women who underwent MD.[13] Among the eight women who underwent MD and had a positive margin, in one case the margin was toward the nipple, and in seven the margin was lateral or deep to the center of the lesion.

Another group of investigators attempted to duplicate the above findings. They performed a prospective study of intraoperative MD in patients undergoing partial mastectomy for breast cancer.[16] Eligible patients underwent MD before partial mastectomy. When an abnormality was identified that was not within the partial mastectomy cavity, an additional MD-directed margin of tissue was removed and analyzed. Nipple aspirate fluid was collected in 19 of 30 (63%) women; MD was successful in all 19. An intraductal abnormality was identified in 15 (79%) women, but in only one case was an occult carcinoma identified by MD outside of the resection cavity. The authors concluded that

routine MD during partial mastectomy was not indicated.

Intraductal Biopsy

The feasibility of intraductal biopsy is limited by technology. With ductoscopes less than 1 mm in diameter, the working channel diameter limits the size of the biopsy tool. Various designs have been and are being tried, including microbrushes, probes with sharp edges to remove a portion of the specimen, and forceps. The simplest method is to abrade the lesion with the tip of the endoscope.[11,12] A recent report of intraductal biopsy (duct abrasion or brushing) provided a specimen for cytologic rather than histologic review.[17]

Perhaps the greatest experience with intraductal biopsy was reported by Matsunaga and associates.[7] They reported 133 biopsies on 69 intraductal papillomas and 28 biopsies on 19 ductal carcinomas. Small portions of tissue or cells were collected through one of three methods. For lesions in a dilated duct, pancreatic duct forceps with an outside diameter of 1 mm were guided next to the ductoscope, and the biopsy was performed under direct vision. For lesions that were in the main ductal system but where the duct was too small for the pancreatic forceps to fit, a metal tube with a side aperture near the tip was advanced along the outside of the ductoscope to the lesion and the lesion was entrapped in the tube under direct vision. The ductoscope was removed and the biopsy collected by applying negative pressure to the end of the tube. For lesions in a ductal branch that could not be reached using the first approach, a 19-gauge elastic tube with a diagonal tip was advanced on the outside of the ductoscope to the branch containing the lesion, the ductoscope was removed, a dura mater tube was advanced toward the lesion through the 19-gauge tube, and ductal fluid was aspirated adjacent to the lesion. In the last method described, the aspiration was not performed under direct vision. Of the 28 biopsies from 19 subjects that were attempted for a lesion that turned out to be cancer, four were insufficient for diagnosis, seven were suspicious for carcinoma, three were false-negative on biopsy but positive on cytology from the same duct, and five had the diagnosis of carcinoma. Of 133 biopsies for lesions that turned out to be intraductal papilloma, 17 were inadequate for diagnosis. Of 46 papillary lesions followed up for over 2 years, nipple discharge ceased after one intraductal biopsy in 28 and after more than two biopsies in 5 additional cases. In the remaining 13 cases, discharge continued. Of these 13, two recurrent papillomas were noted at last follow-up.

Matsunaga and associates[9] have published an updated report of their experience with intraductal biopsy. In this report, they reviewed their experience with biopsy of 193 intraductal papillomas from 107 patients and 30 ductal carcinomas from 27 patients. Intraductal biopsy correctly identified carcinoma in 33.3% of patients (9 of 27) and was therapeutic (no further nipple discharge) in 77.6% of women with papillomas. Further improvements in technology that provide consistently adequate histologic specimens for review will be critical in differentiating atypical ductal hyperplasia from DCIS, and DCIS from invasive breast cancer.

Screening

The potential is great for using MD to screen patients at high risk for breast cancer because of an imaging abnormality, PND, or a strong family history of breast cancer. MD can be performed in an office setting under local anesthesia (topical anesthetic cream plus intradermal local anesthetic injected at the areolar margin) without significant complications. A recent report documents the feasibility of MD in an office setting for women who are *BRCA* mutation carriers, a group with a very high risk for developing breast cancer.[11] Another report evaluated women deemed at high risk either because of nipple discharge or a strong family history of breast cancer.[17] Intraductal abnormalities prompting biopsy through duct abrasion or brushing were performed in 82% of cases, with severe atypia or malignant cells found in 20% of cases. One concern with this approach is that cytologic specimens from women with PND can rarely be interpreted as malignant, when in fact they are benign.[10] As such, atypical or malignant cytology in subjects with PND must be followed by a specimen allowing histologic review before definitive therapy.

Delivery of Diagnostic and Therapeutic Agents

Using the ductoscope to deliver agents into the ductal system is a promising area of current and

future investigation. Intraductal delivery of indigo carmine[7] or methylene blue[18] to guide limited surgical excision (microdochectomy or microductectomy) of the involved duct, rather than the removal of multiple ducts, has been reported. A follow-up study from the second group[19] compared single-duct with multiple-duct excision in women presenting with single-duct nipple discharge. The researchers found that although the percentage of patients with atypical ductal hyperplasia and lobular carcinoma in situ was similar in the two groups (9% versus 10%), only 3% of subjects in the microductectomy group versus 9% in the multiple duct excision group were found to have carcinoma (DCIS or invasive), which they propose is due to the larger size of the latter specimens.

YAG laser irradiation of intraductal papillomas was first reported in 1996 to treat intraductal papillomas that were not successfully removed through intraductal biopsy. Irradiation was successful in 50% of cases.[20] Patients had no adverse sequelae. The authors concluded that the cost of the equipment may not justify its use for treating benign disease. Intraductal instillation of a therapeutic agent is currently possible, and microcatheters small enough to allow directed injection of therapeutic agents into an abnormal area of a duct are under development. The feasibility of this approach has to be balanced against the concern that there could be disease outside of the treated ductal system, as suggested by the report previously outlined[19] documenting malignancy in ducts other than the duct with pathologic nipple discharge. On the other hand, intraductal therapy may be ideal for treating benign lesions such as papillomas that cannot be completely removed through intraductal biopsy.

Conclusion

MD is feasible in most subjects and is an excellent method for evaluating women presenting with PND. Its role in evaluating the breast of women who do not have PND is less clear. MD cytology will not likely be sufficiently sensitive when used alone to become part of routine clinical use, and additional biologic and/or clinical markers will be required to optimize the sensitivity of MD to aid in breast cancer detection or to optimize surgical resection of a breast known to contain disease. Papillomas can present a diagnostic problem, so women presenting with PND and cytologic evidence of malignancy need to have histologic confirmation before the initiation of cancer therapy. Using the ductoscope to aid in the targeted resection of a breast duct containing an intraductal lesion is in current practice, although this limited approach may miss the detection of some cancers. Targeted therapy will become more practical with technologic advances in catheter design and treatment delivery.

Future Perspective

The ability of MD to diagnose breast cancer in women of normal risk and high risk for breast cancer and those with an abnormality suggesting the need for surgery is limited primarily by its ability to reach the site of and biopsy the disease. Limitations due to duct diameter will gradually be overcome by smaller scopes, although ductoscope diameter is limited by the need for an irrigation/biopsy channel and, if a biopsy is required, by the type of biopsy tool that can fit within the channel. Biopsy tools are being tested that will allow biopsy of sufficient size that a reliable histologic diagnosis can be obtained in most cases.[21]

Total resection of intraductal lesions may be possible in the future, but will require the development of better biopsy and extraction tools. For complete resection to be possible, the biopsy must be sufficiently large to include the terminal duct-lobular unit where most breast cancers originate, an area beyond which the MD can generally reach. Treatment delivery may also be possible once a diagnosis of disease has been made, with evaluation of response through repeat MD.

Early breast cancer detection will be optimized through the use of clinical and biologic markers that aid in predicting disease when it is not visualized and sampled through the endoscope. Preliminary evidence with image analysis suggests one potential approach to improve the specificity of breast cancer detection over MD cytology alone. Molecular markers to detect precancer or invasive cancer will require the ability to detect abnormalities in the presence of a benign cell background or will require the use of enrichment techniques to remove benign cells that may limit disease detection.

References

1. Young JL, Jr, Ward KC, Wingo PA, et al: The incidence of malignant non-carcinomas of the female breast. Cancer Causes Control 15(3):313–319, 2004.
2. Wrensch MR, Petrakis NL, Miike R, et al: Breast cancer risk in women with abnormal cytology in nipple aspirates of breast fluid. J Natl Cancer Inst 93(23):1791–1798, 2001.
3. Okazaki A, Okazaki M, Asaishi K, et al: Fiberoptic ductoscopy of the breast: a new diagnostic procedure for nipple discharge. Jpn J Clin Oncol 21(3):188–193, 1991.
4. Teboul M: A new concept in breast investigation: echo-histological acino-ductal analysis or analytic echography. Biomed Pharmacother 42(4):289–295, 1988.
5. Shen KW, Wu J, Lu JS, et al: Fiberoptic ductoscopy for patients with nipple discharge. Cancer 89(7):1512–1519, 2000.
6. Berna JD, Garcia-Medina V, Kuni CC: Ductoscopy: a new technique for ductal exploration. Eur J Radiol 12(2):127–129, 1991.
7. Matsunaga T, Ohta D, Misaka T, et al: Mammary ductoscopy for diagnosis and treatment of intraductal lesions of the breast. Breast Cancer 8(3):213–221, 2001.
8. Dooley WC: Endoscopic visualization of breast tumors. JAMA 284(12):1518, 2000.
9. Matsunaga T, Kawakami Y, Namba K, et al: Intraductal biopsy for diagnosis and treatment of intraductal lesions of the breast. Cancer 101(10):2164–2169, 2004.
10. Sauter ER, Ehya H, Klein-Szanto AJ, et al: Fiberoptic ductoscopy findings in women with and without spontaneous nipple discharge. Cancer 103(5):914–921, 2005.
11. Sauter ER, Ehya H, Schlatter L, et al: Ductoscopic cytology to detect breast cancer. Cancer J 10(1):33–41; discussion 15–16, 2004.
12. Sauter ER, Klein-Szanto A, Ehya H, et al: Ductoscopic cytology and image analysis to detect breast carcinoma. Cancer 101(6):1283–1292, 2004.
13. Dooley WC: Routine operative breast endoscopy during lumpectomy. Ann Surg Oncol 10(1):38–42, 2003.
14. Going JJ, Moffat DF: Escaping from Flatland: clinical and biological aspects of human mammary duct anatomy in three dimensions. J Pathol 203(1):538–544, 2004.
15. Sauter ER, Ehya H, Babb J, et al: Biological markers of risk in nipple aspirate fluid are associated with residual cancer and tumour size. Br J Cancer 81(7):1222–1227, 1999.
16. Kim JA, Crowe JP, Woletz J, et al: Prospective study of intraoperative mammary ductoscopy in patients undergoing partial mastectomy for breast cancer. Am J Surg 188(4):411–414, 2004.
17. Dooley WC, Francescatti D, Clark L, et al: Office-based breast ductoscopy for diagnosis. Am J Surg 188(4):415–418, 2004.
18. Escobar PF, Baynes D, Crowe JP: Ductoscopy-assisted microdochectomy. Int J Fertil Womens Med 49(5):222–224, 2004.
19. Sharma R, Dietz J, Wright H, et al: Comparative analysis of minimally invasive microductectomy versus major duct excision in patients with pathologic nipple discharge. 62nd Annual Meeting, Central Surgical Association, 2005.
20. Okazaki A, Okazaki M, Hirata K: Recent progress of image diagnosis for breast cancer: ductoscopy of the breast. Jap J Breast Cancer 11:262–269, 1996.
21. Hunerbein M, Raubach M, Gebauer B, et al: Ductoscopy and intraductal vacuum assisted biopsy in women with pathologic nipple discharge. Breast Cancer Res Treat 99(3):301–307, 2006.

Conclusion

25

Lisa Jacobs and Christina A. Finlayson

We all know the statistics on the impact that breast cancer has on our population. Today, 1 in 8 women will experience breast cancer in her lifetime, and 1 in 33 women will die of the disease. In addition, in the United States, approximately 2000 men are diagnosed with breast cancer annually. Even more profound is the increase in the number of women living with breast cancer. Currently more than 2 million women in the United States have been successfully treated for breast cancer and are going on to live full and active lives subsequent to their treatment.[1] This statistic represents the tremendous impact that public awareness and education, early detection and diagnosis, and research into improved therapies can have on decreasing the burden of disease and improving quality of life. The impact that grassroots organizations and patient advocacy have had on increasing awareness and directing funding to important research initiatives serves as a model for those wishing to make a similar impact on other diseases that negatively affect the public good.

The importance and impact of well-conducted research trials are seen throughout the chapters of this book. Clinical trials conducted regarding prevention, imaging and early detection, local and systemic therapies, and quality of life have defined and redefined optimal care for patients and providers grappling with this disease. Funding for these clinical trials comes from many sources, including government funding agencies and private foundations. Recent financial reports indicate that annually the National Cancer Institute (NCI) sponsors $573 million in breast cancer research funding, the Department of Defense $138 million,[2] the

Komen Foundation $64 million,[3] and the Avon Foundation $14 million.[4] Many other organizations large and small provide direct and indirect support for breast cancer research as well as additional monies to support education, public awareness, and direct patient care services. A significant portion of these funds comes from the generous donations of private citizens, many of whom have had personal experience with breast cancer and who want to do their part to help others in their community who have been touched by this disease.

The results of these clinical trials have moved breast cancer treatment from the early 1900s, when most patients received a Halsted radical mastectomy for local control, to this century, when many women can preserve their breast with minimal cosmetic change. This has come not at the detriment of survival but with improved survival rates. Most women diagnosed today can expect a greater than 70% 10-year survival rate; for those with the earliest stages of even invasive disease, a 10-year survival rate of over 90% is the norm. Surgeons have a wide armamentarium of options available to provide optimal local control as well as cosmetic outcome. Larger tumors can be converted to smaller tumors amenable to breast conservation with neoadjuvant chemotherapy. Oncoplastic techniques can reshape the breast to improve overall cosmesis in the breast conservation setting. Patients who require or choose mastectomy have a variety of reconstructive options available that can recreate the breast mound in a fashion that offers a very similar size, shape, and texture to the native breast. The future may bring ever more focal destruction and ablation techniques that will further minimize the cosmetic consequences of surgical breast cancer therapy.

As large debilitating surgical procedures have given way to smaller operations, further research has also better defined chemotherapy regimens in a similar vein. Although 40 years ago only one or two chemotherapy regimens were applied to all cases of breast cancer, the focus now is on the patients who are most likely to benefit from a given regimen while minimizing the side effects of these therapies. Substratification of tumor types by molecular characteristics has expanded breast cancer from being defined as one disease to recognizing distinct subsets with individual prognostic and treatment response signatures. Pregnancy-associated breast cancer, luminal or basal-subtype tumors, HER2/neu-positive tumors, triple-negative tumors, and tumors with low oncotype scores are currently recognized as having very distinct behaviors, and specific therapies are being developed to take these variations into consideration for treatment planning. Tailoring therapy to these specific subsets maximizes treatment benefit and further improves the cost-benefit ratio not only in financial terms but also in terms of the mental, physical, emotional, and relationship costs to the patient.

Similarly, radiation therapy is moving from a prolonged course of daily radiation to much shorter, more focused treatment modalities. Six-week courses of external-beam radiation therapy are being replaced with 3- to 4-week courses, brachytherapy radiation is being investigated for an even shorter on-treatment time, and some institutions are investigating single-dose, intraoperative treatment regimens. It is important to recognize, however, that intriguing and novel treatment options can often become available to the general public in advance of the data supporting equivalence or superiority to standard protocols. The application of these new techniques "off-protocol" needs to be carefully considered to prevent the unintentional introduction of less effective therapies in the absence of compelling research results. Carefully conducted research trials are the foundation for a future that will continue to focus on ever more targeted therapies to increase benefit and decrease morbidity.

As the medical management of breast cancer as a disease has improved, the opportunity to focus on risk stratification, prevention, and life-style interventions that can impact and reduce the incidence of breast cancer is receiving more attention. Identifying the women at highest risk for developing breast cancer, even though they currently represent a smaller proportion of all patients affected by this disease, allows targeted intervention either to prevent breast cancer or to identify early the development of breast cancer. Women and men identified as carrying known gene defects such as *BRCA1* and *BRCA2* are at particularly high risk. Earlier and more intensive screening can detect disease at the earliest possible stage, or prophylactic surgery can significantly decrease disease occurrence. Although effective medical therapies for chemoprevention for patients with a known gene defect have not yet been identified, the future will undoubtedly bring focused medical interventions that will correct the underlying defect, returning these family members to a baseline risk profile.

Learning from the experience of these highest-risk individuals, however, will lead to further improvements in risk stratification that will help us define and focus interventions on the women most likely to be affected by breast cancer. Most women who develop breast cancer have no known identifiable risk factors. For these women we currently have a one-size-fits-all approach to screening and early detection. Whatever your response to the recently published U.S. Preventive Services Task Force (USPSTF) recommendations on mammographic screening,[5] the clear message is that most women will never get breast cancer, and identifying the women with an elevated risk will increase the yield and decrease the economic and noneconomic costs of screening. Targets that show promise include proliferative and atypical changes identified on benign breast biopsy, the quantification of breast density, and the influence of lifestyle markers such as obesity and sedentary lifestyle on subsequent breast cancer development.

Further definition of women at risk allows us to institute specific interventions such as chemoprevention and nutritional and lifestyle changes on the women most likely to benefit. Current prevention recommendations have been arbitrarily set at a 1.67% 5-year risk calculated using the Gail model. More specific modeling constructs as well as tailored prevention strategies are needed. Underutilization of currently available chemoprevention indicates that the side-effect profile of future medications must be much smaller than that demonstrated by tamoxifen and raloxifene if women are going to adopt them as part of their prevention strategy. Additional emerging strategies that include exercise and weight control also show promise as providing some reduction in breast cancer incidence, although they face the uphill battle of any intervention that requires significant behavior modification.

Efforts at early diagnosis rely heavily on imaging. Mammography continues to be the gold standard; however, emerging technologies such as magnetic resonance imaging (MRI) and whole-breast ultrasound appear to have important roles to play in a selected high-risk population. The importance of a clinical breast exam is often overlooked but needs to be reinforced because over one third of new breast cancers are diagnosed by the patient's physician on physical exam. Use of image-guided and percutaneous biopsy techniques have tremendously improved the diagnostic quality while decreasing the cost of therapy. Percutaneous image-guided biopsy is becoming a quality measure for centers of excellence in breast disease management.

Imaging is also heavily used in the post-treatment surveillance setting. Again, adherence to established surveillance guidelines provides the optimal care. The importance of the physician, trained in comprehensive history and physical examination skills, cannot be overstated. Overutilization of surveillance imaging and laboratory testing is more likely to yield a false-positive than a true finding, increasing the burden of the emotional as well as the financial cost of care on the individual as well as the community.

As we better understand that breast cancer is not one disease but reflects many types of genetic alteration and phenotypic expression with variable aggression and prognosis, our prevention strategies and treatment therapies will be further honed and targeted to interventions appropriate to the disease process. This is an exciting time for a physician to participate in the care of these wonderful patients. The future holds promise of improved methods of diagnosis, more focused treatment, and improved survival and quality of life.

References

1. NCI Office of Women's Health Research on Cancers in Women. http://women.cancer.gov/research/breast.shtml
2. Priority #2: $150 million for the Department of Defense (DOD) Peer-Reviewed Breast Cancer Research Program (BCRP) for Fiscal Year 2009. National Breast Cancer Coalition. www.stopbreastcancer.org/index.php?option=com_content&task=view&id=333
3. Komen Foundation Annual Report 2006–07. ww5.komen.org/uploadedFiles/Content_Binaries/Komen-AR2007.pdf
4. Avon Foundation 2007 Financial Report. www.avoncompany.com/women/avonfoundation/2007_grants.pdf
5. Screening for Breast Cancer: United States Preventive Services Task Force, Agency for Health Research and Quality. www.ahrq.gov/clinic/USpstf/uspsbrca.htm#summary, published November 19, 2009. Accessed February 20, 2010.

Index

Note: Page numbers followed by f indicate figures; those followed by t indicate tables; and those followed by b indicate boxed material.